MANAGEMENT OF CNS TUMORS

Edited by **Miklos Garami**

Management of CNS Tumors
Edited by Miklos Garami

Published by InTech
Janeza Trdine 9, 51000 Rijeka, Croatia

Publishing Process Manager Iva Simcic

Technical Editor Teodora Smiljanic

Cover Designer InTech Design Team

Additional hard copies can be obtained from orders@intechopen.com

Management of CNS Tumors, Edited by Miklos Garami
p. cm.
978-953-307-646-1

For EU product safety concerns:
IN TECH d.o.o., Prolaz Marije Krucifikse Kozulić 3, 51000 Rijeka, Croatia,
info@intechopen.com or visit our website at intechopen.com.

Meet the editor

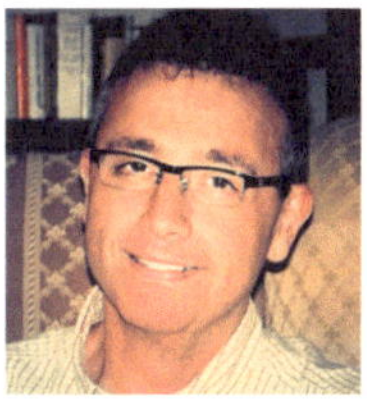

Dr. Miklós Garami, MD., MSc., PhD.; received his MD, Ph.D. and M.Sc. at Semmelweis Medical University (Budapest, Hungary) in 1991.; 2005. and 2007. He also received his Habilitation from Semmelweis Medical University (Budapest, Hungary) in 2010.
Currently he is Associate Professor of Pediatrics; Head of Hungarian Pediatric Cancer Registry; Head of Unit of Pediatric Oncology and Deputy Chairman of 2nd Department of Pediatric, Semmelweis University. Dr. Miklós Garami was awarded by Hungarian Academy of Sciences (Postdoctoral Fellowship Semmelweis University (Budapest, Hungary) in 1991-1992 and by American Heart Association (Postdoctoral Fellowship University of California at San Francisco (UCSF), California, USA) in 1992-1995.
Current research activities include: Pediatric oncology, investigating gene expression profiles in pediatric malignancies (CNS tumors, NBL, Ewing sc.), information systems on microcomputers. He is the author of approximately 70 scientific papers, 9 books / chapters.

Contents

Preface

Brain tumors are classified depending on the exact site of the tumor, the type of tissue involved, whether they are noncancerous (benign) or cancerous (malignant), and other factors. Sometimes, tumors that start out being less invasive can become more invasive.

Tumors may occur at any age, but many types of tumors are most common in a certain age group. In adults, gliomas and meningiomas are most common.

Treatment can involve surgery, radiation therapy, and chemotherapy. Brain tumors are best treated by a team involving a neurosurgeon, radiation oncologist, oncologist, or neuro-oncologist, and other health care providers, such as neurologists and social workers.

Brain tumors present a continuous challenge to the physicians regardless of the patients' age. The goal of this book to provide up-to-date information for physicians based description of the management of selected Central Nervous System (CNS) tumors.

This book is not a textbook; therefore it highlights some importance aspects of selected CNS tumors.

The editor would like to acknowledge the contribution of the authors and the team of the Publishing Process Management at InTech - Open Access Publisher.

Dr. med. habil. Miklos Garami, MD., MSc. PhD., Associate Professor,
Semmelweis University,
Hungary

Part 1

Classification of CNS Tumors

1

Classification of Primary Brain Tumors: Molecular Aspects

Péter Molnár
University of Debrecen, Medical and Health Sciences Center, Department of Pathology
Hungary

1. Introduction

The guiding principle of this chapter is the importance of combining traditional morphological data with the recently acquired knowledge on the genetic and epigenetic signalling pathways which drive the evolution of CNS tumors. The official World Health Organization terminology (WHO, 2007) will be used since it is the source of information for neurooncology, neuroradiology, neurosurgery, etc. It is of outmost importance that new entities have emerged since 2007 and it seems inevitable to see a new classification in the near future. It is beyond the scope if this chapter to dwell on the pitfalls in diagnostic surgical neuropathology, suffice is to say that the classic, traditional case descriptions which are usually presented in textbooks comprise only a fraction of diagnostic dilemmas so often hunting practicing neuro-oncopathologists.

The main focus will be placed on intracranial lesions but it needs to be emphasized that the diagnostic entities which come the way of a surgical neuropathologist broadly overlap with an extensive range of entities which basically belong to hematopathology, soft tissue and bone/chondroid tumors.

In all textbooks on neuropathology the usual way to start is to point out that knowledge of brain and spinal cord anatomy as well as familiarity with the broad range of cellular reactions in diseased CNS are essential for success in understanding pathology reports. There is no way to cover all these details, hence a list of reference books is provided. This chapter is born out of the need to outline unambiguous and consistent terminology of brain tumors. This together with a strong urge to define the use of a universally accepted grading system (be that weak as it is despite of century-old efforts) could help not only all specialists who are involved in treating brain tumor patients but also and of outmost importance the patients themselves.

2. Pathology of brain tumors – A general overview

Brain tumors are not that common (about 1-1.5% of neoplasms in adults) but they still present an often frustrating challenge for oncologists even in developed countries. In contrast to the somewhat limited pathologic variations of adult brain tumors the extreme phenotypic diversity of pediatric brain tumors often results in overwhelming diagnostic problems even for the experienced pediatric pathologist. A recent report from France states that over 5 years, 25 756 cases of newly diagnosed and histologically confirmed primary

CNS tumors (PCNST) have been recorded. Histological diagnoses included glioma 48.9%, all other neuroepithelial tumors 5%, meningioma 28.8%, nerve sheath tumor 8.4%, lymphoma 3.2% and others 5.7%.
Epidemiological data on the most common intracranial tumors are presented in Table 1. The data are from the 2011 CBTRUS Statistical Report (http://www.cbtrus.org/2007-2008/2007-20081.html.)

Tumor type	Grade[a]	Incidence[b]	Male/Female	5-year-survival (%)[c]
Pilocytic astrocytoma	I	0.27	1.0	94
Diffuse astrocytoma	II	0.15	1.2	48
Anaplastic astrocytoma	III	0.48	1.4	27
Glioblastoma	IV	2.60	1.6	5
Oligodendroglioma[d]	II/III	0.38	1.5	80
Ependymoma	II/III	0.24	1.4	82
Medulloblastoma	IV	0.26	1.6	62
Meningeoma[e]	I (II/III)	0.75	0.5	67

a: WHO 2007; b: New case/1 million population/year (1995-2007, CBTRUS; USA); c: observed chance of survival compared to the expected life span („survival") of the reference population (USA). SEER (Survival, Epidemiology and End Results) 2010. d. The five-year-long survival of anaplastic oligodendrogliomata is 49%. e. Intracranial and spinal meningeomata combined.

Table 1.

The direct cause of brain tumors is largely unknown. Inherited tumor-syndromes have helped to shed light on various genetic abnormalities which might play a role in tumor-induction. It is well documented that radiation of the head-and-neck region is associated with an increasing number of meningiomas. Primary CNS lymphomas (PCNSLs) are the most common causes of non-infective intracranial space occupying lesions in immuno-compromised people. The frequency of PCNSL has increased almost by an order of a magnitude (3-10x) and this tendency is present among those with normal immune system. An increased incidence of gliomas has become obvious by the last decade of the 20th century, and this is not due to the advanced sensitivity of diagnostic tools.
Although in most cases the etiology of neoplastic transformation awaits clarification there has been a truly revolutionary explosion of genetic and molecular tools giving new information that has fundamentally changed both basic and translational (clinical) neuro-oncology. Analysis of genetic instability and basic data on invasion and angiogenesis have all became inescapable questions to pursue during routine diagnostic activity. Information on gene expression profiles, application of tissue microarray techniques, follow up on

mRNA splicing patterns, are now considered to be part of the state-of-the-art workup in brain tumor analysis. These inevitably depend on functional genomics and bioinformatics. It is fair to say that the last 2-3 years have fundamentally changed our concept of diagnostic, prognostic and predictive markers in neuro-oncology.

All these changes require a new attitude towards tissue samples: the neurosurgeon must be aware of the importance of sampling that will critically influence the pathologist's ability to outline the major aspects of tailored therapy. Hence it cannot be overemphasized that the decisions on the distribution of various parts of a biopsy between diagnostic labs and research areas (including tumor banks) are the sole and outmost responsibility of the pathologist. This is the only way to ensure that the Hippocratic requirement of "*Salus aegroti suprema lex esto*[1]" is realized. No academic goal may interfere with the proper, individual, personalized diagnosis!

The precise diagnosis (both radiological and pathological) of brain tumors is significantly dependent on the fact that certain entities are linked with specific geographical areas (anatomical locations) within the CNS. Similarly, age does have an almost pathognomonic relevance in most cases. As always, exceptions to this fundamental rule are not infrequent, still it is the combined knowledge of radiological characteristics, exact site of the lesion and the patient's age which is an indispensible guidance for the pathologist.

2.1 Histological classification of various tumor types affecting the central nervous system

It is mentioned above that the last WHO classification was published in 2007. Since then new entities have been recognized. The idea that the pattern of differentiation is reflected by phenotypic features (in other words, phenotype may give a clue about the cell of origin) has been retained in the WHO classification. Despite of a long-lasting dispute it has not been fully decided whether "retrogressive" differentiation (loss of maturity from a mature state) can or cannot result in cancer formation. Meanwhile it has become generally accepted that tumors most often arise from "cancer stem cells". The term tumor initiating cells (TICs) probably describes best the features of these progenitor elements which are assumed to be capable of self-renewal and of divergent differentiation. It is worth noting here that these "stem cells" are hypothesized to strongly interact with their immediate micromilieau (niche). As a result the actual TICs' behavior and chemo- and/or radioresistance will be modified by the niche elements (endothelial cells, microglia, concentration of various signalling molecules, etc.). This explains why these cells which are often of low proliferative activity can maintain tumor growth or recurrence after vigorous treatment.

Table 2. is construed basically on the WHO 2007 classification with some modifications. It is important for oncologists to be aware of new entities which most likely will be included in the next WHO book and already occur in pathology reports. It must repeatedly be stressed that the frequency, location and types of CNS tumors vary with age and to some degree with sex. The largest group of tumors comprises neuroepithelial neoplasms, a significant portion of intracranial tumors are meningeal and metastatic lesions. Gliomas (astrocytomas, oligodendrogliomas and ependymomas) account for circa 40% of all tumors and approximately 80% of malignant tumors. The most comprehensive and up-to-date information on the epidemiology of various CNS tumors is available on the CBTRUS website shown above.

---

[1] In a rather free translation: „Everything is to serve the best interest of the patient."

I. Neuroepithelial tumors

a. **Astrocytic tumors**
   Pilocytic astrocytoma
   Pilomyxoid astrocytoma
   Pleomorphic xanthoastrocytoma
   Diffuse astrocytomas
   Anaplastic astrocytoma
   Glioblastoma
   Glioblastoma with significant oligodendroglial component (GBO)
   Giant cell glioblastoma
   Gliosarcoma
   Gliomatosis cerebri

b. **Oligodendroglial tumors**
   Oligodendroglioma
   Anaplastic oligodendroglioma
   Oligoastrocytoma
   Anaplastic oligoastrocytoma

c. **Ependymal tumors**
   Ependymoma
   Anaplastic ependymoma
   Myxopapillary ependymoma
   Subependymoma

d. **Choroid plexus tumors**
   Choroid plexus papilloma
   Atypical choroid plexus papilloma
   Choroid plexus carcinoma

e. **Other neuroepithelial tumors**
   Astroblastoma
   Chordoid glioma of the third ventricle
   Angiocentric glioma

II. Neuronal and mixed neuronal-glial tumors

a. **Neuronal tumors**
   Gangliocytoma and ganglioglioma
   Dysplastic gangliocytoma of the cerebellum
   Central neurocytoma and variants

b. **Mixed neuronal-glial tumors**
   Ganglioglioma
   Anaplastic ganglioglioma
   Desmoplastic infantile astrocytoma and ganglioglioma (DIA/DIG)
   Central neurocytoma and extraventricular neurocytoma
   Cerebellar liponeurocytoma
   Papillary glioneural tumor (PGNT)
   Rosette-forming glioneural tumor of the 4th ventricle (RGNT)
   Paraganglioma (spinal)
   Dysembryoplastic neuroepithelial tumor

III. Tumors of the pineal region

Pineocytoma
Pineal parenchymal tumor of intermediate differentiation
Pineoblastoma
Papillary tumor of the pineal region

IV. Tumors of the sellar region

Pituitary adenoma
Craniopharyngeoma
Granular cell tumor of the neurohypophysis
Pituicytoma
Spindle cell oncocytoma of the adenohypophysis

V. Embryonal tumors

Medulloblastoma
    Classical medulloblastoma
    Desmoplastic/nodular medulloblastoma
    Medullomyoblastoma
    Melanotic medulloblastoma
CNS primitive neuroectodermal tumor (cPNET)
Medulloepithelioma
Ependymoblastoma
Atypical rhabdoid/teratoid tumor (AT/RT)

VI. Tumors of the cranial nerves

Schwannoma (Neurilemmoma)
Neurofibroma
Perineurioma
Malignant peripheral nerve sheath tumor (MPNST)

VII. Meningeal tumors

Meningiomas
Mesenchymal, non-meningothelial tumors
Hemangiopericytoma
Melanotic lesions
Hemangioblastoma

VIII. Tumors of the hemopoietic system

Malignant lymphomas
Histiocytic tumors

IX. Germ cell tumors

CNS germ cell tumors

X. Familial tumor syndromes

Neurofibromatosis type I. (NF1)
Neurofibromatosis type II. (NF2)
Schwannomatosis

von Hippel-Lindau disease and haemangioblastoma
Tuberous sclerosis complex and subependymal giant cell astrocytoma (SEGA)
Lhermitte-Duclos disease
Cowden disease and dysplastic gangliocytoma of the cerebellum
Turcot syndrome
Li-Fraumeni syndrome and TP53 germline mutations
Rhabdoid tumor predisposition syndrome
Naevoid basal cell carcinoma syndrome

XI. Metastatic tumors of the CNS

Table 2.

The various names date back to the first comprehensive classification of nervous system tumors put together by Percival Bailey and Harvey Cushing in 1926. This was based on presumed parallels between embryologic cell forms and neoplastic elements. This nomenclature is still in use, however much of the terminology has changed fundamentally.
Neoplasia is a genetic disease and now there is abundant information at hand about alterations which occur in key regulatory genes, either inherited in mutant forms or arising sporadically as a result of somatic noxae to growth regulatory genes. Tumors may come about when the function of protein products of key growth regulatory genes is altered or they can develop as a result of random genetic changes which are not properly corrected by DNA repair mechanisms. As it is shown in Fig. 1. current hypotheses drastically overwrite our previous concepts about the origin of neoplastic cells. It has for a long time been held that terminally differentiated cells are incapable to form neoplasms. Recent observations indicate that non-canonical steps, like epithelial-mesenchymal transformation (EMT) or the reverse (MET) may be involved in tumorigenesis and metastatic spread of cancer. In light of these data the hypothetical routes (indicated by dashed lines in the Figure 1) of regressive differentiation become easier to comprehend. This scenario is being actively researched and doubtlessly important role is allocated to cells with pluripotency in the evolution of brain tumors. NB. These cells are often referred to as tumor stem cells, although they do not necessarily fulfill the requirements of *bona fide* stem cells. Figure 1 also shows that there is no common understanding of how ependymal tumors fit into this hypothesis, neither it is clear how exactly mixed glial tumors evolve. The latter phenomenon might be related to clonal selection during the accumulation of genetic damage as tumors progress. In this biological, pathological sense tumor progression is strictly related to dedifferentiation (i. e., increasing grade) and not to the change of total tumor volume, as it is often used in clinical, particularly radiological terminology. Cellular heterogeneity and the almost inevitable progression (accumulation of genetic abnormalities inducing dedifferentiation) are paramount intrinsic features of glial tumors.
The detailed description of histological and cellular features of individual tumor types defies the length of this chapter. Moreover, neither neurosurgeons, nor neuro-oncologists are benefiting from these textbook data. However, if an individual tumor carries unusual features and still needs to be squeezed in an existing category (mainly because health insurance policies often require traditionally "boxed" entities), it is the responsibility of the MDT to come to an agreement about a category which is suitable to fit in treatment protocols. Furthermore, descriptive analysis is bound to be enriched by individualized genetic and molecular data which eventually might carry more relevant information vis-á-vis treatment than the classical histo- and cytopathologic characteristics (*vide infra*).

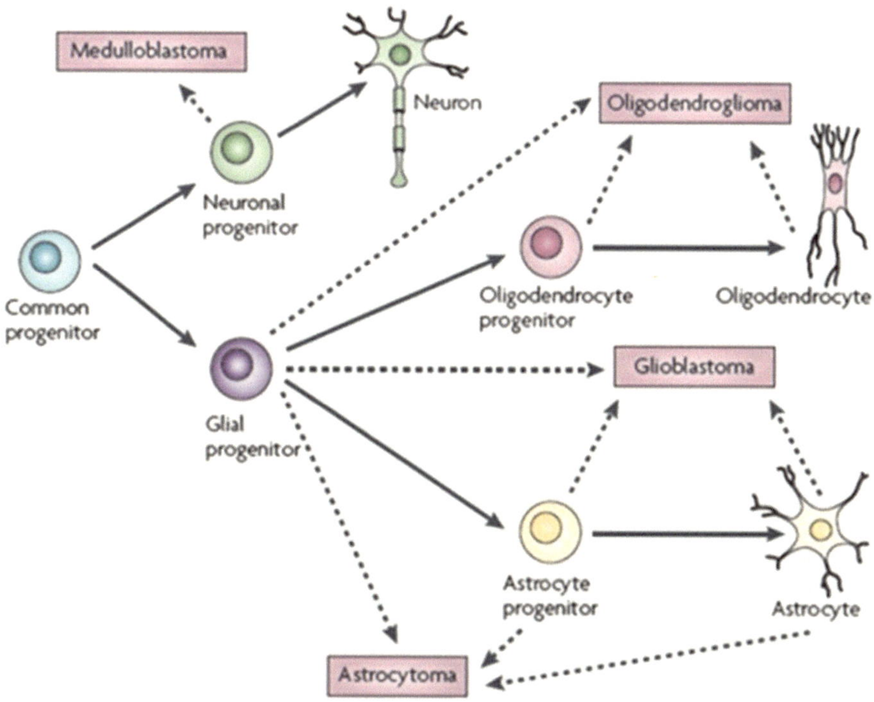

Fig. 1. Origin of neuroglial tumors. Modified after Huse JT and Holland EC. Nature Reviews Cancer **doi:10.1038/nrc2818.**

2.2 Grading of CNS tumors

The WHO classification grades tumors according to their malignant potential on a scale ranging from 1 for "benign" tumors to 4 for the most aggressive and malignant ones. Other grading systems have been used in the past, but the WHO 2007 system is now the one which is the most easy to find and is the one best recognized by pathologists, radiologists, neurosurgeons and oncologists. Modifications of the Kernohan system of grading were adopted by the WHO ever since the publication of the first "blue book" (1979). It was first revised in 1993, then in 2000 and 2007. It is very important to keep in mind that grading criteria are always artificial, arbitrary and despite of all world-wide efforts to avoid it, are always very subjective. Various techniques of the ever growing field of molecular diagnostics are increasingly employed not only in tumor classification but also in tumor grading. At this day and age it is still prudent to state that morphologic findings endure as a golden standard for proper evaluation of genetic and molecular observations.
The original concept of grading was introduced by Broders who first realized that the degree of cellular differentiation does have a reliable value in predicting the biological behavior of cancerous growths of the lip. He hypothesized that the "cell-of-origin" model reflects clinical prognosis: if more than 75% of the cells are "like" the cell of origin (i. e., stratified squamous epithelium) indicating that the neoplastic elements retain significant degree of differentiation then the outlook is favorable. Since it proved to work well for a host of systemic cancers Kernohan introduced the idea to brain tumor analysis and suggested a four-tier grading model.

Four-tier grading scheme		
Grade 1	Low proliferative potential and possibility of surgical cure	Well-differentiated
Grade 2	Diffuse growth, tendency to recur, though only few mitoses	Moderately-differentiated
Grade 3	Histological evidence of malignancy, destructive growth, brisk mitotic activity, anisonucleosis	Poorly-differentiated
Grade 4	Cytologically malignant, mitotically active, necrosis-prone	Anaplastic

Eventually it has become increasingly obvious that the 4-tier-grading can be applied only with significant difficulties even to astrocytic tumors. Ringertz then applied a 3-tiered scheme for astrocytomas.

Three-tier grading scheme		
Grade 1	Low grade	Well-differentiated
Grade 2	Intermediate grade	Moderately differentiated
Grade 3	High grade	Poorly-differentiated

This was replaced by the St.Anne/Mayo classification which was doomed because of the inclusion of a rather elusive and rarely occurring "Grade I." lesion: diffuse astrocytic tumors without atypia. The current concept holds that Grade I. astrocytomas are *relatively circumscribed* (*sic!*), while all other grades by definition comprise diffusely growing tumors. It is obvious from the 2007 WHO classification that certain tumors have only 3 grades, however, the "missing" 4th category may be at the *origo* of the scale (ependymal, oligodendroglial, or mixed glial tumors) and thus the highest (most malignant) grade is Gr. III., which implies that a Gr. III. oligoastrocytoma (OA Gr. III.) often presents all cytological and histological features of the most malignant (Gr. IV.) astrocytoma, i. e., glioblastoma (GBM). Needless to say this often results in confusion, particularly for the oncologist whose decision on therapy is often highly determined by bureaucratic regulations (e. g., financial limitations of treatment options). To complicate issues further several tumors do not have Grade I. forms at all (oligoastrocytic tumors, OAs), while some Gr. I. lesions are strictly related to anatomic location (myxopapillary ependymoma or subependymal giant cell astrocytoma [SEGA]). A firm understanding of the meaning and significance of numerical grading among all people (usually members of the MDT = multidisciplinary team) is quintessential, particularly since the criteria used for assigning diagnoses and grades are different between the various systems in use, sometimes even between the older and newer WHO classifications. Numerical grades do not surmount the need for a fundamental understanding of the histological/cytological criteria for diagnosis of specific types of tumors.

It is important to note that the definition of biological malignancy as reflected by increasing dedifferentiation is not necessary for lethal clinical outcome of a tumor. A highly differentiated meningeal tumor (Gr. I.) may kill a patient if it mechanically compresses vital, eloquent areas (meningioma of the edge of the foramen magnum). By the same token, the general principle of oncology that states that the most important indication of malignancy is metastatic spread does not hold in neuro-oncology. Even GBMs, which are considered to be the most malignant forms of gliomata rarely metastasize outside CNS compartments.

Table 3. summarizes the currently defined WHO grades within the most common CNS tumors. As a general rule staging is not applicable to CNS tumors and grading of non-CNS specific tumors can be found in the proper volume of the WHO series as well as in the 7th Edition of Cancer Staging Handbook. Neither Table 2. nor Table 3. go into details of various subtypes of primary and/or secondary CSN tumors. Everyone should keep in mind that chondrogenic, osteogenic, fibroblastic, etc. tumors may affect the brain or spinal cord either when arising *de novo* within the intracranial or intraspinal compartments or when they directly invade CNS tissue from adjacent structures. Their grading (and staging, for that matter) follows the general principles of systemic pathology. It is noteworthy, however, that the tight and non-compliant intracranial space poses additional biological/clinical problems in the latter cases: increased ic. pressure, brain herniation, etc. complicate treatment of these neoplasms.

2.3 Limitations of morphological grading

To demonstrate the subjectivity of glioma grading it is worth comparing the features of pilocytic tumors (as listed in the WHO fascicle) with those of GBMs. While doing so two definitions need to be taken into account. The highest glioma grade is assigned to tumors which have either endothelial proliferation and/or necrosis in the neoplasm. "Endothelial proliferation" nowadays is more often replaced by "MVP" (=microvascular proliferation). This phenomenon means not solely apparent multilayering of endothelial cells but a complex process that comprises endothelial atypia, endothelial mitotic activity (often accompanied by abnormal p53 immunohistochemical abnormalities, *vide infra*), and endothelial cell (EC) multiplication accompanied by an abnormal deposition of basal lamina (BL) components plus proliferative activity of pericytic elements. This often results in the formation of literally "glomerulum[2]"-like elements (glomeruloid proliferation), but the latter is not a *sine qua non* of Gr. IV. Not infrequently these abnormal vascular structures occur along the edge of the infiltrative zone or partially surrounding necrotic areas ("vasocorona"). Necrosis is another histological feature which often indicates malignant potential. This is not necessarily an indication of the parenchyma's outgrowing the blood supply (as general pathology often states). Glial tumors are known to be very vascular but a heretofore unclarified complex dysregulation results in what is called "*sui generis*" tumor necrosis. The fundamental pathobiology of this phenomenon exceeds the limits of this chapter, it suffices to say that this necrosis (surrounded by palisading tumor cells) is fundamentally different from the "garden variety" infarctions. The latter are also common, since despite of rich neovascularization blood supply to gliomas is often interrupted by thromboses which may affect all sized vessels.
Daily experiences firmly indicate that there is a myth surrounding numerical grades particularly since the problem usually is presented in almost all textbooks in a way that suggests: criteria are strict, obvious, and "self-evident" and their use is only a matter of routine. The following paragraphs are intended to shed light on the complexity of the issue. First I will quote from the last WHO book those sentences which describe features of pilocytic tumors which are the prime examples of a grade I. tumor (WHO 2007, pp15-20). It is worth to think through these quotations keeping in mind what almost everybody considers as *prima facie* evidence of the worst grade, i. e., glioblastoma.

---

[2] The "magic" capillary structure that occupies the Bowman space.

	I	II	III	IV
Astrocytic tumours				
Subependymal giant cell astrocytoma	•			
Pilocytic astrocytoma	•			
Pilomyxoid astrocytoma		•		
Diffuse astrocytoma		•		
Pleomorphic xanthoastrocytoma		•		
Anaplastic astrocytoma			•	
Glioblastoma				•
Giant cell glioblastoma				•
Gliosarcoma				•
Oligodendroglial tumours				
Oligodendroglioma		•		
Anaplastic oligodendroglioma			•	
Oligoastrocytic tumours				
Oligoastrocytoma		•		
Anaplastic oligoastrocytoma			•	
Ependymal tumours				
Subependymoma	•			
Myxopapillary ependymoma	•			
Ependymoma		•		
Anaplastic ependymoma			•	
Choroid plexus tumours				
Choroid plexus papilloma	•			
Atypical choroid plexus papilloma		•		
Choroid plexus carcinoma			•	
Other neuroepithelial tumours				
Angiocentric glioma	•			
Chordoid glioma of the third ventricle		•		
Neuronal and mixed neuronal-glial tumours				
Gangliocytoma	•			
Ganglioglioma	•			
Anaplastic ganglioglioma			•	
Desmoplastic infantile astrocytoma and ganglioglioma	•			
Dysembryoplastic neuroepithelial tumour	•			
Central neurocytoma		•		
Extraventricular neurocytoma		•		
Cerebellar liponeurocytoma		•		
Paraganglioma of the spinal cord	•			
Papillary glioneuronal tumour	•			
Rosette-forming glioneuronal tumour of the fourth ventricle	•			
Pineal tumours				
Pineocytoma	•			
Pineal parenchymal tumour of intermediate differentiation		•	•	
Pineoblastoma				•
Papillary tumour of the pineal region		•	•	
Embryonal tumours				
Medulloblastoma				•
CNS primitive neuroectodermal tumour (PNET)				•
Atypical teratoid / rhabdoid tumour				•
Tumours of the cranial and paraspinal nerves				
Schwannoma	•			
Neurofibroma	•			
Perineurioma	•	•	•	
Malignant peripheral nerve sheath tumour (MPNST)		•	•	•
Meningeal tumours				
Meningioma	•			
Atypical meningioma		•		
Anaplastic / malignant meningioma			•	
Haemangiopericytoma		•		
Anaplastic haemangiopericytoma			•	
Haemangioblastoma	•			
Tumours of the sellar region				
Craniopharyngioma	•			
Granular cell tumour of the neurohypophysis	•			
Pituicytoma	•			
Spindle cell oncocytoma of the adenohypophysis	•			

"...hyperchromatic and pleomorphic nuclei, glomeruloid vascular proliferation, infarct-like necrosis and infiltration of leptomeninges are compatible with the diagnosis of pilocytic astrocytoma"; "....degenerative atypia with pleomorphism, smudgy chromatin, and nuclear-cytoplasmic pseudoinclusions (are) *frequently seen in long-standing lesions"; "enfilades resemble those of what was termed the 'primitive polar spongioblastoma'* (may occur)*"; "one study found the acquisition of atypia, particularly of increased cellularity and occasional mitoses, to be of no prognostic significance". – It is also noted that pilocytic astrocytoma may undergo malignant transformation: "They often feature multiple mitoses per single high power field, endothelial proliferation and palisading necrosis. Such tumors should not be designated glioblastoma..."* – given all these statements from the "horse's mouth" (i. e., the most authoritative book on CNS tumors) it is not surprising that unless there is a firm understanding of the complexity of issues at hand oncologists often are dumbfounded when having read the descriptive part of a report they expect the worst (Gr. IV.) still they are given the best (Gr. I.) possible diagnosis. How is that possible?

One should keep in mind that morphological evaluation is not a black-or-white type of decision forming intellectual activity; it is an analogous thinking process. Pathologists compare a waste amount (in fortunate situations) of mentally stored images to the actual fields in the microscope, they compare images-to-images, complex patterns to complex patterns and then put everything in context (age, sex, imaging features, intraoperative findings, macroscopic features, etc.) – provided they do have all this information. Anyone familiar with the image below can decide how objective and reliable analogous thinking is:

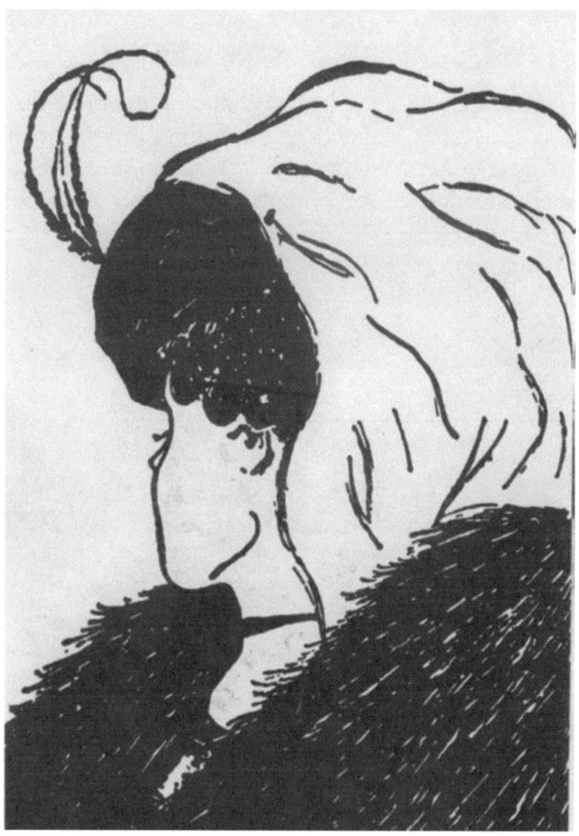

The dilemma is more obvious if one considers the proverbial pathologist's answer to the clinicians' question: *Why is the diagnosis "this" and not "that"? – Because it looks more like "this" than "that"!* And it does not mean that the pathologist is incompetent, the problem is inherent in the psychophysiology of "analogous thinking". There is nothing else that would emphasize MDT work's importance more than realization of this theoretical problem.
To drop another stone into the seemingly quiet pond: there are physical limitations as well, namely, sampling errors. This is demonstrated (in an analogous way) with the help of the following images, which show two sides of the same apple from my kitchen table:

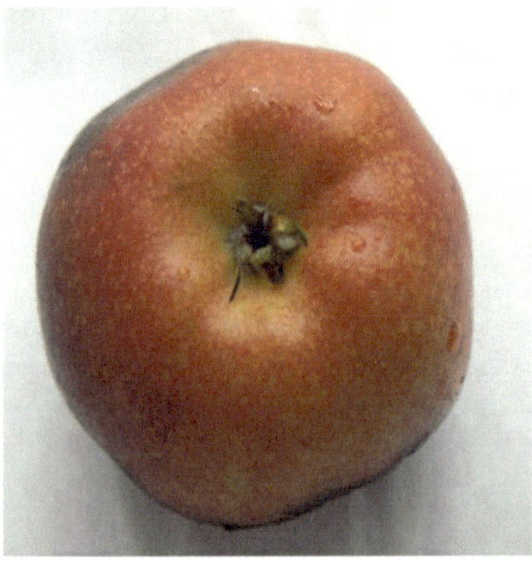

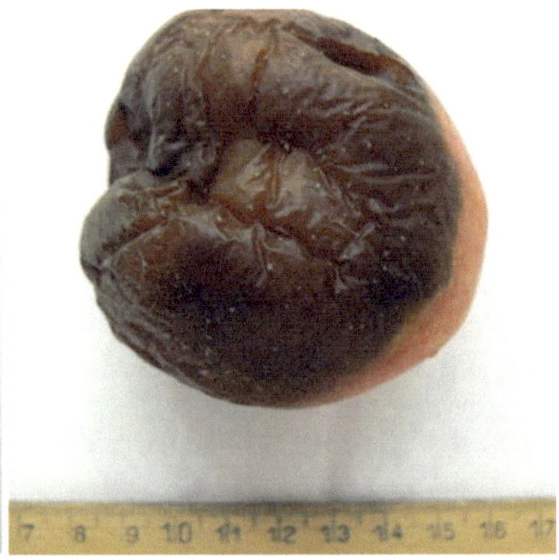

Obviously often the pathologist does not have a chance to evaluate the whole lesion, in 3D, from all aspects. He is absolutely dependent upon the guidance of the neuroradiologist (who may be able to grade tumours in vivo [see Jakab et al]) and the neurosurgeon. Unfortunately the latter's freedom of sampling is often highly limited and that complicates issues further:

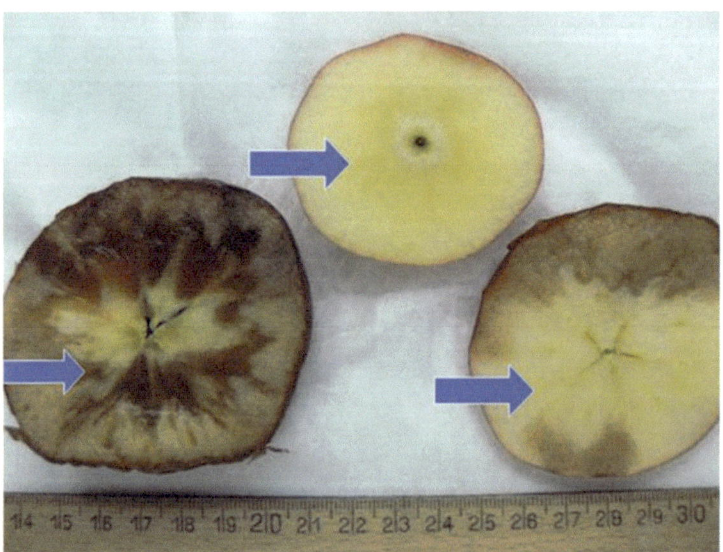

The blue arrows indicate the variability and often non-representative nature of sampling. Imagine the inherent errors in grading when comparing the 3 biopsies from the same apple ("tumor"). Added to the problem is the almost pathognomonic regional heterogeneity of gliomas, particularly of high grade astrocytic tumors. Any neuro-oncopathologist who regularly diagnoses glioma samples could without any specific effort take a series of microphotographs from a GBM demonstrating tumor grades from I through IV.

So, what is the conclusion? Can anyone trust pathologists for any degree of reliability? The answer is yes, but with adjuncts. Unless one is asking for legal and/or ethical problems should only give an opinion only if she or he is convinced that all necessary information is provided plus no part of the tissue has been retained (for scientific reasons or tissue banking). **It is the prerogative of the pathologist** to select the areas which are eventually embedded, sectioned, stained and analyzed by the most advanced techniques (including molecular, genetic, biochemical, etc. methods). The final diagnosis must be discussed at MDT sessions and any controversies must be put in the right context *vis-á-vis* clinical data, imaging information and surgical procedure. There is ample evidence to show how therapy may change the morphology (and grade) of brain tumours (Molnár and Berényi). Experience shows that morphological diagnoses are mostly reliable, problems usually arise when the above outlined theoretical and physical limits are neglected, or, in the worst case, if the pathologist is inexperienced (which unfortunately often is compensated by over-self-confidence). Hence the verdict: every patient has the right for and is entitled to a second (third?) opinion, should the need arise! These requests must not ever be handled as "vanity" issues[3]. The wisdom of a pathologist is reflected by his humble (but not subservient) attitude firstly and outmost towards the patient. The question "Whose tissue is it, after all?" cannot be avoided either. Unfortunately with the dawn of tissue collection second opinions are often hindered by avaricious motivations of tissue banking and block-anxiety.

2.4 Biomarkers in neuro-oncology

In order to indentify the most adequat patient-tailored therapy the pathologist needs to identify 3 basic kinds of factors. These comprise diagnostic, prognostic and predictive markers. There is a standard but ever growing armamentarium of techniques for achieving these goals. Diagnostic markers are those which help to recognize those features which will allow the proper WHO classification of the lesion. Traditional histological stains, immunohistochemistry (IHC) and certain chromosomal and/or genetic characteristics belong to this category. It is mandatory to follow the current literature to realize that certain parameters may get moved from the list of one specific kind of markers to another. This is well exemplified by the chromosomal change commonly referred to as 1p19q status which used to be a predictive marker, nowadays it is one of the most important diagnostic markers while having important prognostic significance as well. Prognostic markers are defined as such that allow formation of an opinion on the "outlook" of the patient. In other words, prognostic markers help to estimate progression free or overall survival of the patient. These again may be histological/cytological features (necrosis, proliferative potential) or genetic alterations. It has only recently been realized that mutation(s) of the cytoplasmic isocytrate-dehydrogenase enzyme, IDH-1/IDH-2 are of prognostic significance in gliomas. Predictive markers are those which help to define the most effective treatment for an individual brain

[3] This author has ample personal experience to the contrary!

tumor and thus help to avoid the application of ineffective therapeutic interventions which would only induce unpleasant and dangerous complications without real therapeutical benefit. The most widely studied such marker is the methylation status of the promoter region of the MGMT gene (MGMT = methylguanine-methyltransferase). Promoter methylation reduces the amount of the enzyme which is encoded by the gene and the smaller the amount of this repair enzyme the more effective are the alkylating drugs. Recently (BNOS meeting, Cambridge, July 1, 2011) the predictive value of the MGMT status has been seriously questioned, although it remains an important prognostic marker. It is thus important to note that there is an overlap between various members of these 3 groups of biological markers.

3. Molecular and genetic background for biomarkers

3.1 Neuroepithelial tumors

In hindsight it seems rightful to say that the work which started with the identification of altered clinical behavior of oligodendroglial tumors with 1p19q co-deletions erupted in an unprecedented way once the study of 206 GBM's genome was published. One can confidently state that a new era in neuro-oncology started with the identification of the 3 major signalling pathways [**RTK/RAS/PI(3)K** (88%), **p53** (87%) and **Rb** (78%)]. Analysis of DNA copy numbers, gene-**e**xpression profiles and DNA-methylation patterns provided a whole new perspective for the proper evaluation of the real role of **ERBB2**, **NF1** and **TP53** genes. Frequent mutations of **PIK3R1** have also been observed. The promoter methylation of the MGMT gene acquired unequivocal and clinically fundamental importance. It is now accepted that in treated cases of GBM the surfacing hypermutator phenotype is due to „mismatch repair deficiency".

Mutations may cause primer sequence-alterations, may be indicated by copy number changes and evidently may cause activation (gene amplification or overexpression) of oncogenes or inactivation (chromosomal loss or gene deletions) of tumor suppressor genes. The data published in Nature summarize the analysis of 97 million base pairs that is the somatic mutations of 601 genes. It became obvious that in GBMs with NF1 mutations RAF or MEK inhibitors may be effective, while CDK inhibitors may prove useful in tumors with **CDKN2A** or **CDKN2C** mutated GBMs.

Parsons et al published data on amplification and/or deletion patterns of 20.661 protein coding genes in 22 human GBMs. New methodologies (aCGH, high density oligonucleotide arrays, next generation sequencing technologies, single nucleotide genomics, massively parallel DNA resequencing) reconfirmed their most unexpected result: the earliest genetic change in most glial tumors affects the gene that encodes the active site of the cytoplasmic form of a carbohydrate-metabolizing enzyme, i. e., IDH = isocytrate dehydrogenase. The enzyme has several isoforms but now it is accepted that IDH-1 mutations are the most common in relatively young patients' secondary GBMs which have a better prognosis. The results have been confirmed by Blass et al, and Yan et al. and it has also been amply shown that IDH-1 mutations are highly specific for glial tumors, they do not occur in systemic forms of malignant diseases (certain types of AML are exceptions to the rule). Zhao et al published their observations in 2009 which showed that the mutations (IDH-1; R132 or IDH-2; R172) reduce the enzyme's affinity towards its substrate plus inactive heterodimers appear which dominantly block the activity of the WT IDH-1 activity. There is a simultaneous induction of HIF-1α. A prime role was played in this work by Professor von

Deimling and his co-workers in Heidelberg who not only showed (by direct gene-sequencing) that the IDH-1 mutation is missing from pilocytic astrocytomas but were also able to identify a BRAF-KIAAA1549 gene fusion which characterizes these tumors. Thus the Heidelberg group for the first time made it routinely possible to separate not only reactive astrocytes from neoplastic ones (reactive cells are IDH-1 negative with the commercially available antibody which they generated) but also solved the haunting problem of reliably identifying pilocytic astrocytomas.

It is not easy to portray this explosive evolution that has so basically changed the routine approach to glioma diagnostics. It has happened so rapidly that in a recent book on "Neuro-Oncology" (published by Elsevier as part of the "Blue Books of Neurology series in 2010) **only one** (yes, only 1) vague sentence is included on the importance of IDH-1 mutations. Meanwhile, in 2011, there is a general agreement amongst neuro-oncopathologists that a treatment-determining routine of glioma diagnostics should include the analysis of IDH-1 mutations (immunohistochemistry), checking of the 1p19q status (FISH) and the mutations of TP53 (p53 IHC). These three steps are the minimum "must" for adequate diagnoses.

The following salient facts support the statement above. Except for the relatively rare primary GBMs it seems that the first step in glioma-genesis is the IDH-1 mutation. If that is followed by the damage of the 1p19q regions then oligodendrogliomas or oligoastrocytic tumors develop. If contrarily, not the 1p19q loci are altered but the TP53 gene is mutated, then progression to secondary GBM is inevitable.

We currently think that primer (*de novo*) GBMs arise from a different progenitor (TIC) cell than all other gliomas, moreover, those genetic alterations which accumulate during the biological progression of the various neoplasms which belong to either group are also different. These differences obviously have an effect on the proper choice of tailored therapy protocols.

The intrinsic significance of IDH-1 mutations is explained by the fact that this cytoplasmic enzyme is a key element in lipid-synthesis, most likely is a regulator of stress-provoked protective mechanisms, definitely is an important factor in oxidative cellular mechanisms and as such functions as an important player in oxygen-sensor transduction signalling. The question whether it is or it is not 2HG (2-hydroxyglutarate; which is a metabolite of the IDH-catalyzed metabolic events) that interferes with cellular processes and thus induces neoplasms awaits further studies and eventual clarification.

It is truly amazing to experience the molecular revolution that has recently changed our concepts about glioma genesis. This process is in the making, as this chapter is being formulated. A very recent publication proves that despite rather similar phenotypic features anaplastic oligodendroglial tumors are biologically and clinically heterogeneous. NB. The problem of classifying and diagnosing oligodendroglial tumors solely based on cytomorphology or immunohistochemistry has been a problem that has haunted neuro-oncopathologists for a long time (just remember an elusive and highly subjective category: glioblastomas with a significant oligodendroglial component). Idbaih et al reported that thirty-three BACs (**B**acterial **A**rtificial **C**hromosome array) with prognostic value were identified which helped to separate 4 genomic subgroups of anaplastic oligodendroglial tumors (AOTs). Type I tumors (25%) also displayed EGFR amplification, higher rate of necrosis and were associated with poor prognosis. Type II tumors were usually frontal tumors with the well known 1p19q loss and also had the usual oligodendroglial appearance. These patients (21.7%) had a longer survival. Type III tumors (11.7%) were characterized with deletion of prognostic BACs (21q) and had short survival. Type IV tumors are defined negatively by the absence of the genomic abnormalities seen in the other 3 groups and this represents 42% of all tumors. It is seriously thought-provoking that this material was comprised of samples of an EORTC trial, meaning, that all tumors were centrally reviewed and validated. What else could more convincingly illustrate the preceding paragraphs on analogous thinking and the issues related to subjectivity of pathological diagnoses? Regardless of some uncertainties associated with this series it is beyond doubt that soon we will see the overwhelming need of molecular sub-classification(s) of brain tumors which will be prerequisite for tailored therapy.

A similar tendency is present with regard to GBMs. Based on molecular analyses already in 2006 GBMs were sub-typed as mesenchymal and proneural. There was one group with a high number of CD133+ cells, with relatively sharp demarcation, cortical location. The lack of a high number of CD133+ cells was associated with a more expressed angiogeneic and proliferative activity. Verhaak et al continued the analysis and currently GBMs seem to belong to 4 subtypes: "classic", mesenchymal, proneural and neural. What is of outmost importance is that the canonical Stupp protocol seems to be effective only in the classic and mesenchymal subtypes. There is no further need to convince anyone that tailored, personalized, individual brain tumor therapy will very soon be more dependent upon molecular/genetic features than on traditional tinctorial and immunohistochemical profiles.

Another recently recognized and increasingly significant observation concerns epigenetic features (hyper-, and hypomethylation) as well as the rapidly growing information on miRNAs' regulatory effects. Suffices to say though that the various molecular analyses cannot replace traditional morphology: the proper candidates for the adequate molecular tests will for a long time to come be chosen based on something like the WHO classification. This is demonstrated in Table 4. Entities are still being identified based on pattern recognition (i. e., *traditional analogous thinking*).

Glioma type	**Genomic abnormality** BRAF alteration	1p19q deletion	IDH1 mutation	MGMT methylation	**WHO grade**
pilocytic astrocytoma	+	neg	neg	neg	I
oligodendroglioma	neg	+	+	+	II
anaplastic ODG	neg	+	+	+	III
oligoastrocytoma OA	neg	+	+	+	II
anaplastic OA	neg	+	+	+	III
diffuse astrocytoma	neg	neg	+	+	II
anaplastic astrocytoma	neg	neg	+	+	III
Secondary GBM	neg	neg	+	+	IV
Primary GBM	neg	neg	+	+	IV

Table 4.

Based upon the data in Table 4 it is obvious that state-of-the-art neuro-oncopathology is inconceivable without those analyses which are indicated in green. Lack of these results is highly counterproductive when it comes to tailored therapy and easily results in inadequate (or even harmful) chemotherapy.

It cannot be overemphasized that the various markers' definition and their clinical significance must from this time on serve as mental charts for neuro-oncologists, much more than the minute descriptions of morphological features. However, the latter are still of outmost importance for the pathologists, and these are easily accessible (a list of relevant reference books are found at the end of the chapter).

It is disappointing that ependymal tumors *en masse* show a much less well established list of easily detectable, well controlled, prospectively analyzed markers of either diagnostic and/or prognostic value. Recent data indicate that 3 groups of ependymomas might be possible to separate which do have significantly different survival rates. The best faring patients (**Group 1**; almost 100% 5-year overall survival: OS) suffered from tumors which were characterized by gains of chromosome 9, 15q, and/or 18, plus loss of chromosome 6. **Group 2** patients with a 5-year OS around 70% had mostly diploid genome. **Group 3** patients harbored ependymomas with the worst prognosis (5-year OS less than 30%) showed 1q gain and/or homozygous deletion of 9p21. It is important to note that often the actual chromosomal portion's function which is involved is not as yet clarified. Suffice it to say here that even for this highly elusive group of tumors there is light at the end of the tunnel and based on the recent past it can be expected that multicenter collaborative work on these entities will bring highly awaited results.

3.2 Embryonal tumors

Parallel to the evolution of molecular markers for gliomas a similar and fundamental change has occurred with regard to some embryonal tumors, namely, medulloblastomas. Similarly to those that apply to gliomas most of the required analyses are available for not only major centers but also for smaller laboratories, mainly due to the availability of immunohistochemical methods (i. e., proper and reliably tested antibodies: IDH-1, β-catenin, etc.)

Recent results indicate that medulloblastomas are highly heterogeneous and complex neoplasms, which require tailored treatment. Unfortunately on a daily basis therapeutic decisions for these patients are still predominantly made on risk group assignment based on clinical parameters and histological assessment takes place mainly of end stage disease. It is encouraging however, that our understanding of the molecular pathways involved in the pathogenesis of the majority of embryonal neoplasms is rapidly increasing. As in the case of systemic malignancies (breast-, lung-, colon cancer, and melanoma) molecular profiling of individual cancer reflects the individuality of each tumour, reveals the presence or absence of distinct disease-associated molecular signatures (see Table 4. and below). Hence these data represent a crucial component for the application of new molecular data obtained within the realm of basic oncology to tailored clinical practice.

Molecular subgroups in medulloblastomas (MBs) are characterized by distinct gene expression profiles. Convincing presentations at the British Neuro-oncology Society (Glasgow, 2010) and at the Salzburg Conference of the ISN (International Society of Neuropathology, 2010) plus several rather recent publications attest to the fact that activation of the WNT or SHH signalling pathway separates two such subgroups. The "WNT subgroup" (cca. 15%) is associated with low-risk disease. New chemotherapeutics are

available to target the SHH pathway (SHH subgroup: approximately 30%). Active research is going on to further characterize the non-SHH/WNT type of medulloblastoma (more than 50% of MBs). Commercially available IHC reagents (GAB1, ß-catenin, filamin A, and YAP1 antibodies) are helpful in distinguishing the various subtypes.
It is important to realize that MBs originate from cerebellar cortical progenitor cells. The first step seems to involve the activation of the WNT and Hedgehog (SHH) pathway. Activation of these two signalling pathways leads to the development of "classic" MB, nodular/desmoplastic MB and medullomyoblastoma. Accumulation of further genetic abnormalities (c-myc and/or N-myc amplification/overexpression, 17p loss, hTERT amplification/overexpression, etc.) results in the phenotypic change that characterizes large cell/anaplastic MBs.
Ellison et al reported the IHC classification of medulloblastomas into 3 groups. Their modified table is presented below as Table 5.

Pathway	IHC decoration of			
	GAB1	β-catenin	Filamin A	YAP1
SHH	cytoplasmic (CP)	CP	CP	nuclear + CP
WNT	negative	nuclear + CP	CP	nuclear + CP
non/SHH/WNT	negative	CP	negative	negative

Table 5.

Northcott et al have furthered this work and divided the **non/SHH/WNT** group into "Group C" and "Group D". Their exon array analysis was supplemented with IHC detection of the related proteins. The differential expression of 4 genes (**DKK1**, **SFRP1**, **NPR3**, and **KCNA1**) seems to correlate with variability of age groups and risk categories. IHC comprised antibodies against *ß-catenin*, *DKK1*, *SFRP1*, *GLI1*, and *KCNA1* proteins. The two papers were published during a 2-months-long period within the last six months. This only goes to show how rapidly this field is changing. It is to be tested on an ever increasing number of patients with proper stratification and statistical analysis but it is already clear that at least part of the late and unfortunate consequences of radical chemo- and radiotherapy of MBs can be avoided.

3.3 Meningiomas

Loss of 22q has long been described in meningeal tumors, however, no prognostic value has been possible to link to this alteration which occurs in about 60% of all meningiomas. It is important that 1p and 14q deletions are of diagnostic value when the not infrequent issue of separating meningiomas from hemangiopericytomas, superficial GBMs or metastatic carcinomas is at stake. It is also documented that allelic losses on 1p are characteristic features of meningiomas with a higher grade. Probably the most important observation is that loss of 14q seems to correlate with not only higher grade but also with an increased frequency of recurrence. Our results (Molnár et al. to be published) indicate that ploidy measurements combined with nuclear digitized morphometry helps to divide meningiomas basically into two major groups with significantly different tendency to recur or progress towards higher grades.

3.4 Primary CNS lymphomas, PCNSLs

Statistically the dominant forms are B-cell derived neoplasms. Determination of the proper treatment is fundamentally dependent on the results of various IHC reactions. It is notable that these data are of both diagnostic-, prognostic- and predictive value. Separation of PCNSLs into germinal center type (GC) or postGC/nonGC subtypes has become the standard procedure. The most widely used IHC panel is comprised of CD10, CD20, Bcl-6, IRF4/MUM1 antibodies. Details of data interpretation are discussed adequately in various handbooks/textbooks on the neoplasms of the hematopoietic-lymphoid tissues.

It is to be kept in mind that the distinctive capillary types of brain tumours (BTB = blood-tumour barrier [Schlageter et al]) have a unique feature in PCNLs: endothelial cells tend to undergo apoptosis as a result of steroid treatment (Molnár et al).

3.5 Metastatic tumors

An often encountered problem is that systemic cancers often present themselves as brain - or less frequently - spinal cord metastases. The thorough discussion of all problems related to clarifying the exact origin of MCUPs (metastatic cancer of unknown primary) exceeds the limits of this chapter.

4. Concluding remarks

1. Traditional histotechniques continue to provide the basis for starting to evaluate neurosurgical samples of neoplastic disease of the CNS.
2. If the lesion is a glial tumor IDH-1/2 analysis is to be complemented with the determination of the 1p19q status and IHC analysis of p53.
3. If the tumor's glial nature is equivocal IDH-1/2 IHC should be decisive and needs to be complemented by EGFR amplification analysis. If EGFR amplification is present with IDH1 mutation then diagnosis of GBM is warranted.
4. Grade determination might be supported and validated by IDH-1/2 analysis, 1p19q, EGFR and p16 FISH. MGMT methylation status is crucial in deciding the actual use of already widely available chemotherapeutic protocols (e. g., Stupp's).
5. Medulloblastomas already are feasible to stratification into low and high risk groups.
6. Primary CNS lymphomas can be grouped as B or T cell neoplasms and the most common type (DLBCL = diffuse large B cell lymphoma) can be separated into GC (Germinal Center) types and post GC types with the conventional IHC panels.
7. Metastatic lesions should be worked up along the lines which are well established in systemic pathology.

Recently, techniques such as next-generation DNA sequencing, massively parallel DNA resequencing and 'single-molecule genomics' have revolutionized cancer genomics. The results are "pouring in" and we can all expect that these will make a huge impact on personalized medicine in the near future. It definitely is an exceedingly exciting time ahead and at last neuro-oncopathologists may have positive intellectual reinforcements when trying to integrate this information into a morpho-functional interpretation.

5. Acknowledgement

The author is grateful for the support of the National Cancer Center, New York, NY (USA) and the VFK Krebsforschung GmbH. (Germany). Research Grant # 516/2010, Dr. Molnár P.

6. References

AJCC Cancer Staging Handbook. From the AJCC Cancer Staging Manual. Edge SB, Byrd DR, Compton CC, Fritz AG, Greene FL, Trotti A. (Eds.) 7th Ed. Springer, New York/Dordrecht/Heidelberg, London. 2010. pp 651-660.

Bailey P, Cushing H: A Classification of the Tumors of the Glioma Group on a Histogenetic Basis with a Correlated Study of Prognosis. Philadelphia: Lippincott, 1926.

Balss J, Meyer J et al: Analysis of the IDH1 codon 132 mutation in brain tumors. Acta Neuropath 116: 597-602, 2008.

Burger PC, Scheithauer BW et al: Surgical Pathology of the Nervous System and Its Coverings. 4th ed. Churchill Livingstone, Philadelphia. 2002.

Carlsson A, Persson O et al: Plasma proteome profiling reveals biomarker patterns associated with prognosis and therapy selection in glioblastoma multiforme patients. Proteomics Clin Appl 4: 591-602, 2010. doi:101002/prca.200900173

CBTRUS. Annual report. Chicago: Central Brain Tumor Registry of the United States, 2010.

Garber K. Oncometabolite? IDH1 discoveries raise possibility of new metabolism targets in brain cancers and leukaemia. JNCI 102: 926-928, 2010.

Goutagny S, Yang HW et al: Genomic Profiling Reveals Alternative Genetic Pathways of Meningioma Malignant Progression Dependent on the Underlying NF2 Status. Clin Cancer Res 16:4155-4164, 2010

Gozé C, Rigau V et al: Lack of complete 1p19q deletion in a consecutive series of 12 WHO grade II gliomas involving the insula: a marker of worse prognosis? J Neuroncol 91: 1-5, 2009. doi:10.1007/s11060-008-9680-8

Huse JT and Holland EC. Targeting brain cancer: advances in the molecular pathology of malignant glioma and medulloblastoma. Nature Reviews Cancer 10: 319-331, 2010. doi:10.1038/nrc2818

Jakab A, Molnár P et al: Glioma grade assessment by using histogram analysis of diffusion tensor imaging-derived maps. Neuroradiology 2010. doi:10.1007/s00234-010-0769-3)

Jeuken JWM, van der Maazen, Wesseling P. Molecular diagnostics as a tool to personalize treatments in adult glioma patients. Technology in Canc Res and Treatment 5: 1-15, 2008.

Joo MH et al. Clinical and biological implications of CD133-positive and CD133-negative cells in glioblastomas. Lab Invest 88: 808-815, 2008.

Kernohan JW, Mabon RF et al: A simplified classification of the gliomas. Mayo Clin Proc 24: 71-75, 1949.

Korshunov A, Meyer J et al: Combined molecular analysis of BRAF and IDH1 distinguishes pilocytic astrocytoma from diffuse astrocytoma. Acta Neuropathol 118: 401-405, 2009. doi:10.1007/s00401-009-0550-z

Korshunov A, Witt H et al: Molecular staging of intracranial ependymoma in children and adults. J Clin Oncol 28: 1-14, 2010. doi:10.1200/JCO.2009.27.3359

Loius DN, Ohgaki H et al: The 2007 WHO Classification of Tumours of the Central Nervous System. Acta Neuropathol 114: 97–109, 2007. doi:10.1007/s00401-007-0243-4

Mawrin Ch and Perry A. Pathological classification and molecular genetics of meningiomas. J Neuro-Oncol. Published online Sept. 01, 2010. doi:10.1007/s11060-010-0342-2

Molnár PP, Berényi E. Therapy-induced morphological alterations in brain tumors. The Open Pathology Journal 3: 81-90, 2009

Molnár PP. O'Neill BP et al: The blood-brain barrier in primary CNS lymphomas: Ultrastructural evidence of endothelial cell death. Neuro-Oncology 1: 89-100, 1998.

Ohgaki H and Kleihues P. Genetic alterations and signalling pathways in the evolution of gliomas. Cancer Science 100: 2235-2241, 2009.

Parsons DW et al. An Integrated Genomic Analysis of Human Glioblastoma Multiforme. Science 321: 1807-1812, 2008.

Perry A and Brat DJ. Practical Surgical Neuropathology. A Diagnostic Approach. Churchill Livingstone/Elsevier. Philadelphia. 2010

Philips HS et al. Molecular subclasses of high-grade glioma predict prognosis, delineate a pattern of disease progression, and resemble stages of neurogenesis. Cancer Cell 9: 157-173, 2006.

Rivera AL and Pelloski ChE. Diagnostic and prognostic molecular markers in common adult gliomas. Expert Rev. Mol Diagn 10: 637-649, 2010.

Schlageter KE, Molnar P et al: Microvessel organization and structure in experimental brain tumors: microvessel populations with distinctive structural and functional properties. Microvasc Res 58: 312-328, 1999

Shete S et al. Genome-wide association study identifies five susceptibility loci for glioma. Nature Gen 41: 899-904, 2009. doi:10.1038/ng.407

Stupp R, Mason WP, et al: Radiotherapy plus concomitant and adjuvant temozolomide for glioblastoma. N Engl J Med. 352: 987-96, 2005.

The Cancer Genome Atlas Research Network. Comprehensive genomic characterization defines human glioblastoma genes and core pathways. Nature 455: 1061-1068, 2008. doi:10.1038/nature07385

UICC (Union for International Cancer Control) http://www.uicc.org Sobin L, Gospodarowicz M, Wittekind Ch. TNM Classification of Malignant Tumours. 7th Ed. UICC. Wiley-Blackwell, Oxford. 2010.

Verhaak RGV et al. Integrated Genomic Analysis Identifies Clinically Relevant Subtypes of Glioblastoma Characterized by Abnormalities in PDGFRA, IDH1, EGFR, and NF1 Cancer Cell 17: 98-110, 2010.

von Deimling A. British Neuro-Oncological Society, BNOS Conference. Glasgow. 2010.

WHO Classification of Tumours of Haematopoietic and Lymphoid tissues. WHO/IARC. Swerdlow SH, Campo E et al, Lyon, 2008. pp 20-241.

WHO Classification of Tumours of the Central Nervous System. Louis DN, Ohgaki H et al: International Agency for Research on Cancer (IARC). Lyon. 2007.

Wibom C, Mörén L et al: Proteomic profiles differ between bone invasive and noninvasive benign meningiomas of fibrous and meningothelial subtype. J Neuro-Oncol 94: 321-331, 2009.

Yan H et al. IDH1 and IDH2 Mutations in Gliomas. NEJM 360: 13-21, 2009.

Yan H, Bigner DD, et al: Mutant metabolic enzymes are at the origin of gliomas. Cancer Res 69: 9157-9159, 2009. doi:10.1158/0008-5472.CAN-09-2650

Zachary JR and Yan H. Isocitrate dehydrogenase 1 and 2 mutations in cancer: alterations at a crossroads of cellular metabolism. JNCI 102: 932-941, 2010.

Zhao Sh et al. Glioma-Derived Mutations in IDH1 Dominantly Inhibit IDH1 Catalytic Activity and Induce HIF-1α. Science 324: 261-265, 2009.

Part 2

Molecular Pathways of CNS Tumors

2

Molecular Pathways of Glioblastoma and Glioblastoma Stem Cells

Cho-Lea Tso
Surgical Oncology, University of California, Los Angeles
United States of America

1. Introduction

Glioblastoma (GBM, WHO grade IV) is a type of highly malignant brain tumor that infiltrates the brain extensively and remains virtually incurable despite being treated with gross total resection and post-operative adjuvant radiation and chemotherapy. The vast majority of patients with GBM will always develop tumor recurrence. The tumor's location, its unique feature of high motility, and its protection by the blood brain barrier make certain therapies that are effective for some other cancers ineffective against brain tumors. Overall, the 5-year survival rate is less than 10%, with a final mortality rate of close to 100 percent. The molecular mechanisms that underlie persistent tumorigenesis and treatment resistance are still poorly understood. A genome-wide expression profile analysis revealed that besides those genes associated with cell proliferation, inflammation, angiogenesis, and extracellular matrix (ECM) remodeling, a series of genes linked with neuroepithelial stem cells, mesenchymal stem cells, skeletal/cartilage development, morphogenesis, and organogenesis, were determined to be overexpressed when compared with normal brain tissue, implicating that a tissue regeneration/repair-like program is constantly activated in GBM tumors. A subset of GBM develops from lower-grade gliomas and can thus be clinically classified as "secondary," whereas some GBM occur with no prior evidence of a lower-grade tumor and can be clinically classified as "primary." Substantial genetic differences between these groups of GBM have been identified. Moreover, a molecular classification study indicated that both treatment-refractory and untreated primary GBM tumors are clustered in a group segregated from treated and untreated secondary GBM tumors, and supports the view that GBM subtypes may have derived from a distinct cell-of-origin, which is resistant to conventional therapy, therefore allowing for re-seeding tumor with molecular properties similar to untreated tumors. Thus, post-treatment tumor recurrence may mimic the scenario of post-injury tissue repair. Many adult tissues undergo renewal after injury, and hence require a new supply of cells originating from specialized tissue stem cells with the capability to undergo self-renewal and differentiation to repair damaged tissue. Recently, glioblastoma stem cells (GSC) or glioblastoma stem-like cells (GSLC), a minor subpopulation within tumor mass, were isolated and characterized as tumor-initiating cells and were hypothesized to be responsible for post-treatment recurrence because of their enhanced radio-/chemo-resistant phenotype and ability to reconstitute the original tumor tissue when grafted into mice. In contrast to the hyperproliferative, inflammatory, and hyperangiogeneic properties seen in GBM tumors, molecular analysis by gene expression profiling revealed that GSC possess neuroectodermal properties and express molecular signatures of radial glial cells (RGC) and neural crest cells (NCC), as well as portray a migratory, quiescent, and slow-growing phenotype that characterizes tumor suppressor properties. Based on the tumor stem cell model and theory, conventional cell cycle-targeted radio-chemotherapy, which aims to kill fast-growing tumor cells, would then be unable to eliminate post-operative remaining tumorigenic cells that possess quiescent stem cell properties. Thus, in order to prevent tumor recurrence, a strategy targeting essential gene pathways of GSC must be identified and incorporated into the standard treatment regimen. Identifying intrinsic and extrinsic cues, by which GSC maintain tumorigenic capacity and antiapoptotic feature to sustain tumorigenesis may highlight novel therapeutic strategies to greatly diminish the recurrence rate of GBM and provide potentially curative strategies for treating brain cancers. In this chapter, we review molecular properties of GBM tumors and GSC. We also summarize molecular signaling pathways that have been relatively well-studied in GSC and are essential for maintaining GSC stemness, tumorigenic capacity, and radio-chemoresistant phenotype.

2. Molecular properties of glioblastoma

2.1 Genetic and clinical pathways to glioblastomas

GBM remains refractory to conventional therapy. The histopathologic features that distinguish it from lower-grade astrocytic tumors are the presence of cellular atypia, mitotic figures, necrotic foci with peripheral cellular pseudopalisading, and microvascular hyperplasia (1). Two subgroups of GBM have been established based on clinical experience and have been affiliated with distinct genetic mechanisms of tumorigenesis. Secondary GBM, also known as progressive GBM, develop slowly through progression from low-grade glial tumors (WHO grade II) or anaplastic glial tumors (WHO grade III) and frequently display p53 mutation (chromosome 17) (~65%) and amplification or overexpression of platelet-derived growth factor receptor (PDGFR), but not epidermal growth factor receptor (EGFR) (2-3). Additionally, progression to secondary GBM often accompanies an allelic loss at chromosome 19q, 17p, and 10q, and a loss of expression of deleted-in-colorectal-carcinoma gene (DCC) (~50%) but rarely include PTEN mutations (5%) (4-6). The p53 mutation is usually found in the low-grade lesions, indicating p53 alteration is an early event in astrocytoma progression (7). PDGFR amplification or overexpression is also present at the early stages suggesting that it may have a role in the progression of these tumors. In contrast, loss of heterozygosity for the retinoblastoma-1 (RB1) gene was found in high-grade astrocytomas (25%) but not in low-grade astrocytomas, indicating disruption of the RB pathway is likely a significant event in the malignant transformation to GBM (8). On the other hand, primary GBM, also known as de novo GBM, seem to develop rapidly and manifest high-grade lesion from the outset and are genetically characterized by EGFR amplification/overexpression (chromosome 7) (~60%), a simultaneous loss of chromosome 10, but rarely a concurrent p53 mutation. The most common EGFR gene mutation in primary GBMs is EGFRvIII, a variant lacking exons 2-7 (corresponding to cDNA nucleotides 275-1075 encoding amino acids 6–273), which results in a truncated cell surface receptor with ligand-independent constitutive tyrosine kinase activity (9-11). This mutation presumably occurs through alternative splicing or gene rearrangements (12-13) and leads to the loss of binding activation by its normal ligand, EGF and TGF-a (14-15). Mouse double minute 2 (MDM2) amplification that neutralizes p53 activity (16), is observed in more than 50% of primary GBM, but rarely in secondary GBM. Additionally, CDKN2A (p16INK4a) deletion, PTEN mutation, Rb protein alterations and loss of all or a portion of chromosome 10 are frequently seen in primary GBM (17-18). p16INK4a deletion is infrequent in secondary GBMs and its deletion and p53 mutation appear to be two mutually exclusive events in GBMs (19). Primary GBMs account for the vast majority of cases (60%) and typically occur in the elderly (>50 years old), whereas secondary GBMs, are less common (40%) and typically develop in younger patients (<45 y) (4). Primary and secondary GBMs are indistinguishable to the neurosurgeon as well as neuropathologist, and the clinical management of these two GBM subtypes is identical. To date, temozolomide (TMZ) administered daily with radiation therapy (RT) for six weeks, followed by adjuvant TMZ for six months, has become standard therapy for patients with newly diagnosed GBM.

2.2 Genetic characteristics of GBM link to prognosis

The overall prognosis for patients with GBM is extremely poor. However, a small proportion of patients show prolonged survival. A study indicates that different glioma-associated genomic aberrations may serve as prognostic markers in combination with histopathological findings (17). The use of comparative genomic hybridization (CGH)-based analysis of 20 primary GBMs suggests that loss of chromosome 10 and gain/amplification in chromosome 7 are most frequently observed in primary GBMs and are associated with microvascularization and poor prognosis (17). In contrast, the combination of chromosome 1p and 17p13-p14 and 19q deletions are associated with a longer survival time (5, 17, 20-21). The analysis of loss of heterozygosity (LOH) on chromosomes 19q, 1p, and 13q, using polymorphic microsatellite markers, however, has indicated that LOH on chromosome 19q was frequently found in secondary GBMs (50%) but rarely detected in primary GBMs (20), suggesting that tumor suppressor gene(s) located on chromosome 19q are frequently involved in the progression from a low-grade astrocytoma to secondary glioblastoma, but do not play a major role in the evolution of primary glioblastomas. Clinical trials indicated that patients whose tumor had a methylated promoter for the gene encoding O-6-methylguanine-DNA methyltransferase (MGMT), were more likely to benefit from the addition of TMZ to RT (22-23). A recent study further showed that pattern of, and time to, recurrence after TMZ concomitant with and adjuvant to radiotherapy are strictly correlated with MGMT methylation status (21). Recently, genomewide mutational analysis of GBM revealed somatic mutations of cytosolic isocitrate dehydrogenase 1 gene (IDH1), which catalyzes the oxidative decarboxylation of isocitrate to α-ketoglutarate, most frequently in WHO grade II and III astrocytomas and secondary GBM but rarely in primary GBM (22-23), and patient tumors with IDH1 or related mitochondrial IDH2 mutations had a improved clinical prognosis than those with wild-type IDH genes (25, 27). It is suggested that IDH mutation is a highly prognosis predictor and selective molecular signature of secondary GBM (28-29).

2.3 Molecular classification of glioblastoma subtypes

Identification of chromosomal abnormalities and cancer-associated genes in solid tumors is becoming easier as genome-wide analysis technologies improve and as the genome sequence is being completed. These technologies allow for genome-wide data acquisition in study of cancer genetics and biology, particularly in analysis of complex expression patterns, in a rapid and efficient fashion. Moreover, since the expression of thousands of genes is analyzed simultaneously, we can expect to obtain more comprehensive information underlying the interactions of genes related to malignant transformation as well as crucial clues about alteration in the relevant genetic and biological networks (30). Since the genetic basis of human cancer is combinatorial, this approach becomes especially important when combined with computational technology (31). Likewise, genomic mutation (e.g. deletions, inversions, chromosome re-arrangement, amplification, promoter mutation) and posttranslational modifications of proteins are the key factors that induce and maintain the malignant transformation of cancer. The success of using gene expression patterns to study cancer will depend largely on how much they reflect genomic changes. If a significant portion of the effects of genomic abnormalities can be reflected at the RNA level, the gene expression patterns will be highly informative and can be analyzed to explain the molecular mechanisms underlying the pathological development and behavior of cancers (32). GBM tumor heterogeneity is likely to play a significant role in explaining the unsuccessful treatment modalities. Therefore, molecular classification with large-scale expression assays will be more prognostically and therapeutically significant (33-34) since comprehensive and unbiased information can be obtained and would allow for the development therapies specifically tailored to each subtype. Multiple studies also indicate that gene expression-based classification of malignant gliomas correlates better with survival than histological classification (35). Successful integration of molecular/genetic data into tumor status must be descriptive and partially explain known tumor behavior, pathology, and resistance to therapy, as well as provide an insight to how the deregulation of multigene networks leads to tumor development, progression and treatment resistance (32, 36-37).

2.3.1 Glioblastoma subtypes express distinct transcription profiles

To identify whether molecular profiling can distinguish GBM subtypes, we and others have performed genome-wide microarray expression profiling and identified molecular subtypes that express distinct genes associated with tumor progression and predict clinical outcome better than histological class (35, 37-38). In general, using molecular profiling, GBM can be classified into three major subtypes include proliferative, mesenchymal and neuronal phenotypes (38-39), and the poor prognosis tumor subtypes are distinguished by the molecular markers of proliferation or mesenchymal/ECM/angiogenesis, which the majority is associated with losses on chromosome 10 that span 10q23.3 and gain on chromosome 7. In particular, most cases of mesechymal GBM had relative losses at all loci on chromosome 10 and gains of all loci on chromosome 7, whereas proliferative tumors had more heterogeneous pattern of losses chromosome 10 (38). However, upon recurrence, GBM tumors tend to shift toward mesenchymal phenotype (38, 40). In order to elucidate whether primary and secondary GBM subgroups use distinct molecular pathways as well as identify gain-of-function genes that are associated with acquisition of malignant features of GBM subtypes, we have performed a large-scale DNA microarray analysis to compare the mean level of normalized transcript levels in each of the two clinically defined GBM groups versus the grade II and III astrocytomas. We have identified shared and non-shared GBM-associated gene (GAGs) over-expressed by respective subtype (40). As anticipated, shared GAGs reflect common characteristics of hyperproliferation, hypervascularity, and apoptotic resistance in both GBM subgroups, whereas GAGs distinct to primary or secondary tumors provided information on the heterogeneous properties and apparently distinct oncogenic mechanisms of these tumors. Secondary GBM-associated GAGs were mostly related to the mitotic cell cycle **(Figure 1A)**, which corresponds to the fact that secondary GBM have high frequencies of TP53 and Rb mutations (2-3). Moreover, secondary GAGs reflect the causes and effects of such genotypic and phenotypic changes. Therefore, the molecular properties of secondary GBM support the notion that mutation or dysfunction of cell cycle regulators would be the major mechanism responsible for the development of malignant phenotype in secondary GBM. In contrast, primary GAGs highlight genes typical of a stromal/inflammatory response and are strongly associated with invasive phenotype, suggesting the importance of extracellular signaling **(Figure 1B)**. The molecular properties of primary GBM thus support the view that the interplay between GBM derived bone/cartilage-associated factors and tumor-associated stromal cells play a key role in the malignant transformation of primary GBMs. To rule out the possibility that the distinct GBM progression-associated genes identified between the two subgroups are due to selection pressure (e.g. radiation or chemotherapy), we further conducted clustering-based analysis of a set of primary GBM (n=13) that are recurrent and had prior treatment and secondary GBM (n=12) samples that had been treated during grade step prior to tumor sampling, using these identified GAGs. The results indicate that both tumor subtypes, regardless of prior treatment, cluster within their clinical grouping based on gene expression of the selected GAGs **(Figure 2)**. Of note, 85% of recurrent primary GBM are clustered to mesenchymal GBM and 83% of secondary GBM are clustered into cell-cycle GBM, indicating that prior treatment is not disrupting this identified gene expression signature of primary and secondary GBM nor driving the selection of the genes. These data therefore support the notion that diverse mechanisms and properties underlying distinct transformation events or perhaps distinct cells of origin of GBM subtypes.

2.3.2 Primary glioblastoma express mesechymal stem cell properties

The most striking observation in the molecular properties of primary GBM among all is the series of genes highly expressed in mesenchymal tissues, but not in neural or glial cells, were identified. These overexpressed genes are related to osteogenesis and chondrogenesis (e.g. cartilage glycoprotein-39/YKL-40, chitinase 3-like 2, glycoprotein nmb, lysyl oxidase, lung type-I cell membrane-associated glycoprotein, collagen type V, VI, biglycan, mesenchyme homeobox 2, and fatty acid-binding protein). These molecular properties characterized a mesenchymal phenotype of these glial tumors. To access gene pathways that are potentially associated with tumor development of primary GBM, a comparative analysis of primary GBM (n = 46) relative to normal brain tissue (n = 10) was performed. As anticipated, genes that were previously identified as primary GBM progression-associated genes reappeared in this gene list, which reflected the status of inflammation, coagulation, immune/complement responses, angiogenesis, and ECM remodeling (40, Figure 1B). Strikingly, a new series of genes linked with neural stem cells (NSC), mesenchymal stem cells (MSC), skeletal/cartilage development, morphogenesis, organogenesis, and embryonic neuroepithelial stem cells was determined. It thus implicates that a tissue regeneration/repair program is constantly activated in GBMs (Figure 3). Furthermore, a subset of primary GBM tumor-derived tumor lines expresses cellular markers that are associated with MSC (CD90, CD105, CD29, and CD44) and that GBM cell cultures can be induced to differentiate into multiple mesenchymal lineage-like cell types, including adipocytes, chondrocytes, and osteocytes (41). These findings suggest

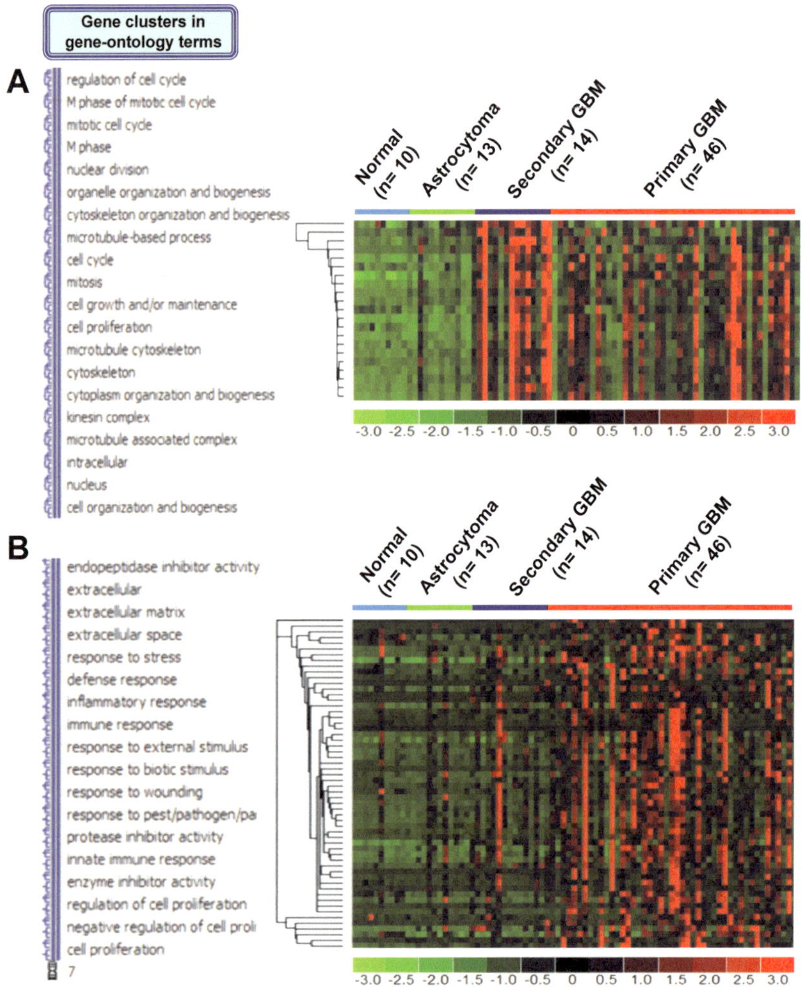

Fig. 1. Glioblastoma-associated genes (GAGs) overexpressed in GBM subtypes relative to lower grade gliomas. All plots show normalized gene expression values converted into a heat map. The log2 of the fold difference is indicated by the heat map scale at the bottom of the Figure. Each column is an individual tissue or tumor sample organized into histologic groups defined at the top of the figure. Each row is a single probe set measurement of transcript abundance for an individual gene. All genes were filtered to select transcripts with 2.5-fold or higher expression in the respective GBM group relative lower grade astrocytomas (P value < 0.05, t-test). **A**. GAGs overexpressed uniquely in secondary glioblastomas: 21 secondary GAGs were defined as being uniquely detected with a >2.5-fold overexpression in the secondary GBM group compared with the lower-grade astrocytomas and not overexpressed within the primary glioblastoma group. **B.** GAGs overexpressed uniquely in primary GBM: 58 primary GAGs were defined as overexpressed 2.5-fold relative to lower-grade astrocytomas and not detected in the secondary glioblastomas comparison using the same criteria. Functional categories of gene clusters in gene-ontology (GO) terms were shown and were analyzed using a GO annotation–based gene function enrichment analysis (d-chip software). Gene description listed in Figure 2.

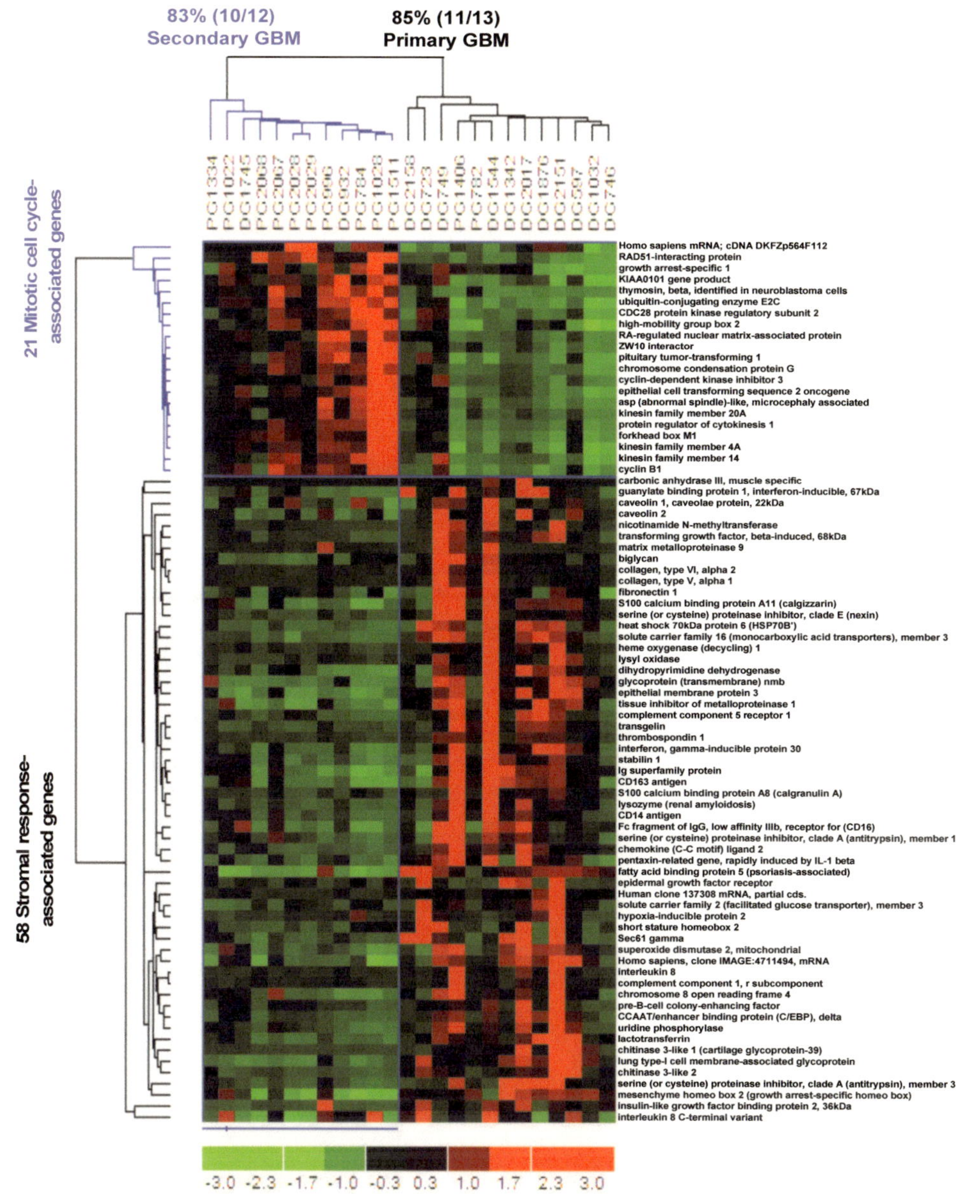

Fig. 2. Unsupervised sample clustering of primary and secondary GBM that are recurrent and had treatment using 21 secondary GAGs (Figure 1A) and 58 primary GAGs (Figure 1B). Distinct GAGs segregated GBM subtypes, suggesting they may be repopulated by GBM stem cells with distinct molecular properties. PG= progressive/secondary GBM. DG= de novo/primary GBM.

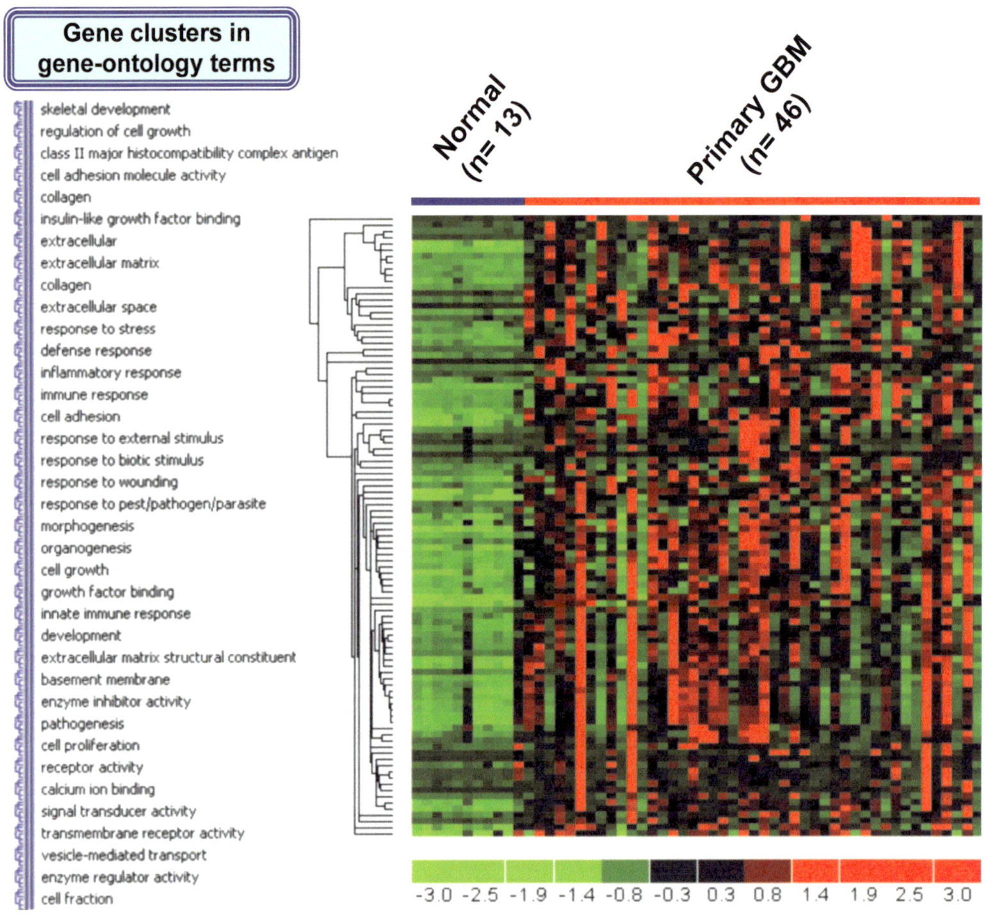

Fig. 3. A comparative analysis of gene expression profiles in primary GBM (n = 46) and normal brain tissue (n = 10). Analysis was based on a cutoff of a 2.5-fold increase in relative expression ($P < 0.05$). Top 100 primary GBM-associated genes expressed at higher levels compared with normal brain tissue were extracted. Functional categories of gene clusters in gene-ontology (GO) terms were shown.

that either a subset of primary glioblastomas derives from transformed stem cells containing MSC-like properties and retains partial phenotypic aspects of a MSC nature in tumors, or that GBMs activate a series of genes resulting in mesenchymal properties of the cancer cells to effect sustained tumor growth and malignant progression. Since primary GBM express both NSC (e.g. nestin, SOX2) and MSC makers, it is hypothesized that a subset of GBM tumors may be derived from neural crest-stem-like cells (41). The lack of MSC-like properties in secondary GBM may suggest that they originate from a different cell type of cellular origin. Further characterization of stem-like cells in GBM tumors would help to identify new targets and subsequently develop new therapeutic strategies to delay tumor progression and prevent tumor regeneration.

3. Glioblastoma stem cells

3.1 Glioblastoma contain tumorigenic stem -like cells

Tumorigenic, stem-like GBM cells, or so-called glioblastoma stem cells (GSC) have been recently isolated and characterized as GBM tumor-initiating cells by multiple groups (42-46). Although CD133/prominin, a normal NSC marker, is not an obligatory marker for GSC (46-47), CD133 was first applied as a surface marker for isolation and enrichment of GSC (42, 44-46, 48-49). Other surface markers are also reported to be used for GSC isolation and enrichment, including Musashi homolog 1 (MSI1) (50), and A2B5 (51). Through studies in both in-vitro and in-vivo GSC functional models, several essential genes and signaling pathways for maintaining tumorigenic potential have been implicated. At the functional level, GSC behave in ways similar to tissue stem cells, are capable of self-renewal and differentiation, and reconstitute the tumor tissue when grafted into mice. GSC possess a multi-lineage differentiation capacity also support for the hypothesis that cancer hierarchy is a result of developmental diversity among cancer cells in different states of differentiation (52-54). However, it is plausible that multiple genetic and/or epigenetic instabilities that take place within tumor stem cells might prevent progeny from undergoing non-proliferative terminal differentiation, leading to uncontrolled tumor growth (55-57). Tumors initiated in mouse brain by injection of patient-derived GSC often recapitulate the histopathological features of the patient tumors from which the cells were derived, indicating the ability to self-renew and reproduce the cellular heterogeneity found in human GBM tumors (44-45, 47-48). Uniquely, we found GSC isolated from treatment-refractory recurrent GBM tumors can spontaneously migrate radially outward from tumor spheres that they initiated and populated in cultures followed by spread out over the surface of the culture dish and form the secondary tumor spheres without additional factors added into the culture to influence the behavior of cells **(Figure 4)**. This in-vitro observation suggests that the migratory nature of GSC is likely to be an intrinsic property that reflects inherently migratory properties of the GBM tumor of origin. Likewise, an intracranial injection of these GSC leads to the development of YKL-40+ infiltrative tumors that display hypervascularity and pseudopalisading necrosis-like features in mouse brain **(Figure 4).** Thus, it is possible that tumor recurrence in the secondary site may be due to tumor stem cells escaping from primary treatment, migrating out of core mass, infiltrating adjacent brain tissue, and continuing seeding a new tumor. Importantly, GSC were shown to resist the effects of ionizing radiation and chemotherapy (58-59) with a marked increase in activation of several checkpoint proteins in response to DNA damage, pointing to they may be responsible for the post-treatment tumor recurrence. Thus, identification of genes and pathways confer the migratory ability, anti-apoptotic features, and tumorigenic capacity of GSC would be essential for better understanding GSC and identifying potential targets in order to eradicate and prevent them from regenerating a new tumor.

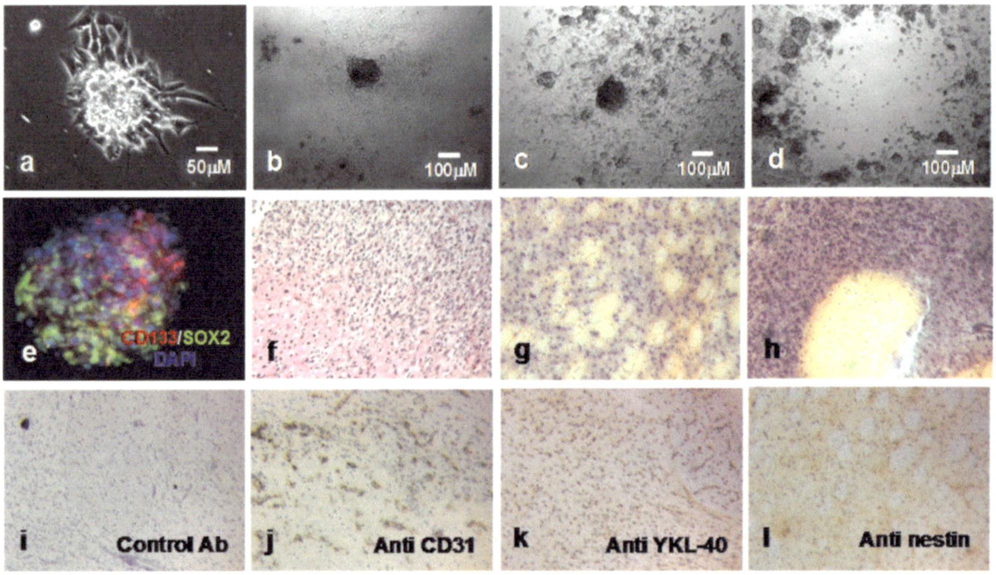

Fig. 4. Patient-derived glioblastoma stem cells (GSC) are highly motile cells and are capable of populating tumor spheres in cultures and initiating an infiltrating tumor in mouse brain. GSC isolated from treated and recurred tumor possess the ability to clonally self-renew, form primary tumor sphere (a), migrate outward (b), form secondary tumor spheres in secondary sites (c), and display pseudopalisading necrosis-like morphology (d). Immunofluorescent staining showed GSC spheres co-express CD133 and SOX2 (e) and can be propagated in cultures for indefinite passages. Brain tissues from mice injected with GSC display invasive growth of gliomas with diffuse infiltration into the surrounding tissue and exhibit hypercellular zones surrounding necrotic foci (f-h). Immunohistochemistry staining showed positivity in CD31/platelet endothelial cell adhesion molecule, YKL-40, and nestin, indicating an angiogenic progression of gliomas (i-l).

3.2 Molecular properties of tumorigeneic glioblastoma stem cells

Isolation and characterization of tumorigenic GSC derived from treatment-refractory GBM tumor may have a clinical implication of identifying innovative molecular targets for the development of a more effective treatment protocol. Particularly, elucidation of essential gene pathways of GSC that confer sustained self-renewal, cell migration and cell survival will be vital important for targeting and preventing of GSC mediated-tumor recurrence. Gene expression profile analysis revealed that purified, tumorigenic CD133+ GSC derived from treatment-refractory recurrent brain tumors possess neuroectodermal properties and portray astrogliogenic and chondrogenic potential. Moreover, CD133+GSC express molecular signatures for multiple adult stem cells, including RGC (e.g. fatty acid binding protein 7, secreted protein acidic and rich in cysteine-like 1), NCC (e.g. endothelial 3, Distal-less homeo box 5/6, v-myc myelocytomatosis viral-related oncogene), NSC (e.g. SOX2, nestin), MSC (e.g. CD44, CD105), and stem cells in the small intestine and colon (e.g. Leucine-rich repeat-containing G protein-coupled receptor 5). More strikingly, in contrast to hyperproliferative and hyperangiogenic phenotype of GBM tumors, purified CD133+ GSC, not CD133+ glioblastoma spheres (containing mostly CD133- progeny), express a tumor-suppressor phenotype, which is characterized by the expression of a series of genes associated with an anti-growing, anti-inflammatory, anti-angiogenic, anti-developmental, and migrating phenotype (42). This observation implicate that these GSC may be clinically indolent/quiescent prior to undergoing proliferative cell division, which would produce proliferative and angiogenic GBM effector progeny. Thus, it is possible that some migratory, tumorigenic GBM-stem like clones may use properties of stem cell quiescence to evade first-line treatment and regrow a new tumor at a secondary site after treatment. The molecular properties of GSC also support the view that genes guarding the pools and tumorigenic potential of GSC may not be in the subgroup of genes directly controlling cell proliferation, but in the subgroup regulating cellular quiescence, development, differentiation, and survival. Analysis of the expression of the CD133 in gliomas found that both the proportion of CD133+ cells and their topological organization in clusters were significant prognostic factors for adverse progression-free survival and overall survival (60). Computational comparisons with a collection of published gene expression profiles further reveal that the CD133 gene signature transcriptionally resembles human embryonic stem cells (ES) and GSC, and this signature successfully distinguishes glioblastoma from lower-grade gliomas, and identify an aggressive glioblastoma subtype with excess mutation (61). To date, most anti-cancer therapies aim to eliminate rapidly proliferating tumor cells; thus, the discovery of treatment-resistant, quiescent GSC (42, 58-59, 62) possessing the enhanced ability to repopulate tumors provides an excellent model to explain our inability to eradicate brain tumors (**Figure 5**). The identification of genes and pathways and performing pre-clinical validation of gene function in animal experiments may facilitate the discovery and development of innovative treatment protocols for the prevention of post-treatment tumor recurrence through the targeting tumorigenic stem-like GBM cells, which is not targeted in any current anti-cancer treatment.

4. Essential gene pathways for GSC

4.1 In-vitro cultivation of tumorigenic GSC

It is plausible that the quiescent, migratory, and tumorigenic properties render GSC an excellent candidate for being responsible for post-treatment tumor recurrence. Based on the in vitro and in vivo characterization of GSC, the GSC population is being considered a dynamic fraction of cells highly sensitive to microenvironmental changes or stimulation (e.g. self-renewal and differentiation). Therefore, identifying both intrinsic and extrinsic signaling pathways by which GSC maintain the tumorigenic capacity to support continuous tumor growth will facilitate the development of novel therapeutic strategies to diminish the recurrence rate of glioblastoma tumors. Current experimental models for the study of GSC in the laboratory have been relatively standardized. In laboratory, GSC are maintained in serum-free media supplemented with epidermal growth factor (EGF) and fibroblast growth factor (FGF) and are able to propagated as a non-adherent or semi-adherent sphere cultures for indefinite passages. More importantly, GSC are capable of clonal self-renewal and proliferative differentiation, thereby allowing populate single cell-derived tumor spheres in cultures. Genome-wide expression microarray analysis of GSC have identified a series of

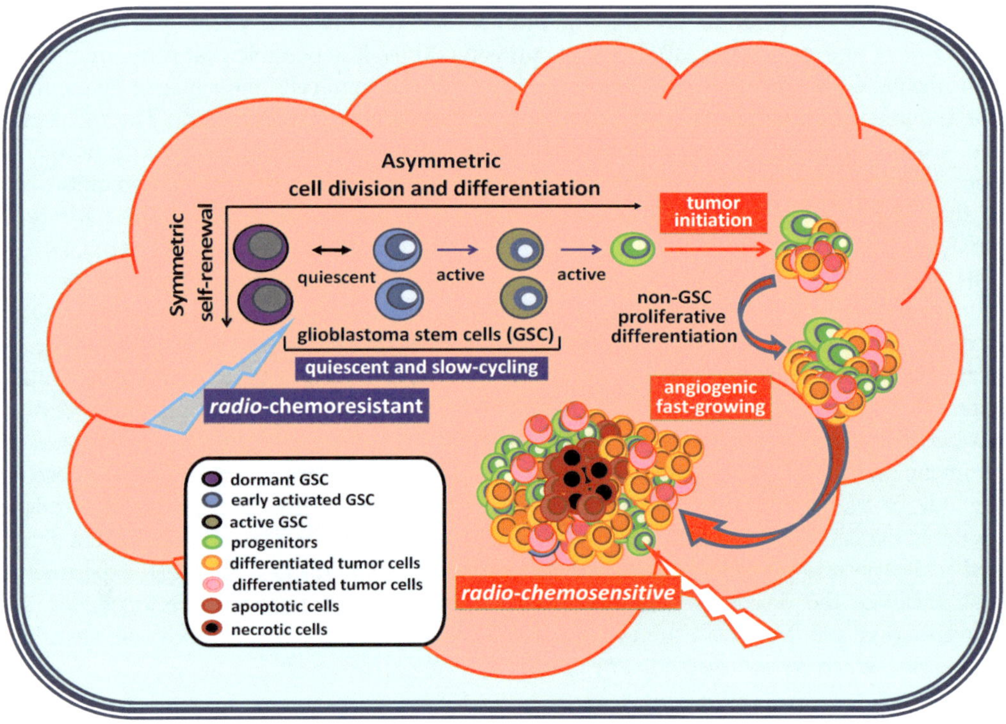

Fig. 5. A theoretical model of glioblastoma stem cells (GSC) contribute to both tumorigenesis and treatment resistance. GSC use both symmetric and asymmetric division to sustain self-renewal and proliferative differentiation to initiate and maintain a tumor. GSC contain both quiescent and active cell types; the quiescent GSC are slow-cycling, radio-chemoresistant, and capable of unlimited self-renewal, whereas the activated GSC can undergo proliferative differentiaion and initiating a tumor. Progeny of GSC populate a tumor containing a heterogeneous population in different states of differentiation, and are fast-growing, angiogenic, and radio-chemosensitive. Quiescent GSC can escape from radio-chemotherapy and continually replenish tumor cells, leading to sustained tumorigenesis.

molecular markers associated with adult stem cells (42) and a recent study further showed that GSC express EC markers which can distinguish GSC from NSC (63). GSC possess tumorigenic potential, and by contrast to regular glioblastoma cell lines cultured in serum-containing media, injection of lower number of GSC into mice with severe combined immune deficiency (SCID) is able to initiate and reconstitute GBM tumors in mouse brains, which recapitulate the histopathological features of the patient tumor from which the GSC were derived (42-47). Thus, by using these well-documented in-vitro and in-vivo functional assays of GSC, which can be visualized, assayed, and quantified, investigators have discovered and established several essential gene pathways by which properties and function of GSC can be maintained; in particular, studies using small interfering RNA (siRNA)-mediated loss-of-function phenotype, a particular gene pathway that is involved in maintaining GSC can be identified and verified. Thus, by both in-vitro and in-vivo GSC functional models, several essential genes and signaling pathways for maintaining GSC stemness, tumorigenic capacity, and anti-apoptotic features have been implicated (64, Review).

4.2 Notch signaling pathway

Several Notch effector genes, including inhibitor of differentiation 4 (ID4) (65), hairy and enhancer of split 1 (HES1) (66), hairy/enhancer-of-split related with YRPW motif 1 (HEY1) (67) and fatty acid binding protein 7 (FABP7) (68), have been detected in GSC by expression microarray analysis, thereby reflecting the prolonged Notch activation (42). Notch signaling controls numerous cell fate specification events, and it has been implicated in the maintenance of cellular quiescence in many adult stem cell pools by retaining self-renewal potential, suppressing cell differentiation, and protecting them from exhaustion of their proliferative capacity (66, 69-70). The Notch signaling network is composed of a family of four Notch receptors (Notch1, Notch2, Notch3, Notch4) and five ligands from the members of the Delta-like (DLL1, DLL3, DLL4) and the Jagged (JAG1, JAG2) families. The signaling permits the gamma secretase-mediated proteolytic release of the Notch intracellular domain (NICD), which translocates into the nucleus and transactivates target genes. Notch signaling regulates NSC differentiation; indication of Notch signaling drives NSC into quiescence, whereas blocking Notch signaling stimulates NSC undergo neurogenesis (69, 71). Moreover, Notch signaling is required to convert the hypoxic stimulus into epithelial-mesenchymal transition (EMT), increased motility, and invasiveness (72). Thus, expression of Notch effector genes in GSC implies abrogation of neurogenesis, promoting a migratory phenotype and enhancing glial-fate specification. Importantly, increased expression of FABP7 was found to be associated with regions of GBM tumor infiltration (73), suggesting that Notch activation in GSC may not only maintain the stemness of GSC, but also promote a infiltrating characteristics of brain tumor. Treatment of GBM sphere cultures with gamma-secretase inhibitors (GSIs) can deplete GSC, downregulate stem cell markers (CD133, nestin, BMI1, Olig2), and inhibit self-renewal of GSC in cultures and growth of xenografts (74). The depletion of tumorigenic GSC by Notch signaling blockade was found to occur via reduced cell proliferation and increased cell apoptosis due to decreased levels of phosphorylated AKT and STAT3 (75). In addition, it has be shown that tumor endothelial cells support GSC maintenance, which is in part via Notch signaling (76) and suggested that inhibition of Notch signaling can target GSC via an endothelial cell intermediate.

4.3 Hypoxia and hypoxia-inducible factors

It has been shown that hypoxia-inducible factors (HIFs) regulate tumorigenic capacity of GSC (77-78). When glioblastoma sphere cultures are grown in 1% oxygen, hypoxic response genes, including HIF-1, HIF-2, lysyl oxidase, and vascular endothelial growth factor (VEGF), are greatly induced, in addidton, both the stem-like side population and CD133+ cells were increased (79). Moreover, GSC respond to hypoxia by enhancing their self-renewal activity and anti-differentiated status (80). Loss of HIF-2α in GSC leads to a significant decrease in both GSC proliferation and self-renewal in cultures, and attenuation of tumorigenic capacity in animals (80). Hypoxia requires Notch signaling for maintaining cells in an undifferentiated state, which occurs by recruiting HIF-1α to the promoters of Notch-responsive target genes (81). The maintenance of GSC by a hypoxic microenvironment via enhancing the activity of other stem cell factors such as Oct4, c-Myc, and Nanog, also partially promotes and stabilizes the stem cell phenotype (77, 82). Thus, HIFs might potentially represent a promising target for depleting GSC populations.

4.4 GLI – Nanog axis

Nanog and Hedgehog (HH) are two essential regulators of stemness in ES. HH proteins act through the Patched (Ptc) and Smoothened (Smo) and ultimately activates the GLI family of transcription factors. HH-GLI signaling modulates neural progenitor proliferation and survival in the developing neural tube, and controls stem cell behavior in the postnatal and adult brain (83-85). Nanog, a pluripotency homeobox gene, is regulated by HH-GLI signaling via binding of HH effectors, Gli1 and Gli2, to the Nanog promoter, thus activating Nanog expression (86). A study shows that HH-GLI signaling regulates glioma growth, GSC self-renewal, and tumorigenic capacity, and the blockade of HH-GLI signaling by treatment with cyclopamine depletes GSC (87). Nanog was recently reported to be a novel HH-GLI mediator for expanding CD133+ GSC and promoting glioblastoma growth (88). More importantly, it was found that loss of tumor suppressor p53 activates HH-GLI signaling, thereby contributing to Nanog upregulation and leading to the promoting of GSC stemness. In contrast, the presence of p53 can negatively regulate the activity and level of GLI1, thus downregulating Nanog expression (86, 88-89). Therefore, the inversely reciprocal levels of GLI1 and p53 are consistently maintained in GSC (88). Concurrently, GLI1 upregulates Notch and downregulates bone morphogenetic protein (BMP) signaling, a pro-differentiative action on stem cells (89), implying an essential role of a functional GLI1-NANOG-p53-Notch network in maintaining stemness and tumorigenic capacity of GSC. Thus, **GLI–Nanog axis** provides a potential treatment target for the prevention of GSC-mediated tumor recurrence.

4.5 Transforming growth factor beta (TGFβ) signaling

The TGF-β signaling pathway plays an essential role in the regulation of embryonic development, cell proliferation, motility and apoptosis, ECM production and modulation of immune function (90). The TGF-β superfamily comprises both growth and differentiation factors including TGF-βs, activins, inhibins, and bone morphogenetic proteins (BMPs). TGFβ signaling by binding to type I and type II receptors on the cell surface. The type II receptor phosphorylates the type I receptor, which propagates the signal by phosphorylating receptor-activated SMAD (R-SMAD) proteins (91) that transduce TGF-β family signals into a transcriptionally regulated developmental program. A recent study showed that the TGFb/activin signaling pathway is essential for the maintenance of ES cells, which is via binding of SMAD2/3 to the NANOG proximal promoter in human ES (92). Alternatively, TGFβ signaling can act through Smad-independent pathways, which activate Ras/extracellular signal-regulated kinase (ERK), TGFβ-activated kinase-1/p38 mitogen-activated protein kinase (MAPK)/c-Jun NH2-terminal kinase (TAK1/P38/JNK), phosphatidylinositol 3-kinase(PI3K)/AKT, and signal transducers and activators of transcription 3 (STAT3) (93-94). A study showed that TGFβ signaling promotes the self-renewal and tumorigenic capacity of GSC by Smad-dependent induction of leukemia inhibitory factor (LIF) (95). Treatment of GSC with recombinant LIF induced a rapid phosphorylation of STAT3. Thus, TGFβ signaling promotes GSC self-renewal through the activation of JAK-STAT pathway by the induction of LIF secretion (95). Mice receiving GSC pre-treated with a TGFβ receptor inhibitor and a JAK inhibitor significantly increased the survival rate compared to the group receiving non-treated GSC, indicating the TGFβ and JAK-STAT signaling pathways play an essential role for maintaining tumorigenic potential of GSC (95).

A direct mechanistic link of STAT3 activation to GSC growth and self-renewal was further evidenced by two separated studies, demonstrating that knockdown of STAT3 signaling by a short hairpin RNA (shRNA) or inhibitors of STAT3-DNA binding, leads to loss of capacity for tumor sphere formation, induction of cell apoptosis, and a decrease in tumor-initiating capacity in animals (96-97). Therefore, these data suggest that the STAT3 signaling pathway may be a potential target for GSC-directed brain tumor therapy. Since STAT3 signaling is a downstream effector of interleukin-6 (IL-6), blockade of IL-6R alpha or IL-6 expression with shRNAs also suppresses tumor sphere formation capacity and increases survival of mice bearing intracranial glioblastoma xenografts (98). Another related study showed that autocrine TGF-beta signaling maintains stemness of GSC by induction of Sry-related HMG-box 2 (SOX2), one of the key transcription factors required in induced pluripotent stem cells, and this induction was mediated by Sox4, a direct TGF-beta target gene (99). Thus, treatment with inhibitors of TGF-beta signaling drastically deplete GSC by promoting their differentiation, and leads to less lethal potency in intracranial transplantation assay. SOX2 silencing or induction of GSC differentiation by treatment with bone morphogenetic protein 4 led to the loss of self-renewal capacity and tumorigenicity of GSC (62, 100-101), indicating the maintenance of the undifferentiated phenotype is one of the key criteria for retaining tumorigenic capacity of GSC.

4.6 Epidermal growth factor receptor (EGFR) and down-stream AKT, MEK (mitogen-activated protein kinase/ERK kinase), and ERK 1/2 signaling

EGFR is commonly amplified and/or mutated in high-grade gliomas. A study showed that EGFR signaling pathway is involved in the maintenance of GSC and is required for gliomagenesis (102). Treatment of GSC with tyrosine kinase inhibitors of EGFR signaling suppresses GSC self-renewal and induces cell apoptosis through the inhibition of phosphorylation of EGFR, AKT kinase, and ERK 1/2 (103-104). Likewise, GSC display preferential sensitivity to Akt inhibition relative to matched non-GSC cells and inhibition of Akt activity in GSC increased the survival of animal bearing human glioma xenografts (105). Similar results are also demonstrated by a targeted inactivation of MEK/ERK signaling, which led to the reduction of sphere-forming capacity of GSC accompanied by their differentiation into neuronal and glial lineages (106). Moreover, combinational blockade of both MEK/ERK and PI3K/mTOR pathways suppressed the tumorigenic capacity of GSC more effectively than blockade of either alone (107). These results therefore indicate that the EGF/EGFR signaling and its downstream effector activation are essential for maintaining GSC, suggesting a potential molecular pathway target for depletion of GSC.

4.7 c-Myc

c-Myc belongs to a family of transcription factors containing basic, helix-loop-helix, and leucine zipper domains and it is an essential factor for normal embryonic development (108). c-Myc is an oncogenic transcription factor commonly overexpressed in a variety of human cancers. In contrast, c-Myc gene inactivation triggers telomere-independent senescence mediated by the cyclin-dependent kinase inhibitor p16INK4a, which is regulated by the polycomb group repressor Bmi-1, a direct transcriptional target of c-Myc (109). High-level of c-Myc expression was found in GSC relative to non-stem glioma cells, and knockdown of c-Myc in GSC induces cell apoptosis and leads to the loss of tumorigenic capacity (110). A recent study further showed that HIF-2α promotes GSC self-renewal and stemness properties via enhancing the expression of c-Myc (82), and inactivation of PTEN and p53 can also lead to the increased expression of c-Myc and promotion of stemness, self-renewal and the tumorigenic capacity of GSC (111). These data suggest that the c-Myc signaling pathway is required for maintaining the self-renewal capability and tumorigenic potential of GSC, and therefore may serve as a potential signaling pathway target for a GSC -directed brain cancer therapy.

4.8 L1 cell adhesion molecule (L1CAM), Olig2, Bmi-1, integrin α6, and A20

L1CAM is a cell adhesion molecule plays an important role in nervous system development, including neuronal migration and differentiation (112). L1CAM expression was found to be preferentially higher in GSC compared to normal neural progenitors, and knockdown of L1CAM expression via shRNA interference can lead to the loss of sphere-forming capacity, induced cell apoptosis, and suppressed tumor growth (113). The induction of GSC apoptosis by decreasing the expression of L1CAM is suggested due to the decreased expression of the basic helix-loop-helix transcription factor Olig2 and the increased expression of the p21WAF1/CIP1 tumor suppressor (113). Correspondingly, it has been shown that an Olig2-regulated lineage-restricted pathway is critical for proliferation and maintenance of tumorigenic GSC through the suppression of p21WAF1/CIP1 (114).

Bmi1 plays an essential part in the self-renewal of hematopoietic stem cells (HSC) and NSC (115-117). Bmi1 is part of the Polycomb group gene family and a member of polycomb-repressing complex 1 (PRC1), which is required to maintain the transcriptionally repressive state of many genes by chromatin remodeling and histone modification (118-119). It has been shown that Bmi-1 is highly expressed in CD133+ GSC and Bmi-1 knockdown resulted in inhibition of self-renewal capacity and induction of both cell apoptosis and cell differentiation, as well as loss of tumorigenic capacity (120). Similarly, disruption of EZH2, the main component of PRC2, robustly impairs self-renewal and tumorigenic capacity of GSC (121). This data thus suggest that PcG proteins are required for maintaining stemness, survival, and tumorigenic capacity of GSC.

Integrins are one of the major families of cell adhesion receptors that cells use to both bind to and respond to the ECM (122). Specifically, integrin α6 subunit is critical for the early development of the nervous system and has been shown to play a role in neuronal migration, neurite outgrowth, and axon guidance during olfactory development (123). A recent study showed that GSC highly express integrin α6 and their interaction with laminin on endothelial cells directly regulates the tumorigenic capacity of GSC (124). Targeting integrin α6 in GSCs inhibits self-renewal, proliferation, and tumor formation capacity (124), indicating integrin α6 is an essential factor for maintaining GSC and can be potentially used as a cellular target for depletion of GSCs.

Tumor necrosis factor, alpha-induced protein 3 (TNFAIP3) or A20, a zinc finger protein, is an NF-κB-inducible gene. A20 can protect the cells from TNF-induced apoptosis by disrupting the recruitment of the death domain signaling molecules TRADD and RIP to the receptor signaling complex (125). A novel anti-apoptotic mechanism of A20 was recently reported and showed that A20 blocks TNF-induced apoptosis through suppression of c-jun N-terminal kinase (JNK) by targeting apoptosis signal-regulating kinase1 (ASK1) (126). A20 was overexpressed in clinical glioma tissue samples and correlates to clinical staging (127). A recent study showed that GSC overexpress A20, relative to non-stem glioma cells, and this protects GSC from cell death (128). Inhibiting A20 expression by shRNA (shRNA) decreased GSC growth and survival through mechanisms associated with decreased cell-cycle progression and decreased phosphorylation of NF-kappaB p65(RelA). By contrast, elevated levels of A20 in GSCs contributed to apoptotic resistance and were less susceptible to TNFalpha-induced cell death than matched non-stem glioma cells. A20 knockdown reduced the self-renewal ability of these cells and decreased tumorigenic potential of GSCs, thereby resulting in increased survival of mice bearing human glioma xenografts. Thus, A20 contributes to glioma maintenance likely through anti-apoptotic effects on GSC.

5. Gene pathways underlying the radio-chemoresistant phenotype of GSC

Concurrent TMZ and RT followed by adjuvant TMZ is standard for patients with newly diagnosed glioblastoma based on a large randomized phase III trial that showed survival benefit (129-130). Studies further showed that patients whose tumor had a methylated promoter for the gene encoding O6-methylguanine-DNA methyltransferase (MGMT), a DNA repair protein, were more likely to benefit from the addition of TMZ (22, 130). Although the survival advantage of combined treatment lasts up to 5 years of follow-up, most patients successfully treated with combined therapy eventually had tumor recurrence and died (130). A significant increase in MGMT expression was found in first recurrence after treatment with RT plus TMZ, indicating either selection of MGMT-expressing cells or induction of the MGMT gene by TMZ (131). Molecular analysis of glioblastoma tumors resistance to the concomitant radio-chemotherapy with TMZ had identified a self-renewal signature dominated by homeobox (HOX) genes, which are comprised of CD133 (132). Of note, tumors with the enhanced expression of HOX genes, high EGFR expression, plus unmethylated MGMT were associated with short survival (132), implicating the association of stem-cell phenotype and radiochemoresistance. It is plausible that the quiescent stem cell nature adopted by GSC may explain the considerable resistance to chemotherapeutic agents (133-136). Moreover, quiescent cells show greater repair capacities than proliferative cells (58, 135), suggesting that slow-cycling GSC may play a key role in the acquired or constitutive resistance to radio-chemotherapy (137).

5.1 Activation of checkpoint proteins

A study indicated a potential role of DNA damage checkpoint protein, Chk1 and Chk2 kinases in the radioresistant phenotype of CSC (58). Particularly, CD133+ GSC isolated from glioblastoma tumors preferentially activated Chk1/2 kinases, and repaired radiation-induced DNA damage more effectively than CD133- non-GSC cells (58), indicting stem-like glioblastoma cell population within tumor mass are likely responsible for the treatment resistance. This notion was further supported by the demonstrating that the radioresistant phenotype of GSC can be reversed by the treatment with a specific inhibitor of the Chk1 and Chk2 checkpoint kinases (58).

5.2 Evasion of cell-death pathway

Evidently, GSC exhibit enhanced chemoresistance to anticancer drugs (59, 138-139). The expression of ATP-binding cassette transporter ABCG2 in a tumorigenic stem-like side population (SP) distinguish them from the non-stem-like cells (138), suggesting a potential mechanism underlying chemoresistance in CSCs. Several anti-apoptotic genes (e.g. BCL-2, BCL2L1a, and MCL1) were also found to be at higher expression levels in TMZ resistant-GSC clones than those in differentiated cell lines (140). Likewise, CD133+ GSC were characterized by the enhanced expression of multidrug resistance 1 (MDR1) compared to CD133- non-stem cells (139). Moreover, the radio-resistance of GSC could be alleviated by treatment with an XIAP inhibitor (141). Thus, the radio-chemoresistance of GSC may be linked to the activation of the DNA damage checkpoint response, MGMT-mediated DNA repair, expression of both drug efflux transporters and anti-apoptotic factors, or abnormalities of cell-death pathways (59, 132,138, 141).

5.3 Constitutively active Notch and PI3K/Akt signaling

Notch signaling promotes radioresistance of GSC by upregulating PI3K/AKT pathway signaling and increasing the expression levels of myeloid cell leukemia-1(MCL1), an anti-apoptotic member of Bcl-2 family. The knockdown of Notch1 or Notch2 signaling in GSC sensitizes GSC to radiation treatment and impairs tumorigenic capacity (142), indicating a critical role of Notch/PI3K/AKT signaling in radioresistance of GSC. Moreover, addition of GSIs enhances TMZ treatment of human gliomas by inhibiting neurosphere repopulation and xenograft recurrence (143), pointing out the essential role of Notch pathway in chemoprotection of GSC.

5.4 Bmi-1-mediated DNA damage response

Bmi-1 plays important roles in histone H2A ubiquitination and HOX gene silencing, and is a potent negative regulator of the Ink4a/Arf locus, which encodes the cell cycle regulators and tumor suppressor p16Ink4a and p19Arf genes (144, 145). BMI1 was enriched at the chromatin after irradiation and colocalized with ataxia-telangiectasia mutated (ATM) kinase and the histone gammaH2AX, an important DNA double strand break (DSB) repair pathway (144). A recent study showed that Bmi-1 preferentially copurified with non-homologous end joining (NHEJ) proteins in CD133+ GSC, suggesting that Bmi-1 confers radioresistance to GSC may through the recruitment of DNA damage response machinery (145).

5.5 Insulin-like growth factor binding protein 2 (IGFBP2)

IGFBP-2 is a member of a family of six highly conserved IGFBPs that are carriers for the IGFs. The heparin-binding domain (HBD) of IGFBP2 has anabolic activity by activating IGF-I/Akt and β-catenin signaling pathways (146). IGFBP2 is known to be overexpressed in a majority of glioblastoma tumors, and its expression is inversely correlated to glioblastoma patient survival (40, 147). IGFBP2 enhances tumor invasion by upregulating matrix metalloproteinase-2 and CD24 (148, 149). Recent studies indicated that IGFBP2 is overexpressed in GSC (42, 150) and autocrine IGFBP2 is required for self-renewal and expansion of GSC (150). The knockdown of IGFBP2 expression downregulated the expression of stemness-associated gene and reduced AKT activation, and treatment with an IGFBP2 neutralizing antibody sensitized GSC to irradiation and multiple anti-neoplastic agents (150). As anticipated, recombinant IGFPB2 substantiated AKT signaling-mediated GSC viability that could be blocked by treatment with PI3K/Akt inhibitors, suggesting that IGFBP2 contributes to anti-apoptotic features of GSC.

6. Final remarks

The isolation and characterization of GSC have not only significantly changed the biological view of tumors, but has also impacted the design of effective therapies, as radio-chemoresistant, stem-like, tumorigenic glioblastoma cells may continue seeding the new tumor, despite local treatment to the tumor mass. Currently, the GSC hypothesis and model are not fully established. However, the accumulated preclinical data generated and established from both in-vitro and in-vivo GSC model systems will certainly facilitate the exploration of new concepts in tumor biology, tumor relapse and the design of potentially more effective treatment protocols that can specifically target GSC with radio-chemoresistant features. Meanwhile, since CSC share many signaling pathways with normal stem cells, exploring differences between normal and tumor stem cells may reveal novel, tumor-specific molecular targets for a safe therapy for brain cancer. Moreover, identifying the extrinsic cues and effects from their niche on GSC is also crucial as they may provide vital signaling to modulate GSC physiology and pathology (151-152). The cure for cancer requires eliminating both GSC and non-GSC populations; thus, it is important to design preclinical studies and clinical trials which evaluate the synergistic benefits of incorporating GSC-targeted therapies into conventional cancer treatments. Based on the molecular pathways of gliblastoma and GSC discussed in this chapter, I designed a therapeutic model for targeting both fast-growing, hyper-angiogenic glioblastoma tumor cells and slow-cycling, quiescent, anti-apoptotic GSC; the model theoretically and ideally, can prevent post-treatment tumor recurrence (Figure 6).

7. Acknowledgments

I thank Jonathan Tso, for the critical review of this chapter. This work was supported by the grants from American Cancer Society (RSG-07-109-01-CCE), National Cancer Institute (1 R21 CA140912-01), National Institute of Health (1DP2OD006444-01), and The Bradley Zankel Foundation to C-L T.

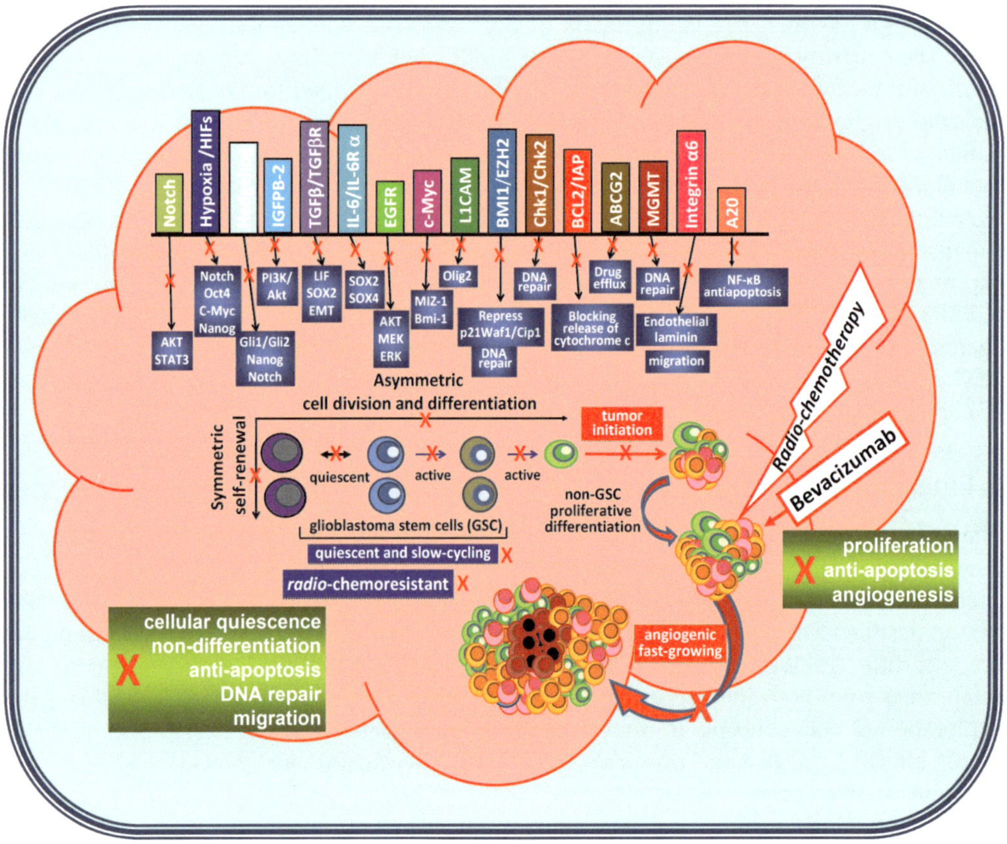

Fig. 6. A model of glioblastoma stem cell (GSC)-targeted brain cancer therapy. GSC utilize multiple stem cell associated-signaling pathways to achieve a radio-chemoresistant phenotype that sustains tumorigenesis. Essential gene pathways as indicated have been determined to be required for maintaining stemness properties, tumorigenic capacity and a radio-chemoresistant phenotype of GSC. Radiochemoresistance may be accomplished via collaboration of constitutive activation of the DNA damage checkpoint response and PI3K-Akt signaling pathway, high expression of both anti-apoptotic proteins and drug efflux transporters, and evasion of both differentiation and irreversible cell cycle arrest (cellular quiescence). In order to eradicate a tumor and prevent post-treatment tumor recurrence, a therapeutic strategy that target essential gene pathways for maintaining GSC must be developed to be fully integrated into radio-chemotherapy and anti-angiogenic therapy in order to target both quiescent GSC and fast-growing, angiogenic non-GSC populations.

8. References

[1] Prat DJ, Van Meir EG. Vaso-occlusive and prothrombotic mechanisms associated with tumor hypoxia, necrosis, and accelerated growth in glioblastoma (review). Lab Invest 2004; 84: 397–405.

[2] Kleihues P, Ohgaki H. Primary and secondary glioblastomas: from concept to clinical diagnosis. Neuro-oncol. 1:44-51, 1999. Review.

[3] Maruno M, Ninomiya H, Ghulam Muhammad AK, Hirata M, Kato A, Yoshimine T. Whole-genome analysis of human astrocytic tumors by comparative genomic hybridization. Brain Tumor Pathol. 17:21-7, 2000.

[4] Brat DJ, Castellano-Sanchez A, Kaur B, Van Meir EG. Genetic and biologic progression in astrocytomas and their relation to angiogenic dysregulation. Adv Anat Pathol. 9:24-36, 2002. Review.

[5] Schmidt MC, Antweiler S, Urban N, Mueller W, Kuklik A, Meyer-Puttlitz B, Wiestler OD, Louis DN, Fimmers R, von Deimling A. Impact of genotype and morphology on the prognosis of glioblastoma. J Neuropathol Exp Neurol. 61:321- 328, 2002.

[6] Watanabe K, Tachibana O, Sata K, Yonekawa Y, Kleihues P, Ohgaki H. Overexpression of the EGF receptor and p53 mutations are mutually exclusive in the evolution of primary and secondary glioblastomas. Brain Pathol. 6:217-223, 1996.

[7] Ohgaki H, Kleihues P. Genetic pathways to primary and secondary glioblastoma. Am J Pathol 170:1445-1453, 2007.

[8] Henson JW, Schnitker BL, Correa KM, von Diemling A, Fassbender F, Xu HJ, Benedict WF, Yandell DW, Louis DN. The retinoblastoma gene is involved in malignant progression of astrocytomas. Ann. Neurol. 36: 714-721, 1994.

[9] Schwechheimer K, Huang S, Cavenee WK. EGFR gene amplification– rearrangement in human glioblastomas. Int. J. Cancer, 62: 145-148, 1995.

[10] Wong AJ, Ruppert JM, Bigner SH, Grzeschik CH, Humphrey PA, Bigner DS, Vogelstein B. Structural alterations of the epidermal growth factor receptor gene in human gliomas. Proc. Natl. Acad. Sci. USA, 89: 2965-2969, 1992.

[11] Ekstrand A J, Sugawa N, James CD, Collins VP. Amplified and rearranged epidermal growth factor receptor genes in human glioblastomas reveal deletions of sequences encoding portions of the N- and/or C-terminal tails. Proc. Natl. Acad. Sci. USA, 89: 4309-4313, 1992.

[12] Chu CT, Everiss KD, Wikstrand CJ, Batra SK, Kung HJ, Bigner DD. Receptor dimerization is not a factor in the signalling activity of a transforming variant epidermal growth factor receptor (EGFRvIII). Biochem. J. 324: 855-861, 1997.

[13] Ekstrand AJ, Longo N, Hamid ML, Olson JJ, Liu L, Collins VP, James CD. Functional characterization of an EGF receptor with a truncated extracellular 19 domain expressed in glioblastomas with EGFR gene amplification. Oncogene. 9: 2313-2320, 1994

[14] Wong AJ, Ruppert JM, Bigner SH, Grzeschik CH, Humphrey PA, Bigner DS, Vogelstein B. Structural alterations of the epidermal growth factor receptor gene in human gliomas. Proc. Natl. Acad. Sci. USA, 89: 2965-2969, 1992.

[15] Frederick L, Wang XY, Eley G, James CD. Diversity and frequency of epidermal growth factor receptor mutations in human glioblastomas. Cancer Res. 60:1383-1387, 2000.

[16] Shieh SY, Ikeda M, Taya Y, Prives C. DNA damage-induced phosphorylation of p53 alleviates inhibition by MDM2. Cell. 91: 325-334, 1997.

[17] Arslantas A, Artan S, Oner U, Müslümanoğlu H, Durmaz R, Cosan E, Atasoy MA, Başaran N, Tel E. The importance of genomic copy number changes in the prognosis of glioblastoma multiforme. Neurosurg Rev. 27(1): 58-64, 2004.

[18] Furnari FB, Fenton T, Bachoo RM, Mukasa A, Stommel JM, Stegh A, Hahn WC, Ligon KL, Louis DN, Brennan C, Chin L, DePinho RA, Cavenee WK. Malignant astrocytic glioma: genetics, biology, and paths to treatment. Genes Dev. 21:2683-2710, 2007.

[19] Fulci G, Labuhn M, Maier D, Lachat Y, Hausmann O, Hegi ME, Janzer RC, Merlo A, Van Meir EG.p53 gene mutation and ink4a-arf deletion appear to be two mutually exclusive events in human glioblastoma. Oncogene. 19:3816-3822, 2000.

[20] Nakamura M, Yang F, Fujisawa H, Yonekawa Y, Kleihues P, Ohgaki H. Loss of heterozygosity on chromosome 19 in secondary glioblastomas. J Neuropathol Exp Neurol. 59:539-543, 2000.

[21] Ino Y, Zlatescu MC, Sasaki H, Macdonald DR, Stemmer-Rachamimov AO, Jhung S, Ramsay DA, von Deimling A, Louis DN, Cairncross JG. Long survival 16 and therapeutic responses in patients with histologically disparate high-grade gliomas demonstrating chromosome 1p loss. J Neurosurg. 92:983-990, 2000.

[22] Hegi ME, Diserens AC, Gorlia T, Hamou MF, de Tribolet N, Weller M, Kros JM, Hainfellner JA, Mason W, Mariani L, Bromberg JE, Hau P, Mirimanoff RO, Cairncross JG, Janzer RC, Stupp R.MGMT gene silencing and benefit from temozolomide in glioblastoma. N Engl J Med. 352(10):997-1003, 2005.

[23] Maurer GD, Tritschler I, Adams B, Tabatabai G, Wick W, Stupp R, Weller M. Cilengitide modulates attachment and viability of human glioma cells, but not sensitivity to irradiation or temozolomide in vitro. Neuro Oncol. 11(6):747-756, 2009.

[24] Brandes AA, Franceschi E, Tosoni A, Benevento F, Scopece L, Mazzocchi V, Bacci A, Agati R, Calbucci F, Ermani M. Temozolomide concomitant and adjuvant to radiotherapy in elderly patients with glioblastoma: correlation with MGMT promoter methylation status.Cancer. 115(15):3512-3518, 2009.

[25] Parsons DW, Jones S, Zhang X, Lin JC, Leary RJ, Angenendt P, Mankoo P, Carter H, Siu IM, Gallia GL, Olivi A, McLendon R, Rasheed BA, Keir S, Nikolskaya T, Nikolsky Y, Busam DA, Tekleab H, Diaz LA Jr, Hartigan J, Smith DR, Strausberg RL, Marie SK, Shinjo SM, Yan H, Riggins GJ, Bigner DD, Karchin R, Papadopoulos N, Parmigiani G, Vogelstein B, Velculescu VE, Kinzler KW. An integrated genomic analysis of human glioblastoma multiforme.Science. 321(5897):1807-1812, 2008.

[26] Ichimura K, Pearson DM, Kocialkowski S, Bäcklund LM, Chan R, Jones DT, Collins VP. IDH1 mutations are present in the majority of common adult gliomas but rare in primary glioblastomas.Neuro Oncol. 11(4):341-347, 2009.

[27] Yan H, Parsons DW, Jin G, McLendon R, Rasheed BA, Yuan W, Kos I, Batinic-Haberle I, Jones S, Riggins GJ, Friedman H, Friedman A, Reardon D, Herndon J, Kinzler

KW, Velculescu VE, Vogelstein B, Bigner DD. IDH1 and IDH2 mutations in gliomas.N Engl J Med. 360(8):765-773, 2009.

[28] Nobusawa S, Watanabe T, Kleihues P, Ohgaki H. IDH1 mutations as molecular signature and predictive factor of secondary glioblastomas. Clin Cancer Res. 15(19):6002-6007, 2009.

[29] Hartmann C, Hentschel B, Wick W, Capper D, Felsberg J, Simon M, Westphal M, Schackert G, Meyermann R, Pietsch T, Reifenberger G, Weller M, Loeffler M, von Deimling A. Patients with IDH1 wild type anaplastic astrocytomas exhibit worse prognosis than IDH1-mutated glioblastomas, and IDH1 mutation status accounts for the unfavorable prognostic effect of higher age: implications for classification of gliomas. Acta Neuropathol. 120(6):707-718, 2010.

[30] Szallasi Z. Bioinformatics. Gene expression patterns and cancer. Nat Biotechnol. 16:1292-1293, 1998.

[31] Loging WT, Lal A, Siu IM, Loney TL, Wikstrand CJ, Marra MA, Prange C, Bigner DD, Strausberg RL, Riggins GJ. Identifying potential tumor markers and antigens by database mining and rapid expression screening. Genome Res. 10:1393-1402, 2000.

[32] Liotta L, Petricoin E. Molecular profiling of human cancer. Nat Rev Genet. 1:48-56, 2000.

[33] Bullinger L, Dohner K, Bair E, Frohling S, Schlenk RF, Tibshirani R, Dohner H, Pollack JR.Use of gene-expression profiling to identify prognostic subclasses in adult acute myeloid leukemia. N Engl J Med. 350:1605-1616, 2004.

[34] Cairncross JG, Ueki K, Zlatescu MC, Lisle DK, Finkelstein DM, Hammond RR, Silver JS, Stark PC, Macdonald DR, Ino Y, Ramsay DA, Louis DN. Specific genetic predictors of chemotherapeutic response and survival in patients with anaplastic oligodendrogliomas. J Natl Cancer Inst. 90:1473-1479, 1998.

[35] Nutt CL, Mani DR, Betensky RA, Tamayo P, Cairncross JG, Ladd C, Pohl U, Hartmann C, McLaughlin ME, Batchelor TT, Black PM, von Deimling A, Pomeroy SL, Golub TR, Louis DN. Gene expression-based classification of malignant gliomas correlates better with survival than histological classification. Cancer Res. 63:1602-1607, 2003.

[36] Albertson DG, Collins C, McCormick F, Gray JW. Chromosome aberrations in solid tumors. Nat Genet. 34:369-376, 2003.

[37] Zhu Y, Parada LF. The molecular and genetic basis of neurological tumours. Nat Rev Cancer. 2:616-626, 2002.

[38] Phillips HS, Kharbanda S, Chen R, Forrest WF, Soriano RH, Wu TD, Misra A, Nigro JM, Colman H, Soroceanu L, Williams PM, Modrusan Z, Feuerstein BG, Aldape K.Molecular subclasses of high-grade glioma predict prognosis, delineate a pattern of disease progression, and resemble stages in neurogenesis. Cancer Cell. 9(3):157-173, 2006.

[39] Freije WA, Castro-Vargas FE, Fang Z, et al. Gene expression profiling of gliomas strongly predicts survival. Cancer Res. 64: 6503-6510, 2004.

[40] Tso CL, Freije WA, Day A, Chen Z, Merriman B, Perlina A, Lee Y, Dia EQ, Yoshimoto K, Mischel PS, Liau LM, Cloughesy TF, Nelson SF.Distinct transcription profiles of primary and secondary glioblastoma subgroups. Cancer Res. 66(1):159-67, 2006.

[41] Tso CL, Shintaku P, Chen J, Liu Q, Liu J, Chen Z, Yoshimoto K, Mischel PS, Cloughesy TF, Liau LM, Nelson SF.Primary glioblastomas express mesenchymal stem-like properties. Mol Cancer Res. 4(9):607-619, 2006.

[42] Liu Q, Nguyen DH, Dong Q, Shitaku P, Chung K, Liu OY, Tso JL, Liu JY, Konkankit V, Cloughesy TF, Mischel PS, Lane TF, Liau LM, Nelson SF, Tso CL.Molecular properties of CD133+ glioblastoma stem cells derived from treatment-refractory recurrent brain tumors. J Neurooncol. 94(1):1-19, 2009.

[43] Yuan X, Curtin J, Xiong Y, Liu G, Waschsmann-Hogiu S, Farkas DL, Black KL, Yu JS. Isolation of cancer stem cells from adult glioblastoma multiforme. Oncogene 23:9392–9400, 2004.

[44] Hemmati HD, Nakano I, Lazareff JA, Masterman-Smith M, Geschwind DH, Bronner-Fraser M, Kornblum HI. Cancerous stem cells can arise from pediatric brain tumors. Proc Natl Acad Sci USA. 100:15178–15183, 2003.

[45] Singh SK, Hawkins C, Clarke ID, Squire JA, Bayani J, Hide T, Henkelman RM, Cusimano MD, Dirks PB.Identification of human brain tumour initiating cells. Nature. 432:396–401, 2004.

[46] Galli R, Binda E, Orfanelli U. Isolation and characterization of tumorigenic, stem-like neural precursors from human glioblastoma. Cancer Res. 64:7011–7021, 2004.

[47] Wang J, Sakariassen PØ, Tsinkalovsky O, Immervoll H, Bøe SO, Svendsen A, Prestegarden L, Røsland G, Thorsen F, Stuhr L, Molven A, Bjerkvig R, Enger PØ.CD133 negative glioma cells form tumors in nude rats and give rise to CD133 positive cells. Int J Cancer. 122(4):761-8, 2008.

[48] Beier D, Hau P, Proescholdt M, Lohmeier A, Wischhusen J, Oefner PJ, Aigner L, Brawanski A, Bogdahn U, Beier CP. Cancer Res. 67: 4010-4015, 2007.

[49] Günther HS, Schmidt NO, Phillips HS, Kemming D, Kharbanda S, Soriano R, Modrusan Z, Meissner H, Westphal M, Lamszus K. Oncogene. 27: 2897-2909, 2008.

[50] Son MJ, Woolard K, Nam DH, Lee J, Fine HA. SSEA-1 is an enrichment marker for tumor-initiating cells in human glioblastoma. Cell Stem Cell. 4:440-452, 2009.

[51] Tchoghandjian A, Baeza N, Colin C, Cayre M, Metellus P, Beclin C, Ouafik L, Figarella-Branger D. A2B5 cells from human glioblastoma have cancer stem cell properties. Brain Pathol. 20:211-221, 2010.

[52] Bonnet D, Dick JE.Human acute myeloid leukemia is organized as a hierarchy that originates from a primitive hematopoietic cell. Nat Med. 3(7):730-737, 1997.

[53] Vermeulen L, Todaro M, de Sousa Mello F, Sprick MR, Kemper K, Perez Alea M, Richel DJ, Stassi G, Medema JP. Single-cell cloning of colon cancer stem cells reveals a multi-lineage differentiation capacity. Proc Natl Acad Sci U S A. 105(36):13427-32, 2008.

[54] Dalerba P, Cho RW, Clarke MF. Cancer stem cells: models and concepts. Annu Rev Med. 58:267–284, 2007.

[55] Beachy PA, Karhadkar SS, Berman DM. (2004) Tissue repair and stem cell renewal in carcinogenesis. Nature. 432:324–331, 2004.

[56] Zhang QB, Ji XY, Huang Q, Dong J, Zhu YD, Lan Q. Differentiation profile of brain tumor stem cells: a comparative study with neural stem cells. Cell Res. 16:909–915, 2006.

[57] Clarke MF, Dick JE, Dirks PB, Eaves CJ, Jamieson CH, Jones DL, Visvader J, Weissman IL, Wahl GM. Cancer stem cells—perspectives on current status and future directions: AACR workshop on cancer stem cells. Cancer Res. 66:9339–9344, 2006.
[58] Bao S, Wu Q, McLendon RE, Hao Y, Shi Q, Hjelmeland AB, Dewhirst MW, Bigner DD, Rich JN.Glioma stem cells promote radioresistance by preferential activation of the DNA damage response. Nature. 444: 756-760, 2006.
[59] Eramo A, Ricci-Vitiani L, Zeuner A, Pallini R, Lotti F, Sette G, Pilozzi E, Larocca LM, Peschle C, De Maria R.Chemotherapy resistance of glioblastoma stem cells. Cell Death Differ. 13(7):1238-1241, 2006.
[60] Zeppernick F, Ahmadi R, Campos B, Dictus C, Helmke BM, Becker N, Lichter P, Unterberg A, Radlwimmer B, Herold-Mende CC.Stem cell marker CD133 affects clinical outcome in glioma patients. Clin Cancer Res. 14(1):123-129, 2008.
[61] Yan X, Ma L, Yi D, Yoon JG, Diercks A, Foltz G, Price ND, Hood LE, Tian Q. A CD133-related gene expression signature identifies an aggressive glioblastoma subtype with excessive mutations. Proc Natl Acad Sci U S A. 108(4):1591-1596, 2011.
[62] Piccirillo SG, Reynolds BA, Zanetti N, Lamorte G, Binda E, Broggi G, Brem H, Olivi A, Dimeco F, Vescovi AL. Bone morphogenetic proteins inhibit the tumorigenic potential of human brain tumour-initiating cells. Nature. 444(7120):761-765, 2006.
[63] Field M, Alvarez A, Bushnev S, Sugaya K. Embryonic stem cell markers distinguishing cancer stem cells from normal human neuronal stem cell populations in malignant glioma patients. Clin Neurosurg. 57:151-159, 2010.
[64] Yamada K, Tso J, Ye F, Choe J, Liu Y, Liau LM, Tso CL. Essential Gene Pathways for Glioblastoma Stem Cells: Clinical Implications for Prevention of Tumor Recurrence. Cancers. 3(2):1975-1995, 2011. doi: 10.3390/cancers3021975
[65] Jeon HM, Jin X, Lee JS, Oh SY, Sohn YW, Park HJ, Joo KM, Park WY, Nam DH, DePinho RA, Chin L, Kim H. Inhibitor of differentiation 4 drives brain tumor-initiating cell genesis through cyclin E and notch signaling. Genes Dev. 22:2028-2033, 2008.
[66] Sang L, Coller HA, Roberts JM. Control of the reversibility of cellular quiescence by the transcriptional repressor HES1. Science. 321:1095-1100, 2008.
[67] Sakamoto M, Hirata H, Ohtsuka T, Bessho Y, Kageyama R. The basic helix-loop-helix genes Hesr1/Hey1 and Hesr2/Hey2 regulate maintenance of neural precursor cells in the brain. J Biol Chem. 278:44808-44815, 2003.
[68] Liang Y, Bollen AW, Nicholas MK, Gupta N. Id4 and FABP7 are preferentially expressed in cells with astrocytic features in oligodendrogliomas and oligoastrocytomas. BMC Clin Pathol. 5:6, 2005.
[69] Chapouton P, Skupien P, Hesl B, Coolen M, Moore JC, Madelaine R, Kremmer E, Faus-Kessler T, Blader P, Lawson ND, Bally-Cuif L. Notch activity levels control the balance between quiescence and recruitment of adult neural stem cells. J Neurosci. 30:7961-7974, 2010.
[70] Bray SJ. Notch signalling: a simple pathway becomes complex. Nat Rev Mol Cell Biol. 7:678-689, 2006.

[71] Mizutani K, Yoon K, Dang L, Tokunaga A, Gaiano N. Differential Notch signalling distinguishes neural stem cells from intermediate progenitors. Nature. 449:351-355, 2007.

[72] Sahlgren C, Gustafsson MV, Jin S, Poellinger L, Lendahl U. Notch signaling mediates hypoxia-induced tumor cell migration and invasion. Proc Natl Acad Sci U S A. 105(17):6392-6397, 2008.

[73] Kaloshi G, Mokhtari K, Carpentier C, Taillibert S, Lejeune J, Marie Y, Delattre JY, Godbout R, Sanson M. FABP7 expression in glioblastomas: relation to prognosis, invasion and EGFR status. J Neurooncol. 84:245-248, 2007.

[74] Anthony TE, Mason HA, Gridley T, Fishell G, Heintz N. Brain lipid-binding protein is a direct target of Notch signaling in radial glial cells. Genes Dev. 19:1028-1033, 2005.

[75] Fan X, Khaki L, Zhu TS, Soules ME, Talsma CE, Gul N, Koh C, Zhang J, Li YM, Maciaczyk J, Nikkhah G, Dimeco F, Piccirillo S, Vescovi AL, Eberhart CG. NOTCH pathway blockade depletes CD133-positive glioblastoma cells and inhibits growth of tumor neurospheres and xenografts. Stem Cells. 28:5-16, 2010.

[76] Hovinga KE, Shimizu F, Wang R, Panagiotakos G, Van Der Heijden M, Moayedpardazi H, Correia AS, Soulet D, Major T, Menon J, Tabar V. Inhibition of notch signaling in glioblastoma targets cancer stem cells via an endothelial cell intermediate. Stem Cells. 28:1019-1029, 2010.

[77] Li Z, Bao S, Wu Q, Wang H, Eyler C, Sathornsumetee S, Shi Q, Cao Y, Lathia J, McLendon RE, Hjelmeland AB, Rich JN. Hypoxia-inducible factors regulate tumorigenic capacity of glioma stem cells. Cancer Cell. 15(6):501-513, 2009.

[78] Seidel S, Garvalov BK, Wirta V, von Stechow L, Schänzer A, Meletis K, Wolter M, Sommerlad D, Henze AT, Nistér M, Reifenberger G, Lundeberg J, Frisén J, Acker T. A hypoxic niche regulates glioblastoma stem cells through hypoxia inducible factor 2 alpha. Brain. 133(Pt 4):983-995, 2010.

[79] Bar EE, Lin A, Mahairaki V, Matsui W, Eberhart CG. Hypoxia increases the expression of stem-cell markers and promotes clonogenicity in glioblastoma neurospheres. Am J Pathol. 177:1491-1502, 2010.

[80] Soeda A, Park M, Lee D, Mintz A, Androutsellis-Theotokis A, McKay RD, Engh J, Iwama T, Kunisada T, Kassam AB, Pollack IF, Park DM. Hypoxia promotes expansion of the CD133-positive glioma stem cells through activation of HIF-1alpha. Oncogene. 28: 3949-3959, 2009.

[81] Gustafsson MV, Zheng X, Pereira T, Gradin K, Jin S, Lundkvist J, Ruas JL, Poellinger L, Lendahl U, Bondesson M. Hypoxia requires notch signaling to maintain the undifferentiated cell state. Dev Cell.9:617-628, 2005.

[82] Heddleston JM, Li Z, McLendon RE, Hjelmeland AB, Rich JN. The hypoxic microenvironment maintains glioblastoma stem cells and promotes reprogramming towards a cancer stem cell phenotype. Cell Cycle. 8:3274-3284, 2009.

[83] Cayuso J, Ulloa F, Cox B, Briscoe J, Martí E. The Sonic hedgehog pathway independently controls the patterning, proliferation and survival of neuroepithelial cells by regulating Gli activity. Development. 133(3):517-528, 2006.

[84] Fuccillo M, Joyner AL, Fishell G. Morphogen to mitogen: the multiple roles of hedgehog signalling in vertebrate neural development. Nat Rev Neurosci. 7(10):772-783, 2006.

[85] Palma V, Lim DA, Dahmane N, Sánchez P, Brionne TC, Herzberg CD, Gitton Y, Carleton A, Alvarez-Buylla A. Ruiz i Altaba A. Sonic hedgehog controls stem cell behavior in the postnatal and adult brain. Development 132(2):335-344, 2005.

[86] Po A, Ferretti E, Miele E, De Smaele E, Paganelli A, Canettieri G, Coni S, Di Marcotullio L, Biffoni M, Massimi L, Di Rocco C, Screpanti I, Gulino A. Hedgehog controls neural stem cells through p53-independent regulation of Nanog. Embo J. 29:2646-2658, 2010.

[87] Clement V, Sanchez P, de Tribolet N, Radovanovic I, Ruiz i Altaba A. HEDGEHOG-GLI1 signaling regulates human glioma growth, cancer stem cell self-renewal, and tumorigenicity. Curr Biol. 17:165-172, 2007.

[88] Zbinden M, Duquet A, Lorente-Trigos A, Ngwabyt SN, Borges I, Ruiz i Altaba, A. NANOG regulates glioma stem cells and is essential in vivo acting in a cross-functional network with GLI1 and p53. Embo J. 29:2659-2674, 2010.

[89] Stecca B, Ruiz i Altaba, A. A GLI1-p53 inhibitory loop controls neural stem cell and tumour cell numbers. Embo J. 28:663-676, 2009.

[90] MassaguéJ. (2008). TGFbeta in cancer. Cell. 134:215–230.

[91] Shi Y, Massagué J. Mechanisms of TGF-beta signaling from cell membrane to the nucleus. Cell. 113:685-700, 2003.

[92] Xu RH, Sampsell-Barron TL, Gu F, Root S, Peck RM, Pan G, Yu J, Antosiewicz-Bourget J, Tian S, Stewart R, Thomson JA. NANOG is a direct target of GFbeta/activin-mediated SMAD signaling in human ESCs. Cell Stem Cell. 3(2):196-206, 2008.

[93] Moustakas A, Heldin CH. Non-Smad TGF-beta signals. J Cell Sci. 118:3573-3584, 2005.

[94] Zhao S, Venkatasubbarao K, Lazor JW, Sperry J, Jin C, Cao L, Freeman JW. Inhibition of STAT3 Tyr705 phosphorylation by Smad4 suppresses transforming growth factor beta-mediated invasion and metastasis in pancreatic cancer cells. Cancer Res. 68:4221-4228, 2008.

[95] Penuelas S, Anido J, Prieto-Sanchez RM, Folch G, Barba I, Cuartas I, Garcia-Dorado D, Poca MA, Sahuquillo J, Baselga J, Seoane J. TGF-beta increases glioma-initiating cell self-renewal through the induction of LIF in human glioblastoma. Cancer Cell. 15:315-327, 2009.

[96] Sherry MM, Reeves A, Wu JK, Cochran BH. STAT3 is required for proliferation and maintenance of multipotency in glioblastoma stem cells. Stem Cells. 27:2383-2392, 2009.

[97] Li GH, Wei H, Lv SQ, Ji H, Wang DL. Knockdown of STAT3 expression by RNAi suppresses growth and induces apoptosis and differentiation in glioblastoma stem cells. Int J Oncol. 37:103-110, 2010.

[98] Wang H, Lathia JD, Wu Q, WangJ, Li Z, Heddleston JM, Eyler CE, Elderbroom J, Gallagher J, Schuschu J, MacSwords J, Cao Y, McLendon RE, Wang XF, Hjelmeland AB, Rich JN. Targeting interleukin 6 signaling suppresses glioma stem cell survival and tumor growth. Stem Cells. 27:2393-2404, 2009.

[99] Ikushima H, Todo T, Ino Y, Takahashi M, Miyazawa K, Miyazono K. Autocrine TGF-beta signaling maintains tumorigenicity of glioma-initiating cells through Sry-related HMG-box factors. Cell Stem Cell. 5:504-514, 2009.

[100] Gangemi RM, Griffero F, Marubbi D, Perera M, Capra MC, Malatesta P, Ravetti GL, Zona GL, Daga A, Corte G. SOX2 silencing in glioblastoma tumor-initiating cells causes stop of proliferation and loss of tumorigenicity. Stem Cells. 27:40-48, 2009.

[101] Lee J, Son MJ, Woolard K, Donin NM, Li A, Cheng CH, Kotliarova S, Kotliarov Y, Walling J, Ahn S, Kim M, Totonchy M, Cusack T, Ene C, Ma H, Su Q, Zenklusen JC, Zhang W, Maric D, Fine HA. Epigenetic-mediated dysfunction of the bone morphogenetic protein pathway inhibits differentiation of glioblastoma-initiating cells. Cancer Cell. 13:69-80, 2008.

[102] Mazzoleni S, Politi LS, Pala M, Cominelli M, Franzin A, Sergi Sergi L, Falini A, De Palma M, Bulfone A, Poliani PL, Galli R. Epidermal growth factor receptor expression identifies functionally and molecularly distinct tumor-initiating cells in human glioblastoma multiforme and is required for gliomagenesis. Cancer Res. 70:7500-7513, 2010.

[103] Soeda A, Inagaki A, Oka N, Ikegame Y, Aoki H, Yoshimura S, Nakashima S, Kunisada T, Iwama T. Epidermal growth factor plays a crucial role in mitogenic regulation of human brain tumor stem cells. J Biol Chem. 283:10958-10966, 2008.

[104] Griffero F, Daga A, Marubbi D, Capra MC, Melotti A, Pattarozzi A, Gatti M, Bajetto A, Porcile C, Barbieri F, Favoni RE, Lo Casto M, Zona G, Spaziante R, Florio T, Corte G. Different response of human glioma tumor-initiating cells to epidermal growth factor receptor kinase inhibitors. J Biol Chem. 284:7138-7148, 2009.

[105] Eyler CE, Foo WC, LaFiura KM, McLendon RE, Hjelmeland AB, Rich JN. Brain cancer stem cells display preferential sensitivity to Akt inhibition. Stem Cells. 26:3027-3036, 2008.

[106] Sunayama J, Matsuda K, Sato A, Tachibana K, Suzuki K, Narita Y, Shibui S, Sakurada K, Kayama T, Tomiyama A, Kitanaka C. Crosstalk between the PI3K/mTOR and MEK/ERK pathways involved in the maintenance of self-renewal and tumorigenicity of glioblastoma stem-like cells. Stem Cells. 28:1930-1939, 2010.

[107] Levens DL. Reconstructing MYC. Genes Dev. 17:1071-1077, 2003.

[108] Davis AC, Wims M, Spotts GD, Hann SR, Bradley A. A null c-myc mutation causes lethality before 10.5 days of gestation in homozygotes and reduced fertility in heterozygous female mice. Genes Dev. 7(4):671-682, 1993.

[109] Guney I, Wu S, Sedivy JM. Reduced c-Myc signaling triggers telomere-independent senescence by regulating Bmi-1 and p16(INK4a). Proc Natl Acad Sci U S A. 103:3645-3650, 2006.

[110] Wang J, Wang H, LiZ, Wu Q, Lathia JD, McLendon RE, Hjelmeland AB, Rich JN. c-Myc is required for maintenance of glioma cancer stem cells. PLoS One. 3:e3769, 2008.

[111] Zheng H, Ying H, Yan H, Kimmelman AC, Hiller DJ, Chen AJ, Perry SR, Tonon G, Chu GC, Ding Z, Stommel JM, Dunn KL, Wiedemeyer R, You MJ, Brennan C, Wang YA, Ligon KL, Wong WH, Chin L, DePinho RA. p53 and Pten control neural and glioma stem/progenitor cell renewal and differentiation. Nature. 455:1129-1133, 2008.

[112] Schafer MK, Altevogt P. L1CAM malfunction in the nervous system and human carcinomas. Cell Mol Life Sci.67:2425-2437, 2010.

[113] Bao S, Wu Q, Li Z, Sathornsumetee S, Wang H, McLendon RE, Hjelmeland AB, Rich JN. Targeting cancer stem cells through L1CAM suppresses glioma growth. Cancer Res. 68:6043-6048, 2008.

[114] Ligon KL, Huillard E, Mehta S, Kesari S, Liu H, Alberta JA, Bachoo RM, Kane M, Louis DN, Depinho RA, Anderson DJ, Stiles CD, Rowitch DH. Olig2-regulated lineage-restricted pathway controls replication competence in neural stem cells and malignant glioma. Neuron. 53:503-517, 2007.

[115] Lessard J, Sauvageau G. Bmi-1 determines the proliferative capacity of normal and leukaemic stem cells. Nature. 423:255–260, 2003.

[116] Leung C, Lingbeek M, Shakhova O, Liu J, Tanger E, Saremaslani P, Van Lohuizen M, Marino S. Bmi1 is essential for cerebellar development and is overexpressed in human medulloblastomas. Nature. 428:337–341, 2004.

[117] Molofsky AV, Pardal R, Iwashita T, Park IK, Clarke MF, Morrison SJ. Bmi-1 dependence distinguishes neural stem cell self-renewal from progenitor proliferation. Nature. 425:962–967, 2003.

[118] Valk-Lingbeek ME, Bruggeman SWM, van Lohuizen M. Stem cells and cancer: the Polycomb connection. Cell. 118:409–418, 2004.

[119] Widschwendter M, Fiegl H, Egle D, Mueller-Holzner E, Spizzo G, Marth C, Weisenberger DJ, Campan M, Young J, Jacobs I, Laird PW. Epigenetic stem cell signature in cancer. Nat Genet. 39:157–158, 2007.

[120] Abdouh M, Facchino S, Chatoo W, Balasingam V, Ferreira J, Bernier G. BMI1 sustains human glioblastoma multiforme stem cell renewal. J Neurosci. 29:8884-8896, 2009.

[121] Suva ML, Riggi N, Janiszewska M, Radovanovic I, Provero P, Stehle JC, Baumer K, Le Bitoux MA, Marino D, Cironi L, Marquez VE, Clement V, Stamenkovic I. EZH2 is essential for glioblastoma cancer stem cell maintenance. Cancer Res. 69:9211-9218, 2009.

[122] Hynes RO. Integrins: bidirectional, allosteric signaling machines. Cell. 110: 673-687, 2002.

[123] Whitley M, Treloar H, De Arcangelis A, Georges Labouesse E, Greer CA. The alpha6 integrin subunit in the developing mouse olfactory bulb. J Neurocytol. 34:81-96, 2005.

[124] Lathia JD, Gallagher J, Heddleston JM, Wang J, Eyler CE, Macswords J, Wu Q, Vasanji A, McLendon RE, Hjelmeland AB, Rich JN. Integrin alpha 6 regulates glioblastoma stem cells. Cell Stem Cell. 6:421-432, 2010.

[125] He KL, Ting AT. A20 inhibits tumor necrosis factor (TNF) alpha-induced apoptosis by disrupting recruitment of TRADD and RIP to the TNF receptor 1 complex in Jurkat T cells. Mol Cell Biol. 22(17):6034-6045, 2002.

[126] Won M, Park KA, Byun HS, Sohn KC, Kim YR, Jeon J, Hong JH, Park J, Seok JH, Kim JM, Yoon WH, Jang IS, Shen HM, Liu ZG, Hur GM. Novel anti-apoptotic mechanism of A20 through targeting ASK1 to suppress TNF-induced JNK activation. Cell Death Differ. 17(12):1830-1841, 2010.

[127] Guo Q, Dong H, Liu X, Wang C, Liu N, Zhang J, Li B, Cao W, Ding T, Yang Z, Zhang X. A20 is overexpressed in glioma cells and may serve as a potential therapeutic target. Expert Opin Ther Targets. 13(7):733-741, 2009.

[128] Hjelmeland AB, Wu Q, Wickman S, Eyler C, Heddleston J, Shi Q, Lathia JD, Macswords J, Lee J, McLendon RE, Rich JN. Targeting A20 decreases glioma stem cell survival and tumor growth. PLoS Biol. 8(2):e1000319, 2010.

[129] Stupp R, Mason WP, van den Bent MJ, Weller M, Fisher B, Taphoorn MJ, Belanger K, Brandes AA, Marosi C, Bogdahn U, Curschmann J, Janzer RC, Ludwin SK, Gorlia T, Allgeier A, Lacombe D, Cairncross JG, Eisenhauer E, Mirimanoff RO. Radiotherapy plus concomitant and adjuvant temozolomide for glioblastoma. N Engl J Med. 352: 987-996, 2005.

[130] Stupp R, Hegi ME, Mason WP, van den Bent MJ, Taphoorn MJ, Janzer RC, Ludwin SK, Allgeier A, Fisher B, Belanger K, Hau P, Brandes AA, Gijtenbeek J, Marosi C, Vecht CJ, Mokhtari K, Wesseling P, Villa S, Eisenhauer E, Gorlia T, Weller M, Lacombe D, Cairncross JG, Mirimanoff RO. Effects of radiotherapy with concomitant and adjuvant temozolomide versus radiotherapy alone on survival in glioblastoma in a randomised phase III study: 5-year analysis of the EORTC-NCIC trial. Lancet Oncol. 10:459-466, 2009.

[131] Wiewrodt D, Nagel G, Dreimuller N, Hundsberger T, Perneczky A, Kaina B. MGMT in primary and recurrent human glioblastomas after radiation and chemotherapy and comparison with p53 status and clinical outcome. Int J Cancer. 122:1391-1399, 2008.

[132] Murat A, Migliavacca E, Gorlia T, Lambiv WL, Shay T, Hamou MF, de Tribolet N, Regli L, Wick W, Kouwenhoven MC, Hainfellner JA, Heppner FL, Dietrich PY, Zimmer Y, Cairncross JG, Janzer RC, Domany E, Delorenzi M, Stupp R, Hegi ME. Stem cell-related "self-renewal" signature and high epidermal growth factor receptor expression associated with resistance to concomitant chemoradiotherapy in glioblastoma. J Clin Oncol. 26:3015-3024, 2008.

[133] Mellor HR, Ferguson DJ, Callaghan R. A model of quiescent tumour microregions for evaluating multicellular resistance to chemotherapeutic drugs. Br J Cancer. 93:302-309, 2005.

[134] Liu Y, Perdreau SA, Chatterjee P, Wang L, Kuan SF, Duensing A. Imatinib mesylate induces quiescence in gastrointestinal stromal tumor cells through the CDH1-SKP2-p27Kip1 signaling axis. Cancer Res. 68:9015-9023, 2008.

[135] Masunaga S, Ono K, Hori H, Suzuki M, Kinashi Y, Takagaki M, Kasai S, Nagasawa H, Uto Y. Potentially lethal damage repair by total and quiescent tumor cells following various DNA-damaging treatments. Radiat Med. 17:259-264, 1999.

[136] Ito K, Bernardi R, Morotti A, Matsuoka S, Saglio G, Ikeda Y, Rosenblatt J, Avigan DE, Teruya-Feldstein J, Pandolfi PP. PML targeting eradicates quiescent leukaemia-initiating cells. Nature. 453:1072-1078, 2008.

[137] Guo W, Lasky JL, Chang CJ, Mosessian S, Lewis X, Xiao Y,Yeh JE, Chen JY, Iruela-Arispe ML, Varella-Garcia M, Wu, H. Multi-genetic events collaboratively contribute to Pten-null leukaemia stem-cell formation. Nature. 453:529-533, 2008.

[138] Bleau AM, Hambardzumyan D, Ozawa T, Fomchenko EI, Huse JT, Brennan CW, Holland EC. PTEN/PI3K/Akt pathway regulates the side population phenotype and ABCG2 activity in glioma tumor stem-like cells. Cell Stem Cell. 4:226-235, 2009.

[139] Nakai E, Park K, Yawata T, Chihara T, Kumazawa A, Nakabayashi H, Shimizu K. Enhanced MDR1 expression and chemoresistance of cancer stem cells derived from glioblastoma. Cancer Invest. 27:901-908, 2009.

[140] Hsieh A, Ellsworth R, Hsieh D. Hedgehog/GLI1 regulates IGF dependent malignant behaviors in glioma stem cells. J Cell Physiol. 226:1118-1127, 2011.

[141] Vellanki SH, Grabrucker A, Liebau S, Proepper C, Eramo A, Braun V, Boeckers T, Debatin KM, Fulda S. Small-molecule XIAP inhibitors enhance gamma-irradiation-induced apoptosis in glioblastoma. Neoplasia. 11:743-752, 2009.

[142] Wang J, Wakeman TP, Lathia JD, Hjelmeland AB, Wang XF, White RR, Rich JN, Sullenger BA. Notch promotes radioresistance of glioma stem cells. Stem Cells. 28:17-28, 2010.

[143] Gilbert CA, Daou MC, Moser RP, Ross AH. Gamma-secretase inhibitors enhance temozolomide treatment of human gliomas by inhibiting neurosphere repopulation and xenograft recurrence. Cancer Res. 70:6870-6879, 2010.

[144] Cao R, Tsukada Y, Zhang Y. Role of Bmi-1 and Ring1A in H2A ubiquitylation and Hox gene silencing. Mol Cell. 20:845-854, 2005.

[145] Facchino S, Abdouh M, Chatoo W, Bernier G. BMI1 confers radioresistance to normal and cancerous neural stem cells through recruitment of the DNA damage response machinery. J Neurosci. 30:10096-10111, 2010.

[146] Kawai M, Breggia AC, Demambro VE, Shen X, Canalis E, Bouxsein ML, Beamer WG, Clemmons DR, Rosen CJ. The Heparin-binding Domain of IGFBP-2 Has Insulin-like Growth Factor Binding-independent Biologic Activity in the Growing Skeleton. J Biol Chem. 286(16):14670-14680, 2011.

[147] Lin Y, Jiang T, Zhou K, Xu L, Chen B, Li G, Qiu X, Zhang W, Song SW. Plasma IGFBP-2 levels predict clinical outcomes of patients with high-grade gliomas. Neuro Oncol. 11:468-476, 2009.

[148] Wang H, Shen W, Huang H, Hu L, Ramdas L, Zhou Y.H, Liao WS, Fuller GN, Zhang W. Insulin-like growth factor binding protein 2 enhances glioblastoma invasion by activating invasion-enhancing genes. Cancer Res. 63:4315-4321, 2003.

[149] Fukushima T, Tezuka T, Shimomura T, Nakano S, Kataoka H. Silencing of insulin-like growth factor-binding protein-2 in human glioblastoma cells reduces both invasiveness and expression of progression-associated gene CD24. J Biol Chem. 282:18634-18644, 2007.

[150] Hsieh D, Hsieh A, Stea B, Ellsworth R. IGFBP2 promotes gliomatumor stem cell expansion and survival. Biochem Biophys Res Commun. 397:367-372, 2010.

[151] Evers P, Lee PP, DeMarco J, Agazaryan N, Sayre JW, Selch M, Pajonk F. Irradiation of the potential cancer stem cell niches in the adult brain improves progression-free survival of patients with malignant glioma. BMC Cancer. 10:384, 2010.

[152] Sneddon JB, Werb Z. Location, location, location: the cancer stem cell niche. Cell Stem Cell. 1:607-611, 2007.

3

Midkine Signaling in Glioblastoma: A Novel Developmental Drug Target?

Ayhan Bilir[1] and Mine Erguven[2]
[1]*Istanbul University, Istanbul Faculty of Medicine, Department of Histology and Embryology,*
[2]*Yeni Yüzyıl University, Faculty of Medicine, Department of Clinical Biochemistry, Turkey*

1. Introduction

Glioblastoma (GBM) is the most common primary malignant brain tumor in adults and is a complicated disease to treat. The current standard therapy includes surgical resection, followed by a combination of radiation and chemotherapy with several drugs. However, resistance and recurrence are quite common, so we continue to investigate more effective treatments both for initial therapy and recurrence by searching novel neglected molecular targets as midkine. This article will review the significance of midkine in therapy for newly-diagnosed and recurrent glioblastomas.

2. Glioblastoma

In adults, GBMs are the most lethal and most frequent malignant brain tumors. Approximately, half of all primary brain tumors are gliomas. Gliomas arise from glial cells, the building-block cells of the connective and supportive, tissues in the central nervous system. The common gliomas are diffuse gliomas which infiltrate throughout the brain parenchyma. These are classified histologically and/or ultrastructurally as astrocytomas, oligodendrogliomas, and oligoastrocytomas. They are graded on a World Health Organization (WHO) classification system scale of I to IV according to their degree of malignancy based on different histological features and genetic alterations. Grade I tumors are benign and can be cured if they can be surgically resected; grade II tumors are incurable with surgery because of their early diffuse infiltration of the surrounding brain, and long treatment regimens are needed to treat this disease completely; grade III tumors have increased anaplasia and proliferate over grade IV tumors and are more rapidly fatal; grade IV tumors possess advanced features of malignancy, and are resistant to radio/chemotherapy. Hence, they are characterized with poor prognosis resulting in the death within ~9-12 months. Grade I, II, III, and IV designation are pilocytic astrocytoma, low grade astrocytoma (LGA), anaplastic astrocytoma, and GBM, respectively. The most frequent subtypes are glioblastoma (47%) and grade II–III astrocytoma (23%), followed by oligodendroglioma and mixed glioma (Furnari et al., 2007; Krakstad and Chekenya, 2010).

Patients suffred from GBM generally have a dismal prognosis, with an average survival time of only 9-12 months from their diagnosis, and thus GBMs can be named as "terminator". GBM accounts for ~ 50% of adult gliomas; and up to 10% of pediatric gliomas are either anaplastic astrocytomas or GBMs. Cases of GBMs are distributed over a broad range of ages, with an average age of 53 years at diagnosis. Prognostic factors include age and post-operative physical performance status. The tumors of older patients are more aggressive and more resistant to treatment. The patients who are alive just 3 to 5 years following diagnosis are defined as "long-term survivors" and they are rare. Younger age than the average of 53 years is usually the only common feature of long-term survivors (Furnari et al., 2007; Krakstad and Chekenya, 2010; Ouant and Wen, 2010).

Important characteristics of GBMs are aberrant cellular proliferation, diffuse infiltration, prospensity for necrosis, robust angiogenesis, high resistance to apoptosis, and genomic instability. The intratumoral heterogenity combined with a putative cancer stem cell (CSC) subpopulation and incomplete atlas of epigenetic lesions are the reasons of poor prognosis/high tumoral resistance against chemotherapeutics and recurrence. GBMs have been subdivided into the primary *(de novo)* and secondary (progessive) GBMs according to their clinical evaluation. Primary GBMs are commonly detected as subtypes, and tend to occur in older patients above the age of 45 years. Primary GBMs presents in an acute *de novo* manner without any evidence of prior clinical disease. In contrast, secondary GBMs are quite rare and commonly detected in younger patients below the age of 45 years. In addition, the latter initially present with lower grade astrocytomas and latterly ~70% of grade II gliomas transform into GBMs within 5-10 years of the initial diagnosis, regardless of prior therapy. Primary and secondary GBMs show differences in their clinical characteristics and genetic profiles [different transcriptional patterns and frequency of specific mutations as the mutations of tumour supressor genes retinoblastoma (Rb) and p53 result in DNA copy number aberrations]. However, they also have similarities, which are morphologically indistinguishable and show poor prognosis (Furnari et al., 2007; Cheng et al., 2010; Ouant and Wen, 2010).

Glioblastomas circumvent the blockage of tumour supressor genes [p53, phosphatase and tensin homolog deleted on choromosome 10 (PTEN), and Rb] on positive regulators of cell division, survival and motility. These positive regulators are receptor tyrosine kinases [RTKs, i.e. Platelet derived growth factor receptor (PDGFR), Epidermal growth factor receptor (EGFR), Vascular endothelial growth factor receptor (VEGFR)], growth factors [i.e. platelet derived growth factor (PDGF), vascular endothelial growth factor (VEGF)], cell adhesion molecules (i.e. integrins) and their two major downstream signaling pathways [i.e. mitogen activated protein kinase (MAPK), phosphoinositide-3 kinases (PI3Ks)]. Molecular pathogenesis of primary GBMs present (1) mutations of INK4aARF, PTEN, EGFR, loss of heterozygosity (LOH) of chromosome 10p and 10q, (2) amplications of EGFR, Cyclin D1/3, murine double minute 2 and 4 (MDM2 and MDM4), and (3) overexpressions of Bcl2-like-12 (Bcl2L 12) (~95 %), cyclin D 1/3. In contrast, molecular pathogenesis of secondary GBMs present (1) mutations of tumor supressors p53, Rb, PTEN (~10 %), loss of chromosomes 10q, 11p, 19q, (2) amplications of cyclin dependent kinases 4/6 (CDK4/6), and (3) overexpressions of PDGFR, PDGF, CDK4/6 (Furnari et al., 2007; Krakstad and Chekenya, 2010).

Glioblastomas, the most highly vascular of all solid tumors and microvascular hyperplasia, define both the histological phenotype of primary and secondary GBM. Although primary and secondary GBMs possess different genomic profiles, they form a final common angiogenesis pathway involving hypoxia inducible factor (HIF) and non-HIF-dependent downstream effectors such as VEGF, PDGF, stromal cell-derived factor-1 (SDF-1), endostatin, and thrompospondin 1 and 2 (TSP-1 and TSP-2). Because of their significant roles in GBMs' molecular pathogenesis, these molecules/pathways are accepted as "major targets" for the treatment of GBMs (Furnari et al., 2007; Krakstad and Chekenya, 2010). The poor prognosis despite aggressive treatment indicates the need to establish novel targets for molecular intervention.

3. Midkine

Midkine also known as MDK, FLJ27379, and NEGF2 is a heparin-binding cytokine or a growth factor or an angiogenic factor with a molecular weight of 13 kDa. Midkine binds to oversulfated structures in heparan sulfate and chondroitin sulfate. MDK is the founding member of a family, which is composed of only two members in humans. The other member is pleiotrophin (PTN), also called HB-GAM (Deuel et al., 2002; Rauvala and Peng, 1997) MDK is 50% homologous to PTN at the amino acid level and shares with PTN the genomic organization (Rauvala and Peng, 1997; Muramatsu et al., 1993; Owada et al. 1999) and predicted protein structure (Maeda et al., 1999; Sato et al., 2001).

The structure of MDK is mainly composed of two domains linked by disulfide bonds (Fabri et al., 1993) The C-domain possess basic heparin-binding activity which is responsible for the mechanism of action (Muramatsu et al., 1994). Each domain of MDK has also homology to the thrombospondin Type I repeat (Kilpelainen et al., 2000). Two domains are composed of three anti-parallel β-sheets (Iwasaki et al.,1997). The C-domain has two clusters of basic amino acids named as Cluster-1 and -2. These clusters are required for heparin-binding activity (Asai et al., 1997; Iwasaki et al., 1997; Akhter et al., 1998). MDK forms dimers via spontaneous association and transglutaminase stabilize dimers through crosslinking process 35). MDK is seemed to require dimerization for its activity (Kojima et al.,1997). After dimerization, Cluster-2 forms a fused strong binding site (Iwasaki et al., 1997).

Midkine was originally reported to be the product of a retinoic acid-responsive gene during embryogenesis (Takei et al., 2001). The expression of MDK was high during embryogenesis, but interestingly, MDK is not detectable in healthy adults and only re-appears in the body as a part of the pathogenesis of diseases (Muramatsu et al.2010). MDK promotes proliferation (Muramatsu et al., 2006), migration (Maeda et al., 1999), anti-apoptotic manner (Quin et al., 2011), mitogenesis (Dai 2009) , transforming (Nobata et al., 2005), and angiogenesis (Gustavsson et al., 2008) various cells. It has significant roles in reproduction, repair and in epidemiology of many diseases as rheumatoid arthritis (Maruyama et al.,2004), multiple sclerosis (Wang et al., 2008), hypertension and renal disease (Kodamatsu 2010), and cancer (Gustavsson et al., 2008)). The most intriguing feature of MDK is its massive expression in advanced tumors with high frequency (Qin Li et al., 2011; Kemik et al.,2010). Previous reports showed that the blood MDK level is frequently elevated with advance of human carcinomas, decreased after surgical removal of the tumors (Kemik et al.,2010; Ota et al., 2008; Lucas et al.,2010).

Glycosaminoglycan-recognizing activity of human MDK through its C-domain as heparan sulfate trisulfated unit and chondroitin sulfate E unit is important in its mechanism of action. Heparin inhibits MDK activiy. Proteoglycans like receptor-like protein tyrosine phosphatase-z (PTPz) (Maeda et al. 1999) syndecans (Mitsiadis et al., 1995), glypican-2

(Kurosawa et al., 2001), PG-M/versican (Zou et al.,2000) and neuroglycan C (Ichihara-Tanaka et al., 2006) have strong affinity to MDK. Chondroitin sulfate proteoglycan PTPz is a component of the MDK receptor. Low density lipoprotein receptor-related protein (LRP) (Muramatsu et al., 2000), α4β1-integrin and α6β1-integrin (Muramatsu et al., 2004) also serve as MDK receptors. These proteins and PTPz form a receptor complex of MDK. After the complex formation with PTPz and integrins, MDK starts downstream signaling systems as Src family kinases and tyrosine phosphorylation,respectively (Muramatsu et al., 2000;. Maeda et al. 1999). Increased tyrosine phosphorylation of paxillin leads to migration at osteoblast like cells and followed by suppression of caspases, activation of PI3 kinase and mitogen activated protein (MAP) kinase takes part in survival (Muramatsu et al., 2000;. Maeda et al. 1999; Owada et al.,1999; Ohuchida et al., 2004). The previous reports showed that when MDK binds to a6b1-integrin and tetraspanin, and induces tyrosine phosphorylation of focal adhesion kinase (FAK) followed by activation of paxillin and **s**ignal **t**ransducer and **a**ctivator of **t**ranscription alpha (STAT1α) pathway, it increases migration and invasion at human head and neck squamous cell carcinoma cells in vitro (Huang et al., 2008). Due to phosphorylation of STAT3 by MDK, the proliferation of postconfluent 3T3-L1 cells are stimulated and this leads to adipogenesis (Cernkovich et al., 2007). Notch2 reserves an another receptor for MDK and acting through the janus kinase 2 (Jak2)/STAT3 signalling pathway, MDK leads to epithelial-mesenchymal transition (EMT) in immortalized keratinocytes. Both MDK and PTN plays important role in EMT and neurogenesis during organogenesis process in embryonal development (Huang et al.,2008) Previous reports proposed that Anaplastic lymphoma kinase (ALK) can be included in the receptor group of MDK (Stoica et al., 2002). Unpublished observations of Muramatsu and coworkers, ALK also involves in the MDK complex with LRP and integrins that it is recruited to the receptor complex and plays roles in MDK signaling (Muramatsu 2010). After activation by MDK, ALK phosphorylates insulin receptor substrate-1, activates MAP kinase and PI3 kinase leading to transcriptional activation of nuclear factor kappa-light-chain-enhancer of activated B cells (NF-κB) (Stoica et al., 2002).

MDK binds to nucleolin, a nuclear protein which is also located at the cell surface and functions as a shuttle to the nucleus (Take et al, 1994; Dai 2009). A component of the MDK receptor LRP has major function as endocytose and delivering its ligands to lysosomes for degradation or catabolism (Hussain et al., 1999;Krieger et al., 1994). LRP takes part in internalization of MDK (Shibata et al.,2002). MDK is not internalized in LRP-deficient cells, whereas transfection of a LRP expression vector can restore MDK internalization and subsequent nuclear translocation, suggesting that LRP binds to heparin-binding growth factor, MDK, and mediates nuclear targeting by MDK. After this internalization, nucleolin transfer cytoplasmic MDK to the nucleus (Shibata et al.,2002). With respect to nuclear targeting by MDK, laminin-binding protein precursor (LBP) binds to MDK and is cotranslocated with MDK into nuclei (Owada et al., 1999). MDK may use both nucleolin and LBP precursor as shuttle proteins, revealing a novel role of LRP in intracellular signaling by its ligand, and the importance of nucleolin and LBP in the process of nuclear target of MDK. MDK transferred to the nucleolus is involved in the synthesis of ribosomal RNA (Dai et al., 2008). Unpublished observation by Muramatsu, H. and coworkers, translation initiation factor (eIF3) is can be an MDK-binding protein in the embryonic brain (Muramatsu 2010).

4. Midkine and glioblastoma

In the central nervous system, MDK is expressed by astrocytes in the fetal brain (Satoh et al.,1993), and its expression is developmentally regulated, decreasing progressively to an undetectable level as the fetus matures (Kodamatsu et al., 1990; Mitsiadis, et al.,1995) Previous reports showed that increased levels of MDK expression correlate with the progression of human astrocytomas, MDK mRNA and protein expression levels were higher in high-grade astrocytomas as anaplastic astrocytomas and GBMs than in low-grade astrocytomas (oligodendroglioma,ependioma, schwannoma, meningioma and pituitary adenoma) (Mishima et al., 1997). These reports conclude that MDK correlates with the poor prognosis of GBM. Stoica et al showed that MDK activates PI3-kinase and MAP kinase signal transduction in U87MG human glioblastoma cells which express ALK protein (Stoica et al., 2002). They showed that MDK is also unable to stimulate Akt phosphorylation upon reduction of ALK. In their report they revealed that in contrast with the diminished PTN and MDK signals after reduction of ALK, Akt phosphorylation in the same cells via a different tyrosine kinase receptor, the platelet-derived growth factor receptor (PDGF-R), was not altered by the reduction of ALK levels (Powers et al., 2002). Interestingly, in the U87MG cells mitogen activated protein kinase (MAPK) is activated constitutively and remains unaffected by the ALK reduction or by MDK addition.

In contrast to Stoica and coworkers, Grzelinski and coworkers determined no mRNA levels of ALK and RPTP β/ς levels, but high mRNA levels of MDK and PTN were determined in another human glioblastoma cell lines named T98G (Stoica et al., 2002; Grzelinski et al., 2009). This condition is also same for human glioblastoma cell lines named G55T2. U118 GBM cells possess high mRNA levels of ALK, low mRNA levels of MDK and RPTP β/ς but no mRNA levels of PTN are detected. All cell lines derived from human GBMs are different. In the light of report by Grzelinski and coworkers we can conclude that MDK levels at GBM may not only affected by activity of ALK.

GBM has a complex tumor structure consisting of accumulating tumors cells, abnormal vessel and necrotic debris. The increasing tumor mass leads to increased capillary and venous collapse (Merlo, 2003). The new formed vessels are structurally and functionally abnormal, and leaky, leading to edema, and low oxygen tension (Bani-Yaghoub et al., 2006). High O_2 tension degrades hypoxia inducible factor-1 alpha (HIF-1α) and consequently promotes differentiation or apoptosis, HIF-1α maintains at lower O_2 tension this augments signal transduction pathways leading to promote self-renewal (Panchision, 2009). Hypoxia induces MDK expression through the binding of to a hypoxia responsive element in the MDK promoter.

Survivin, an antiapoptotic protein, has been found to be overexpressed in up to 79% of astrocytic tumors (Kajiwara et al., 2003; Yamada et al., 2003; Chakravarti et al., 2002). The expression of this gene correlates with grade and is present in 90% of GBMs.The activity of this promoter is also enhanced by hypoxia, commonly found in rapidly growing tumors like high grade gliomas (Yang et al., 2004). Survivin seems to play an important role in the oncogenesis and progression of these tumors (Kleinschmidt - DeMasters et al., 2003; Das et al., 2002)This is suggested by its expression pattern and by the fact that patients with survivin positive astrocytic tumors have significantly shorter overall survival times compared with patients who have survivin negative tumors. Ulasov and coworkers showed that Survivin, CXCR4 and midkine mRNAs are overexpressed in brain tumors compared to normal tissue (Ulusov et al., 2007). Although hypoxia activation both on survivin and MDK, high survivin expression detected human GBM cell lines (U87MG and U373MG) showed significantly decreased the expression of MDK mRNA in comparison to others (U118). We can conclude that hypoxia induced activation depends on the genetic profile of tumour and this also strengthen the reason of GBM complexicity during therapies.

Notch2 has been suggested to drive embryonic brain tumor growth, however Notch3 has been implicated in choroid plexus tumors (Solecki et al.,2001;Dang et al., 2006). The frequency and the intensity of Notch2 expression is higher than that of Notch1 in GBM and in medulloblastoma (Sivasankaran et al., 2009; Fan et al., 2004). As a consequence of local genomic amplifications at the Notch2 locus in both brain tumor types, this may also be linked to the later persistence of Notch2 expression in postnatal mouse brain (Tanaka et al.,1999). Previous report showed that Notch1 regulates transcription of the epidermal growth factor receptor gene EGFR, known to be overexpressed or amplified in GBM, through TP53 (Purow et al.,2008). Reports showed that there is a direct correlation between p53 and MDK levels. Consistently, transcription of Notch signaling mediator genes are significantly overexpressed in the molecular subset of GBM with EGFR amplification (Brennan et al., 2009). Notch signaling activates the major GBM signalling pathway. Subsets of gliomas (even with distinct histologies) with impaired Notch signaling result in slower progression.

The most frequent genetic alteration occurring in GBM is genomic amplification of EGFR (Liebermann et al 1985a, 1985b). Consistently, EGF is the major proliferation pathway in GBM, mediated by activation of the RAS-RAF-MEK-ERK and the PI3K-AKT-mTOR cascades (Merlo 2003). Interestingly, mTOR has recently been shown to activate Notch signaling in lung and kidney tumor cells through induction of the Stat3/p63/Jagged signaling cascade (Ma et al.,2010). Lino and coworkers proposed this cross-talk for GBM that this suggests potential creation of a positive feedback loop between Notch and EGF signalling (Lino et al.,2010). The most frequent GBM subset consists of the association of EGFR amplification, homozygous deletions at the cyclin dependent kinase 2A (CDKN2A) locus, and TP53 mutations (Ohgaki et al., 2004). Notch activates expression of EGFR via TP53 (Purow et al., 2008), thus Notch is expected to stimulate the main GBM proliferation pathway. In addition, Notch also transactivates the gene for the EGFR-related ERBB2 in a DTX1-dependent manner (Patten et al.,2006). Notch-2 serves another receptor for MDK and so cross-talk between MDK and Notch-2 has been also shown to be a mediator of chemotherapy resistance to neighboring cells in GBM (Ikushima et al., 2009).

Tumors resistance to chemotherapy occured when a subset of cells overexpress drug transport proteins, possess receptor changes for the commitment of drug bounding and lack of ability to commit apoptosis. Mirkin and coworkers investigate the cytoprotective relationship between resistant and nonresistant cells in tumors which both accomplish to survive against drug cytotoxicity in human neuroblastoma (SKN-SH) and osteosarcoma (Saos2) (Mirkin et al., 2005). They hypothized that drug-resistant cells may secrete in their culture medium factors able to protect sensitive cells from cytotoxicity of drug. They showed that expression of MDK was only detected in drug resistant cells and midkine-enriched fractions exert a significant cytoprotective effect against doxorubicin in the wild-type drug-sensitive cells. In addition, they transfected these cells with MDK gene resulting in decreased response to DXR due to activation of AKT pathway and supression of caspase pathway. They concluded that the existence of intercellular cytoprotective signals such as the one mediated by MDK, originating from cells with acquired drug resistance to protect neighboring drug-sensitive cells and thus contribute to development of resistance to chemotherapy. They didn't mention about the direct effect of MDK on drug efflux transporters.

Hu and coworkers explored the possible effects of MDK gene on the chemotherapeutic drugs efflux and they concluded that there was powerful drug efflux ability in lymphoblastic leukemia cells with high MDK gene expression (Hu et al., 2010). They proposed that MDK gene expression regulates drug efflux upstream of the p-glycoprotein (P-gp) and the other transporter proteins in this cell line. Previous reports showed that the expression of is higher than expression of p-gp in T98G (Rosenbaum et al., 2005). In our study, we investigated whether the combination of an antineoplastic imatinib mesylate (IM) and an antitussive noscapine (Nos) with new identified chemotherapeutic effects, can be an effective GBM treatment and the possible role of midkine (MDK) in this treatment by using human GBM cells named T98G cells (Unpublished data by Erguven et al.). The lowest MRP-1 levels, but highest MDK levels were detected in the combination group. The lowest MDK levels were detected in IM group especially at the 72nd hr ($p<0.05$), but IM takes second place at MRP-1 inhibition. The highest and the lowest p-170 levels were detected at the IM group ($p<0.05$) and the Nos group ($p<0.05$), respectively. Thus, we can conclude that drug efflux ability was not correlated with MDK levels in this experiment.

Yao and coworkers revealed that MDK is expressed in mouse embryonic stem cells (mESCs), human embryonic stem cells (hESCs) and mouse embryonic fibroblasts (MEFs) (Yao et al., 2010). In their study, MDK promotes proliferation and self-renewal of both mESCs and hESCs. Further study by Yao and coworkers showed that the promoted growth of mESCs by MDK is occured through inhibiting apoptosis while accelerating the progression toward the S phase, and MDK leads to enhancement of mESC self-renewal through PI3K/Akt signaling pathway. They concluded that MDK plays profound roles in ESCs and MDK/PTPzeta signaling pathway is a novel pathway in the signal network maintaining pluripotency of ESCs. Their results extend gives information about the pluripotency control of ESCs and the relationship between ESCs and cancers. Huang and coworkers and the others demonstrated that a highly tumorigenic subpopulation of cancer cells called GBM stem cells (GSCs) promotes therapeutic resistance (Huang et al., 2010). Huang and co-workers showed that GSCs stimulate tumor angiogenesis by expressing elevated levels of VEGF and contribute to tumor growth. In addition, stem cell-like cancer cells (cancer stem cells) have been shown to promote metastasis. MDK was found to be expressed in neural precursor cells, which consist of neural stem cells and the progenitor cells which has been translated into a useful therapeutic strategy in the treatment of recurrent or progressive GBMs (Zhou et al., 2006).

5. Midkine inhibitors

After the determination of significant role of MDK in carcinogenesis, the inhibition of MDK through the synthesis or action become a highlighting target for investigators. Previous report by Dai and coworkers showed that MDK inhibitors as antisense oligonucleotides potentiated the cytotoxicity of drugs and decreased their inhibition concentration value 50 (IC_{50}) in hepatocellular carcinoma cells and in situ hepatocarcinoma models (Dai 2009). Other reports showed that antisense oligonucleotides to MDK inhibit the growth of mouse colorectal carcinoma cells in vitro and suppress the growth of the tumor in nude mice (Takei et al., 2001). Takei and coworkers showed combinational antitumor effect of siRNA against midkine and paclitaxel on growth of human prostate cancer xenografts (Takei et al., 2006).

Polyclonal anti-MDK antibodies inhibit the growth of tumor cells in vitro, however many monoclonal antibodies to MDK effected weakly due to internalization MDK. Another type of inhibitors tested for MDK inhibition are aptamers and like monoclonal antibodies, they don't inhibit growth of tumor cells efficiently (Wang et al., 2008). A low molecular weight compounds were seemed promising MDK inhibitors. Matsui and coworkers found two trifluoro compounds: one (PubChem 4603792) is 2-(2,6-dimethylpiperidin-1-yl)-4-thiophen-2-yl-6-(trifluorometh)pyrimidine, and the other has a related structure that inhibits MDK effectively without cytotoxic effects at osteoblast-like cells not at cancer cells (Matsui et al., 2010). Last report by Sakamoto and coworkers in 2011 showed that the premature ligand-receptor interaction during biosynthesis limits the production of MDK and its receptor LDL receptor-related protein 1 (LRP1) (Sakamoto et al.,2011). They utilized an endoplasmic reticulum (ER)-retrieval signal and a LRP1 fragment, which strongly bound to midkine and the LRP1-specialized chaperone RAP, to construct an ER-trapper. The ER-trapper efficiently trapped midkine and RAP, and mimicked the premature ligand-receptor interaction (maturation supresion of the ligand and receptor) and also diminished the inhibitory function of LRP1 on cell migration by PDGF in human colorectal carcinomas. Up to date, we have not seen any application of these therapeutic approaches metioned above for GBM.

In addition to these therapeutic applications, antineoplastic and non-antineoplastic drugs which were used in clinic efficiently for many years, were investigated for their role as MDK inhibitor (Erguven et al., 2011; Bilir et al., 2010). In our another study, we combined a well known microtubule inhibitor drug vinorelbine with antiphysciotic drug lithium chloride and antidepressant drug clomipramine for neuroblastoma treatment in vitro and showed their novel mechanism of action as MDK inhibitor (Bilir et al., 2010). Rawnaq and coworkers showed that IM, a well known tyrosine kinase inhibitor,decreases MDK levels in the serums of patients with GIST (Rawnaq et al., 2010). In concomitant with these result we showed that IM also decreased MDK levels in human GBM cell lines T98G (Erguven et al., 2011). In addition we also revealed novel mechanism of action of an antitussive drug with new antineoplastic effects Nos as MDK inhibitor and effect of MDK in the antagonism of IM with Nos in T98G cells (Erguven et al., 2011)

6. Concluding remarks and discussion

Glioblastoma is the most common and the most aggressive primary brain tumor against conventional therapies, that is, radiotherapy, chemotherapy, surgery and their combinations which have been being resulted in only transient clinical response followed by tumor resistance/recurrence, without any significant improvement of patient survival and life quality. MDK with significant roles at proliferation, survival and resistance, invasion, neovascularization and recurrence holds a promise of being a particularly appropriate target to fight against GBM. Recent studies indicate that cancer stem cells share core signaling pathways with normal somatic or embryonic stem cells, but also display critical distinctions that provide important clues into useful therapeutic targets. High MDK levels also plays critical role in this distinction (Yao et al., 2010). These are very highly infiltrative cancers often invade into normal brain tissues preventing surgical resection, and GSCs are responsible for this aggressive invasive phenotype, so targeting GSCs can effectively reduce tumor resistance and recurrence. All together patient outcome can be improved with the future development of novel therapies interfering with identified MDK signalling pathways. Novel therapies applied with MDK inhibitors can serve more selective and less cytotoxic manner with maximum efficiency and without resistance and/or recurrence as we mentioned above for low molecular weight compounds. All these are needed further investigations. Complexicity of GBM can be seen basicly in different human GBM cell lines derived from patients belonging to different populations in terms of MDK levels and its receptors. Therefore, individual based therapy should be administered.

7. References

Akhter, S., Ichihara-Tanaka, K., Kojima, S., Muramatsu, H., Inui, T. et al. (1998). Clusters of basic amino acids in midkine: roles in neurite-promoting activity and plasminogen activator enhancing activity. The Journal of Biochemistry, Vol. 123, No.6, (June 1998), pp. 1127-1136.

Erguven, M., Bilir, A., Yazihan, N., Ermis, E., Sabanci, A., Aktas, E., Aras, Y., Alpman, V. (2011) Decreased therapeutic effects of noscapine combined with imatinib mesylate on human glioblastoma in vitro and the effect of midkine. Cancer Cell International, Vol.11,No.1, (Jun 2011), pp. 18.

Asai, T., Watanabe, K., Ichihara-Tanaka, K., Kaneda, N., Kojima, S. et al. (1997) Identification of heparin-binding sites in midkine and their role in neurite-promotion. Biochemical and Biophysical Research Communications,Vol. 236, No 1., (July 1997), pp.66-70.

Bani-Yaghoub, M., Tremblay, R.G., Lei, J.X., Zhang, D., Zurakowski, B., et al. (2006).Role of Sox2 in the development of the mouse neocortex. Developmental Biology, Vol. 295, No.1, (July 2006), pp.52-66.

Bilir, A., Erguven, M., Yazihan, N., Aktas, E., Oktem, G. et al. 2010).Enhancement of vinorelbine-induced cytotoxicity and apoptosis by clomipramine and lithium chloride in human neuroblastoma cancer cell line SH-SY5Y. Journal of Neurooncology., Vol.100, No.3, (December 2010), pp.385-95.

Brennan, C., Momota, H., Hambardzumyan, D., Ozawa, T., Tandon, A., et al. (2009). Glioblastoma subclasses can be defined by activity among signal transduction pathways and associated genomic alterations. Public Library of Science since, Vol. 4, No. 11, (November 2009), pp. e7752.

Cernkovich, E. R., Deng, J., Hua, K., Harp, J. B.(2007). Midkine is an autocrine activator of signal transducer and activator of transcription 3 in 3T3-L1 cells. Endocrinology, Vol.148, No.4, (April 2007), pp.1598-1604.

Chakravarti, A., Noll, E., Black, P.M., Finkelstein, D.F., Finkelstein, D.M. et al.(2002) Quantitatively determined survivin expression levels are of prognostic value in human gliomas. Journal of Clinical Oncology, Vol. 20, No.4 (February 2002), pp.1063-8.

Cheng, L., Bao, S., Rich, J.N. (2010). Potential therapeutic implications of cancer stem cells in glioblastoma. Biochemical Pharmacology,Vol.80,No.5,(September 2010),pp.654-65.

Dai,L.C. (2009). Midkine translocated to nucleoli and involved in carcinogenesis. World Journal of Gastroenterology, Vol.15, No.4,(January 2009),pp.412-6.

Dai, L.C., Shao, J. Z., Min, L. S., Xiao, Y. T., Xiang, L. X. et al. (2008) Midkine accumulated in nucleolus of HepG2 cells involved in rRNA transcription. The World Journal of Gastroenterology, Vol. 14, No. 40, (October 2008), pp.6249-6253.

Dang, L., Fan, X., Chaudhry, A., Wang, M., Gaiano,N., Eberhart, C.G.(2006). Notch3 signaling initiates choroid plexus tumor formation. Oncogene,Vol. 25, No.3, (January 2006), pp.487-491.

Das, A., Tan, W.L, Teo, J., Smith, D.R. (2002). Expression of survivin in primary glioblastomas. Journal of Cancer Research& Clinical Oncology, Vol. 128, No.6, (January 2002), pp.302-6.

Deuel, T. F., Zhang, N., Yeh, H. J., Silos-Santiago, I., Wang, Z. Y. (2002) Pleiotrophin: a cytokine with diverse functions and a novel signaling pathway. Archieves Biochemistry and Biophysics,Vol.397, No. 2, (January 2002), pp. 162-167.

Fabri, L., Maruta, H., Muramatsu, H., Muramatsu,T., Simpson, R. J. et al. (1993) Structural characterisation of native and recombinantforms of the neurotrophic cytokine MK. The Journal of Chromatography, Vol.646, No.1 (August 1993), pp. 213-225.

Fan, X., Mikolaenko, I., Elhassan, I., Ni, X., Wang, Y. et al. (2004). Notch1 and notch2 have opposite effects on embryonal brain tumor growth. Cancer Research,Vol. 64,No.21, (November 2004), pp.7787-7793.

Furnari, F.B, Fenton, T., Bachoo, R.M, Mukasa, A., Stommel, J.M et al. (2007). Malignant astrocytic glioma: genetics, biology, and paths to treatment. Genes Development, Vol.21,No. 21, (November 2007), pp.2683-710.

Grzelinski, M., Steinberg, F., Martens, T., Czubayko, F., Lamszus, K. et al. (2009).Enhanced antitumorigenic effects in glioblastoma on double targeting of pleiotrophin and its receptor ALK. Neoplasia, Vol.11, No.2,(February 2009), pp.145-56.

Gustavsson, H., Jennbacken, K., Welén, K., Damber, J.E.(2008). Altered expression of genes regulating angiogenesis in experimental androgen-independent prostate cancer. Prostate, Vol.68,No.2,(February 2008),pp.161-70.

Hu, R., Yan, Y., Li, Q., Lin, Y., Jin, W. et al.(2010). Increased drug efflux along with midkine gene high expression in childhood B-lineage acutelymphoblastic leukemia cells. International Journal of Hematology, Vol. 92,No.1,(July 2010), pp.105-10.

Huang, Y., Hoque, M. O., Wu, F., Trink, B., Sidransky, D. et al.(2008) Midkine induces epithelial-mesenchymal transition through Notch2/Jak2-Stat3 signaling in human keratinocytes. Cell Cycle ,Vol.7, No.11, (June 2008), pp. 1613-1622.

Huang, Y., Sook-Kim, M. and Ratovitski, E. (2008) Midkine promotes tetraspanin-integrin interaction and induces FAK-Stat1a pathway contributing to migration/invasiveness of human head and neck squamous cell carcinoma cells. Biochemical and Biophysical Research Communications,Vol.377, No.2, (December 2008), pp. 474-478.

Huang, Z., Cheng, L., Guryanova, O.A., Wu, Q., Bao, S.(2010). Cancer stem cells in glioblastoma-molecular signaling and therapeutic targeting. Protein and Cell, Vol.1, No.7,(July 2010), pp.638-55.

Hussain, M.M., Strickland, D.K., Bakillah, A. (1999).The mammalian low-density lipoprotein receptor family. The Annual Review of Nutrition. Vol.19,pp.141–172.

Ichihara-Tanaka, K., Oohira, A., Rumsby, M. And Muramatsu, T. (2006) Neuroglycan C is a novel midkine receptor involved in process elongation of oligodendroglial precursor-like cells. The Journal of Biological Chemistry.,Vol.281,No. 41, (October 2006), pp.30857-30864.

Ikushima, H., Todo, T., Ino, Y., Takahashi, M., Miyazawa, K. et al. (2009).Autocrine TGF-beta signaling maintains tumorigenicity of glioma-initiating cells through Sry-related HMG-box factors. Cell Stem Cell, Vol. 5,No.5, (November 2009), pp.504-514.

Iwasaki, W.., Nagata, K.., Hatanaka, H., Inui, T.,Kimura, T. et al. (1997) Solution structure of midkine, a new heparin-binding growth factor. The EMBO Journal, Vol.16, No. 23, (December 1997), pp. 6936-6946.

Kadomatsu K.(2010). Midkine regulation of the renin-angiotensin system. Current Hypertension Reports, Vol.12, No.2,(April 2010),pp.74-9.

Kadomatsu, K., Huang, R.-P., Suganuma, T., Murata, F., Muramatsu, T.(1990), A retinoic acid responsive gene MK found in the teratocarcinoma system is expressed in spatially and temporally controlled manner during mouse embryogenesis. The Journal of Cell Biology, Vol. 110, No.3, (March 1990), pp. 607–616

Kajiwara, Y., Yamasaki, F., Hama, S., Yahara, K., Yoshioka, H. et al.(2003) Expression of survivin in astrocytic tumors: Correlation with malignant grade and prognosis. Cancer, Vol. 97, No.4, (February 2003), pp.1077-83.

Kilpelainen, I., Kaksonen, M., Kinnunen, T., Avikainen,H., Fath, M. et al. (2000) Heparin binding growth-associated molecule contains two heparin-binding b-sheet domains that are homologous to the thrombospondin type I repeat. Journal of Biological Chemistry,Vol. 275, No.18., (May 200), pp. 13564-13570.

Kemik, O., Sumer, A., Kemik, A.S., Hasirci, I., Purisa, S. et al. (2010).The relationship among acute-phase response proteins, cytokines and hormones in cachectic patients with colon cancer. World Journal of Surgical Oncology, Vol.8,(September 2010),pp. 85.

Kleinschmidt-DeMasters, B.K., Heinz, D., McCarthy, P.J., Bobak, J.B., Lillehei, K.O. et al. (2003) Survivin in glioblastomas: Protein and messenger RNA expression and comparison with telomerase levels. Archives of Pathology&Laboratory Medicine, Vol.127, No.7, (July 2003),pp. 826-33.

Kojima, S., Inui, T., Muramatsu, H., Suzuki, Y.,Kadomatsu, K. et al. (1997). Dimerization of midkine by tissue transglutaminase and its functional implication. The Journal of Biochemistry, Vol. 272,No. 14, (April 1997), pp.9410-9416.

Krakstad, C., Chekenya, M.(2010). Survival signalling and apoptosis resistance in glioblastomas: opportunities for targeted therapeutics, Molecular Cancer. Vol.9, (June 2010),pp.135.

Krieger, M., Herz, J.(1994). Structures and functions of multiligand lipoprotein receptors: macrophage scavenger receptors and LDL receptor-related protein (LRP) .The Annual Review of Biochemistry, Vol.63, pp.601–637.

Kurosawa, N., Chen, G. Y., Kadomatsu, K., Ikematsu,S., Sakuma, S. et al. (2001). Glypican-2 binds to midkine: the role of glypican-2 in neuronal cell adhesion and neurite outgrowth. Glycoconjugate Journal, Vol.18,No. 6, (June 2001), pp. 499-507.

Libermann, T.A., Nusbaum, H.R., Razon, N., Kris, R., Lax, I. et al. (1985a). Amplification, enhanced expression and possible rearrangement of EGF receptor gene in primary human brain tumours of glial origin. Nature, Vol. 313, No. 5998, (January 1985),pp.144-147.

Libermann, T.A., Nusbaum, H.R., Razon, N., Kris, R., Lax, I. et al. (1985b). Amplification and overexpression of the EGF receptor gene in primary human glioblastomas. Journal of Cell Science Supplement, Vol.3, pp.161-172.

Lino, M.M, Merlo, A., Boulay, J.L.(2010). Notch signaling in glioblastoma: a developmental drug target? BMC Medicine, Vol.8, (November 2010), pp.72.

Lucas S., Henze G., Schnabel D., Barthlen W., Sakuma S. et al. (2010).Serum levels of Midkine in children and adolescents without malignant disease. Pediatrics International,Vol.52,No.1,(February 2010),pp.75-9.

Ma, J., Meng, Y., Kwiatkowski, D.J., Chen, X., Peng, H. et al. (2010). Mammalian target of rapamycin regulates murine and human cell differentiation through STAT3/p63/Jagged/Notch cascade. The Journal of Clinical Investigation,Vol.120, No. 1, (January 2010), pp.103-114.

Maeda, N., Ichihara-Tanaka, K., Kimura, T., Kadomatsu, K., Muramatsu, T. et al. (1999) A receptor-like protein-tyrosine phosphatase PTPz/ RPTPb binds a heparin-binding growth factor midkine. Involvement of arginine 78 of midkine in the high af_nity binding to PTPz. Journal of Biological. Chemistry Vol. 274, No. 18, (April 1999), pp12474-12479.

Maruyama, K., Muramatsu ,H., Ishiguro, N., Muramatsu, T. (2004). Midkine, a heparin-binding growth factor, is fundamentally involved in the pathogenesis of rheumatoid arthritis. Arthritis & Rheumatism, Vol.50,No.5,(May 2004),pp.1420-9.

Matsui, T., Ichihara-Tanaka, K., Lan, C., Muramatsu, H., Kondou, T. et al.(2010). Midkine inhibitors: application of a simple assay procedure to screening of inhibitory compounds. International Archives of Medicine, Vol.3,(June 2010), pp.12.

Merlo, A.(2003). Genes and pathways driving glioblastomas in humans and murine disease models. Neurosurgical Review,Vol.26,(July 2003), pp.145-158.

Mirkin, BL., Clark, S., Zheng, X., Chu, F., White, BD. et al.(2005).Identification of midkine as a mediator for intercellular transfer of drug resistance. Oncogene. Vol.24, No.31,(July 2005), pp.4965-74.

Mishima, K., Asai, A., Kadomatsu, K., Ino, Y., Nomura, K., et al.(1997). Increased expression of midkine during the progression of human astrocytomas. Neuroscience Letters,Vol 233,No.1,(September 1997), pp.29-32.

Mitsiadis, TA., Salmivirta, M., Muramatsu, T., Muramatsu, H., Rauvala, H., et al.(1995) Expression of the heparin-binding cytokines, midkine (MK) and HB-GAM (pleiotrophin) is associated with epithelial-mesenchymal interactions during fetal development and organogenesis. Development, Vol.121, No.1,(January 1995), pp. 37-51.

Muramatsu, T.(2010). Midkine, a heparin-binding cytokine with multiple roles in development, repair and diseases. Proceedings of the Japan Academy, Ser. B, Physical and Biological Sciences,Vol. 86, No.4, pp. 410-425.

Muramatsu, H., Zou, K., Sakaguchi, N., Ikematsu, S., Sakuma, S. et al. (2000) .LDL receptor-related protein as a component of the midkine receptor. Biochemical and Biophysical Research Communication,Vol. 270,(April 2000), pp. 936-941.

Muramatsu, H., Inui, T., Kimura, T., Sakakibara, S., Song, XJ., et al. (1994) Localization of heparin-binding, neurite outgrowth and antigenic regions in midkine molecule. Biochemical and Biophysical Research Communications,Vol. 203,(September 1994), pp.1131-1139.

Muramatsu, H., Zou, P., Suzuki, H., Oda, Y., Chen, G. Y., et al. (2004) .a4b1- and a6b1-integrins are functional receptors for midkine, a heparin-binding growth factor. Journal of Cell Science, Vol.117,(October 2004),pp.5405-5415.

Muramatsu, H., Shirahama, H., Yonezawa, S.,Maruta, H. and Muramatsu, T. (1993) Midkine, a retinoic acid-inducible growth/di_erentiation factor: immunochemical evidence for the function and distribution. Developmental Biology, Vol.159,(October 1993),pp. 392-402.

Muramatsu, H., Zou, P., Kurosawa, N., Ichihara-Tanaka, K., Maruyama, K., et al. (2006) Female infertility in mice de_cient in midkine and pleiotrophin, which form a distinct family of growth factors. Genes to Cells ,Vol.11,(December 2006),pp. 1405-1417.

Nobata, S., Shinozawa, T., Sakanishi, A.(2005). Truncated midkine induces transformation of cultured cells and short latency of tumorigenesis in nude mice. Cancer Letters,Vol.219,No.1,(February 2005),pp. 83-9.

Ohgaki, H., Dessen, P., Jourde, B., Horstmann, S., Nishikawa, T.et al.(2004).Genetic pathways to glioblastoma: a population-based study. Cancer Research ,Vol. 64, (October 2004), pp.6892-6899.

Ohuchida, T., Okamoto, K., Akahane, K., Higure, A., Todoroki, H. et al. (2004) Midkine protects hepatocellular carcinoma cells against TRAILmediated apoptosis through down-regulation ofcaspase-3 activity. Cancer, Vol.100, (june 2004),pp.2430-2436.

Ota, K., Fujimori, H., Ueda, M., Shiniriki, S., Kudo, M. Et al.(2008). Midkine as a prognostic biomarker in oral squamous cell carcinoma. British Journal of Cancer, Vol.99, No.4,(Augst 2008), pp. 655-62.

Owada, K., Sanjo, N., Kobayashi, T., Mizusawa, H.,Muramatsu, H.et al. (1999) Midkine inhibits caspase-dependent apoptosis via the activation of mitogen-activated protein kinase and phosphatidylinositol 3-kinase in cultured neurons. Journal of Neurochemistry, Vol.73,(November 1999),pp.2084-2092.

Panchision, D.M.(2009).The role of oxygen in regulating neural stem cells in development and disease. J Cell Physiol,Vol.220,(September 2009), pp.562-568.

Patten, BA., Sardi, SP., Koirala, S., Nakafuku, M., Corfas, G.(2006). Notch1 signaling regulates radial glia differentiation through multiple transcriptional mechanisms. The Journal of Neuroscince, Vol.26, (March 2006),pp.3102-3108.

Powers, C., Aigner, A., Stoica, GE., McDonnell, K., Wellstein, A.(2002). Pleiotrophin signaling through anaplastic lymphoma kinase is rate-limiting for glioblastoma growth. The Journal of Biological Chemistry, Vol.277, No.16,(April 2002),pp.14153-8.

Purow, B.W., Sundaresan, T.K., Burdick, M.J., Kefas, B.A., Comeau, L.D. et al.(2008).Notch-1 regulates transcription of the epidermal growth factor receptor through p53. Carcinogenesis, Vol. 29,(May 2008), pp.918-925.

Rauvala, H., Peng, H.B. (1997). HB-GAM (heparin-binding growth-associated molecule) and heparin-type glycans in the development and placiticity of neuron-target contacts. Progress in Neurobiology,Vol 52, (June 1997),pp.127-144.

Rawnaq, T., Kunkel, M., Bachmann, K., Simon, R., Zander, H. et al.(2010). Serum Midkine Correlates with Tumor Progression and Imatinib Response in Gastrointestinal Stromal Tumors. Annals of Surgical Oncology, (Jun 2010) , [Epub ahead of print] PubMed.

Rosenbaum, C., Röhrs, S., Müller, O., Waldmann, H. Modulation of MRP-1-mediated multidrug resistance by indomethacin analogues. (2005).Journal of Medicinal Chemistry,Vol.48, No.4,(February 2005), pp.1179-87.

Qin, Li, L., Lian Huang, H., Liang Ping, J., Xu, W., Li, J. et al.(2011). Expression of midkine and endoglin in breast carcinomas with different immunohistochemical profiles. Acta Pathologica, Microbiologica et Immunologica Scandinavica, Vol.119,No.2, (February 2011), pp.103-10.

Quant, E.C., Wen P.Y.(2010). Novel medical therapeutics in glioblastomas, including targeted molecular therapies, current and future clinical trials, Neuroimaging Clinics North America. Vol.20, No.3, (August 2010),pp.425-448.

Sakamoto, K., Bu, G., Chen, S., Takei, Y., Hibi, K.et al.(2011),The premature ligand-receptor interactionduring biosynthesis limits the production of growth factor midkine and its receptor LDL receptor-related protein 1(LRP1).The Journal of Biological Chemistry (January 2011) [Epub ahead of print]

Sato, W., Kadomatsu, K., Yuzawa, Y., Muramatsu, H., Hotta, N. et al. (2001) Midkine is involved in neutrophil in_ltration into the tubulointerstitium in ischemic renal injury. The Journal of Immunology. Vol.167, (September 2001),pp.3463-3469.

Satoh, H., Muramatsu, G., Moretto, T., Muramatsu, H.J., Chang, ST. et al. (1993). Midkine that promotes survival of fetal human neurons is produced by fetal human astrocytes in culture. Brain Research,Vol. 75 , pp. 201–205.

Shibata, Y., Muramatsu T., Hirai M., Inui, T., Kimura, T.et al. (2002).Nuclear targeting by the growth factor midkine. Molecular and Cellular Biology,Vol.22,No.19,(October 2002),pp.6788-96.

Sivasankaran, B., Degen, M., Ghaffari, A., Hegi,M.E., Hamou, M.F.et al.(2009).Tenascin-C is a novel RBPJk-induced target gene for Notch signaling in gliomas. Cancer Research,Vol. 69,(January 2009),pp.458-465.

Solecki, D.J., Liu, X.L., Tomoda, T., Fang, Y., Hatten, M.E. (2001). Activated Notch2 signaling inhibits differentiation of cerebellar granule neuron precursors by maintaining proliferation. Neuron, Vol.31,(August 2001), pp.557-568.

Stoica, G E., Kuo, A., Powers, C., Bowden, E T., Sale, E B. et al. (2002) Midkine binds to anaplastic lymphoma kinase (ALK) and acts as a growth factor for different cell types. The Journal of Biological Chemistry, Vol. 277, (September 2002), pp.35990-35998.

Mitsiadis, TA., Salmivirta, T., Muramatsu, H., Muramatsu, H., Rauvala, E.et al.(1995). Thesleff, Expression of the heparin-binding cytokines, midkine (MK) and HB-GAM (pleiotrophin) is associated with epithelial-mesenchymal interactions during fetal development and organogenesis. Development ,Vol.121, (January 1995),pp. 37–51.

Takei, Y., Kadomatsu, K., Matsuo, S., Itoh, H., Nakazawa, K. et al. (2001). Antisense oligodeoxynucleotide targeted to Midkine, a heparinbinding growth factor, suppresses tumorigenicityof mouse rectal carcinoma cells. Cancer Research, Vol. 61, (December 2001),pp.8486-8491.

Takei, Y., Kadomatsu, K., Goto, T., Muramatsu, T. (2006).Combinational antitumor effect of siRNA against midkine and paclitaxel on growth of human prostate cancer xenografts. Cancer, Vol.107, No.4,(August 2006), pp.864-73.

Take, M., Tsutsui, J., Obama, H., Ozawa, M., Nakayama, T. et al.(1994). Identification of nucleolin as a binding protein for midkine (MK) and heparin-binding growth associated molecule (HB-GAM). The Journal of Biochemistry,Vol.116,(November 1994), pp.1063-1068.

Tanaka M, Kadokawa Y, Hamada Y, Marunouchi T (1999) Notch2 expression negatively correlates with glial differentiation in the postnatal mouse brain. J Neurobiol, Vol. 41, No. 4 (December 1999),pp. 524-539.

Ulasov, IV., Rivera, AA., Sonabend, AM., Rivera, LB., Wang, M. et al. (2007). Comparative evaluation of survivin, midkine and CXCR4 promoters for transcriptional targeting of glioma gene therapy. Cancer Biology& Therapy, Vol.6, No.5, (May 2007), pp. 679-85.

Wang, J., Takeuchi, H., Sonobe, Y., Jin, S., Mizuno, T. et al.(2008). Inhibition of midkine alleviates experimental autoimmune encephalomyelitis through the expansion of regulatory T cell population. Proceedings of the National Academy Sciences online U S A, Vol.105, No. 10, (March 2008), pp.3915-20.

Wang, J., Takeuchi, H., Sonobe, Y., Jin, S., Mizuno, T.et al.(2008). Inhibition of midkine alleviates experimental autoimmune encephalomyelitis through the expansion of regulatory T cell population. Proceedings of the National Academy of Sciences of the United States of America, Vol.105, No.10,(March 2008), pp.3915-20.

Yamada, Y., Kuroiwa, T., Nakagawa, T., Kajimoto, Y., Dohi, T. et al.(2003) Transcriptional expression of survivin and its splice variants in brain tumors in humans. Journal of Neurosurgery Vol.99, No. (October 2003), pp.738-45.

Yang, L., Cao, Z., Li, F., Post, DE., Van Meir, E.G. et al. (2004) Tumor-specific gene expression using the survivin promoter is further increased by hypoxia. Gene Therapy, Vol. 11, No.15, (August 2004), pp.1215-23.

Yao, X., Tan, Z., Gu, B., Wu, R.R., Liu, Y.K. et al.(2010). Promotion of self-renewal of embryonic stem cells by midkine. Acta Pharmacologica Sinica, Vol.31, No.5,(May 2010), pp.629-37.

Zou, K., Muramatsu, H., Ikematsu, S., Sakuma, S., Salama, RH.et al. (2000). A heparin-binding growth factor, midkine, binds to a chondroitin sulfate proteoglycan, PG-M/versican. European Journal of Biochemistry, Vol. 267,(July 2000), pp.4046-4053.

Zou, P., Muramatsu, H., Miyata, T., Muramatsu, T.(2006). Midkine, a heparin-binding growth factor, is expressed in neural precursor cells and promotes their growth. Journal of Neurochemistry, Vol.99, No.6,(December 2006), pp.1470-9.

Part 3

Importance of Blood - Brain Barrier in CNS Tumors

4

The Blood-Brain Barrier in Brain Tumours

Susan Noell[1], Karen Wolburg-Buchholz[2], Andreas F. Mack[3], Hartwig Wolburg[2] and Petra Fallier-Becker[2]
[1]*Department of Neurosurgery, University of Tübingen*
[2]*Institute of Pathology and Neuropathology, University of Tübingen*
[3]*Institute of Anatomy, University of Tübingen*
Germany

1. Introduction

The literature on glioblastoma is increasingly concerned with genetic pathways to and genomic analyses of glioblastoma (Ohgaki et al., 2004; Parsons et al., 2008). Mutations of numerous genes were demonstrated to be involved in the development of brain tumours; however, in most cases the mechanistic roles of these mutated genes in the dysregulation of the cells of tumour origin are not understood in functional terms, but are used for molecular diagnostics (Riemenschneider et al., 2010). Moreover, several potential biomarkers of glioblastoma were identified and classified for clinical prognosis without precise knowledge of their function (Sreekanthreddy et al., 2010). A new dimension of brain tumour research has been reached by the detection of cancer stem cells in glioblastoma which were identified as a small subpopulation of brain tumour propagating cells (Huang et al., 2010; Tabatabai & Weller, 2011). A link between glioblastoma stem cells and tumour vascularization has been established by the first description of the possibility that tumour vessels can be recruited from glioblastoma stem cells (Ricci-Vitiani et al., 2010). This opens a new field concerning the plasticity of tumour vessel endothelial cells including their lost or undifferentiated barrier properties. Since the clinical signs of the glioblastoma are connected to the intracerebral pressure due to edemas, understanding the alterations of the blood-brain barrier (BBB) is of central importance. For this reason, we will begin this chapter on the blood-tumour barrier with the description of cell biological aspects of the healthy BBB.

The BBB is responsible for the homeostasis of the microenvironment in the neural parenchyma and essential for normal function of the brain. In the strict sense, it is located in the endothelial cells and restricts the paracellular diffusion of hydrophilic molecules by both complex tight junctions (Reese & Karnovsky, 1967; Brightman & Reese, 1969) and a low degree of transcytosis (Peters et al., 1991). This implies the necessity of various specific transporters for providing the brain with compounds essential for brain energy metabolism (Begley, 2004).

It is generally accepted now that astrocytes play a decisive role in the maintenance if not induction of the BBB (Abbott et al., 2006; Wolburg et al., 2009). But we have to be aware that the mechanism by which this maintenance or induction of the BBB is performed, is not understood so far. In any case, in the mature brain, the astrocytes embrace the vessels by sending an endfoot towards the perivascular basal lamina (Mathiisen et al., 2010). It has been well-known for many years that the astroglial membranes contacting the subendothelial or pericytic basal lamina are characterized by the occurrence of orthogonal arrays of particles (OAPs). These arrays can, up to now, exclusively be demonstrated by the freeze-fracturing technique (for a recent survey, see Wolburg et al., 2011), but it is known that they consist of the water channel protein aquaporin-4 (AQP4). Where the glial membrane loses the contact with the basal lamina by diving into the neuropil for making contacts with other astroglial cells, oligodendrocytes, neurons and synapses, the density of OAPs drops dramatically. The distribution of OAPs in both astroglial membrane domains, the perivascular endfoot membrane and the non-endfoot membrane, can be described as a polarization of the astrocyte. Interestingly, this polarity of astrocytes arises concomitantly with the maturation of the BBB, and is not maintained by cultured astrocytes (Nico et al., 2001). In the context of this chapter, it is important that the polarity of glioma cells heavily decreases (Neuhaus, 1990; Noell et al., submitted). It will take some space in this review to describe the circumstances under which the polarity is decreased and which consequences will arise for the pathophysiology of brain tumours.

2. The healthy blood-brain barrier

2.1 Endothelial cells

The endothelial cells of the BBB have been shown to form the most complex tight junction networks among all endothelial cells of the entire vasculature of the body (Nagy et al., 1984). Previously, the complexity of the network of tight junction strands has been used for the prediction of the physiological parameters, permeability and transepithelial electrical resistance (Claude, 1978). However, this relationship between morphological and physiological parameters has originally been established for epithelial cells: its validity for endothelial cells was confirmed on the basis of Claude's paradigm. In the last years, many details of the molecular composition of tight junctions have been published. Most of these results have been obtained from studies on epithelial cells, and only few publications have tried to compare molecular aspects of endothelial, and in particular BBB endothelial, tight junctions with those of epithelial cells (Wolburg & Lippoldt, 2002). ZO-1 was the first protein identified and characterized as a tight junction-associated protein (Stevenson et al., 1986). ZO-1 is a cytoplasmic 220 kDa phosphoprotein of the membrane associated guanylate kinase homologues (MAGUK) family. The localization of ZO-1 to the tight junction is not exclusive (Itoh et al., 1993), as in cellular systems with less elaborate or no tight junctions, ZO-1 is found enriched in regions of the adherens or gap junctions (Giepmans & Moolenaar, 1998; Itoh et al., 1993). ZO-2, a 160kDa protein of the same MAGUK family, turned out to be a ubiquitous component of epithelial and endothelial tight junctions (Jesaitis & Goodenough, 1994). Independently of ZO-1, ZO-2 can determine claudin polymerization in the tight junction strands (Umeda et al., 2006). The family of claudins turned out to be the most important molecules of tight junctions, because they are the permeability-restricting molecules proper (Furuse et al., 1998; Morita et al., 1999a). Prior to the discovery of claudins, occludin was detected by the Tsukita group as well (Furuse et al., 1993). Both occludin and the claudins are membrane proteins with four transmembrane domains, which are nevertheless not homologue. Initially, occludin has been assumed to be essential for tight junction integrity, but the occludin-knock out mouse is viable and has no essential morphological phenotype and normally structured tight junctions in all organs (Saitou et al., 2000). Accordingly, occludin is presently believed to act in a yet undefined regulatory context rather than as a major structural tight junction protein. The same is true for the recently detected tight junction molecule MarvelD3 which has been described as a new occludin family member not essential for the formation of functional tight junctions but determining paracellular permeability (Steed et al., 2009). In addition to the four-span transmembrane proteins, another family of single-span proteins occur at tight junctions, the junctional adhesion molecules (JAMs) including JAM-A,-B,-C, the coxsackie and adenovirus-associated receptor (CAR) and the endothelial selective adhesion molecule (ESAM) (Ebnet et al., 2004).

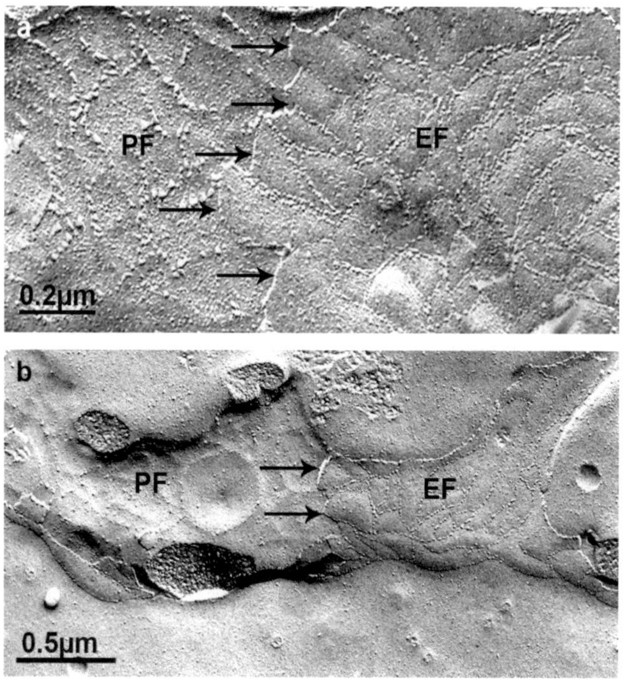

Fig. 1. Freeze-fracture replicas of endothelial cells in vivo (a) and in vitro (b). In vivo, BBB tight junctional strands have the highest degree of P-face (protoplasmic fracture face, PF) association found in the whole vasculature in the body. The most impressive alteration in vitro when compared with in vivo is the reduction of this association of the tight junctional strands with the PF. EF external fracture face or E-face. Arrows point to the switch from the P-face of the one cell to the E-face of the connected cell.

The molecular complexity of the tight junctions including the junctional scaffolding proteins such as ZO-1-3, cingulin, PAR-3, PAR-6, AF-6, MUPP1 or symplekin which are regulating the tight junctions are comprehensively described in a number of recent overviews (see, for example, Ebnet, 2008; Angelow et al., 2008; Krause et al., 2008; Balda & Matter, 2009; Steed et al., 2010).

In order to observe and describe tight junctions in terms of morphology, the freeze-fracture method still is most valuable (Fig. 1). The advantage of this method is that the two membranous lipidic bilayers are cleaved and shadowed with platinum/carbon vapour to replicate the molecular details of the fracture planes. Two aspects of the membrane can be distinguished: if the observer looks from outside the cell, the inner leaflet of the membrane is displayed which is called the protoplasmic fracture face or P-face. If the observer looks from inside the cell, the outer leaflet of the membrane is displayed which is called the external fracture face or E-face. Concerning the tight junctions, two parameters can be visualized by freeze-fracture electron microscopy: the complexity of strands and the association of the particles with the P- or E-face. The complexity of the tight junction network was recognized to be related to the transepithelial electrical resistance (Claude, 1978). Nagy et al. (1984) investigated the tight junctions of the BBB and found them the most complex ones in the whole vasculature of the body. An additional parameter to describe the quality of the BBB tight junctions turned out to be the association of the tight junction particles with the P- or the E-face of the endothelial membrane (Wolburg et al., 1994). The BBB tight junctions are unique among all endothelial tight junctions in that their P-face association is as high as or even slightly higher than their E-face association (Fig. 1a). Interestingly, the P-face/E-face-ratio of BBB tight junctions continuously increases during development (Kniesel et al., 1996). In cell culture, the BBB endothelial cell tight junctions are mainly E-face-associated (Fig. 1b), and this is similar to non-BBB endothelial cells *in situ* (Wolburg et al., 1994) indirectly indicating that the association of the strand particles within the membrane leaflets is under the close control of the brain microenvironment. In our context, it is of particular interest that Claudin-1 and Claudin-3 led to the formation of tight junctions almost completely associated with the P-face when transfected into fibroblasts. In contrast, claudin-2 and claudin-5 transfected fibroblasts showed particles associated with the E-face (Tsukita & Furuse, 1999; Morita et al., 1999b). Therefore, the particle association with either the P- or E-face is believed to be a consequence of the stoichiometry of claudins within the tight junction. The dominant P-face-association is a particular feature of the BBB (Wolburg et al., 1994; Liebner et al., 2011).

The brain is faced with the dilemma between the necessary protection against neurotoxic compounds in the blood and against continuous variations of the blood composition on the one hand, and the delivery of energy-rich compounds to fuel the extremely demanding metabolism of the brain on the other hand. The second demand requires the presence of a lot of different transporters such as glucose transporters, amino acid transporters, anionic transporters or multidrug resistance transporters (for an overview, see Begley, 2004). The endothelial cells express a high density of glucose transporter molecules (which provides for glucose transport into the brain neuropil). The density of glucose transporters in the luminal membrane is three to four times lower than in the abluminal membrane (Farrell & Pardridge, 1991). Moreover, many Na^+, K^+ pump molecules are localized asymmetrically in the abluminal membrane which facilitates the clearance of excess K^+ ions into the blood vessels, and is involved into the generation of osmotical forces for transendothelial water transport.

2.2 Astrocytes

The brain is the location where the interaction between vessels and surrounding tissue is extremely close. In no other organ, perhaps with the exception of the lung alveoles, endothelial cells are so intimately connected to non-endothelial cells. In the brain, these cells are the astrocytes which form so-called endfeet beneath the basal lamina around vessels and at the surface of the brain. Where the astrocyte processes touch the basal lamina, OAPs are inserted into the membrane: where the contact is lost, the OAP density drops sharply. The OAPs were described to contain the water channel protein aquaporin-4 (AQP4; Fig. 2; for reviews, see Rash et al., 2004; Rash, 2010; Wolburg et al., 2011). Aquaporins mediate water movements between the intracellular, interstitial, vascular and ventricular compartments which are under the strict control of osmotic and hydrostatic pressure gradients (Amiry-Moghaddam &

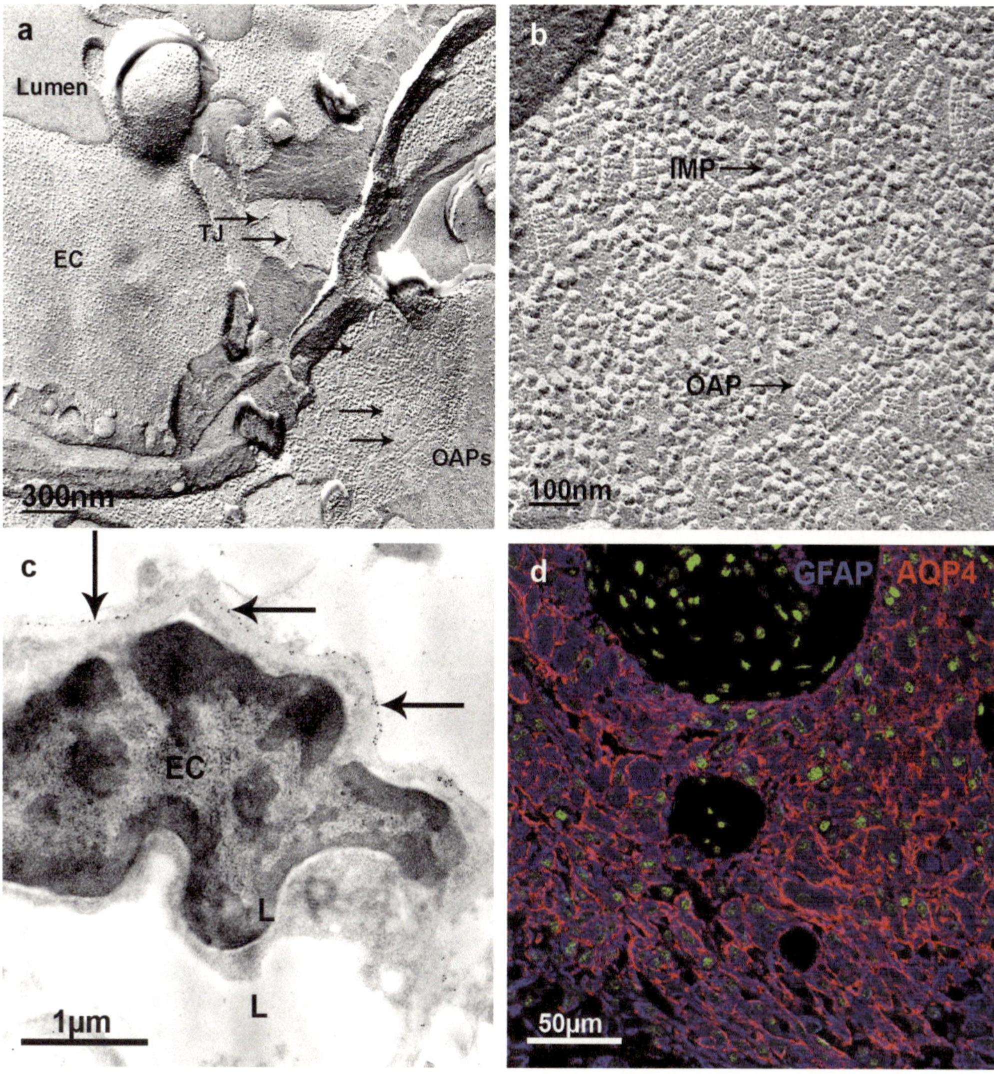

Fig. 2. Freeze-fracture replica (a,b; b is a detail of a) of the glio-vascular unit of the normal mouse brain, EC endothelial cell, TJ tight junction, OAPs orthogonal arrays of particles in the astroglial endfoot membrane, IMP intramembrane particles. The OAPs are located at and restricted to astroglial endfeet (from a collaboration with Christer Betsholtz, Karolinska Institute, Stockholm, Sweden). c: immunogold labeling of AQP4 in the astroglial membrane (arrows) around an endothelial cell (EC). L lumen of a microcapillary blood vessel. d: Immunohistochemical double labeling of AQP4 (red) and the glial fibrillary acidic protein (GFAP) in human glioblastoma. AQP4 is no more restricted to glial (or glioma cell) endfeet, but distributed over the whole surface of the cell.

Ottersen, 2003; Benfenati & Ferroni, 2010; Pasantes-Morales & Cruz-Rangel, 2010; MacAulay & Zeuthen, 2010). The composition of the OAPs by AQP4 molecules is now generally accepted and was shown by several lines of evidence: the absence of OAPs in astrocytes of AQP4-deficient mice (Verbavatz et al., 1997), the formation of OAPs in chinese hamster ovary (CHO) cells stably transfected with AQP4 (Yang et al., 1996), and the immunogold fracture-labeling technique directly showing that AQP4 is a component of the arrays (Rash et al., 1998). Moreover, Nielsen et al. (1997) were able to demonstrate by immunogold labeling that the distribution of the AQP4-related immunoreactivity in the retinal Müller glial cells was identical to that of the OAPs and was restricted to glial membranes.

Aquaporins in general form tetrameric protein complexes within the membrane plane (King et al., 2004). On the molecular level, each monomer represents a water channel proper (Tani et al., 2009). On the electron microscopical level, a structural subunit of the OAP measuring about 7x7nm represents a tetramer. The number of subunits (tetramers) per OAP can change between four and more than one hundred. AQP4 was described to occur as heterotetramers (Nicchia et al., 2010) reflecting the relative expression level of the different splice variants (M1 and M23; Neely et al., 1999, see below). The distribution of the inward rectifier potassium channel Kir 4.1 and the K^+ conductivity is similar to that of AQP4 and the dystrophin-dystroglycan complex (DDC) (Blake & Kröger, 2000; Amiry-Moghaddam & Ottersen, 2003; Connors et al., 2004; Nagelhus et al., 2004; Warth et al., 2005; MacAulay & Zeuthen, 2010). These molecules participate in the spatial buffering process of the extracellular space: synaptic activity and neuronal conductance evoke increase of the concentration of extracellular K^+ ions which are taken up by astrocytes. This K^+ uptake is followed osmotically by water entry through water channels of the type AQP4 (which are not absent in synaptic regions, but reduced in comparison with endfeet). In order to avoid swelling of astrocytes the water must be released into large extracellular spaces, and these are available around vessels and at the surface of the brain. It is exactly at this location, where AQP4 and also the inward rectifier potassium channel Kir4.1 are present for the directed extrusion of water and K^+ ions.

If this directed water flow is so essential for brain physiology, it may be expected to be closely regulated. Indeed, novel insights speak in favor of the hypothesis that the extracellular matrix heparansulfate proteoglycans have an important role for the insertion of AQP4 into the correct membrane domain. At present, at least two components of the BBB-ECM have been identified to be expressed during maturation of the BBB and which are not expressed by peripheral vessels, suggesting a specific role for the induction of the BBB: agrin (Barber and Lieth, 1997) and laminin (Hunter et al., 1992). The HSPG agrin was initially found to cluster acetylcholine receptors at the motor endplate (Nitkin et al., 1987; Bezakova and Ruegg, 2003) and described to participate also in maintaining the integrity of the BBB (Barber and Lieth, 1997; Berzin et al, 2000). Agrin is present in the subendothelial basal lamina (Barber and Lieth, 1997) and has a binding site to α-dystroglycan (Gee et al., 1994), like laminin. Laminin is deposited in the basal lamina of CNS vessels, upregulated at the onset of BBB-maturation, and it is also localised in the neuromuscular endplate (Sanes et al., 1990). Furthermore, it is expressed by astrocytes and secreted as a soluble factor into the medium by cultured cells (Chiu et al., 1991). In addition, laminin participates in the correct positioning of the K^+ channel Kir4.1 and AQP4 in the astrocyte endfoot membrane (Guadagno and Moukhles, 2004).

3. The BBB in gliomas

3.1 General alterations of the BBB in gliomas

Brain tumours, in particular the most malignant human glioblastoma, are characterized by pronounced hypercellularity, pleomorphism, numerous mitoses, foci of central necrosis, and excessive vascularization (Fig. 3a,b, 4a,b).

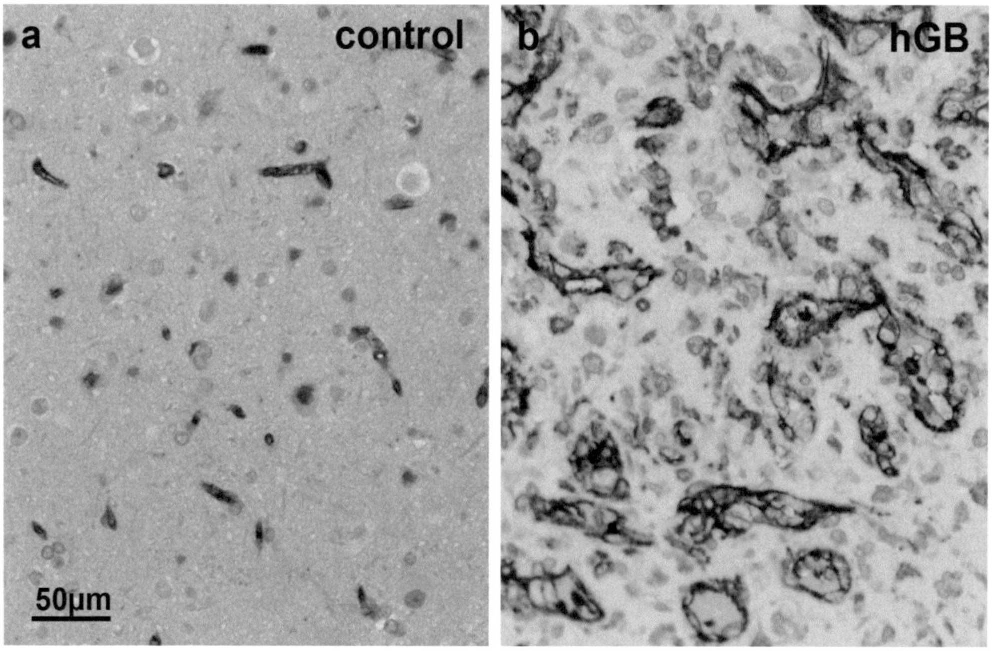

Fig. 3. Immunohistochemical staining of control (a) and glioblastoma tissue (b) of human brain (hGB) with an antibody against PECAM. Note the extreme difference of blood vessel structure in both tissues.

The literature on morphological alterations of the tumour blood vessels is extremely extensive (Hirano and Matsui, 1975; Dinda et al., 1993; Bertossi et al., 1997) but mainly related to the formation of fenestrations, the alterations in the number of caveolae and mitochondria, the thickness of the subendothelial basal lamina, the increase of the perivascular space, and to the pericytes. Previously, barrier-related molecular alterations in the capillary endothelial cells vascularising glioblastoma have been described (Liebner et al., 2000). The lost barrier function could be seen in magnetic resonance imaging (MRI) by contrast medium (CM) application (Sage & Wilson, 1994). The standard CM gadolinium is not able to cross the intact BBB, but the compromised barrier in glioblastoma. Low grade astrocytomas (WHO Grade II and III) are less aggressive than glioblastomas (WHO grade IV). Vessels of astrocytomas appear mostly normal and show rarely dysfunction of the BBB, which can be seen at MRI images. WHO grade II astrocytomas show no or little CM enhancement. WHO III grade astrocytomas enrich more CM than WHO grade II, but mostly less than glioblastomas. WHO III grade astrocytomas enrich more CM than WHO grade II tumours but much less than glioblastomas (Larsson et al. 1990). Pronin et al. (1997) found that edema production is quantitatively related to the degree of breakdown of the BBB as determined by gadolinium enhancement. The results of this group implied that the origin of the edema is in the area of the impaired BBB. Some drugs for example hypericin which normally can't cross the intact BBB are able to reach the main bulk of gliomas in rats through the disturbed BBB (Noell et al. 2011). The difficulty of treatment is how to reach single tumour cells in the infiltration zone where the BBB is not or less altered. It is easier to get drugs into the main centre of a high grade tumour than into the brain with an intact or less altered BBB.

3.2 Tight junctions in glioblastoma

As we have seen, the healthy BBB is dependent on a complex composition of tight junction molecules which obviously must be steadily maintained by the microenvironment, first of all by the highly polarized astrocytes. The astrocyte polarization in turn is evoked by local clustering of water and K^+ channels in endfoot membranes by means of ECM compounds such as agrin. There is a mutual interrelationship between glial polarity and endothelial barrier, but it is not clear whether the endothelial TJs evoke glial polarity or *vice versa*. In an *in vitro* study, Tao-Cheng et al. (1990) were able to co-culture astrocytes and endothelial cells and to observe an accumulation of OAPs in the astrocyte membranes where they contacted endothelial cells. In human glioblastoma, Wolburg et al. (2003) described a loss of claudin-3 from the BBB (Fig. 5). In addition, we observed a thinning of the tight junction network which, in addition, was associated with the E-face (Liebner et al., 2000). Up to date, there is insufficient knowledge about the link between the detachment of astrocytes from the vessels and the vessel basal lamina, and down-regulation of tight junction components. Rascher et al. (2002) reported on a loss of the anti-agrin immunoreactivity in glioma vessels. Furthermore, a strict correlation of the expression patterns of occludin and agrin was described: Vessels without agrin-immunoreactivity revealed a loss of occludin from the tight junctions. This supported the suggestion that occludin as an important regulatory tight junction component is dependent on the presence of agrin.

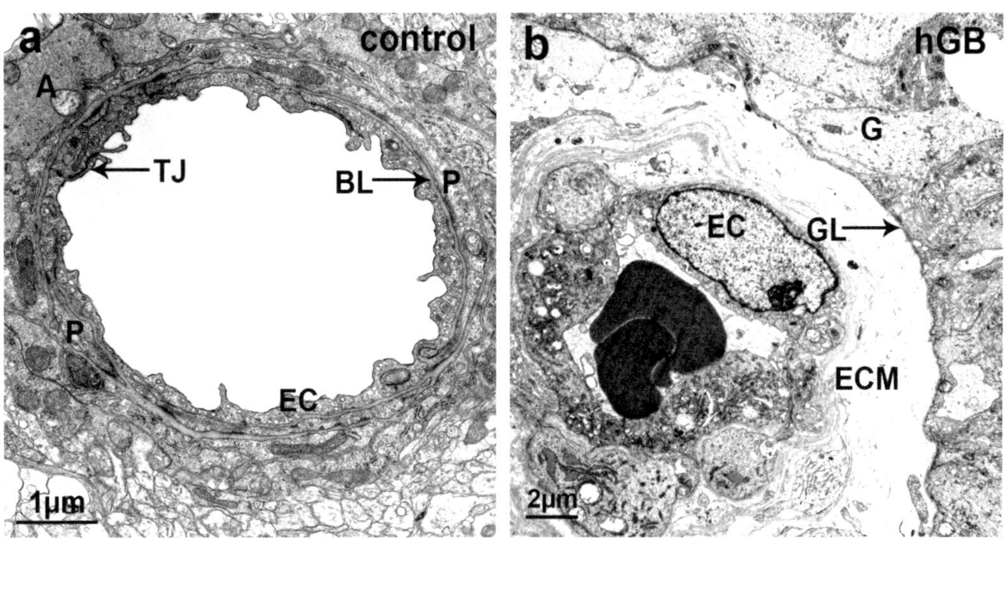

Fig. 4. Conventional electron microscopy of healthy brain (a) and human glioblastoma (b; hGB). Whereas normal blood vessels are intimately integrated into the neuropil, in brain tumour they are separated by a large extracellular space filled with extracellular matrix (ECM) substances. A astrocyte, BL basal lamina, EC endothelial cell, G glioma cell, GL glial limiting membrane, P pericyte, TJ tight junction

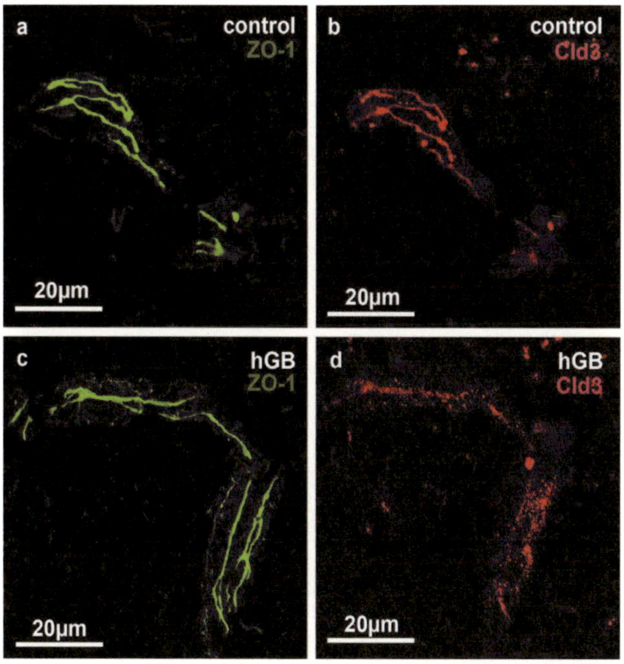

Fig. 5. Immunohistochemical stainings of tight junctional proteins ZO-1 (green) and claudin-3 (Cld3; red) in normal brain tissue (a,b) and in human glioblastoma (hGB; c,d). Note that the staining of claudin 3, but not of ZO-1, is disturbed, at places even missing, in glioblastoma.

3.3 Aquaporin 4 in glioblastoma

In human brain tumours, we see an increase of the perivascular ECM (Liebner et al., 2000). Absence of agrin (in the agrin-knockout mouse) has been described to evoke redistribution of AQP4 over the cellular surface (Noell et al., 2009), and loss of agrin (in the tumour) has the same consequence: AQP4 was no more restricted to vessel-directed membrane domains, but visible in all other membrane domains as well (Noell et al., submitted; Figs. 2, 6). Correspondingly, OAPs could be detected not only in membranes directed to blood vessels, but also in parenchymal membranes. In addition, AQP4 was described several times to be up-regulated in brain tumours (Saadoun et al., 2002; Warth et al., 2004). There is a remarkable inconsistency in the occurrence of AQP4 immunoreactivity and OAPs: In healthy brain tissue, only the OAP-crowded endfoot membrane is immunoreactive against AQP4. The parenchymal membrane is immunonegative. In the tumour, the whole glioma cell is strongly AQP4-immunopositive but the density of OAPs, even near vessels, is far below the density in the normal endfoot membrane. Therefore, there is only one conclusion: in glioma cells, AQP4 must also occur as a non-OAP molecule. We are far from understanding the functional difference between AQP4 in the form of arrays and AQP4 not in the form of arrays. Furman et al. (2003) have shown the freeze-fractured membranes of cells transfected with the AQP4 isoform M23, M1 and a mixture of M1 and M23. At the N-terminus of the protein, M1 is 22 amino acids longer than M23 (Jung et al., 1994). The M23 transfected cells formed huge lattices, whereas M1 transfected cells formed no arrays. Only the transfection of both isoforms resulted in the formation of OAPs resembling those in astrocytes. However, the expectation that in glioma the M1 isoform would be specifically upregulated to explain up-regulation of AQP4 along with the down-regulation of OAPs was not verified: western blotting did not show any alteration of the ratio between both isoforms (Noell et al., submitted). A relationship between AQP4 expression and migration of astrocytomas cells has been postulated (Auguste et al., 2007). AQP4 was described to facilitate the infiltration of malignant cells in glioblastoma. This may suggest that an inhibition of AQP4 would limit this infiltration rate. However, there is no validated study to prove the specific pharmacological inhibition of AQP4. As well, there is neither any information on the influence of putative inhibitors on the AQP4 isoforms M1 and M23, nor on the link between water transport inhibition and the inhibition of migration of tumour cells (Zelenina, 2010).

3.4 Agrin in glioblastoma and its regulation by matrix metalloproteinases

In this section, we focus on the loss of agrin in brain tumour more closely (Fig. 6). One possible explananation is the gene-controlled down-regulation of agrin, however, there is no evidence for this assumption. More likely, agrin loss is a result of its degradation by matrix metalloproteinase 3 (MMP3; see below).

The MMPs are a growing family of degrading enzymes, which are associated with tumour cell invasion and blood vessel transmigration (for review see Nelson et al., 2000). MMP-2 (gelatinase A, type IV collagenase, 72kDa gelatinase), MMP-9 (gelatinase B, type V collagenase, 92 kDa gelatinase) and MMP-12 (metalloelastase, macrophage elastase) have been found to be upregulated by glioma cells, and MMP-9 and MMP-2 are secreted by proliferating glioma endothelial cells (Raithatha et al., 2000; Forsyth et al., 1999, Kachra et al., 1999). Basic fibroblast growth factor and vascular endothelial growth factor induce the release of MMP-9 in glioma cells *in vitro* in a dose- and cell density-dependent manner, implicating possible effects on these growth factors to enhance MMP-9 expression levels in gliomas (Tamaki et al., 1998).

Proteases may be involved in BBB-impairment in three different ways. 1. Shedding of growth factors which have been stored in the vessel ECM contributing to angiogenic processes. 2. Remodeling of the vessel ECM via stimulation of integrin receptors by binding to RGD binding sites. $\alpha_v\beta_3$ integrin was demonstrated to be upregulated in glioma endothelial cells (Gladson, 1996), and its binding to these domains is able to induce cell spreading, migration, and angiogenesis. 3. The cleavage of the basal lamina which destroys the functionality of certain ECM-components (including agrin) which are thought to be important for the BBB integrity (Candelario-Jalil et al., 2009). Interestingly, we have found that laminin, in contrast to agrin, was not degraded in different gliomas (Fig. 6a,b).

Although it has been well-known for a long time that MMPs cleave all compounds of the extracellular matrix including agrin, reports by VanSaun and Werle (2000) in the muscular system and of Solé et al. (2004) in the CNS are still the only studies that have focused on the cleavage of agrin by MMP-3 (also called stromelysin-1). In the context of this review concerned with the role of agrin in BBB and absence of agrin in BBB deterioration in human brain tumours, the presence or regulation of MMP-3 within the perivascular complex seems to be of eminent importance (Fig. 7). Indeed, in cerebral ischemia (Candelario-Jalil et al., 2009), and in multiple sclerosis patients (Rosenberg et al., 1996; Kanesaka et al., 2006), MMP-3 was found to be upregulated and its level increased in the serum. In addition, an inhibitor of MMPs prevented MMP-induced tight junction degradation (Yang et al., 2007). Finally, in the MMP-3 knockout mouse, the lipopolysaccharide-induced opening of the BBB was less pronounced and the tight junction proteins claudin-5 and occludin were less degraded than in the wild-type mouse (Gurney et al., 2006) suggesting that not only agrin is a substrate of MMP3, but tight junction molecules as well.

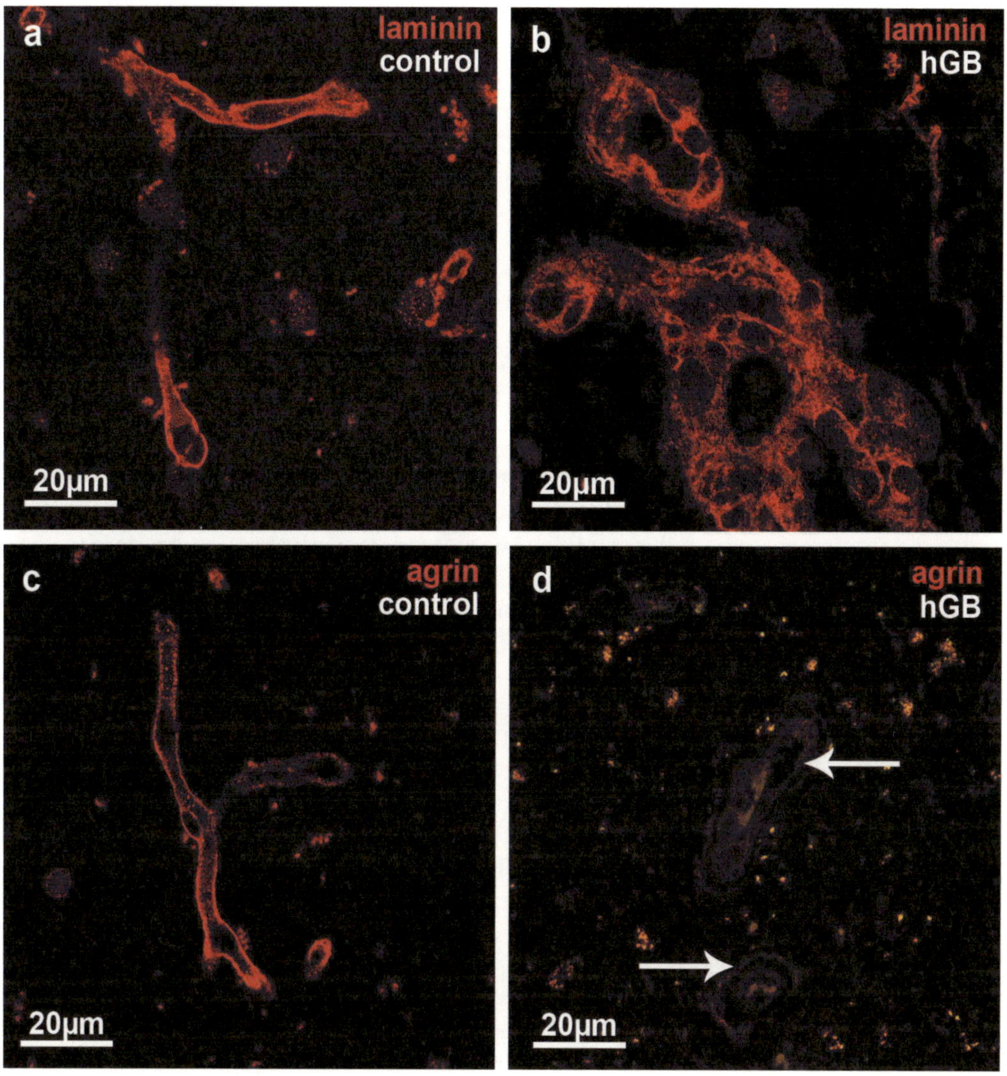

Fig. 6. Immunohistochemical staining of blood vessels in normal (a,c) and human glioblastoma (hGB; b,d) using antibodies against laminin (a,b) and agrin (c,d). Whereas laminin was not degraded in hGB in relation to control (a,b), agrin is heavily expressed around blood vessels under normal conditions (c), but the immunoreactivity has partially lost or reduced under glioma conditions (arrows in d).

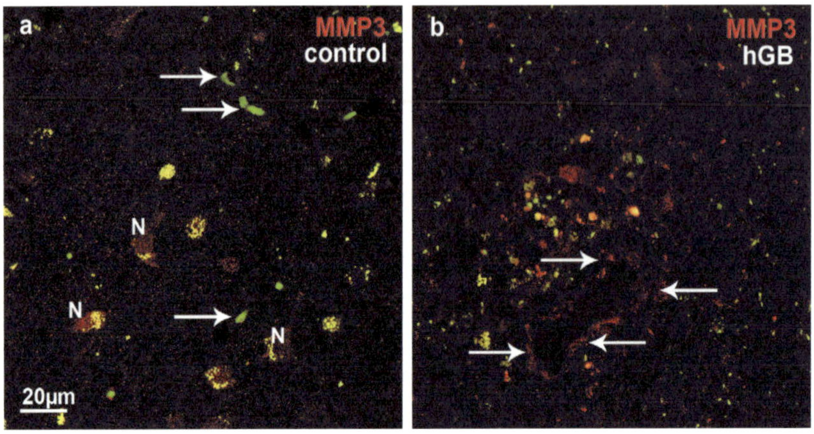

Fig. 7. Immunohistochemical staining of control (a) and glioblastoma tissue (b) of human brain (hGB) using an antibody against the matrix metalloproteinase 3 (MMP3, red). In normal tissue, MMP3 is expressed by neurons (N) and not by endothelial cells (white arrows in a, showing green autofluorescence), in glioblastoma MMP3 is upregulated by endothelial cells (arrows in b).

Interestingly, we have found in glioblastoma a mutual expression pattern of agrin and MMP3. Thus, the loss of agrin in the glioblastoma (Fig. 6c,d) may be explained as a degradation process dependent on the up-regulation of MMP3. Whereas MMP3 normally is expressed in neurons and, under conditions of ischemia/reperfusion, in oligodendrocytes, microvessels and microglia as well (Solé et al., 2003; Candelario-Jalil et al., 2009), we found in primary tumour a positive staining of MMP3 around blood vessels suggesting release of MMP3 into the perivascular space (Noell et al., submitted). Accordingly, where MMP3 was highly expressed the MMP3-substrate agrin could not be detected. The MMP3-inhibitor TIMP1 was detectable in NeuN-positive neurons, not in GFAP-positive glial cells. In normal tissue, there is an equilibrium between MMP3- and TIMP1-expression. This equilibrium which is carried by neurons is assumed to be disturbed in the glioblastoma, because neuronal loss leads to a decline of TIMP-1, but not of MMP3. It should be stressed that "the exact molecular mechanisms through which active MMP3 activates microglial cells remain to be clarified" (Candelario-Jalil et al., 2009). The disturbance of the MMP3/TIMP1-equilibrium in glioblastoma may be one of the factors leading to an increased degradation of agrin.

The concept that at least agrin is responsible for the correct targeting of AQP4-based OAPs to endfeet membranes has to be scrutinized for its validity in the *in vivo* situation. As described above, agrin has an effect on the assembly of AQP4 molecules in the membrane (Noell et al., 2007, 2009). Therefore, loss and degradation of agrin in glioblastoma must have disastrous consequences such as polarity loss and consecutive edema formation.

4. Conclusions

The present overview is characterized by the detailed description of two systems bridged by a not well-defined and still shaky connection: the tight junction molecules of the brain microvessel endothelial cells representing the barrier proper, and the non-endothelial and extracellular molecules which are responsible for the regulation of the endothelial barrier.

Both systems are extremely complicated *sui generis* and increase their complexity by a crosstalk which, however, is poorly understood at present. Nobody knows the differential impact leading to barrier commitment, nothing is known about the links between extracellular matrix and barrier regulation, the pathway from integrins to the claudins or the precise role of astrocytes or astrocytoma cells in barrier formation or dysregulation, respectively. There is no doubt that the molecular analysis of the BBB is of outstanding clinical relevance, since insight into regulatory mechanisms of the paracellular barrier in the brain are of primary significance for the development of new therapeutic strategies. Treatment of brain tumours has to consider both tumour angiogenesis and the permeability of tumour vessels. The essential point of this contribution was the role of the extracellular matrix for the polarity of astrocytes, the loss of this polarity in glioma cells due to the increased activity of MMP3 followed by the degradation of agrin, and the resulting incapability of the glioma cell to directed release of water out of the interstitial space. Both are intimately dependent on the brain microenvironment, and in future research the analysis of this microenvironment will be the greatest challenge in understanding the blood-brain and blood-tumour barrier.

5. Acknowledgement

The studies as far cited in this overview were supported by grants of the Deutsche Krebshilfe (Mildred Scheel foundation; grant numbers 107686 and 109219) and the Hertie-foundation (grant number 1.01.1/07/003) to HW. The last grant was given to HW together with Prof. Britta Engelhardt (Theodor Kocher-Institute, University of Bern, Switzerland). Ria Knittel is thanked for skilful help with freeze-fracturing experiments.

6. References

Abbott, N.J.; Rönnbäck, L. & Hansson, E. (2006). Astrocyte-endothelial interactions at the blood-brain barrier. *Nature Review Neuroscience* Vol. 7, No. 1, (January 2006), pp. 41-53

Amiry-Moghaddam, M. & Ottersen, O.P. (2003). The molecular basis of water transport in the brain. *Nature Review Neuroscience Vol.* 4, No.12, (December 2003), pp. 991-1001

Angelow, S.; Ahlstrom, R. & Yu, A.S.L. (2008). Biology of claudins. *American Journal of Physiol*ogy Vol. 295, No. 4 (October 2008), pp. F867-F876

Auguste, K.I.; Jin, S.; Uchida K.; Yan, D., Manley, G.T.; Papadopoulos, M.C. & Verkman, A.S. (2007). Greatly impaired migration of implanted aquaporin-4-deficient astroglial cells in mouse brain toward a site of injury. *FASEB Journal* Vol. 21, No. 1, (January 2007), pp. 108-116

Balda, M.S. & Matter, K. (2009). Tight junctions and the regulation of gene expression. *Biochimica and Biophysica Acta* Vol. 1788, No. 4, (December 2008), pp. 761-767

Barber, A.J. & Lieth, E. (1997). Agrin accumulates in the brain microvascular basal lamina during development of the blood-brain barrier. *Developmental Dynamics* Vol. 208, No. 1, (January 2008), pp. 62-74

Begley, D.J. (2004). ABC transporters and the blood-brain barrier. *Current Pharmaceutical Design* Vol. 10, No. 12, (2004), pp. 1295-1312

Benfenati, V. & Ferroni,S. (2010). Water transport between CNS compartments: Functional and molecular interactions between aquaporins and ion channels. *Neuroscience* Vol. 168, No. 4 ,(July 2010), pp. 926-940

Bertossi, M.; Virgintino, D.; Maiorano, E.; Occhiogrosso, M. & Roncali, L. (1997) Ultrastructural and morphometric investigation of human brain capillaries in normal and peritumoural tissues. *Ultrastructural Pathology* Vol. 21, No. 1, (January - February 1997), pp. 41-49

Berzin, T.M.; Zipser, B.D.; Rafii, M.S.; Kuo-Leblanc, V.; Yancopoulos, G.D.; Glass, D.J.; Fallon, J.R. & Stopa, E.G. (2000). Agrin and microvascular damage in Alzheimer's disease. *Neurobiology of Aging* Vol. 21, No. 2 (March/April 2000), pp. 349-355

Bezakova, G. & Ruegg, M.A. (2003) New insights into the roles of agrin. *Nature Reviews Molecular Cell Biology* Vol. 4, No. 4 (April 2003), pp. 295-308

Blake, D.J.& Kröger, S. (2000). The neurobiology of Duchenne muscular dystrophy: learning lessons from muscle? *Trends in Neuroscience* Vol. 23, No. 3 (November 1999), pp. 92-99

Brightman, M.W. & Reese, T.S. (1969). Junctions between intimately apposed cell membranes in the vertebrate brain. *Journal of Cell Biology* Vol. 40, No.3, (March 1969), pp. 648-677

Candelario-Jalil, E.; Yang, Y. & Rosenberg, G.A. (2009). Diverse roles of matrix metalloproteinases and tissue inhibitors of metalloproteinases in neuroinflammation and cerebral ischemia. *Neuroscience* Vol. 158, No. 3 (February 2009), pp. 983-994

Chiu, A.Y.; Espinosa de los Monteros, A.; Cole, A.R.; Loera, S. & De Vellis, J. (1991). Laminin and s-laminin are produced and released by astrocytes, Schwann cells, in schwannomas in culture. *Glia* Vol. 4, No. 1 (January 1991), pp. 11-24

Claude, P. (1978). Morphologic factors influencing transepithelial permeability.A model for the resistance of the zonula occludens. *Journal of Membrane Biology* Vol. 39, No. 3, (March 1978), pp. 219-232

Connors, N. C.; Adams, M. E.; Froehner, S.C. & Kofuji, P. (2004). The potassium channel Kir4.1 associates with the dystrophin glycoprotein complex via alpha-syntrophin in glia. *Journal of Biological Chemistry* Vol. 279, No. 27 (July 2004), pp. 28387-28392

Dinda, A.K.; Sarkar, C.; Roy, S.; Kharbanda, K.; Mathur, M.; Khosla, A.K. & Banerji, A.K. (1993).A transmission and scanning electron microscopic study of tumoural and peritumoural microblood vessels in human gliomas. *Journal of Neurooncology* Vol. 16, No. 2 (May 1993), pp. 149-158

Ebnet, K.; Suzuki, A.; Ohno, S. & Vestweber D. (2004). Junctional adhesion molecules (JAMs): more molecules with dual functions? *Journal of Cell Science* Vo. 117, No. 1, (January 2004), pp. 19-29

Ebnet, K. (2008). Organization of multiprotein complexes at cell-cell junctions. *Histochemistry and Cell Biology* Vol. 130, No. 1 (July 2008), pp. 1-20

Farrell, C.L. & Pardridge, W.M. (1991). Blood-brain barrier glucose transporter is asymmetrically distributed on brain capillary endothelial lumenal and ablumenal plasma membranes: an electron microscopic immunogold study. *Proceedings of the National Academy of Science of the United States of America* Vol. 885, No. 13 (July 1991), pp. 779-783

Forsyth, P.A.; Wong, H.; Laing, T.D.; Rewcastle, N.B.; Morris, D.G.; Muzik, H.; Leco, K.J.; Johnston, R.N.; Brasher, P.M.; Sutherland, G. & Edwards, D.R. (1999). Gelatinase-A (MMP-2), gelatinase-B (MMP-9) and membrane type matrix metalloproteinase-1

(MT1-MMP) are involved in different aspects of the pathophysiology of malignant gliomas. *British Journal of Cancer* Vol. 79, No. 11-12, (April 1999), pp. 1828-1835

Furman, C.S.; Gorelick-Feldman, D.A.; Davidson, K.G.; Yasumura, T.; Neely, J.D.; Agre, P. & Rash, J.E. (2003). *Proceedings of the National Academy of Science of the United States of America* Vol. 100, No. 23, (November 2003), pp. 13609-13614

Furuse, M.; Fujita, K.; Hiiragi ,T.; Fujimoto, K. & Tsukita, S. (1998). Claudin-1 and -2: novel integral membrane proteins localizing at tight junctions. *Journal of Cell Biology* Vol. 141, No. 7, (June 1998), pp. 1539-1550

Furuse, M.; Hirase, T.; Itoh, M.; Nagafuchi, A.; Yonemura, S.; Tsukita, S. & Tsukita, S. (1993). Occludin: a novel integral membrane protein localizing at tight junctions. *Journal of Cell Biology* Vol. 123, No. 6 pt 2, (December 1993), pp. 1777-1788

Gee, S.H.; Montanaro, F.; Lindenbaum, M.H. & Carbonetto, S. (1994). Dystroglycan-α: a dystrophin-associated glyoprotein, is a functional agrin receptor. *Cell* Vol.77, No. 5, (June 1994), pp. 675-686

Giepmans, B.N. & Moolenaar, W.H. (1998). The gap junction protein connexin 43 interacts with the second PDZ domain of the zona occludens-1 protein. *Current Biology* Vol. 8, No. 14, (July - August 1998), pp. 931-934

Gladson, C.L. (1996) Expression of integrin alpha v beta 3 in small blood vessels of glioblastoma tumours. *Journal of Neuropathology and Experimental Neurology* Vol. 55, No. 11 (November 1996),pp. 1143-1149

Guadagno, E. & Moukhles, H. (2004) Laminin-induced aggregation of the inwardly rectifying potassium channel, Kir4.1, and the water-permeable channel, AQP4, via a dystroglycan-containing complex in astrocytes. *Glia* Vol. 47, No. 2, (August 2004), pp.138-149

Gurney, K.J.; Estrada, E.Y. & Rosenberg, G.A. (2006). Blood-brain barrier disruption by stromelysin-1 facilitates neutrophil infiltration in neuroinflammation. *Neurobiology of Disease* Vol. 23, No,. 1, (July 2006), pp. 87-96

Hirano, A. & Matsui, T. (1975). Vascular structures in brain tumours. *Human Pathology* Vol. 6, No. 5, (September 1975), pp. 199-208

Huang, Z.; Cheng, L.; Guryanova, O.A.; Wu, Q. & Bao, S. (2010). Cancer stem cells in glioblastoma - molecular signaling and therapeutic targeting. *Protein Cell*, Vol. 1, No. 7 (July, 2010), pp. 638-655

Hunter, D.D.; Llinas, R.; Ard, M.; Merlie, J.P. & Sanes, J.R. (1992). Expression of s-laminin and laminin in the developing rat central nervous system. *Journal of Comparitive Neurology* Vol. 323, No. 2, (September 1992), pp. 238-251

Itoh, M.; Nagafuchi, A.; Yonemura, S.; Kitaniyasuda, T. & Tsukita, S. (1993). The 220 kD protein colocalizing with cadherins in non-epithelial cells - cDNA cloning and immunoelectron microscopy. *Journal of Cell Biology* Vol. 121, No. 3 (May 1993), pp. 491-502

Jesaitis, L.A. & Goodenough, D.A. (1994). Molecular characterization and tissue distribution of ZO-2, a tight junction protein homologous to ZO-1 and the Drosophila discs-large tumour suppressor protein. *Journal of Cell Biology* Vol. 124, No. 6, (March 1994), pp. 949-962

Jung, J.S.; Bhat, R.V.; Preston, G.M.; Guggino, W.B.; Baraban, J.M. & Agre, P. (1994). Molecular characterization of an aquaporin cDNA from brain: candidate osmoreceptor and regulator of water balance. *Proceedings of the National Academy of Sciences U S A* Vol. 91, No. 26 (December 1994), pp. 13052-13056

Kachra, Z.; Beaulieu, E.; Delbecchi, L.; Mousseau ,N.; Berthelet, F.; Moumdjian, R.; Del Maestro, R. & Beliveau, R. (1999). Expression of matrix metalloproteinases and their inhibitors in human brain tumours. *Clinical and Experimental Metastasis* Vol. 17, No. 7, (1999), pp. 555-566

Kanesaka, T.; Mori, M.; Hattori, T.; Oki, T. & Kuwabara, S. (2006). Serum matrix metalloproteinase-3 levels correlate with disease activity in relapsing-remitting multiple sclerosis. *Journal of Neurology, Neurosurgery and Psychiatry* Vol. 77, No. 2, (February 2006), pp. 185-188

King, L.S.; Kozono, D. & Agre, P. (2004). From structure to disease: the evolving tale of aquaporin biology. *Nature Review of Molecular Cell Biology* Vol. 5, No. 9, (September 2004), pp. 687-698

Kniesel, U.; Risau, W. & Wolburg, H. (1996). Development of blood-brain barrier tight junctions in the rat cortex. *Developmental Brain Research* Vol. 96, No. 1-2, (October 1996), pp. 229-240

Krause, G.; Winkler, L.; Mueller, S.L.; Haseloff, R.F.; Piontek, J. & Blasig, I.E. (2008) Structure and function of claudins. *Biochimica and Biophysica Acta* Vol. 1778, No. 3, (March 2008), pp. 631-645

Larsson, H.B.; Stubgaard, M.; Frederiksen, JL.; Jensen, M.; Henriksen, O. & Paulson, OB. (1990). Quantitation of blood-brain barrier defect by magnetic resonance imaging and gadolinium-DTPA in patients with multiple sclerosis and brain tumours. *Magnetic Resonance Medicine* Vol. 16, No.1, (October 1990), pp. 117-133

Liebner, S.; Fischmann, A.; Rascher, G.; Duffner, F.; Grote, E.H.; Kalbacher, H. & Wolburg, H. (2000) Claudin-1 and claudin-5 expression and tight junction morphology are altered in blood vessels of human glioblastoma multiforme. *Acta Neuropathologica* Vol. 100, No. 3 (September 2000), pp. 323-331

Liebner, S.; Czupalla, C.J. & Wolburg, H. (2011) Current concepts of blood-brain barrier development. *International Journal of Developmental Biology*, in press

MacAulay, N. & Zeuthen, T. (2010). Water transport between CNS compartments: contributions of aquaporins and cotransporters. *Neuroscience* Vol. 168, No. 4 ,(July 2010), pp. 941-956

Mathiisen, T.M.; Lehre, K.P.; Danbolt, N.C. & Ottersen, O.P. (2010) The perivascular astroglial sheath provides a complete covering of the brain microvessels: an electron microscopic 3D reconstruction. *Glia* Vol. 58, No. 9, (July 2010), pp. 1094-1103.

Morita, K.; Furuse, M.; Fujimoto, K. & Tsukita, S. (1999a). Claudin multigene family encoding four-transmembrane domain protein components of tight junction strands. Proceedings of the *National Academy of Science of the United States of America* Vol. 96, No. 2, (January 1999), pp. 511-516

Morita, K.; Sasaki, H.; Furuse, M. & Tsukita, S. (1999b). Endothelial Claudin: Claudin-5/TMVCF constitutes tight junction strands in endothelial cells. *Journal of Cell Biology* Vol. 147, No.1, (October 1999), pp. 185-194

Nagelhus, E.A.; Mathiisen, T.M. & Ottersen, O.P. (2004). Aquaporin-4 in the central nervous system: cellular and subcellular distribution and coexpression with Kir4.1. *Neuroscience* Vol. 129, No. 4, (December 2004), pp. 905-913

Nagy, Z.; Peters, H. & Hüttner, I. (1984). Fracture faces of cell junctions in cerebral endothelium during normal and hyperosmotic conditions. *Laboratory Investigation* Vol. 50, No. 3, (March 1984), pp. 313-322

Neely, J.D.; Christensen, B.M.; Nielsen, S &, Agre, P. (1999). Heterotetrameric composition of aquaporin-4 water channels. *Biochemistry* Vol. 38, No. 34 (August 1999), pp. 11156-11163

Nelson, A.R.; Fingleton, B.; Rothenberg, M.L. & Matrisian, L.M. (2000). Matrix metalloproteinases: biologic activity and clinical implications. *Journal of Clinical Oncology* Vol. 18, No. 5 (March 2000), pp. 1135-1149

Nicchia, G.P.; Rossi, A.; Mola, M.G.; Pisani, F.; Stigliano, C.; Basco, D.; Mastrototaro, M.; Svelto, M. & Frigeri, A, (2010). Higher order structure of aquaporin-4. *Neuroscience* Vol. 168 No. 4, (July 2010), pp. 903-914

Nico, B.; Frigeri, A.; Nicchia, G.P.; Quondamatteo, F.; Herken, R.; Errede, M.; Ribatti, D.; Svelto, M. & Roncali, L. (2001). Role of aquaporin-4 water channel in the development and integrity of the blood-brain barrier. *Journal of Cell Science* Vol. 114, No. 7 (April 2001), pp. 1297-1307

Nico, B.; Nicchia, G.P.; Frigeri, A.; Corsi, P.; Mangieri, D.; Ribatti, D.; Svelto, M. & Roncali, L. (2004). Altered blood-brain barrier development in dystrophic mdx mice. *Neuroscience* Vol. 125, No. 4, (2004), pp. 921-935

Neuhaus, J. (1990). Orthogonal arrays of particles in astroglial cells: quantitative analysis of their density, size, and correlation with intramembranous particles. *Glia* Vol. 3, No. 4, (1990), pp. 241-251

Nielsen, S.; Nagelhus, E.A.; Amiry-Moghaddam, M.; Bourque, C.; Agre, P. & Ottersen, O.P. (1997). Specialized membrane domains for water transport in glial cells: high-resolution immunogold cytochemistry of aquaporin-4 in rat brain. *Journal of Neuroscience* Vol. 17, No. 1, (January 1997), pp. 171-180

Nitkin, R.M.; Smith, M.A.; Magill, C.; Fallon, J.R.; Yao, Y.M.; Wallace, B.G. & McMahan, U.J. (1987). Identification of agrin, a synaptic organizing protein from Torpedo electric organ. *Journal of Cell Biology* Vol. 105, No. 6 (December 1987), pp. 2471-2478

Noell, S.; Fallier-Becker, P.; Beyer, C.; Kröger, S.; Mack, A.F. & Wolburg, H. (2007). Effects of agrin on the expression and distribution of the water channel protein aquaporin-4 and volume regulation in cultured astrocytes. *European Journal of Neuroscience* Vol. 26, No. 8, (October 2007), pp. 2109-2118

Noell, S.; Fallier-Becker, P.; Deutsch, U.; Mack, A.F. & Wolburg, H. (2009). Agrin defines polarized distribution of orthogonal arrays of particles in astrocytes. *Cell & Tissue Research* Vol. 337, No. 2 (August 2009), pp. 185-195

Noell, S.; Mayer, D.; Strauss, W.S.; Tatagiba, M.S. & Ritz, R. (2011). Selective enrichment of hypericin in malignant glioma: pioneering in vivo results. *International Journal of Oncology* Vol. 38, No. 5 (May 2011), pp. 1343-1348

Ohgaki, H.; Dessen, P.; Jourde, B.; Horstmann, S.; Nishikawa, T.; Di Patre, P.-L.; Burkhard, C.; Schüler, D.; Probst-Hensch, N.M.; Maiorka, P.C.; Baeza, N.; Pisani, P.; Yonekawa, Y.; Yasargil, M.G.; Lütolf, U.M. & Kleihues, P. (2004). Genetic pathways to glioblastoma: a population-based study. *Cancer Research* Vol. 64, No. 19,(October 2004), pp. 6892-6899

Pasantes-Morales, H. & Cruz-Rangel, S. (2010). Brain volume regulation: osmolytes and aquaporin perspectives. *Neuroscience* Vol. 168, No.4, (July 2010), pp. 871-884

Parsons, D.W.; Jones, S.; Zhang, X.; Lin, J.C.-H.; Leary, R.J.; Angenendt, P.; Mankoo, P.; Carter, H.; Siu, I.-M.; Gallia, G.L.; Olivi, A.; McLendon, R.; Rasheed, B.A.; Keir, S.; Nikolskaya, T.; Nikolsky, Y.; Busam, D.A.; Tekleab, H.; Diaz, L.A. Jr.; Hartigan, J.; Smith, D.R.; Strausberg, R.L.; Marie, S.K.N.; Shinjo, S.M.O.; Yan, H.; Riggins, G.J.; Bigner, D.D.; Karchin, R.; Papadopoulos, N.; Parmigiani, G.; Vogelstein, B.;

Velculescu, V.E. & Kinzler, K.W. (2008). An integrated genomic analysis of human glioblastoma multiforme. *Science* Vol. 321, No. 5897, (September 2008), pp. 1807-1812

Peters, A.; Palay, S.L. & Webster, H. (1991). *The fine structure of the nervous system* (second edition), Oxford University Press, ISBN 0-19-506571-9, New York

Pronin, I.N.; Holodny, A.I. & Petraikin, A.V. (1997). MRI of high-grade glial tumours: correlation between the degree of contrast enhancement and the volume of surrounding edema. *Neuroradiology* Vol. 39, No. 5, (May 1997), pp. 348-350

Raithatha, S.A.; Muzik, H.; Muzik, H.; Rewcastle, N.B.; Johnston, R.N.; Edwards, D.R. & Forsyth, P.A .(2000). Localization of gelatinase-A and gelatinase-B mRNA and protein in human gliomas. *Neuro-Oncology* Vol. 2, No. 3, (July 2000), pp. 145-150

Rascher, G.; Fischmann, A.; Kröger, S.; Duffner, F.; Grote, E.-H. & Wolburg, H. (2002). Extracellular matrix and the blood-brain barrier in glioblastoma multiforme: spatial segregation of tenascin and agrin. *Acta Neuropathologica* Vol. 104, No. 1, (July 2002), pp. 85-91

Rash, J.E.; Yasumura, T.; Hudson, C.S.; Agre, P. & Nielsen, S. (1998). Direct immunogold labeling of aquaporin-4 in square arrays of astrocyte and ependymocyte plasma membranes in rat brain and spinal cord. *Proceedings of the National Academy of Sciences of theUnited States of America*Vol. 95, No. 20, (September 2010), pp. 11981-11986

Rash, J.E.; Davidson, K.G.V.; Yasumura, T. & Furman, C.S. (2004) Freeze fractureand immunogold analysis of aquaporin-4 (AQP4) square arrays,with models of AQP4 lattice assembly. *Neuroscience* Vol. 129, No. 4, (December 2004), pp. 915–934.

Rash, J.E. (2010). Molecular disruptions of the panglial syncytium block potassium siphoning and axonal saltatory conduction: pertinence to neuromyelitis optica and other demyelinating diseases of the central nervous system. *Neuroascience* Vol. 168, No. 4 , (July 2010), pp. 982-1008

Reese, T.S. & Karnovsky, M.J. (1967). Fine structural localization of a blood-brain barrier to exogenous peroxidase. *Journal of. Cell Biology* Vol. 34, No. 1, (July 1967), pp. 207-217

Ricci-Vitiani, L.; Pallini R.; Biffoni, M.; Todaro, M.; Invernici, G.; Cenci, T.; Maira, G.; Parati, E.A.; Stassi, G.; Larocca, L.M. & De Maria, R. (2010). Tumour vascularization via endothelial differentiation of glioblastoma stem-like cells. *Nature* Vol. 468, No. 7325, (December 2010), pp. 824-828

Riemenschneider MJ, Jeuken JWM, Wesseling P, Reifenberger G (2010) Molecular diagnostics of gliomas: state of the art. Acta Neuropathol 120: 567-584

Rosenberg, G.A.; Navratilm M.; Baronem F. & Feuerstein, G. (1996). Proteolytic cascade enzyme increase in focal cerebral ischemia in rat. *Journal of Cerebral Blood Flow & Metabolism* Vol. 16, No. 3, (May 1996), pp. 360-366

Saadoun, S.; Papadopoulos, M.C.; Davies, D.C.; Krishna, S. & Bell, B.A. (2002). Aquaporin-4 expression is increased in oedematous human brain tumours. *Journal of Neurology, Neurosurgery, Psychiatry* Vol. 72, No. 2, (February 2002), pp. 262-265

Sage, M.R. & Wilson, A.J. (1994). The blood-brain barrier: an important concept in neuroimaging. *American Journal of Neuroradiology* Vol. 15, No. 4, (April 1994), pp. 601-622

Saitou, M.; Furuse, M.M.; Sasaki, H.; Schulzke, J.-D.; Fromm, M.; Takano, H.; Noda, T. & Tsukita, S. (2000). Complex phenotype of mice lacking occludin, a component of tight junction strands. *Molecular Biology of the Cell* Vol. 11, No. 12, (December 2000), pp. 4131-4142

Sanes, J.R.; Engvall, E.; Butkowski, R. & Hunter, D.D. (1990). Molecular heterogeneity of basal laminae: isoforms of laminin and collagen IV at the neuromuscular junction and elsewhere. *Journal of Cellular Biolology* Vol. 111, No. 4, (October 1990), pp. 1685-1699

Solé, S.; Petegnief, V.; Gorina, R.; Chamorro, Á. & Planas, A.M. (2004). Activation of matrix metalloproteinase-3 and agrin cleavage in cerebral ischemia/reperfusion. *Journal of Neuropathology and experimental Neurology* Vol. 63, No. 4, (April 2004), pp. 338-349

Sreekanthreddy, P.; Srinivasan, H.; Kumar, D.M.; Nijaguna, M.B.; Sridevi, S.; Vrinda, M.; Arivazhagan, A.; Balasubramaniam, A.; Hegde, A.S.; Chandramouli, B.A.; Santosh, V.; Rao, M.R.S.; Kondaiah, P. & Somasundaram, K. (2010). Identification of potential serum biomarkers of glioblastoma: serum osteopontin levels correlate with poor prognosis. *Cancer Epidemiology, Biomarkers & Prevention* Vol. 19, No. 6, (June 2010), pp. 1409-1422

Steed, E.; Rodrigues, N.T.L.; Balda, M.S. & Matter, K. (2009). Identification of MarvelD3 as a tight junction-associated transmembrane protein of the occludin family. *BioMed Central Cell Biology* Vol. 10, (December 2009), doi: 10.1186/1471-2121-10-95

Steed, E.; Balda, M.S. & Matter, K. (2010) Dynamics and functions of tight junctions. *Trends in Cell Biology* Vol. 20, No. 3, (March 2010), pp. 142-149

Stevenson, B.R.; Siliciano, J.D.; Mooseker, M.S. & Goodenough,D.A. (1986) Identification of ZO-1: a higher molecular weight polypeptide associated with the tight junction (zonula occludens) in a variety of epithelia. *Journal of Cell Biology* Vol. 103, No. 3, (September 1986), pp. 755-766

Tabatabai, G. & Weller, M. (2011). Glioblastoma stem cells. *Cell & Tissue Research*, Vol. 343, No. 3 (March 2011), pp. 459-465

Tamaki, M.; McDonald, W. & Del Maestro, R.F. (1998). The importance of cell density in the interpretation of growth factor effects on collagenase IV activity release and extracellular matrix production from C6 astrocytoma cells. *Journal of Neurooncology* Vol. 39, No. 3, (September 1998), pp. 205-216

Tani, K.; Mitsuma, T.; Hiroaki, Y.; Kamegawa, A.; Nishikawa, K.; Tanimura, Y. & Fujiyoshi, Y. (2009). Mechanism of aquaporin-4's fast and highly selective water conduction and proton exclusion. *Journal of Molecular Biology* Vol. 389, No. 4, (June 2009), pp. 694-706

Tao-Cheng, J.-H.; Nagy, Z. & Brightman, M.W. (1990). Astrocytic orthogonal arrays of intramembranouis assemblies are modulated by brain endothelial cells. *Journal of Neurocytology* Vol. 19, No. 2, (July 1990), pp. 143-153

Tsukita, S. & Furuse, M. (1999). Occludin and claudins in tight-junction strands: leading or supporting players? *Trends Cell Biol* Vol. 9, No.7 (July 1999), pp. 268-273

Umeda, K.; Ikenouchi, J.; Katahira-Tayama, S.; Furuse, K.; Sasaki, H.; Nakayama, M.; Matsui, T.; Tsukita, S.; Furuse, M. & Tsukita, S. (2006). ZO-1 and ZO-2 independently determine where claudins are polymerized in tight-junction strand formation. *Cell* Vol. 126, No. 4, (August 2006), pp. 741-754

Van Saun, M. & Werle, M.J. (2000). Matrix metalloproteinase-3 removes agrin from synaptic basal lamina. *Journal of Neurobiology* Vol. 44, No. 3, (September 2000), pp. 140-149

Verbavatz, J.-M.; Ma, T.; Gobin, R. & Verkman, A.S. (1997) Absence of orthogonal arrays in kidney, brain and muscle from transgenic knockout mice lacking water channel aquaporin-4. *Journal of Cell Science* Vol. 110, No. 22), pp. 2855-2860

Warth, A.; Kröger, S. & Wolburg, H. (2004). Redistribution of aquaporin-4 in human glioblastoma correlates with loss of agrin immunoreactivity from brain capillary basal laminae. *Acta Neuropathologica* Vol. 107, No. 4,(April 2004), pp. 311-318

Warth, A.; Mittelbronn, M. & Wolburg, H. (2005). Redistribution of the water channel protein aquaporin-4 and the K^+ channel protein Kir4.1 differs in low- and high-grade human brain tumours. *Acta Neuropathologica* Vol. 109, No. 4, (April 2005), pp. 418-426

Wolburg, H. & Lippoldt, A. (2002). Tight junctions of the blood-brain barrier: Development, composition and regulation. *Vascular Pharmacology* Vol. 38, No. 6, (June 2002), pp. 323-337

Wolburg, H.; Neuhaus, J.; Kniesel, U.; Krauss, B.; Schmid, E.-M.; Öcalan, M.; Farrell, C. & Risau, W. (1994). Modulation of tight junction structure in blood-brain barrier endothelial cells. Effects of tissue culture, second messengers and cocultured astrocytes. *Journal of Cell Science* Vol. 107, No. 5 (May 1994), pp. 1347-1357

Wolburg, H.; Wolburg-Buchholz, K.; Kraus, J.; Rascher-Eggstein, G.; Liebner, S.; Hamm, S.; Duffner, F.; Grote, E.-H.; Risau, W. & Engelhardt, B. (2003). Localization of claudin-3 in tight junctions of the blood-brain barrier is selectively lost during experimental autoimmune encephalomyelitis and human glioblastoma multiforme. *Acta Neuropathologica* Vol. 105, No. 6 (June 2003), pp. 586-592

Wolburg, H.; Noell, S.; Wolburg-Buchholz, K.; Mack, A.F. & Fallier-Becker, P. (2009). Agrin, aquaporin-4, and astrocyte polarity as an important feature of the blood-brain barrier. *The Neuroscientist* Vol.15, No. 2, (April 2009), pp. 180-193

Wolburg, H.; Wolburg-Buchholz, K.; Fallier-Becker, P.; Noell, S. & Mack, A. (2011). Structure and functions of aquaporin-4-based orthogonal arrays of particles. *International Review of Cellular & Molecular Biology* Vol. 287, pp. 1-41

Yang, B.; Brown, D. & Verkman, A.S. (1996). The mercurial insensitive water channel (AQP-4) forms orthogonal arrays in stably transfected chinese hamster ovary cells. *Journal of Biological Chemistry* Vol. 271, No. 9, (March 1996), pp. 4577-4580

Yang, Y.; Estrada, E.Y.; Thompson, J.F.; Liu, W. & Rosenberg, G.A. (2007). Matrix metalloproteinase-mediated disruption of tight junction proteins in cerebral vessels is reversed by synthetic matrix metalloproteinase inhibitor in focal ischemia in rat. *Journal of Cerebral Blood Flow & Metabolism* Vol. 27, No. 4, (April 2007), pp. 698-709

Zelenina, M. (2010). Regulation of brain aquaporins. *Neurochemical International* Vol. 57, No. 4, (April 2010), pp. 468-488

Part 4

Management of Pediatric CNS Tumors

5

Childhood Brain Tumors

Sri Gururangan
*The Preston Robert Tisch Brain Tumor Center At Duke,
Duke University Medical Center, Durham, North Carolina,
USA*

1. Introduction

Central nervous system (CNS) cancers are the second most frequent malignancy in childhood and the most common solid tumor in this age group. In recent years, significant advances in surgery, radiotherapy, and chemotherapy have favorably impacted survival for children with these tumors. However, a significant proportion of patients with CNS tumors suffer progress disease despite such treatment. Advances in the understanding the nature of the blood-brain/tumor barrier, chemotherapy resistance, tumor biology, and the role of angiogenesis and other signaling pathways in tumor progression and metastases have led to the advent of newer therapeutic strategies that circumvent these obstacles or target specific receptors that control signal transduction and/or angiogenesis in tumor cells. Ongoing clinical trials will determine if these novel modalities of treatment will improve the outcome of children with brain tumors.

1.1 Epidemiology of pediatric brain tumors

An estimated 2400 children between the ages of 0-19 years are diagnosed with invasive primary central nervous system (CNS) tumors in the United States each year. (Bleyer 1999; Gurney, Smith et al. 1999) The incidence of CNS tumor in children < 20 years is 4.58 per 100,000 person years (CBTRUS report, 2009). Brain tumors are second only in frequency to acute lymphoblastic leukemia (ALL) in children. Pilocytic astrocytomas ((0.79 per 100,000 person-years) malignant glioma (0.51 per 100,000 person-years), and medulloblastoma (0.49 per 100, 000 person-years) are the commonest tumors (Figure 1) (Gurney, Smith et al. 1999). The incidence of low-grade astrocytomas, PNET, and ependymoma is inversely proportional to age while that of malignant glioma is relatively constant between birth to < 20 years (Bleyer 1999). The incidence of CNS tumors in children was found to have increased by 35% between the years 1975-84 (Smith, Freidlin et al. 1998). This increase has been mainly attributed to the introduction of magnetic resonance imaging (MRI) in the 1980s that improved detection of low grade tumors previously unidentifiable by other less optimal imaging modalities (Smith, Freidlin et al. 1998). Brain growth occurs rapidly during early gestation and peaks around 4 months after birth but continues until 2-3 years thereafter (Baldwin and Preston-Martin 2004). Hence, it is more vulnerable to genotoxic damage and neoplastic transformation than any other organ in the body due to its relatively longer course of development both in utero and post -natal life during which the rapidly dividing cells become susceptible to exposure to potential environment toxins and DNA damage (Baldwin and Preston-Martin 2004).

In addition, it appears that fetal brain is less able to efficiently repair DNA alkylation induced by various mutagenic agents. The blood-brain barrier (discussed further below) is also not complete in the fetal brain and facilitates free transfer of carcinogens into the vulnerable neural tissue (Baldwin and Preston-Martin 2004). While hereditary genetic syndromes do cause a proportion of pediatric brain tumors, it is distinctly rare. Only about 5% of CNS malignancies are the direct consequence of a specific gene defect (Table 1). However, in the majority of sporadic brain tumors, the factors that incite neoplastic transformation are largely unknown but are likely to be multi-factorial due to an inter play of both genes and the environment. One known environmental cause of brain tumors is ionizing radiation and can induce both benign and malignant gliomas or occasionally primitive neuro-ectodermal tumors (PNET) (Ron, Modan et al. 1988) (Hader, Drovini-Zis et al. 2003). Ron et al., reported a 33.1 relative risk (RR) of developing nerve sheath tumors of the head and neck in children who had received up to 600 cGy of irradiation for *tinea captis* infection in the 1950s (Ron, Modan et al. 1988). There was a lower but excess incidence of both meningiomas (RR 9.5) and malignant gliomas (RR 2.6) as well in this cohort. In recent years, radiation exposure is solely due to therapeutic irradiation of the brain for CNS leukemia or brain tumors and has been associated with a 22-fold risk of developing secondary brain tumors (mostly glioblastoma multiforme) especially in children less than 5 years at diagnosis (Neglia, Meadows et al. 1991). The role of other environmental toxins is relatively unclear (Gurney, Smith et al. 1999).

2. Factors that contribute to treatment failure in children with brain tumors

Although the annual mortality rate for pediatric cancers has steadily decreased over the last two decades, the proportion of deaths from CNS tumors in the same population has increased from 18% to 30% (Bleyer 1999). These figures clearly highlight the suboptimal outcomes in children with CNS malignancies compared to other pediatric tumors.

Surgery, chemotherapy, and radiotherapy have long been established as treatment modalities for patients with brain tumors. It has also become obvious that a significant proportion of brain tumor patients suffer progressive disease during or following cytotoxic therapy. The causes for such therapeutic failure have been have been attributed to the presence of the blood-tumor barrier and drug or radio- resistance.(Groothuis 2000; Bredel 2001)The refractoriness of brain tumors to cytotoxic therapy stems from a multitude of factors that can be broadly classified as apparent or inherent cellular resistance (Bredel 2001; Scotto and Bertino 2001). Apparent resistance to a cytotoxic agent is usually due to the presence of the blood-brain barrier (BBB) (Groothuis 2000), the cell kinetics of a large tumor that has a smaller growth fraction (larger number of cells in the G_0 fraction of the cell cycle), and hypoxic areas that limits the effect of cytotoxic therapy (Scotto and Bertino 2001). Inherent resistance can be either *de novo* or acquired. The various mechanisms of resistance to cytotoxic agents that are typically used in brain tumors are listed in Table 2.

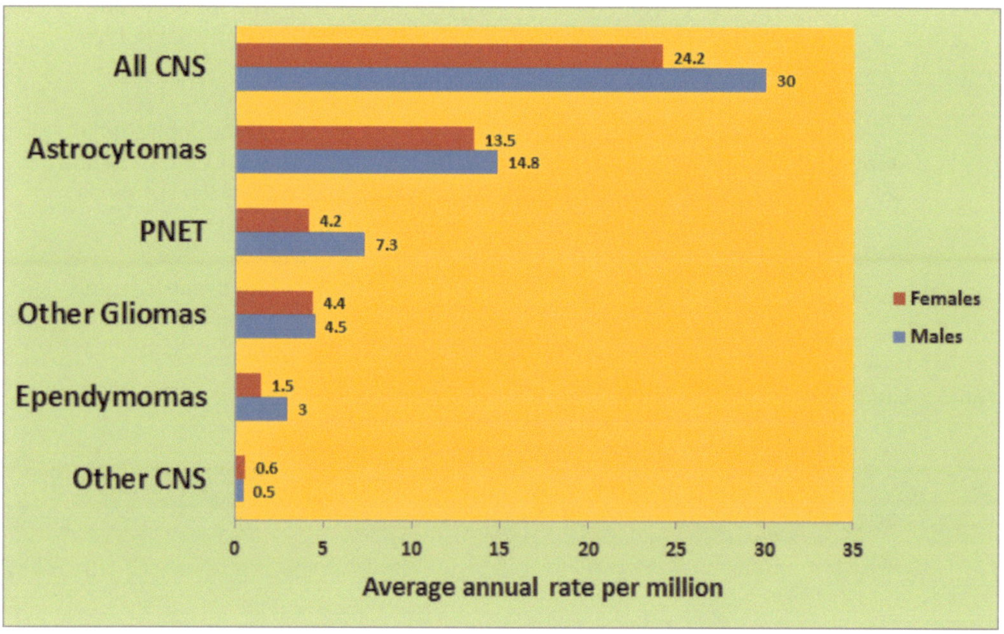

*incidence rates by histologic group and sexage <20, all races, SEER1990-95

Fig. 1. Malignant CNS tumor age-adjusted

SYNDROME	GENE	CHROMOSOME	TUMORS
Neurofibromatosis Type I	*NF-1*	17q11	Optic Gliomas Astrocytomas Neurofibromas
Neurofibromatosis Type II	*NF-2*	22q12	Vestibular schwannomas Meningiomas Spinal cord ependymomas
Von Hippel Lindau	*VHL*	3p25	Cerebellar hemangioblastomas
Tuberous Sclerosis	*TSC1 and TSC2*	9q34 and 16p13	Subependymal Giant Cell Astrocytoma
Turcot	*APC* *MLH1* *PMS-2*	5q21 3p21 7p22	Medulloblastoma Colorectal polyps Glioblastoma multiforme Colorectal polyps
Gorlin	*PTCH*	9q31	Medulloblastoma Basal Cell Carcinoma Ovarian Fibromas
Li- Fraumeni	*P53*	17p13	Astrocytoma PNET Soft tissue sarcoma Breast Carcinoma Leukemia

Table 1. Common Genetic Syndromes and associated tumors

Mechanism of resistance	Drug	Cellular Enzyme/protein involved in resistance
Decreased entry into cell Increased efflux	Vinca alkaloids Etoposide Anthracyclines Trimetrexate	↑ p-glycoprotein expression
Increased inactivation	Cyclophosphamide Cisplatin Camptothecins	↑ aldehyde dehydrogenase ↑ glutathione and metallothioneins ↑ Cytochrome P-450 (e.g., CYP3A4)
Increased DNA repair following DNA damage	Nitrosoureas Temozolomide Cyclophosphamide Platinum compounds	↑ alkyl guanine alkyltransferase ↑ poly-ADP ribonucleotide polymerase (PARP)
Decreased topoisomerase binding	Etoposide Anthracyclines Campothecins	Topoisomerase I and II
Mismatch repair deficiency	Temozolomide Platinum compounds Busulfan	MSH-2, 3, and 6; MLH1

Table 2. Mechanisms of cellular drug resistance in brain tumors.

Distribution	No. of patients (%) (of n = 713)*
Tumor location	
Cerebellar hemisphere	**225 (32%)**
Cerebral hemisphere	**197 (28%)**
Midline (basal ganglia, thalamus, brain stem)	**135 (19%)**
Cerebellar vermis	**128 (18%)**
Chiasmatic-hypothalamic	**28 (4%)**
Tumor histology	
Juvenile pilocytic astrocytoma	**396 (76%)**
Fibrillary astrocytoma	**43 (8%)**
Ganglioglioma	**32 (6%)**
Oligodendroglioma	**28 (5%)**
Pleomorphic xanthoastroctyoma	**8 (1.5%)**
Other gliomas	**7 (1.3%)**
Mixed gliomas	**6 (1.2%)**

* Tumor location and histology in 713 children enrolled on CCG 9891/ POG 9130 low grade glioma study (adapted from Wisoff, J. H., J. M. Boyett, et al. (1998)

Table 3. Distribution of low-grade gliomas in children based on location and histology

2.1 The blood-brain barrier

The BBB is composed of endothelium that covers almost the entire capillary network supplying the brain. The endothelium in the BBB is non-fenestrated with high-resistance tight junctions. Other components of the BBB include the astroglial processes, basement membrane, and pericytes (Gururangan and Friedman 2002) (Gururangan and Friedman 2004). The foot processes of the astrocytes cover the entire capillary endothelium and are essentially interposed between the endothelium and the neurons (Gururangan and Friedman 2004). There is minimal pinocytotic activity across the endothelial cells. Hence, in a physiologic state, the BBB functions as a diffusion barrier preventing hydrophilic molecules less than 180 kilo Daltons from passively entering the brain, and is intended to keep noxious substances from damaging the neuronal cells (Englehard and Groothuis 1999). The BBB serves to transport nutrients and water soluble substances between the blood and the CNS (Engelhard 2000). It also serves as a conduit for carrier mediated, energy-dependent specialized transport systems that enable specific molecules in the blood to cross the endothelium into the neurons (e.g., the glucose transporter, GLUT-1) or from the cell back to blood (e.g., p-glycoprotein efflux pump) (Englehard and Groothuis 1999). The endothelium is fenestrated and permits free exchange of large molecules in some areas of the brain including pituitary and pineal glands, the median eminence, area postrema, subfornicial organ, and the lamina terminalis. The absence of the BBB is reflected by the appearance of normal contrast enhancement in these areas in neuroimaging studies.

2.1.1 Brain tumors cause disruption of the blood-brain barrier

The proliferation and invasion of tumor cells in the brain generally results in the disruption of the brain microvasculature, breach of the BBB, and development of vasogenic edema even in small tumors (Gururangan and Friedman 2002). The BBB is histologically abnormal in the presence of a tumor with thickened basement membrane, increased pinocytotic activity within the endothelial cells, and diminished interaction between the pericytes and astrocytic foot processes causing increased fenestrations between endothelial cells and exudation of plasma into the tumor. This interstitial edema can in turn influence cerebral blood flow, brain metabolism, and intracranial pressure. Tumor cells also secrete pro-angiogenic factors including basic fibroblast growth factor (b-FGF) and vascular endothelial growth factor (VEGF) resulting in the influx of new blood vessels into the tumor, a process called tumor angiogenesis (Folkman 2007). These tumor capillaries are different from the capillaries of the normal brain in that they are hyperplastic, have frequent fenestrations, lax intercellular junctions, and less well developed glial processes abutting on the abluminal surface of the endothelium (Groothuis 2000). Thus the continuing proliferation of the tumor cells in the brain actually results in disruption of the BBB (Stewart 1994). However, it is possible that such disruption can be variable between tumors and even within a given tumor. Also, it is likely that small tumors (for e.g., the infiltrative edge of a malignant glioma) might have a relatively intact BBB that might lead to chemotherapy failure (Stewart 1994).

2.1.2 Blood-brain barrier and efficacy of brain tumor chemotherapy

In the ongoing search for more effective chemotherapeutic agents for patients with brain tumors, there is a general bias towards choosing lipophilic agents with a high octanol-water partition coefficient (a measure of the lipid solubility of the drug) to enable rapid transfer of these drugs from the blood to the tumor cells despite an intact BBB (Englehard and Groothuis 1999). However, as indicated in the previous section, it appears that the BBB might be disrupted even in small tumors allowing drug entry. Also, studies have shown that the average concentration of chemotherapeutic agents in brain tumors does not significantly differ from their extra cranial counterparts, although the homogeneity of drug distribution varies both within and between brain tumor deposits (Stewart 1994; Gururangan and Friedman 2002). Also, it must be remembered that while lipophilic drugs do penetrate the blood-brain barrier better, it does not necessarily translate into equal efficacy in all patients with brain tumors (Stewart 1994). There are clearly other reasons for chemotherapy failure in such patients besides the BBB (Groothuis 2000; Gururangan and Friedman 2002). Nevertheless, it is possible that disruption of the BBB may not be uniform in brain tumors and areas of the brain surrounding the main tumor may have a relatively intact BBB. This notion has led to an increasing trend towards devising methods that further disrupt the blood-tumor barrier to facilitate entry of chemotherapy into brain tumors. Such increased disruption could potentially increase drug concentration in areas where the barrier has not been completely disrupted by the tumor (Stewart 1994) and help chemotherapy reach areas of adjacent tumor infiltration wherein the barrier may be relatively intact (Stewart 1994; Englehard and Groothuis 1999). Alternatively, the BBB can be by-passed using strategies like intra-arterial or intra-thecal delivery of chemotherapeutic agents; convection-enhanced delivery of large molecules like toxins directly into the tumor;

or intracavitary administration of chemotherapy wafers (e.g., Gliadel™ wafers, Eisai Pharmaceuticals, Woodcliff Lake, NJ) (Gururangan and Friedman 2002).

3. Angiogenesis and brain tumors

In 1971, Dr. Judah Folkman proposed that continued tumor growth after the initial tumor take (up to a 2 mm^3 size) is dependent on growth of new blood vessels into the tumor (Folkman 2007). This influx of new capillaries was termed 'tumor angiogenesis'. This initial hypothesis has since been confirmed in several studies and has led to the discovery of several pro angiogenesis and anti-angiogenesis factors (Folkman 2007). The principal pro-angiogenesis mediators are α and β fibroblast growth factors (b-FGF), vascular endothelial growth factor (VEGF), angiogenin, and other factors (Folkman 2007). The principal negative regulators of new capillary growth are endostatin, thrombospondin-1 and 2, and angiostatin (Folkman 2007). While tumor dormancy is generally dependent on a balance between positive and negative regulators of angiogenesis, an excess of stimulators results in the "angiogenic switch" and exponential tumor growth (Hanahan and Folkman 1996). These pro-angiogenic factors can be produced by the tumor cells, mobilized from the extracellular matrix through matrix metalloproteases (MMP), or released by macrophages or neutrophils attracted to the tumor through elaboration of VEGF (Folkman 2007). The angiogenic process also leads to tumor invasion and ultimately metastasis to other body sites (Folkman 2007). This induction of angiogenesis is the reason why neovascularization is present in most brain tumors (Li, Folkerth et al. 1994). Immunohistochemical studies have demonstrated the presence of angiogenic factors including b-FGF in high concentrations in brain tumors (Li, Folkerth et al. 1994). This peptide stimulates vascular endothelial cell proliferation and such cells either produce or possess receptors for b-FGF. Li et al. have detected b-FGF in the cerebrospinal fluid (CSF) in 62% of children with brain tumors but none in controls (Li, Folkerth et al. 1994). The CSF specimens with elevated b-FGF increased the DNA synthesis of capillary endothelial cells *in vitro* and such activity was blocked by neutralizing antibody to b-FGF. The concentration of b-FGF in CSF was also correlated with increased micro vessel density (MVD) in histologic sections of the brain tumors and negatively correlated with prognosis. While b-FGF was the only proangiogenic factor studied in this report, it is possible that other angiogenic peptides could mediate growth of brain tumors including VEGF, integrins ($\alpha_v\beta_3$, $\alpha_v\beta_5$, $\alpha_3\beta_1$), Platelet derived growth factor (PDGF), plasminogen activator, cyclooxygenases, and copper. VEGF is highly expressed in several types of primary brain tumors (Leung, Chan et al. 1997; Huang, Held-Feindt et al. 2005) and is an important growth factor that sustains endothelial proliferation, survival, and motility (Kerbel 2008). There are four cognate VEGF receptors including VEGFR-1 (flt-1), VEGFR-2 (KDR), VEGFR-3, and VEGFR-4. However, VEGFR-2 is the most important receptor that mediates the effects of VEGF on the endothelial cells (Kerbel 2008). The level of VEGF expression has also been correlated with outcome in patients with glioblastoma multiforme (Kim, Li et al. 1993).

The demonstration of the role of angiogenesis in sustaining tumor growth has led to the exploration of inhibitors of angiogenesis as a means of curtailing tumor progression. Elegant pre-clinical studies in mouse tumor xenograft models have shown dramatic tumor regression and cure of animals bearing tumors (Boehm, Folkman et al. 1997). There are at least 40 such inhibitors in various stages of clinical development in a wide variety of tumors in centers in the U.S and Europe, and should help our understanding of the toxicity, dose schedules, and possibly the usefulness of these agents in these malignancies.(Folkman 2007). Three of these agents have received FDA approval, including Bevacizumab (Avastin™, Genentech Corporation, San Francisco, USA) (for colorectal cancer, lung cancer, glioblastoma mulitforme), Sorafenib (Nexavar™, Bayer Pharmaceuticals, Berlin, Germany)(for renal carcinoma), and Sunitinib (Sutent™, Pfizer Corporation, USA) (for renal carcinoma) (Folkman 2007). In particular, Bevacizumab (a humanized antibody against VEGF), AZD2171 (Cediranib, Astra Zeneca, U.K.) (VEGF-R2 inhibitor), and Cilengitide (an integrin $\alpha_v\beta_3$, $\alpha_v\beta_5$ inhibitor) (EMD121974; Merck KGaA, Darmstadt, Germany) have undergone extensive evaluation in adults with malignant glioma and are currently being tested in phase III trials against standard therapy (Reardon, Desjardins et al. 2008).

4. Advances in the treatment of pediatric brain tumors

4.1 Low-grade gliomas

Pediatric low-grade gliomas (LGG) are a heterogeneous group of tumors and constitute the most frequent CNS neoplasia encountered in children (30-40% of all CNS tumors diagnosed in the United States) (Watson, Kadota et al. 2001). They can be classified based on histology or location (Table 3). Pilocytic astrocytoma is the commonest LGG in children with an incidence of 0.79 per 100,000 person-years. The commonest neuro-cutaneous syndrome associated with LGG is Neurofibromatosis Type I (NF-1). The genetic mutation is NF-1 is located on chromosome 17q and results in loss of the GTP-ase activating protein (GAP), Neurofibromin. Lack of Neurofibromin activity results in increased activity of the RAS- MAPK, cyclic AMP, and mTOR signaling pathways, and cellular proliferation (Rubin and Gutmann 2005). About 15% of patients with NF-1 develop LGG (typically piloyctic astrocytoma, WHO grade I) and less commonly, other gliomas (Reed and Gutmann 2001). NF-1 patients with LGG have a more favorable prognosis than those with sporadic tumors (Gururangan, Cavazos et al. 2002). The risk factors for development of non-NF-1 LGG is largely unknown although one case-control study identified an increased risk of developing low grade brain stem gliomas in the offspring of mothers who ingested an excessive amount of cured meats during pregnancy (Preston-Martin, Pogoda et al. 1996).

The pathology of pilocytic astrocytoma is one of low cellularity and a biphasic pattern of solid sheets of bipolar cells and Rosenthal fibers along with areas of micro and macro cysts (Burger, Scheithauer et al. 2000). The tumor nuclei typically lack anaplasia. The tumor demonstrates hyalinized glomerular blood vessels that are quite leaky and hence cause intense contrast enhancement on neuroimaging studies. The pilomyxoid astrocytoma is a closely related tumor type that occurs predominantly in the hypothalamic/chiasmatic region and is characterized by the presence of a myxoid matrix and angiocentric arrangement of monomorphous bipolar cells, and has a high predilection for leptomeningeal spread (Louis, Ohgaki et al. 2007).

4.2 Treatment

Since these tumors only rarely metastasize through the neuraxis, local control using surgery and/or radiotherapy have been the traditional components of therapy for patients with LGG. Due to a direct positive correlation between extent of resection and progression-free and overall survival (PFS and OS), aggressive surgery of tumor should be attempted in tumor locations where feasible (Watson, Kadota et al. 2001). The cystic cerebellar astrocytoma is an example of a LGG that can be resected completely without causing neurologic deficits and results in cure rates of over 90% (Figure 2) (Watson, Kadota et al. 2001). Similarly, exophytic tumors of the brain stem including the cervico-medullary region are typically pilocytic astrocytomas, amenable to complete surgical removal, and have an excellent prognosis (Watson, Kadota et al. 2001). Tectal plate gliomas usually present with hydrocephalus due to early compression of the cerebral aqueduct. Patients with these tumors are observed without any treatment after controlling hydrocephalus with a third ventriculostomy. The operating microscope and ultrasonic surgical aspirator allows the surgeon to perform an adequate tumor resection without compromising adjacent normal brain. Pre-operative imaging can be correlated with intra-operative observation using frame-based or frameless stereotactic system that also help in guiding the surgeon with trajectories to deep-seated lesions. Functional magnetic resonance imaging, positron emission tomography, and electrode grids for mapping areas of the cerebral cortex have helped the surgeon to accurately delineate tumor margins and improve post -surgical morbidity in these patients. However, tumors in certain areas of the brain (about 30% of all LGG) are still unsafe for surgical resection and include the optic pathway, diencephalon (hypothalamus and thalamus), and intrinsic portion of the brain stem. For tumors in such locations and those that recur after initial surgical resection and/or cause functional impairment, chemotherapy and/or radiotherapy (RT) can be used for disease control. There are no reported prospective randomized trials assessing the benefits of adjuvant radiotherapy in children with LGG (Watson, Kadota et al. 2001). Extrapolating data from adult phase III trials, it seems appropriate to use focal radiotherapy in doses of 45-54 Gy in 1.8 to 2.0 Gy fractions. Three-D conformal RT, intensity modulated RT, and proton-beam therapy are new radiation delivery techniques that are designed to minimize damage to normal brain but await validation in larger studies (Watson, Kadota et al. 2001). A preliminary report from St. Jude Children's Hospital explored the usefulness of 3-D conformal RT in patients with localized LGG (Merchant, Happersett et al. 1999). Thirty eight patients (median age 8.7 years, range 2.2 -18.7) with LGG (JPA, 25) were enrolled on this phase II trial. With a median follow-up of 17 months (range, 3-44), four patients have suffered local failures, 3 within the clinical target volume (CTV) and one just outside the CTV. While data from this study is encouraging for limited field radiotherapy, long-term follow up is required to assess the impact of field reduction on long-term complications and outcome. In view of the deleterious effect of radiotherapy on the growing brain in young children, chemotherapy agents including vincristine, actinomycin-D, cyclophosphamide, carboplatin, lomustine, and etoposide have been employed individually or in combination in patients with progressive LGG to delay or avoid irradiation (Gururangan, Cavazos et al. 2002). Following preliminary clinical evidence of activity, carboplatin, a second-generation cisplatin analog, either alone or in combination with vincristine, has been used as a frontline therapy for children with low-grade glioma, particularly for those with optic pathway tumors (Friedman, Krischer et al. 1992; Packer, Ater et al. 1997; Gururangan, Cavazos et al. 2002). Objective responses and disease stabilization have been observed in 25-58% and 80-90% of patients respectively in these studies. The three-year PFS in patients with recurrent low-grade glioma following this chemotherapy regimen has been reported to be 64-68% (Packer, Ater et al. 1997; Gururangan, Cavazos et al. 2002). Myelosuppression is the main toxicity related to carboplatin followed by allergic reactions in about 10-30% of patients (Gururangan, Cavazos et al. 2002). An alternative nitrosourea - based chemotherapy regimen [6-Thioguanine, Procarbazine, Lomustine (CCNU), Vincristine, and Dibromodulcitol] was reported by Prados et al., and was shown to produce prolonged disease stabilization in children with progressive LGG (Prados, Edwards et al. 1997). This treatment combination without Dibromodulcitol (TPCV regimen) was evaluated in comparison with the carboplatin + vincristine combination in a Children's Oncology Group phase III trial in 401 eligible children with progressive or symptomatic LGG (Ater, Holmes et al. 2008). The results of this study, available in abstract form, showed that both regimens were efficacious in prolonging disease-free survival (median time to progression of 3.2 and 4.9 years for carboplatin + vincristine and TPCV regimens respectively) and enabled delaying radiotherapy. The overall survival was 86% for non- NF-1 children and 98% for those with NF-1 (p= 0.0017), again demonstrating that NF-1 patients with recurrent LGG have a better prognosis than those without NF-1. Recently, we and others have also reported on the efficacy of Temozolomide (an oral methylating imadazole tetrazinone compound) in both adults and children with LGG (Kuo, Weiner et al. 2003; Quinn, Reardon et al. 2003; Gururangan, Fisher et al. 2007). In a phase II trial of 26 children with progressive/recurrent optic pathway or juvenile pilocytic astrocytoma, the disease stabilization rate was over 50% for a median interval of 34 months (Gururangan, Fisher et al. 2007).

4.3 Molecular alterations in pediatric LGG and novel therapies

While *Nf-1* loss is clearly related to the genesis of tumors in patients with NF-1, the molecular events in sporadic LGG had not been well characterized until recently. Several groups have now identified tandem duplication of 7q34 that contains the *BRAF* gene in about 60-80% of sporadic pilocytic astrocytomas resulting in a fusion product between *KIAA1549* and *BRAF* that includes the *BRAF* kinase domain without the auto-inhibitory N-terminus (Pfister, Janzarik et al. 2008; Yu, Deshmukh et al. 2009). This is an activating mutation that is also present in 50% of fibrillary astrocytomas. On the other hand, an activating point mutation in Exon 15 position 600 of the *BRAF* gene (BRAF V600E) is found in over 40% of gangliogliomas but only rarely in pilocytic astrocytomas (Dougherty, Santi et al. 2010). BRAF is a member of the RAF family of serine-threonine protein kinases and is a key intermediary in the RAS-RAF-MEK-ERK- MAP kinase pathway(Yu, Deshmukh et al. 2009). Activation of BRAF would signal downstream via MEK-ERK and finally MAP-kinase resulting in cellular proliferation. In fact, tumors with activating mutations of BRAF were found to have overexpression of MAP-K (Kolb, Gorlick et al. 2010).

In contrast to sporadic tumors, *BRAF* mutations are not found in NF-1 associated pilocytic astrocytomas (Yu, Deshmukh et al. 2009). It is therefore possible that this mutation is an initiating event only in non- NF-1 tumors. Interestingly, this activating mutation seems to be preferentially expressed in posterior fossa tumors (Yu, Deshmukh et al. 2009). In addition to *BRAF* mutations, *HIPK2* (Homeo-box interfering protein kinase 2) amplifications have been identified in a proportion of sporadic pilocytic astrocytomas that also harbor *BRAF* rearrangements (Yu, Deshmukh et al. 2009). The significance of this molecular event is unknown. In addition, VEGF overexpression has also been observed in pilocytic astrocytomas and might explain the intense vascular proliferation seen in these tumors (Leung, Chan et al. 1997).

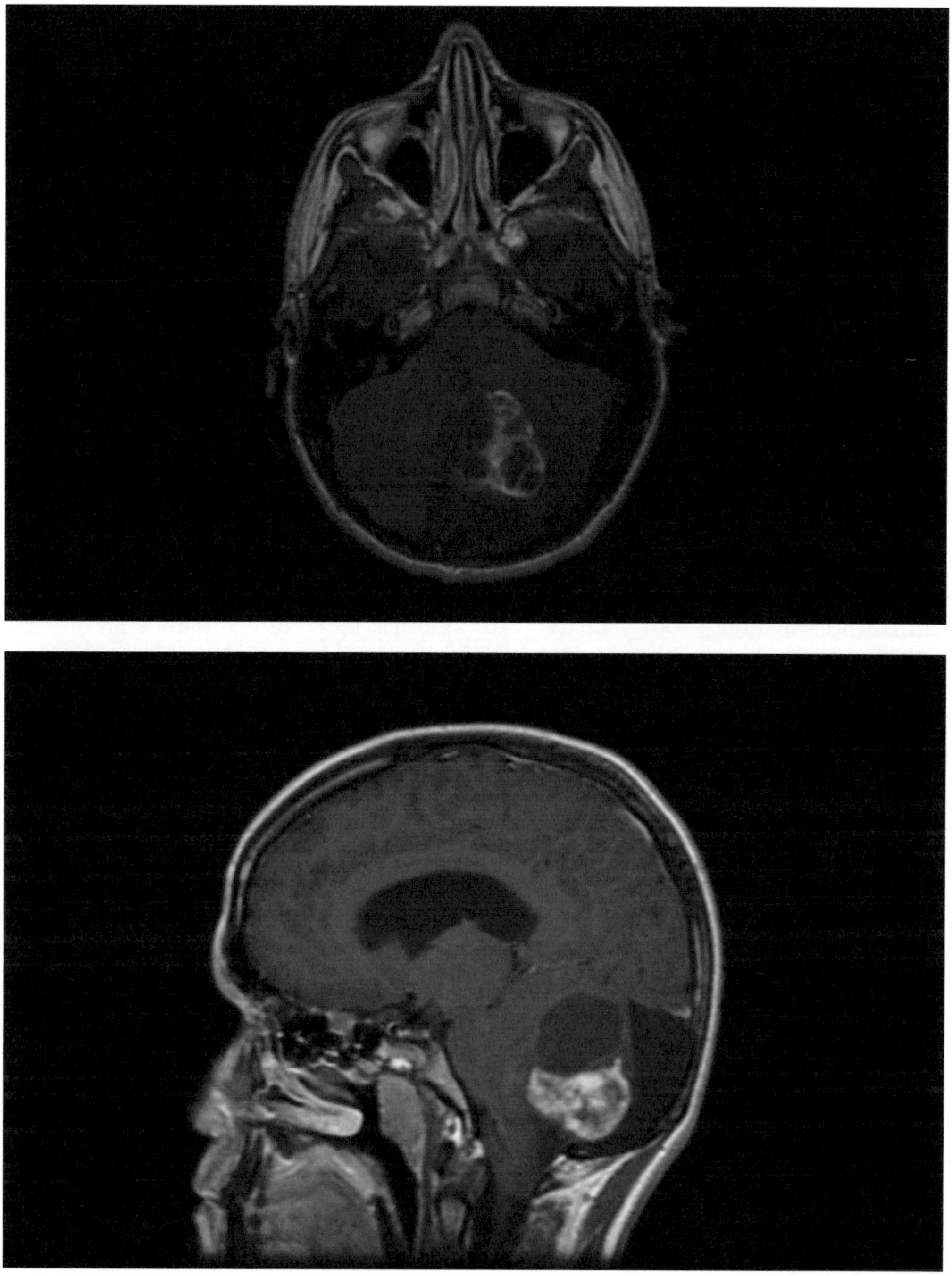

Fig. 2. T-1 weighted axial and sagittal gadolinium enhanced images of the brain in a 4-year old male demonstrating an enhancing cystic lesion in the cerebellum that is compressing the IV ventricle and causing hydrocephalus. Histology of this mass was a pilocytic astrocytoma.

Biologic therapies are being increasingly used in children with recurrent LGG using information on expression of specific targets in these tumors. The intense vascularity of pilocytic astrocytoma implies that these tumors might be susceptible to anti-angiogenic therapies. Using the principle of metronomic chemotherapy that preferentially kills tumor endothelial cells rather than tumor (Kerbel, Viloria-Petit et al. 2000), Bouffet et al., conducted a phase II study of intravenous vinblastine 6 mg/m²/week administered for up to 52 weeks in 51 patients with recurrent LGG (Bouffet, Jakacki et al. 2008). Disease stabilization was obtained in 42% of patients at a median follow up of 31 months from starting treatment. In a recent phase I study of Lenalidomide (an immune modulating drug and angiogenesis inhibitor) in children with recurrent brain tumors, Warren et al., reported objective responses in 2 patients with an optic pathway glioma and pilocytic astrocytoma respectively (Warren, Goldman et al. 2011). Similarly, Packer et al., have observed sustained objective responses or disease stabilization and improvement in neurologic deficits in 7 of 9 children with multiply recurrent LGG treated with Bevacizumab plus irinotecan (Camptosar™, Pfizer corporation, USA) (Packer, Jakacki et al. 2009). A multi-institutional phase II trial of the same combination in children with recurrent LGG has just been completed and results of this study should be available soon.

Since about 70% of sporadic pilocytic astrocytomas express activating BRAF mutations, there has been an interest in using targeted inhibitors of the BRAF pathway. In the pediatric pre-clinical testing program (PPTP), AZD6244, a potent and selective inhibitor of MEK1/2 kinases, demonstrated significant activity in one of two JPA xenografts that carried the activating V600E mutation (Kolb, Gorlick et al. 2010). There is an ongoing multi-institutional phase I trial in the United States through the National Cancer Institute sponsored Pediatric Brain Tumor Consortium (PBTC) using AZD6244 in older children with recurrent low-grade gliomas testing the toxicity, pharmacokinetics, and preliminary assessment of efficacy of this agent in this population (Larry Kun M.D., Memphis, TN; personal communication 2011).

5. Primitive neuroectodermal tumors

Primitive neuroectodermal tumors (PNET) of the central nervous system (CNS) are a group of aggressive embryonal neoplasia that occurs both in adults and children. Under this broad rubric, three tumors are mainly recognized based on their location - medulloblastoma, which occurs exclusively in the cerebellum, pineoblastoma in the pineal gland, and supratentorial PNET in the cerebral hemispheres or suprasellar region. Although histologically similar with a propensity for aggressive neuraxis dissemination, these tumors markedly differ in terms of genetic makeup and prognosis. In recent years, much controversy has been generated in the histologic classification of PNET (Rorke 1983). Simultaneously, considerable progress has been made in identifying the molecular characteristics of these tumors, particularly medulloblastoma (Pomeroy, Tamayo et al. 2002 ; Gilbertson 2004). Also, significant strides have been made in the treatment of patients with these malignancies.

5.1 Medulloblastoma

Medulloblastoma is the most common malignant brain tumor in children. About 400 children are diagnosed with this tumor each year in the United States (Gurney, Smith et al. 1999). The peak age of onset is between 5-9 years of age. Over 90% of medulloblastoma typically arise from the superior medullary velum, grows and fills the cavity of the fourth ventricle (Figure 3a) (Mclendon, Enterline et al. 1998). The tumor mass can encroach on to

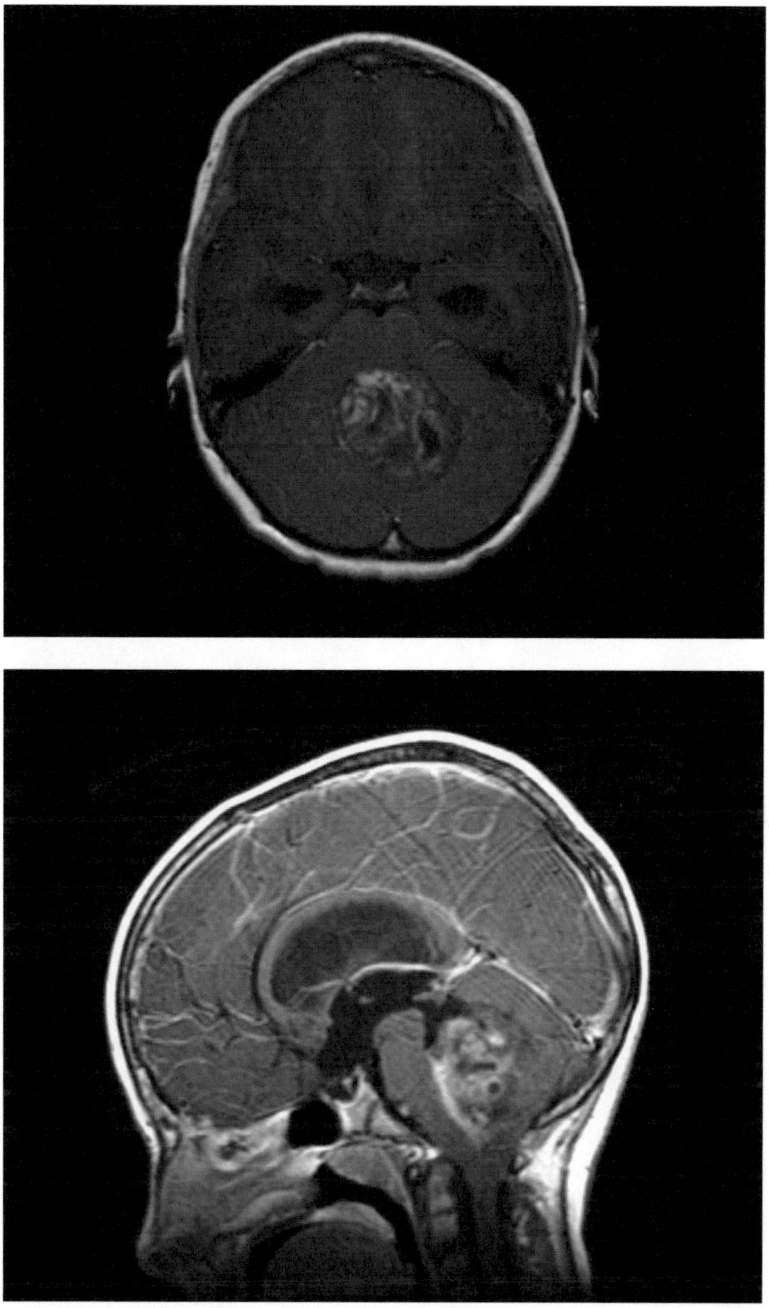

Fig. 3. a: Figure: T-1 weighted axial and sagittal gadolinium enhanced images of the brain in a 16-year old black female that demonstrates a heterogeneously enhancing mass filling the IV ventricle and causing obstructive hydrocephalus

the cisterna magna and sometimes infiltrates the floor of the fourth ventricle or brain stem. A minority of tumors, particularly in patients over 16 years of age, arises more laterally in the cerebellar hemispheres (Mclendon, Enterline et al. 1998). Macroscopically, these tumors are soft, friable, and moderately demarcated from the cerebellar tissue. Areas of central necrosis may be present. The microscopic structure of medulloblastoma is characterized by densely packed cells with round to oval carrot -shaped highly hyperchromatic nuclei surrounded by scanty cytoplasm. Neuroblastic rosettes are a typical but not constant feature. The main pathologic subtypes of medulloblastoma recognized in the 2000 World Health Organization (WHO) classification of brain tumors include classic, desmoplastic, extensive nodularity with advanced neuronal differentiation, and the large cell/anaplastic varieties (Giangaspero, Perilongo et al. 1999; Giangaspero, Bigner et al. 2000; Leonard, Cai et al. 2001; Louis, Ohgaki et al. 2007). The predominant presenting symptoms in patients with this tumor are those of raised intracranial pressure including irritability, headache, lethargy, vomiting, and poor school performance (Packer, Cogen et al. 1999). Additional symptoms due to invasion of other local structures include truncal ataxia, nystagmus, neck stiffness, and cranial nerve palsies. Dissemination of tumor to the leptomeninges (Figure 3b) occurs in about 10-30% of cases, with infants suffering this complication more frequently than older children. In less than 10% of cases, the tumor can spread outside of the neuraxis (Packer, Cogen et al. 1999). Patients with certain genetic disorders including Gorlin's (nevoid-basal cell carcinoma syndrome), p-53 germline mutation, and Turcot's syndromes have a higher risk of developing medulloblastoma (Packer, Cogen et al. 1999).

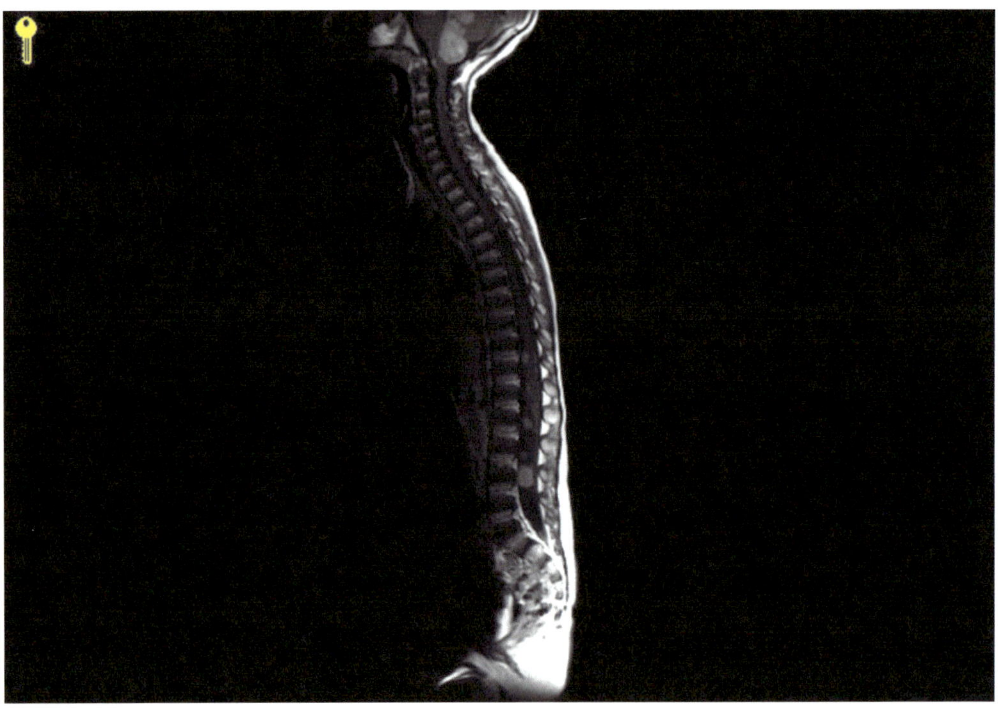

Fig. 3. b: T-1 weighted sagittal gadolinium enhanced image of the spine in a 2-year old black female with posterior fossa medulloblastoma demonstrating multiple nodular metastatic lesions along the spinal cord

5.2 Treatment

Patients with medulloblastoma are classified as average or high-risk to enable assignment of appropriate treatment based on the extent of tumor following surgery. Those with average risk disease are over > 3 years of age and have ≤ 1.5 cm^2 of tumor in the primary site and no brain stem involvement or metastatic disease (Packer, Cogen et al. 1999). Patients with high-risk medulloblastoma include children < 3 years at the time of diagnosis, and those who have gross residual disease post-surgery or metastatic disease (Packer, Cogen et al. 1999). Conventional therapy for patients with low-risk medulloblastoma is complete surgical resection followed by craniospinal irradiation (24-36 Gy) and a focal boost to the primary site (54 - 56 Gy) with a 5-year event-free survival rate of approximately 60% (Packer, Cogen et al. 1999; Freeman, Taylor et al. 2002). The addition of chemotherapy (vincristine, cisplatin, and lomustine or cyclophosphamide) appears to benefit patients with high-risk features and might help to decrease the dose of neuraxis irradiation in patients with average risk disease (Packer, Cogen et al. 1999; Freeman, Taylor et al. 2002). Infants with medulloblastoma fare poorly with standard chemotherapy and irradiation and have a higher incidence of neuro-cognitive deficits following radiotherapy (Duffner, Horowitz et al. 1993; Walter, Mulhern et al. 1999). There is evidence that some infants can be successfully treated with high-dose chemotherapy alone without neuraxis irradiation (Mason, Grovas et al. 1998). 3-D conformal radiotherapy is currently being utilized in children with medulloblastoma in an attempt to delivery radiation boost to the tumor bed and residual tumor and decrease radiation scatter to the cochlea, supratentorial brain, and hypothalamus. Preliminary results from single- institution studies appear promising with no increased failures documented in the posterior fossa (Merchant, Happersett et al. 1999; Wolden, Dunkel et al. 2003) and lesser risk of oto-toxicity and neuro-cognitive deficits. The validity of these results will be further tested in a randomized fashion in the ongoing Children's Oncology Group (COG) phase III trial (ACNS 0331) for average- risk medulloblastoma in children.

Patients with recurrent tumors fare very poorly despite conventional retrieval therapy with few or no long-term survivors. The use of high-dose chemotherapy (HDC) with stem cell rescue has been useful in prolonging PFS in a proportion of patients with tumors that are localized and sensitive to standard chemotherapy, relapse following chemotherapy only, and hence can also receive standard doses of radiotherapy in addition to HDC (Dunkel, Boyett et al. 1998; Guruangan, Dunkel et al. 1998; Gururangan, Krauser et al. 2008). In contrast, studies at Duke University Medical Center and others have shown that this strategy does not seem to be efficacious in those patients who relapse after receiving standard chemotherapy and radiotherapy (Gururangan, Krauser et al. 2008). Recurrent medulloblastoma is invariably associated with leptomeningeal dissemination (LMD) at some point in its disease course. Treatment for LMD with currently available options is suboptimal. Intrathecal chemotherapy with thiotepa, mafosfamide, or busulfan has been tested in phase I/II clinical trials in patients with LMD (Gururangan and Friedman 2002). However, benefits are transient since the delivered chemotherapy is unable to penetrate beyond a few millimeters into the tumor tissue from CSF due to the high interstitial pressure within the tumor. More innovative therapies are needed to improve outcome for patients with recurrent medulloblastoma through a better understanding of the biology of the tumor.

5.3 Molecular characteristics and biologic therapy

There has been a profusion of studies describing the molecular characteristics of medulloblastoma including the Sonic-Hedgehog and WNT signaling pathways, Trk-C expression, c-Myc amplification, OTX-2 amplification, presence of isochromosome 17q, erBB-2 and 4 over-expression, and PDGFR α and RAS/MAP-kinase activation, that can predict the biologic behavior and outcome independent of clinical characteristics (Packer, Cogen et al. 1999; MacDonald, Brown et al. 2001; Gilbertson 2004; Di, Liao et al. 2005). At least one clinical trial has prospectively validated the usefulness of some of these molecular markers and, in future, could potentially help to decrease therapy for those patients with favorable biologic features (Gajjar, Chintagumpala et al. 2006). Whereas patients with WNT pathway activation identified by beta-catenin point mutations on residue S33 and S37 have a 100% survival with standard risk adapted therapy, those with either SHH or non-SHH/non-WNT tumors have an inferior survival (Gajjar, Chintagumpala et al. 2006; Schwalbe, Lindsey et al. 2011). More recently, gene expression profiling of medulloblastoma has revealed that tumors cluster within four distinct molecular groups; WNT, SHH, Group C, and D (Northcott, Korshunov et al. 2010). Interestingly, each group could be identified by immunohistochemistry or mRNA based expression potentially allowing for easy categorization of prospective patients at diagnosis (Northcott, Korshunov et al. 2010; Schwalbe, Lindsey et al. 2011). Such classification has potential advantages of allowing for stratification of intensity of standard therapy based on the known prognosis of each group and possibly using specific small molecule kinase inhibitors specific for that group. An activating mutation of the Smoothened gene is present in about 10% of sporadic medulloblastoma and tumors harboring this mutation would be responsive to Smoothened inhibitors. GDC 0449 (Genentech Corporation, San Francisco, USA) is one such inhibitor that has shown excellent activity in transgenic PATCH mouse models of medulloblastoma (Romer, Kimura et al. 2004) and in one patient with metastatic medulloblastoma (Rudin, Hann et al. 2009). Recently, retinoids including All Trans Retinoic Acid (ATRA) and 13-cis retinoic acid have been found to mediate apoptosis in medulloblastoma cells and decrease tumor growth in xenograft mouse models, especially those bearing anaplastic medulloblastoma with OTX-2 amplification (Hallahan, Pritchard et al. 2003) (Di, Liao et al. 2005). On this basis, an ongoing COG trial will test the efficacy of 13 cis-retinoic acid in a randomized fashion along with maintenance chemotherapy in children with high-risk medulloblastoma. A recent pre-clinical study demonstrated that while 9-cis retinoic acid reduced growth of an OTX-2 overexpressing D425 medulloblastoma xenograft implanted in the flanks of athymic mice but failed to do so in intracranial implants of the same tumor (Bai, Siu et al. 2010). Fibroblast growth factor (FGF) expression was implicated in the failure of retinoic acid therapy in the intracranial tumor model and resistance can be abrogated by combining 9- cis retinoic acid with a specific FGF inhibitor (Bai, Siu et al. 2010).

5.4 Pineoblastoma and other supratentorial PNET

The incidence of pineoblastoma is approximately 3-10% of all primary malignant brain tumors in all age groups (Jakacki 1999) They constitute approximately 45% of all pineal parenchymal tumors. They usually occur in the first 2 decades of life with most cases occurring in the within 10 years. A familial tendency for occurrence of PNET in pineal or suprasellar region has been observed in patients with familial retinoblastoma, also called the trilateral retinoblastoma syndrome (Paulino 1999; Singh, Shields et al. 1999). Other supratentorial PNETs including cerebral neuroblastoma, ependymoblastoma, and medulloepithelioma constitute 1-2% of all CNS tumors and about 6% of all CNS PNETs. These tumors occur commonly in the cerebral hemispheres, periventricular region, thalamus, hypothalamus, basal ganglia, and rarely as diffuse leptomeningeal disease without a evidence of a primary tumor (Jennings, Slatkin et al. 1993; Dai, Backstrom et al. 2003). These tumors mostly occur in young children with a median age at diagnosis of 5.5 years (range, 4 weeks to 10 years) and a male predominance (Jakacki 1999). Supratentorial PNETs have been known to occur following cranial irradiation as a second malignancy (Hader, Drovini-Zis et al. 2003). No specific genetic associations have been noted in patients with these tumors. The histologic features of these tumors are similar to that of medulloblastoma.

The clinical features of pineoblastoma include those due to hydrocephalus due early compression of the aqueduct and pressure on the tectum of the mid-brain which produces the Parinaud's syndrome. Cerebral PNETs typically cause headache, vomiting, and seizures depending upon the location of the tumor (Berger, Edwards et al. 1983; Dai, Backstrom et al. 2003).

5.4.1 Treatment

The treatment of these tumors includes surgical resection, chemotherapy, and radiotherapy (Jakacki 1999; Gururangan, McLaughlin et al. 2003). However, survival for patients with these tumors is far inferior compared to those with medulloblastoma. Infants with supratentorial PNET have a dismal prognosis with standard chemotherapy and irradiation (Duffner, Horowitz et al. 1993; Jakacki 1999). In contrast, a PFS of over 60% has been observed in older children with pineoblastoma treated with lomustine (CCNU), vincristine, and prednisone or the "8 in 1" drug regimen following neuraxis irradiation and a focal boost to the pineal region (Jakacki 1999). The use of HDC with stem cell rescue plus radiotherapy has also resulted in improved survival in some children with these tumors especially for those with metastatic disease (Mason, Grovas et al. 1998; Gururangan, McLaughlin et al. 2003; Gururangan, Driscoll et al. 2008; Chintagumpala, Hassall et al. 2009). The efficacy of HDC in infants with pineoblastoma has been encouraging even without the need for radiotherapy (Gururangan, McLaughlin et al. 2003). Optimal management of children with pineoblastoma and other supra-tentorial PNETs continues to be a challenge and further therapeutic refinements are needed especially for those with recurrent disease.

5.4.2 Molecular characteristics

Although supratentorial PNETs resemble medulloblastoma histologically, the inferior survival seen in this group despite using intensive therapies as used for metastatic medulloblastoma suggest that there are intrinsic biologic differences between these two tumors. The most common non-random chromosomal abnormality is 4q loss occurring in 50% of cases (Li, Bouffet et al. 2005). In contrast to medulloblastoma, none of the supratentorial PNETs expresses isochromosome 17q. Other molecular characteristics include high NOTCH2 expression, and p53 dysfunction (as indicated by p53 immunopositivity) (Li, Bouffet et al. 2005). In addition, heritable loss of the mismatch repair gene PMS2 (homozygous missense mutation in exon 14) results in learning difficulties, café-au-lait spots, and early onset of supratentorial PNETs has been described in two siblings of a heavily consanguineous family (De Vos, Hayward et al. 2006). It appears that supratentorial PNETs might arise due to impaired DNA repair mechanisms as evidenced by the presence of high p53 immunopositivity, occurrence following exposure to radiotherapy, and in the context of mismatch repair mutations (Li, Bouffet et al. 2005).

6. High-grade glioma

High-grade glioma (HGG) including anaplastic astrocytoma (AA, WHO grade III) and glioblastoma multiforme (GBM, WHO Grade IV) constitutes about 14% of CNS tumors in children. These tumors can occur anywhere in the brain. In a recent Children's Cancer Group study report of 131 evaluable children with HGG, over 90% of tumors occurred in a supratentorial location (63% in the superficial cerebral hemisphere (Figure 4a and 4b) and 38% in the deep or midline cerebrum and only 8% occurred in the posterior fossa (including brain stem and cerebellum) (Wisoff, Boyett et al. 1998). The principal histologic features of AA are increased cellularity, nuclear atypia, and marked mitotic activity. The neoplastic cells are consistently positive for glial fibrillary acidic protein and have a proliferative index of around 5-10%. GBM on the other hand is made up of pleomorphic astrocytic cells with brisk mitotic activity, nuclear atypia, vascular proliferation, and areas of necrosis.

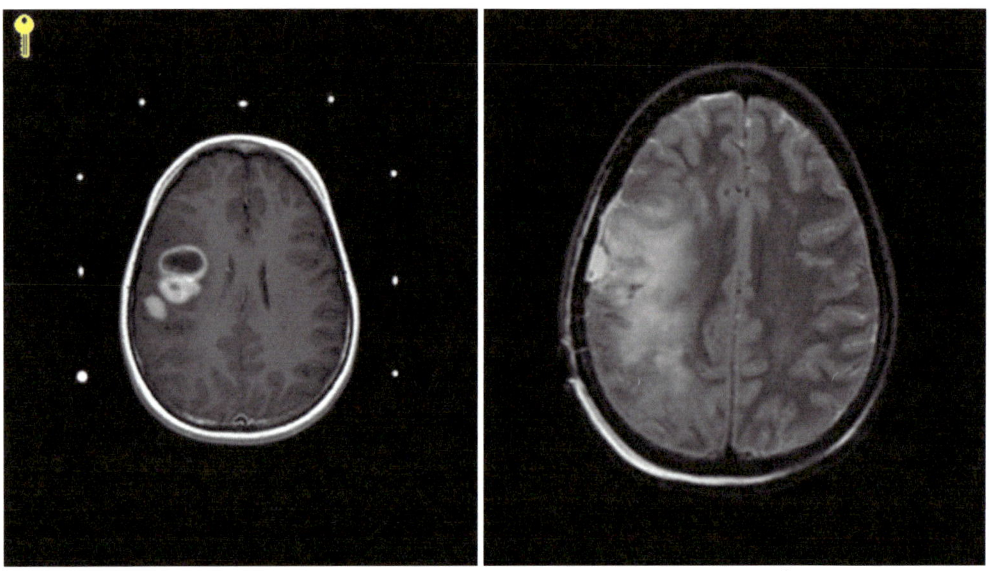

4a 4b

Fig. 4. a and b: Axial T-1 weighted gadolinium enhanced and T-2 weighted images of the brain in a 13-year old boy who presented with seizures. Biopsy of the enhancing lesion revealed an anaplastic astrocytoma. Note the satellite lesion posterior to the main tumor mass and the extensive T-2 signal abnormality that extends beyond the enhancing lesion and indicates peritumoral edema and potentially non-enhancing tumor

6.1 Treatment

Treatment of HGG in any site includes adequate surgical resection, radiotherapy, and chemotherapy. The efficacy of this combined modality approach was recently demonstrated in a Children's Cancer Group phase III randomized study (CCG-945) in which children with HGG received surgical resection followed by either vincristine, lomustine (CCNU), and prednisone (control arm) or the "8 in 1" chemotherapy regimen (experimental arm) (Finlay, Boyett et al. 1995; Wisoff, Boyett et al. 1998). While there was no difference in 5-year PFS between the two arms of the study, the extent of surgical resection (> 90% *vs.* ≤ 90% resection) as assessed by post-operative imaging, was highly predictive of outcome with patients who had complete resection (> 90%) having a significantly better 5-year PFS as compared to those with less extensive resection (≤ 90%) [AA + GBM, 35% *vs.* 17%, p = 0.006; AA, 44% *vs.* 22% and GBM, 29% *vs.* 4%]. Based on the favorable outcome and FDA approval of using Temozolomide (Temodar™, Schering Plough Corporation, Kenilworth, New Jersey) concurrently with radiotherapy in adults with newly diagnosed glioblastoma multiforme especially those with methylation of the MGMT promoter (Cohen, Johnson et al. 2005), a pediatric phase II study was done in children with newly diagnosed malignant glioma in conjunction with radiotherapy followed by maintenance treatment for one year (Cohen, Pollack et al. 2011). The outcome for children with either Grade III or IV astrocytoma was no different compared to those who were treated on CCG-945 but over expression of MGMT was associated with poorer survival (Cohen, Pollack et al. 2011). Temozolomide does not provide the same benefit in children as it does for adults with HGG either at diagnosis or relapse (Gilbert, Friedman et al. 2002; Lashford, Thiesse et al. 2002). Other chemotherapeutic agents including irinotecan (CPT-11) have been utilized in children with HGG with only modest benefit (Turner, Gururangan et al. 2002). The combination of BCNU or Temozolomide with topoisomerase I inhibitors like CPT-11 has demonstrated synergism in pre-clinical studies (Gururangan and Friedman 2002). These combinations have been tested in adult clinical trials at our institution but with only modest benefits (Reardon, Quinn et al. 2004; Quinn, Jiang et al. 2009). Although mismatch repair defects in the tumor is a putative mechanism for resistance in tumors that do not respond to methylating agents like Temozolomide despite low AGAT expression, very few such tumors have been noted to harbor MMR deficiency (Pollack, Hamilton et al. 2010). Alternatively, excessive base excision repair (BER) could be operative in the face of overexpression of the enzyme poly (ADP-Ribose) polymerase (PARP) in these tumors. Inhibition of PARP prior to treatment with Temozolomide would prevent BER and make the tumor sensitive to the drug again. ABT -888 (Olaparib™, Abbot Laboratories, USA) is an effective PARP inhibitor that has been shown to effectively deplete PARP in tumors and is undergoing clinical testing both as a single agent and in combination with chemotherapy and other cytotoxics. Temozolomide + ABT-888 is currently being evaluated both in adults with malignant glioma and children with recurrent brain tumors.

Children with midline HGG including those in the thalamus and diffuse intrinsic lesions within the brain stem (e.g., diffuse pontine glioma) are unresectable based on location and have a grave prognosis (Reardon, Gajjar et al. 1998; Mandell, Kadota et al. 1999). While patients with thalamic tumors undergo biopsy to confirm histology of HGG, it is no longer deemed necessary in patients with MRI findings of a diffuse intrinsic brain stem glioma. The use of radiotherapy and chemotherapy has had little impact on the dismal outcome of these patients in recent years (Mandell, Kadota et al. 1999; Cohen, Heideman et al. 2011).

Since drug resistance and the blood-brain barrier are considered to be the most important impediments to effective chemotherapy in brain tumors, strategies have been devised to circumvent these barriers (Gururangan and Friedman 2002). For locally invasive tumors like HGG, therapies that circumvent the BBB include intra-cavitary implantation of BCNU wafers (Gliadel™ wafers, Aventis Corporation, USA), use of agents that disrupt the BBB, intra-arterial chemotherapy with or without BBB disruption, and convection-enhanced delivery (CED) (Gururangan and Friedman 2002). A modest but significant efficacy was noted with the use of polymers impregnated with BCNU (Gliadel™ wafers, Aventis Corporation, USA) in a phase III randomized double-blind trial in adults with malignant glioma (Brem, Piantadosi et al. 1995; Westphal, Hilt et al. 2003). Intra-arterial chemotherapy using agents like carmustine, cisplatin, and etoposide, despite some theoretical advantages, has not proven to be useful but has some prohibitive neuro-toxicities (Gururangan and Friedman 2002). Transient disruption of the BBB can be achieved with chemical agents including mannitol, prostaglandin, histamine, and bradykinin that then facilitate chemotherapy entry into the brain tumor (Gururangan and Friedman 2002). Recently, Labridimil (Cereport™), a bradykinin analogue, has been used as a BBB disrupting agent prior to carboplatin chemotherapy (Warren, Patel et al. 2001). However, preliminary trials using this combination have had disappointing results.

Convection-enhanced delivery is a recently described method of delivering large molecules via a micro infusion pump directly into the tumor using strategically placed catheters (Kunwar 2003; Sampson, Akabani et al. 2003). Using a pressure gradient, the solution containing the large molecules (typically a tumor toxin) penetrates directly through the tumor by convection and reaches several centimeters beyond the tumor (Gururangan and Friedman 2002). Toxins used have been fusion proteins made up of pseudomonas exotoxin and either Transforming growth factor or interleukin -13 (IL-13 PE38QQR) (Kunwar, Prados et al. 2007). The latter molecules are designed to target the cognate receptors expressed selectively on glioma cells and spare normal brain tissue. Once the glioma cells are targeted, the exotoxin is internalized and causes cytotoxicity (Kunwar, Prados et al. 2007) This strategy has undergone extensive testing in the clinic and has been proven to be reasonably safe (Kunwar, Prados et al. 2007). However, a recent phase III trial (PRECISE) comparing outcome of adults with recurrent GBM who received CED of IL-13PE38QQR with those who were treated with BCNU wafers showed no difference in outcome (Kunwar, Chang et al. 2010). The reasons for lack of better benefit from this promising strategy could be due to poor catheter placement, inadequate expression of target receptors in the tumor, or other unknown factors.

The problem of drug resistance to alkylating agents has been extensively addressed at Duke University Medical Center and is predominantly due to overexpression of alkyl guanine alkyltransferase (AGAT) in tumor cells. The cellular enzyme, O^6 guanine DNA alkyl transferase (AGAT), is responsible for removing the alkyl groups from the O^6 -position of deoxyguanosine and prevents cross-linking of DNA (Dolan and Pegg 1997). Increased expression of this DNA repair protein is the major mechanism of resistance to nitrosoureas and other alkylating agents (Dolan and Pegg 1997). O^6-Benzylguanine (O^6-BG) is a modulating agent that demonstrates high affinity for AGAT and effectively enhances nitrosourea activity *in vitro* and *in vivo* (Dolan and Pegg 1997). Friedman et al. at Duke University Medical Center conducted a phase I trial of O^6-BG in patients with malignant glioma and determined the optimum biologic dose that depletes tumor tissue of AGAT to be 100 mg/m^2(Friedman, McLendon et al. 1998). This dose of O^6-BG has been subsequently used in combination with BCNU in a phase I trial in adults with recurrent HGG (Friedman, Pluda et al. 2000). The MTD of BCNU when used in this combination was 40 mg/m^2 given every 6 weeks. However, a phase II trial of this combination in adults with recurrent malignant glioma did not demonstrate any objective response, suggesting that elevation of

AGAT is not the only mechanism for treatment failure in these patients (Quinn, Dolan et al. 2001). Treatment failure in this setting could also be related to limitations of achieving adequate intratumor drug concentrations due to the lower dose of BCNU. For similar reasons, the combination of oral Temozolomide plus O^6BG in the clinic has met with limited success in both adults and children with recurrent malignant glioma (Warren, Aikin et al. 2005; Quinn, Jiang et al. 2009). Since high concentration of a chemotherapeutic agent like BCNU can be achieved in tumor through intracavitary application with minimal systemic exposure, a recent phase II study at Duke University Medical center explored the use of O^6BG prior to implantation of Gliadel™ wafers with some improvement in survival (Quinn, Jiang et al. 2009). Although defective mismatch repair (MMR) is a putative mechanism for resistance to methylating agents like Temozolomide, very few human tumors exhibit MMR deficiency (Pollack, Hamilton et al. 2010). Alternatively, excessive base excision repair (BER) mediated by overexpression of the enzyme Poly (ADP- Ribose) Polymerase (PARP) is another resistance mechanism than can cause failure of Temozolomide therapy irrespective of AGAT expression (Palma, Wang et al. 2009). ABT-888 (Olgaparib™, Abbott Laboratories, Abbott Park, Illinois, USA) is a potent PARP inhibitor that has shown effective PARP depletion in tumors and restores sensitivity to Temozolomide (Palma, Rodriguez et al. 2008; Palma, Wang et al. 2009). It is currently undergoing evaluation in combination with Temozolomide in adults with malignant glioma and children with recurrent brain tumors.

6.2 Molecular characteristics and specific biologic therapies

The molecular characteristics of pediatric HGG is quite different from its adult counterpart. Isocitrate dehydrogenase (IDH) 1 and 2 mutations that characterize secondary GBM in adults are almost unknown in pediatric tumors (Yan, Parsons et al. 2009; Paugh, Qu et al. 2010). Focal PDGFR amplification is a common event as is chromosome 1q gain (Paugh, Qu et al. 2010). However, EGFR amplification, EGFR vIII mutation, and PTEN loss are less common (Bax, Gaspar et al. 2009; Paugh, Qu et al. 2010). Some of these molecular markers of disease have been chosen as targets for inhibition using small molecule protein kinase inhibitors including ZD1839 (Iressa™, Astra Zeneca Pharmaceuticals, New Jersey, USA) targeting EGFR and STI571 (Gleevec™, Novartis Pharmaceuticals, USA) the PDGF receptor (Pollack, Jakacki et al. 2007). It is likely that these small molecule inhibitors might have some indirect negative effect on tumor angiogenesis by affecting downstream targets that are involved in new blood vessel formation (Folkman 2007). Phase I trials of these two drugs have been completed in children with newly diagnosed and recurrent HGG (including diffuse pontine glioma) through the PBTC but no specific efficacy was observed with either drug (Pollack, Jakacki et al. 2007). Bevacizumab, a humanized monoclonal antibody against VEGF, recently gained approval by the FDA for treatment of GBM in adults on the basis of impressive responses and improvement in overall survival noted in adults with recurrent GBM treated with Bevacizumab alone or Bevacizumab plus CPT-11 (Cohen, Shen et al. 2009; Friedman, Prados et al. 2009). A PBTC phase II trial of this combination in children with recurrent malignant glioma and diffuse pontine glioma however failed to show efficacy in either tumor type (Gururangan, Chi et al. 2010). The reasons for the lack of efficacy of Bevacizumab in pediatric malignant gliomas are unknown. It is possible that VEGF is not the prime mediator of angiogenesis in these tumors. It is also likely that angiogenesis inhibition might be better if it is used in newly diagnosed patients and in the setting of minimal disease following initial surgical resection. The Children's Oncology Group is currently doing a phase III study exploring the efficacy of Bevacizumab, vorinostat (Zolinza™, Merck Pharmaceuticals, USA), a histone deacetylase inhibitor, or Temozolomide concurrently with radiotherapy followed by Bevacizumab plus Temozolomide for 6 months in children newly diagnosed malignant glioma (Fouladi M., Cincinnati, OH; 2011; personal communication). Since it is unlikely that these drugs will be efficacious as single agents, future studies will address whether small molecule protein kinase inhibitors can work additively or synergistically with cytotoxics, other kinase inhibitors, and anti-angiogenic agents.

7. Ependymoma

Ependymomas are the third most common CNS neoplasm and occur in about 10% of all children with brain tumors. The tumor typically arises from the neuroepithelial cells lining the ventricles. The incidence of ependymomas is inversely related to age, with the peak incidence occurring in children less than 6 years of age (Allen, Siffert et al. 1998). Over 90% of all childhood ependymomas are intracranial in location and less than 10% occur in the spinal cord. Of the intrancranial tumors, 66% are infratentorial (Figure 5) and 34% supratentorial in location. No specific risk factors are associated with ependymomas except for the increased frequency of spinal cord ependymomas in patients with neurofibromatosis type II. Ependymomas are soft and friable and grayish-red in appearance. Microscopically, they are extremely cellular with the tumor cells forming pseudo-rosettes around blood vessels. Specific histologic variants include the clear-cell, papillary, myxopapillary, and anaplastic (WHO grade III). About 20% of patients with ependymomas have metastatic spread of disease either at the time of diagnosis or relapse.

7.1 Treatment

The current standard of care for patients with non-metastatic ependymoma includes adequate surgical resection followed by focal radiotherapy to the tumor site. Patients who present with metastatic disease would require neuraxis irradiation as well. Complete surgical resection alone could cure a proportion of patients with grade II ependymoma arising in the cerebral hemispheres (Awaad, Allen et al. 1996). Extent of surgical resection is directly correlated with outcome and hence a complete resection should be attempted either at diagnosis or following initial cytotoxic therapy. Young children with disease confined to the infratentorial compartment especially in the cerebello-pontine angle are at high risk for post-surgical complications as the tumor encompasses blood vessels and cranial nerves in this region (Morris, Li et al. 2009). Aggressive surgery in inexperienced hands can result in severe dysphagia, vocal cord paralysis, and ataxia but is usually associated with neurologic recovery over a period of several months (Morris, Li et al. 2009). Focal radiotherapy is usually directed at the tumor bed (gross tumor volume, GTV) plus a 1-cm margin (clinical target volume, CTV) with additional corrections for day to day variations in patient positioning (planned target volume, PTV) (Merchant, Li et al. 2009).The dose of radiotherapy should be between 45-60 Gy with conventional fractionation and administered over 6 weeks (Merchant, Li et al. 2009). Proton, intensity-modulated, or 3-D conformal radiotherapy is being increasingly used to avoid injury to normal structures including hearing and cognition. Since the majority of recurrences are local, there is no specific advantage to using craniospinal radiotherapy in patients with non-metastatic disease including those with anaplastic histology (Taylor 2004). The use of

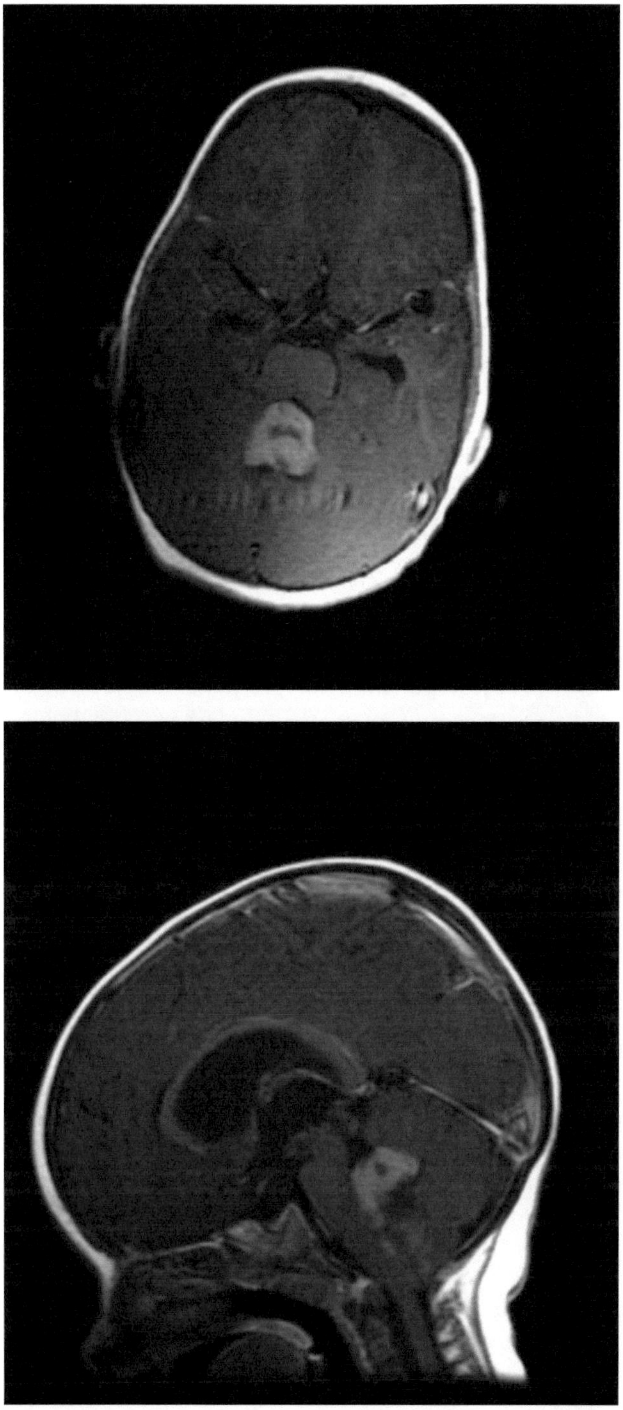

Fig. 5. T-1 weighted axial and sagittal images of the brain following gadolinium administration in a 15 month old boy showing a uniformly enhancing lesion within the fourth ventricle that on histology was found to be a well-differentiated ependymoma.

chemotherapy has been found to be ineffective in patients with ependymomas and might be explained partly by the over-expression of p-glycoprotein in over 80% of these tumors (Chou, Barquin et al. 1996; Bouffet and Foreman 1999). Currently, this modality is used mainly in infants (children < 4 years of age) in whom even focal radiotherapy to areas of the brain can have devastating consequences on neuro- cognitive function (Duffner, Horowitz et al. 1993). Platinum compounds (cisplatin or carboplatin) and cyclophosphamide are the most commonly used agents against ependymoma (Duffner, Horowitz et al. 1993; Bouffet and Foreman 1999). Although objective responses have been observed in some studies, outcome for those who receive chemotherapy plus irradiation is similar to those following radiotherapy alone. It is possible that chemotherapy can be used upfront in some children to allow for more radical second look surgery following tumor shrinkage. Survival for children with ependymoma is between 40-77% at 5 years post-treatment. Outcome for children with recurrent tumors remains poor despite salvage chemotherapy (Bouffet, Capra et al. 2009).

The most important prognostic factor in children with ependymoma is the extent of surgical resection. Patients who have inadequate tumor resection experience a worse outcome. Other poor prognostic factors include young age, infratentorial location of tumor, and avoidance of radiotherapy (Kilday, Rahman et al. 2009). Anaplastic tumors have been found to confer an independently worse prognosis in a recent meta-analysis of over 2000 patients (Rodriguez, Scheithauer et al. 2008) but not in other studies (Messahel, Ashley et al. 2009). It is possible that the impact of histopathology on prognosis might be dependent on the inter-observer differences in assessment of anaplasia amongst neuropathologists (Puget, Grill et al. 2009).

7.2 Molecular characteristics

It is also worth noting that about 50% of patients relapse after focal radiotherapy for localized grade II ependymoma following a gross total resection (Kilday, Rahman et al. 2009). It is clear that tumor biology plays an important part in determining prognosis in such apparently low-risk patients. Recent studies have noted that over-expression of ERBB-2/4 and nucleolin, gain of chromosome 1q, and homozygous deletion of the CDKN2A gene are associated with a worse prognosis independent of clinical factors (Gilbertson, Bentley et al. 2002; Kilday, Rahman et al. 2009; Puget, Grill et al. 2009). On the other hand, gains of chromosomes 9, 15q, and 18, and loss of chromosome 6 were associated with excellent survival. Such molecular alterations need to be validated in larger studies and might serve as targets for future novel biologic therapies and also facilitate identification of a group of patients who have a good prognosis who could be successfully managed with conservative treatment

8. Germ cell tumors

CNS germ cell tumors in children are rare and constitute about 2-5% of all pediatric brain tumors. Intracranial germ cell tumors are typically classified as either germinomas or non-germinomatous germ cell tumors (NGGCT). The former includes pure germinomas and germinomas with syncytiotrophoblastic cells and the latter yolk-sac tumors (secreting alpha-fetoprotein, AFP), choriocarcinomas (secreting beta subunit of human chorionic gonadotropins, β-HCG), embryonal carcinoma (secreting carcinoembryonic antigen, CEA), teratomas (mature and immature), and mixed germ cell tumors (including varying components of germinoma and NGGCT) (Rosenblum, Matsutani et al. 2000). The incidence of these tumors is higher in the Asian population (15-18% of all childhood brain tumors) compared to western countries (Rosenblum, Matsutani et al. 2000). The peak age of onset is 10-12 years of age and occasionally in the second to third decade of life (Rosenblum, Matsutani et al. 2000). There is a sex predilection for tumor site and histologic type with female predominance for tumors that originate in the suprasellar region and NGGCT. CNS germ cell tumors occur commonly in the pineal region (45%), suprasellar region (35%), both (10%), and other sites including intraventricular, basal ganglia, thalamus, medulla oblongata, and cerebral hemispheres (10%) (Rosenblum, Matsutani et al. 2000). Presentation of bifocal tumors is not uncommon and represents development of tumors in two independent sites and not metastasis (Figure 6). Presenting symptoms in patients with germ cell tumors depend on the location of tumor. Suprasellar germ cell tumors can present with isolated diabetes insipidus caused by pituitary stalk thickening, hydrocephalus, visual disturbances, delayed growth, or precocious puberty (Diez, Balmaceda et al. 1999; Rosenblum, Matsutani et al. 2000). Pineal tumors can cause hydrocephalus due to early compression of the aqueduct and paralysis of upward gaze and convergence due to pressure on the tectum of the mid-brain (Parinaud's syndrome). Leptomeningeal seeding occurs in about 10-15% of patients and can cause symptoms of spinal cord compression due to block disease (Diez, Balmaceda et al. 1999). It is important to remember that patients with germinoma can have isolated cerebrospinal fluid positivity for malignant cells without any evidence of spinal cord dissemination on neuroimaging.

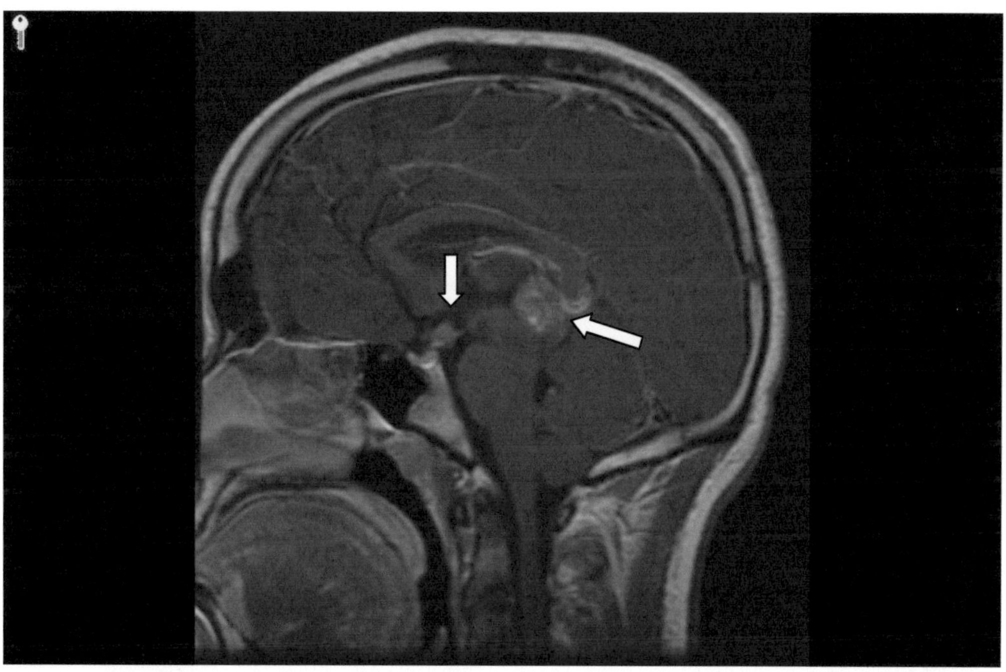

Fig. 6. T-1 weighted sagittal image of the brain following gadolinium in an 18-year old black male showing enhancing lesions in the suprasellar and pineal region (white arrows) that was found to be a pure germinoma on biopsy of the pineal mass

Histologically, germinoma consists of a uniform sheet of cells that have vesicular nuclei, prominent nucleoli, and a glycogen-rich cytoplasm. Additional features include lymphocytic infiltration, and scattered syncytiotrophoblastic cells (Rosenblum, Matsutani et al. 2000). Teratomas recapitulate somatic development from the three embryonic germ layers with mature forms demonstrating adult tissue including cartilage, bone, and teeth and the immature variety composed of primitive neuro-epithelial cells arranged in an abortive formation of neural tubes (Rosenblum, Matsutani et al. 2000). Yolk-sac tumors are composed of primitive appearing epithelial cells in a loose myxoid matrix and eosinophilic hyaline globules immunoreactive for AFP (Rosenblum, Matsutani et al. 2000). The histologic diagnosis of a choriocarcinoma requires the identification of cytotrophoblastic and syncytiotrophoblastic giant cells that are positive for beta-HCG and human placental lactogen (Rosenblum, Matsutani et al. 2000). Embryonal carcinoma consists of large cells that proliferate in nests and sheets, forming abortive papillae and embryoid bodies with germinal discs and miniature amniotic cavities, large nucleoli, and high mitotic index. The cells are positive for cytokeratin and human placental alkaline phosphatase (Rosenblum, Matsutani et al. 2000).

In addition to neuro-imaging studies and biopsy confirmation, patients with intracranial germ cell tumors usually have serum and CSF estimated for protein markers including AFP and beta-HCG, for diagnosis and assessment of tumor response (Gregory and Finlay 1999). If the markers are elevated in CSF samples, diagnosis can be made and treatment initiated without the need for a biopsy (Gregory and Finlay 1999).

8.1 Treatment

The standard treatment for patients with pure germinoma is radiotherapy (Diez, Balmaceda et al. 1999). This tumor is exquisitely sensitive to irradiation and excellent survival has been obtained with this modality alone. Germinomas typically spread via the ventricular wall and it is extremely important to include the whole ventricular volume (radiotherapy dose up to 24 Gy) in addition to the primary site (up to 45 Gy) in the radiation field for patients with localized disease and the craniospinal axis (up to 24 Gy) in those with metastatic disease (Diez, Balmaceda et al. 1999). The use of 3-D conformal radiotherapy technique can minimize long-term side effects of irradiation (Diez, Balmaceda et al. 1999). Using this strategy, cure can be achieved in over 90% of these patients (Diez, Balmaceda et al. 1999). Germinoma is very responsive to chemotherapy as well with excellent objective responses (>90%)reported with single agent cyclophosphamide or carboplatin (Diez, Balmaceda et al. 1999). In recent years there have been several clinical trials in the United States, Japan, and Europe that have attempted to use chemotherapy combinations (carboplatin + etoposide, carboplatin + etoposide + bleomycin ± cyclophosphamide, or ifosfamide + carboplatin + etoposide) with the aim of avoiding or reducing the dose and extent of radiotherapy and its associated neuro-psychologic sequelae on the brain. This strategy has been reasonably successful although the progression-free survival with chemotherapy alone is only 50-60% (Diez, Balmaceda et al. 1999). However, most of the patients who fail chemotherapy can be salvaged with radiotherapy underscoring the importance of the latter modality in the cure of patients with germinoma. While some series have indicated that patients with germinoma with beta-HCG elevation up to 50 I.U have an inferior outcome, recent reports have demonstrated that with adequate doses of radiotherapy these patients do just as well as those with pure germinoma (Shibamoto, Takahashi et al. 1997). It must be emphasized that the use of chemotherapy alone in patients with germinoma is effective in only a proportion of patients and is not the standard of care (Diez, Balmaceda et al. 1999). Only large randomized trials of standard radiotherapy alone *vs.* chemotherapy plus reduced dose irradiation will clearly establish the efficacy of chemotherapy in safely allowing dose and field reductions in radiotherapy and whether patients who receive the chemotherapy plus reduced dose irradiation will have fewer neuro-cognitive deficits.

Patients with NGGCT do very poorly with radiotherapy alone with only 20-60% surviving progression-free with this modality alone (Diez, Balmaceda et al. 1999). The addition of chemotherapy as used for patients with germinoma has improved the survival to around 45 - 80% (Diez, Balmaceda et al. 1999). Patients with recurrent germ cell tumors have a poor prognosis. A proportion of patients with chemo sensitive disease have been salvaged with high-dose chemotherapy and autologous stem cell rescue (Modak, Gardner et al. 1997; Tada, Takizawa et al. 1999).

9. Choroid plexus tumors

Choroid plexus tumors are rare in children and comprise 2-4% of brain tumors in this population (Greenberg 1999) Choroid plexus tumors can either be a choroid plexus papilloma (60% - 80%) or carcinoma (20% -40%).(Greenberg 1999). The predominant location of these tumors is in the lateral ventricles and less commonly in the III and IV ventricles. Choroid plexus tumors that occur in the lateral ventricles are invariably found in infants or young children with a median age of diagnosis of 24 months (Greenberg 1999). These tumors typically arise from the choroid plexus epithelium and are extremely vascular. The histologic findings in a choroid plexus papilloma include a papillomatous component lined by single layer of columnar or cuboidal epithelium and a central core of vascular stromal tissue and the absence of mitosis and normal tissue invasion. In contrast, choroid plexus carcinoma consists of sheets of cells without papillary formation, nuclear atypia and pleomorphism, frequent mitoses, and invasion of sub ependymal brain tissue. Children with choroid plexus tumors frequently present with hydrocephalus due to mechanical obstruction and/or CSF overproduction (Figure 7) (Greenberg 1999). Up to 30% of children present with metastatic disease at diagnosis.

9.1 Treatment

Surgical resection of choroid plexus papilloma frequently results in long-term cure (Greenberg 1999). The management of choroid plexus carcinoma is more complex. While adequate surgical resection is the most important determinant of long-term disease control, tumors can be extremely large and vascular at diagnosis precluding adequate resection without causing excessive blood loss or neurologic damage (Greenberg 1999). In these situations, it might be more beneficial to confirm the diagnosis on a limited stereotactic biopsy and treat patients with chemotherapy prior to definitive surgical resection (Greenberg 1999). The standard chemotherapy regimen used in infants and young includes vincristine, cisplatin/carboplatin, cyclophosphamide, and etoposide and can be used in a neoadjuvant or adjuvant setting (Greenberg 1999).

The efficacy of post-operative radiotherapy in patients with choroid plexus carcinoma is unclear (Greenberg 1999; Fitzpatrick, Aronson et al. 2002). The need for craniospinal irradiation for this disease with a high predilection for neuraxis dissemination argues against the use of this modality in young children due to the risk of neuro-cognitive deficits and endocrine sequelae. In general, it appears that the degree of surgical resection seems to determine the outcome of patients with choroid plexus carcinoma irrespective of the adjuvant chemo/radiotherapy received post-surgery (Fitzpatrick, Aronson et al. 2002)

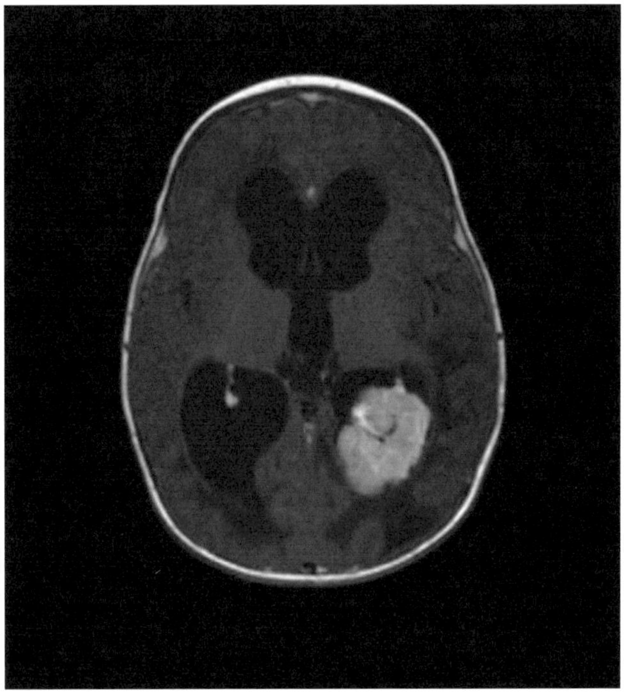

Fig. 7. T-1 weighted axial image of the brain following gadolinium in a 4-month old male showing a large uniformly enhancing lesion in the left occipital horn that on biopsy was found to be a choroid plexus papilloma with some features of anaplasia

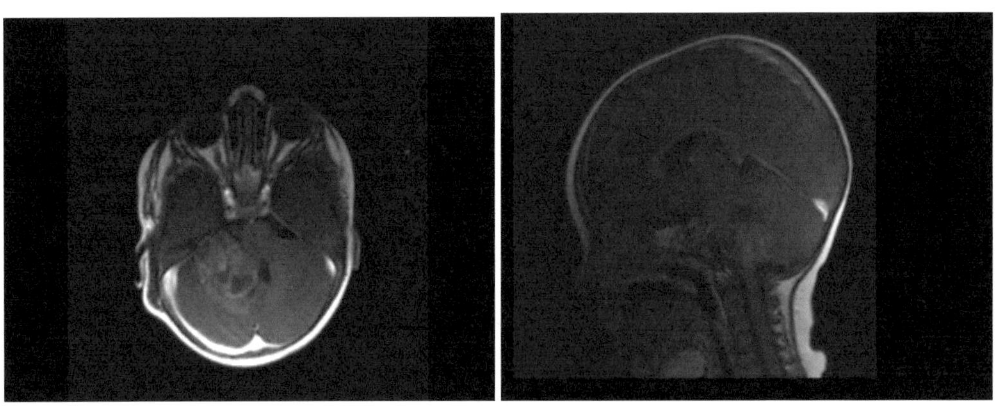

Fig. 8. T-1 weighted axial and saggital images following gadolinium contrast in a 4 month old white male showing a heterogeneously enhancing cystic solid mass in the region of the right foramen of Lushka and cerebello-pontine angle causing mass effect on the brain stem and IV ventricle. Tumor resection revealed an atypical teratoid rhabdoid tumor

10. Atypical teratoid rhabdoid tumors

Atypical Teratoid Rhabdoid tumor (ATRT) of the CNS is a rare embryonal tumor that occurs predominantly in children less than 5 years of age (Rorke, Packer et al. 1996; Oka and Scheithauer 1999). Originally described in 1987, this tumor, in the past, had been mistaken for and treated as a PNET of the nervous system (Packer, Biegel et al. 2002). In recent years, there has been an explosion in knowledge regarding criteria for histologic diagnosis and molecular characteristics of the tumor (Packer, Biegel et al. 2002). ATRT constitutes 1-2% of CNS malignancies in children with a reported incidence of 1.38 per 100,000 children/year (Woehrer, Slavc et al. 2010). The tumors can occasionally be familial due to a rhabdoid tumor predisposition syndrome (Janson, Nedzi et al. 2006). The median age at diagnosis is 2.1 years and 90% of patients are less than 5 years at diagnosis (Oka and Scheithauer 1999). Less than 10% of patients are in older children up to the ages of 10-15 years (Oka and Scheithauer 1999) (figure 8). The commonest location is in the posterior fossa in over 60% of cases; other sites include the cerebral hemispheres, suprasellar region, third ventricle, pineal region, and spinal cord (Rorke, Packer et al. 1996; Oka and Scheithauer 1999). There is a high predilection for CSF dissemination in about 30% of cases (Oka and Scheithauer 1999). Histologically the tumor consists of sheets of rhabdoid cells, areas that resemble classic PNET along with mesenchymal and epithelial differentiation (Rorke, Packer et al. 1996). The rhabdoid cell has an eccentric round nucleus, prominent nucleolus, and a plump cell body. Immunohistochemical staining is positive for vimentin, cytokeratin, and epithelial membrane antigen. Staining for INI-1 gene product can be done using the BAF-47 antibody and absence of INI-1 expression in the nucleus is confirmatory for the presence of ATRT.

10.1 Treatment

Treatment of ATRT has traditionally been surgical resection followed by intensive chemotherapy and irradiation. However, most infants with ATRT have been reported to succumb to the disease with progression-free survival of < 20% despite treatment. However, a recent study from Dana Farber Cancer Institute in Boston, MA, has reported a more favorable outcome of 53% 2-year PFS with intensive chemotherapy plus irradiation in young children with ATRT (Chi, Zimmerman et al. 2009). Older patients with ATRT seem to do better than infants with the same intensive multimodality treatment (Tekautz, Fuller et al. 2005).

10.2 Molecular characteristics and biologic therapies

The molecular characteristic of this tumor has been well delineated in recent years. The tumor typically demonstrates monosomy of chromosome 22 that results in deletion of the tumor suppressor gene HSN5-INI1 located on chromosome 22q11.2 (Biegel, Kalpana et al. 2002). Robust pre-clinical models have clearly demonstrated that deletion of the HSN5-INI1 gene is directly responsible for tumor development and restoration of the gene in the tumor cells can cause tumor regression. INI1 mediates tumor suppression by recruiting HDAC to the cyclin D-1 promoter and preventing cyclin D1 expression (Tsikitis, Zhang et al. 2005). Cyclin D-1 overexpression is commonly seen in CNS ATRTs and the combination of Fenretinide plus Tamoxifen has been shown to synergistically down regulate cyclin D-1 expression and cause tumor regression in animals bearing ATRT xenografts (Alarcon-Vargas, Zhang et al. 2006). It remains to be seen if this strategy would work in children with CNS ATRT.

11. References

Alarcon-Vargas, D., Z. Zhang, et al. (2006). "Targeting cyclin D1, a downstream effector of INI1/hSNF5, in rhabdoid tumors." Oncogene 25(5): 722-734.

Allen, J. C., J. Siffert, et al. (1998). "Clinical manifestations of childhood ependymoma: a multitude of syndromes." Pediatr Neurosurg 28(1): 49-55.

Ater, J., E. Holmes, et al. (2008). "Results of COG Protocol A9952: A Randomized Phase 3 study of two chemotherapy regimens for incompletely resected low-grade glioma in young children (LGG 18)." Neuro-oncology: 451.

Awaad, Y. M., J. C. Allen, et al. (1996). "Deferring adjuvant therapy for totally resected intracranial ependymoma." Pediatric neurology 14(3): 216-219.

Bai, R., I. M. Siu, et al. (2010). "Evaluation of retinoic acid therapy for OTX2-positive medulloblastomas." Neuro-oncology.

Baldwin, R. T. and S. Preston-Martin (2004). "Epidemiology of brain tumors in childhood--a review." Toxicology and applied pharmacology 199(2): 118-131.

Bax, D. A., N. Gaspar, et al. (2009). "EGFRvIII deletion mutations in pediatric high-grade glioma and response to targeted therapy in pediatric glioma cell lines." Clinical cancer research : an official journal of the American Association for Cancer Research 15(18): 5753-5761.

Berger, M. S., M. S. Edwards, et al. (1983). "Primary cerebral neuroblastoma. Long-term follow-up review and therapeutic guidelines." Journal of neurosurgery 59(3): 418-423.

Biegel, J. A., G. Kalpana, et al. (2002). "The role of INI1 and the SWI/SNF complex in the development of rhabdoid tumors: meeting summary from the workshop on childhood atypical teratoid/rhabdoid tumors." Cancer research 62(1): 323-328.

Bleyer, W. A. (1999). "Epidemiologic impact of children with brain tumors." Childs Nerv Syst 15(11-12): 758-763.

Boehm, T., J. Folkman, et al. (1997). "Antiangiogenic therapy of experimental cancer does not induce acquired drug resistance." Nature 390(6658): 404-407.

Bouffet, E., M. Capra, et al. (2009). "Salvage chemotherapy for metastatic and recurrent ependymoma of childhood." Child's nervous system : ChNS : official journal of the International Society for Pediatric Neurosurgery 25(10): 1293-1301.

Bouffet, E. and N. Foreman (1999). "Chemotherapy for intracranial ependymomas." Child's nervous system : ChNS : official journal of the International Society for Pediatric Neurosurgery 15(10): 563-570.

Bouffet, E., R. Jakacki, et al. (2008). "Phase II study of weekly vinblastine in recurrent/refractory pediatric low-grade gliomas (abstr# LGG13)." Neuro-Oncology: 450.

Bredel, M. (2001). "Anticancer drug resistance in primary human brain tumors." Brain Res Brain Res Rev 35(2): 161-204.

Brem, H., S. Piantadosi, et al. (1995). "Placebo-controlled trial of safety and efficacy of intraoperative controlled delivery by biodegradable polymers of chemotherapy for recurrent gliomas. The Polymer-brain Tumor Treatment Group." Lancet 345(8956): 1008-1012.

Burger, P. C., B. W. Scheithauer, et al. (2000). Pilocytic Astrocytoma. Pathology &Genetics: Tumors of the Nervous System. P. Kleihues and W. K. Cavenee. Lyon, IARC Press: 45-51.

CBTRUS. (2009). "CBTRUS (2009). CBTRUS Statistical Report: Primary Brain and Central Nervous System Tumors Diagnosed in the United States in 2004-2005. Source: Central Brain Tumor Registry of the United States, Hinsdale, IL." from www.cbtrus.org.

Chi, S. N., M. A. Zimmerman, et al. (2009). "Intensive multimodality treatment for children with newly diagnosed CNS atypical teratoid rhabdoid tumor." Journal of clinical oncology : official journal of the American Society of Clinical Oncology 27(3): 385-389.

Chintagumpala, M., T. Hassall, et al. (2009). "A pilot study of risk-adapted radiotherapy and chemotherapy in patients with supratentorial PNET." Neuro-oncology 11(1): 33-40.

Chou, P. M., N. Barquin, et al. (1996). "Ependymomas in children express the multidrug resistance gene: immunohistochemical and molecular biologic study." Pediatr Pathol Lab Med 16(4): 551-561.

Cohen, K. J., R. L. Heideman, et al. (2011). "Temozolomide in the treatment of children with newly diagnosed diffuse intrinsic pontine gliomas: a report from the Children's Oncology Group." Neuro-oncology 13(4): 410-416.

Cohen, K. J., I. F. Pollack, et al. (2011). "Temozolomide in the treatment of high-grade gliomas in children: a report from the Children's Oncology Group." Neuro-oncology 13(3): 317-323.

Cohen, M. H., J. R. Johnson, et al. (2005). "Food and Drug Administration Drug approval summary: temozolomide plus radiation therapy for the treatment of newly diagnosed glioblastoma multiforme." Clinical cancer research : an official journal of the American Association for Cancer Research 11(19 Pt 1): 6767-6771.

Cohen, M. H., Y. L. Shen, et al. (2009). "FDA drug approval summary: bevacizumab (Avastin) as treatment of recurrent glioblastoma multiforme." The oncologist 14(11): 1131-1138.

Dai, A. I., J. W. Backstrom, et al. (2003). "Supratentorial primitive neuroectodermal tumors of infancy: clinical and radiologic findings." Pediatric neurology 29(5): 430-434.

De Vos, M., B. E. Hayward, et al. (2006). "PMS2 mutations in childhood cancer." Journal of the National Cancer Institute 98(5): 358-361.

Di, C., S. Liao, et al. (2005). "Identification of OTX2 as a medulloblastoma oncogene whose product can be targeted by all-trans retinoic acid." Cancer research 65(3): 919-924.

Diez, B., C. Balmaceda, et al. (1999). "Germ cell tumors of the CNS in children: recent advances in therapy." Childs Nerv Syst 15(10): 578-585.

Dolan, M. E. and A. E. Pegg (1997). "O6-benzylguanine and its role in chemotherapy." Clin Cancer Res 3(6): 837-847.

Dougherty, M. J., M. Santi, et al. (2010). "Activating mutations in BRAF characterize a spectrum of pediatric low-grade gliomas." Neuro-oncology.

Duffner, P. K., M. E. Horowitz, et al. (1993). "Postoperative chemotherapy and delayed radiation in children less than three years of age with malignant brain tumors." N Engl J Med 328(24): 1725-1731.

Dunkel, I. J., J. M. Boyett, et al. (1998). "High-dose carboplatin, thiotepa, and etoposide with autologous stem- cell rescue for patients with recurrent medulloblastoma. Children's Cancer Group." J Clin Oncol 16(1): 222-228.

Engelhard, H. H. (2000). Brain Tumors and the blood brain barrier. Neuro-Oncology, The essentials. M. S. Berger and M. Bernstein. New York, NY, Thieme Publishers.

Englehard, H. H. and D. G. Groothuis (1999). The Blood-Brain barrier: Structure, Function, and response to neoplasia. The Gliomas. M. S. Berger and C. B. Wilson. Philadelphia, PA, W.B. Saunders Company: 115-120.

Finlay, J. L., J. M. Boyett, et al. (1995). "Randomized phase III trial in childhood high-grade astrocytoma comparing vincristine, lomustine, and prednisone with the eight-drugs- in-1-day regimen. Childrens Cancer Group." J Clin Oncol 13(1): 112-123.

Fitzpatrick, L. K., L. J. Aronson, et al. (2002). "Is there a requirement for adjuvant therapy for choroid plexus carcinoma that has been completely resected?" J Neurooncol 57(2): 123-126.

Folkman, J. (2007). "Angiogenesis: an organizing principle for drug discovery?" Nature reviews. Drug discovery 6(4): 273-286.

Freeman, C. R., R. E. Taylor, et al. (2002). "Radiotherapy for medulloblastoma in children: a perspective on current international clinical research efforts." Med Pediatr Oncol 39(2): 99-108.

Friedman, H. S., J. P. Krischer, et al. (1992). "Treatment of children with progressive or recurrent brain tumors with carboplatin or iproplatin: a Pediatric Oncology Group randomized phase II study." J Clin Oncol 10(2): 249-256.

Friedman, H. S., R. E. McLendon, et al. (1998). "DNA mismatch repair and O6-alkylguanine-DNA alkyltransferase analysis and response to Temodal in newly diagnosed malignant glioma." J Clin Oncol 16(12): 3851-3857.

Friedman, H. S., J. Pluda, et al. (2000). "Phase I trial of carmustine plus O6-benzylguanine for patients with recurrent or progressive malignant glioma." J Clin Oncol 18(20): 3522-3528.

Friedman, H. S., M. D. Prados, et al. (2009). "Bevacizumab alone and in combination with irinotecan in recurrent glioblastoma." Journal of clinical oncology : official journal of the American Society of Clinical Oncology 27(28): 4733-4740.

Gajjar, A., M. Chintagumpala, et al. (2006). "Risk-adapted craniospinal radiotherapy followed by high-dose chemotherapy and stem-cell rescue in children with newly diagnosed medulloblastoma (St Jude Medulloblastoma-96): long-term results from a prospective, multicentre trial." Lancet Oncol 7(10): 813-820.

Giangaspero, F., S. H. Bigner, et al. (2000). Medulloblastoma. Pathlogy & Genetics Tumors of the Nervous System. P. Kleihues and W. K. Cavenee. Lyon, IARC Press: 129-137.

Giangaspero, F., G. Perilongo, et al. (1999). "Medulloblastoma with extensive nodularity: a variant with favorable prognosis." J Neurosurg 91(6): 971-977.

Gilbert, M. R., H. S. Friedman, et al. (2002). "A phase II study of temozolomide in patients with newly diagnosed supratentorial malignant glioma before radiation therapy." Neuro-oncol 4(4): 261-267.

Gilbertson, R. J. (2004). "Medulloblastoma: signalling a change in treatment." Lancet Oncol 5(4): 209-218.

Gilbertson, R. J., L. Bentley, et al. (2002). "ERBB receptor signaling promotes ependymoma cell proliferation and represents a potential novel therapeutic target for this disease." Clin Cancer Res 8(10): 3054-3064.

Greenberg, M. L. (1999). "Chemotherapy of choroid plexus carcinoma." Childs Nerv Syst 15(10): 571-577.

Gregory, J. J., Jr. and J. L. Finlay (1999). "Alpha-fetoprotein and beta-human chorionic gonadotropin: their clinical significance as tumour markers." Drugs 57(4): 463-467.

Groothuis, D. R. (2000). "The blood-brain and blood-tumor barriers: a review of strategies for increasing drug delivery." Neuro-oncol 2(1): 45-59.

Gurney, J. G., M. A. Smith, et al. (1999). CNS and miscellaneous intracranial and intraspinal neoplasms. Bethesda, MD, National Cancer Institute.

Guruangan, S., I. J. Dunkel, et al. (1998). "Myeloablative chemotherapy with autologous bone marrow rescue in young children with recurrent malignant brain tumors." J Clin Oncol 16(7): 2486-2493.

Gururangan, S., C. M. Cavazos, et al. (2002). "Phase II study of carboplatin in children with progressive low-grade gliomas." J Clin Oncol 20(13): 2951-2958.

Gururangan, S., S. N. Chi, et al. (2010). "Lack of efficacy of bevacizumab plus irinotecan in children with recurrent malignant glioma and diffuse brainstem glioma: a Pediatric Brain Tumor Consortium study." Journal of clinical oncology : official journal of the American Society of Clinical Oncology 28(18): 3069-3075.

Gururangan, S., T. Driscoll, et al. (2008). "A Retrospective Study of High-dose Chemotherapy (HDC) With Autologous Stem Cell Rescue (ASCR) in Children and Adults with Supratentorial Primitive Neuroectodermal Tumors (S-PNET): The Duke Experience 1991-2004 (Abstr# PNET-MED 3)." Neuro-oncology: 476.

Gururangan, S., M. J. Fisher, et al. (2007). "Temozolomide in children with progressive low-grade glioma." Neuro-oncology 9(2): 161-168.

Gururangan, S. and H. S. Friedman (2002). "Innovations in design and delivery of chemotherapy for brain tumors." Neuroimaging Clin N Am 12(4): 583-597.

Gururangan, S. and H. S. Friedman (2004). "Recent advances in the treatment of pediatric brain tumors." Oncology 18(13): 1649-1661; discussion 1662, 1665-1646, 1668.

Gururangan, S., J. Krauser, et al. (2008). "Efficacy of high-dose chemotherapy or standard salvage therapy in patients with recurrent medulloblastoma." Neuro Oncol 10(5): 745-751.

Gururangan, S., C. McLaughlin, et al. (2003). "High-dose chemotherapy with autologous stem-cell rescue in children and adults with newly diagnosed pineoblastomas." J Clin Oncol 21(11): 2187-2191.

Hader, W. J., K. Drovini-Zis, et al. (2003). "Primitive neuroectodermal tumors in the central nervous system following cranial irradiation: a report of four cases." Cancer 97(4): 1072-1076.

Hallahan, A. R., J. I. Pritchard, et al. (2003). "BMP-2 mediates retinoid-induced apoptosis in medulloblastoma cells through a paracrine effect." Nat Med 9(8): 1033-1038.

Hanahan, D. and J. Folkman (1996). "Patterns and emerging mechanisms of the angiogenic switch during tumorigenesis." Cell 86(3): 353-364.

Huang, H., J. Held-Feindt, et al. (2005). "Expression of VEGF and its receptors in different brain tumors." Neurological research 27(4): 371-377.

Jakacki, R. I. (1999). "Pineal and nonpineal supratentorial primitive neuroectodermal tumors." Childs Nerv Syst 15(10): 586-591.

Janson, K., L. A. Nedzi, et al. (2006). "Predisposition to atypical teratoid/rhabdoid tumor due to an inherited INI1 mutation." Pediatric blood & cancer 47(3): 279-284.

Jennings, M. T., N. Slatkin, et al. (1993). "Neoplastic meningitis as the presentation of occult primitive neuroectodermal tumors." Journal of child neurology 8(4): 306-312.

Kerbel, R. S. (2008). "Tumor angiogenesis." The New England journal of medicine 358(19): 2039-2049.

Kerbel, R. S., A. Viloria-Petit, et al. (2000). "'Accidental' anti-angiogenic drugs. anti-oncogene directed signal transduction inhibitors and conventional chemotherapeutic agents as examples." Eur J Cancer 36(10): 1248-1257.

Kilday, J. P., R. Rahman, et al. (2009). "Pediatric ependymoma: biological perspectives." Molecular cancer research : MCR 7(6): 765-786.

Kim, K. J., B. Li, et al. (1993). "Inhibition of vascular endothelial growth factor-induced angiogenesis suppresses tumour growth in vivo." Nature 362(6423): 841-844.

Kolb, E. A., R. Gorlick, et al. (2010). "Initial testing (stage 1) of AZD6244 (ARRY-142886) by the Pediatric Preclinical Testing Program." Pediatric blood & cancer 55(4): 668-677.

Kunwar, S. (2003). "Convection enhanced delivery of IL13-PE38QQR for treatment of recurrent malignant glioma: presentation of interim findings from ongoing phase 1 studies." Acta Neurochir Suppl 88: 105-111.

Kunwar, S., S. Chang, et al. (2010). "Phase III randomized trial of CED of IL13-PE38QQR vs Gliadel wafers for recurrent glioblastoma." Neuro-oncology 12(8): 871-881.

Kunwar, S., M. D. Prados, et al. (2007). "Direct intracerebral delivery of cintredekin besudotox (IL13-PE38QQR) in recurrent malignant glioma: a report by the Cintredekin Besudotox Intraparenchymal Study Group." Journal of clinical oncology : official journal of the American Society of Clinical Oncology 25(7): 837-844.

Kuo, D. J., H. L. Weiner, et al. (2003). "Temozolomide is active in childhood, progressive, unresectable, low-grade gliomas." J Pediatr Hematol Oncol 25(5): 372-378.

Lashford, L. S., P. Thiesse, et al. (2002). "Temozolomide in malignant gliomas of childhood: a United Kingdom Children's Cancer Study Group and French Society for Pediatric Oncology Intergroup Study." J Clin Oncol 20(24): 4684-4691.

Leonard, J. R., D. X. Cai, et al. (2001). "Large cell/anaplastic medulloblastomas and medullomyoblastomas: clinicopathological and genetic features." J Neurosurg 95: 82-88.

Leung, S. Y., A. S. Chan, et al. (1997). "Expression of vascular endothelial growth factor and its receptors in pilocytic astrocytoma." The American journal of surgical pathology 21(8): 941-950.

Li, M. H., E. Bouffet, et al. (2005). "Molecular genetics of supratentorial primitive neuroectodermal tumors and pineoblastoma." Neurosurgical focus 19(5): E3.

Li, V. W., R. D. Folkerth, et al. (1994). "Microvessel count and cerebrospinal fluid basic fibroblast growth factor in children with brain tumours." Lancet 344(8915): 82-86.

Louis, D. N., H. Ohgaki, et al. (2007). "The 2007 WHO classification of tumours of the central nervous system." Acta neuropathologica 114(2): 97-109.

MacDonald, T. J., K. M. Brown, et al. (2001). "Expression profiling of medulloblastoma: PDGFRA and the RAS/MAPK pathway as therapeutic targets for metastatic disease." Nat Genet 29(2): 143-152.

Mandell, L. R., R. Kadota, et al. (1999). "There is no role for hyperfractionated radiotherapy in the management of children with newly diagnosed diffuse intrinsic brainstem tumors: results of a Pediatric Oncology Group phase III trial comparing conventional vs. hyperfractionated radiotherapy." Int J Radiat Oncol Biol Phys 43(5): 959-964.

Mason, W. P., A. Grovas, et al. (1998). "Intensive chemotherapy and bone marrow rescue for young children with newly diagnosed malignant brain tumors." J Clin Oncol 16(1): 210-221.

Mclendon, R. E., D. S. Enterline, et al. (1998). Tumors of central neuroepithelial origin. Russell & Rubinstein's Pathology of Tumors of the Nervous System. D. D. Bigner, R. E. McLendon and J. M. Bruner. London, Arnold. I: 308-571.

Merchant, T. E., L. Happersett, et al. (1999). "Preliminary results of conformal radiation therapy for medulloblastoma." Neuro-oncol 1(3): 177-187.

Merchant, T. E., C. Li, et al. (2009). "Conformal radiotherapy after surgery for paediatric ependymoma: a prospective study." The lancet oncology 10(3): 258-266.

Messahel, B., S. Ashley, et al. (2009). "Relapsed intracranial ependymoma in children in the UK: patterns of relapse, survival and therapeutic outcome." European journal of cancer 45(10): 1815-1823.

Modak, S., S. Gardner, et al. (1997). High dose chemotherapy with autologous stem cell rescue in patients with recurrent central nervous system germ cell tumors. Childhood Cancer into the 21st century: An international conference to mark the 20th anniversary of the UKCCSG,, London, United Kingdom.

Morris, E. B., C. Li, et al. (2009). "Evolution of neurological impairment in pediatric infratentorial ependymoma patients." Journal of neuro-oncology 94(3): 391-398.

Neglia, J. P., A. T. Meadows, et al. (1991). "Second neoplasms after acute lymphoblastic leukemia in childhood." The New England journal of medicine 325(19): 1330-1336.

Northcott, P. A., A. Korshunov, et al. (2010). "Medulloblastoma Comprises Four Distinct Molecular Variants." J Clin Oncol.

Oka, H. and B. W. Scheithauer (1999). "Clinicopathological characteristics of atypical teratoid/rhabdoid tumor." Neurologia medico-chirurgica 39(7): 510-517; discussion 517-518.

Packer, R. J., J. Ater, et al. (1997). "Carboplatin and vincristine chemotherapy for children with newly diagnosed progressive low-grade gliomas." Journal of neurosurgery 86(5): 747-754.

Packer, R. J., J. A. Biegel, et al. (2002). "Atypical teratoid/rhabdoid tumor of the central nervous system: report on workshop." Journal of pediatric hematology/oncology : official journal of the American Society of Pediatric Hematology/Oncology 24(5): 337-342.

Packer, R. J., P. Cogen, et al. (1999). "Medulloblastoma: clinical and biologic aspects." Neuro-oncol 1(3): 232-250.

Packer, R. J., R. Jakacki, et al. (2009). "Objective response of multiply recurrent low-grade gliomas to bevacizumab and irinotecan." Pediatric blood & cancer 52(7): 791-795.

Palma, J. P., L. E. Rodriguez, et al. (2008). "The PARP inhibitor, ABT-888 potentiates temozolomide: correlation with drug levels and reduction in PARP activity in vivo." Anticancer Res 28(5A): 2625-2635.

Palma, J. P., Y. C. Wang, et al. (2009). "ABT-888 confers broad in vivo activity in combination with temozolomide in diverse tumors." Clin Cancer Res 15(23): 7277-7290.

Paugh, B. S., C. Qu, et al. (2010). "Integrated molecular genetic profiling of pediatric high-grade gliomas reveals key differences with the adult disease." Journal of clinical oncology : official journal of the American Society of Clinical Oncology 28(18): 3061-3068.

Paulino, A. C. (1999). "Trilateral retinoblastoma: is the location of the intracranial tumor important?" Cancer 86(1): 135-141.

Pfister, S., W. G. Janzarik, et al. (2008). "BRAF gene duplication constitutes a mechanism of MAPK pathway activation in low-grade astrocytomas." The Journal of clinical investigation 118(5): 1739-1749.

Pollack, I. F., R. L. Hamilton, et al. (2010). "Mismatch repair deficiency is an uncommon mechanism of alkylator resistance in pediatric malignant gliomas: a report from the Children's Oncology Group." Pediatric blood & cancer 55(6): 1066-1071.

Pollack, I. F., R. I. Jakacki, et al. (2007). "Phase I trial of imatinib in children with newly diagnosed brainstem and recurrent malignant gliomas: a Pediatric Brain Tumor Consortium report." Neuro-oncology 9(2): 145-160.

Pomeroy, S. L., P. Tamayo, et al. (2002). "Prediction of central nervous system embryonal tumour outcome based on gene expression." Nature 415(6870): 436-442.

Prados, M. D., M. S. Edwards, et al. (1997). "Treatment of pediatric low-grade gliomas with a nitrosourea-based multiagent chemotherapy regimen." J Neurooncol 32(3): 235-241.

Preston-Martin, S., J. M. Pogoda, et al. (1996). "Maternal consumption of cured meats and vitamins in relation to pediatric brain tumors." Cancer epidemiology, biomarkers & prevention : a publication of the American Association for Cancer Research, cosponsored by the American Society of Preventive Oncology 5(8): 599-605.

Puget, S., J. Grill, et al. (2009). "Candidate genes on chromosome 9q33-34 involved in the progression of childhood ependymomas." Journal of clinical oncology : official journal of the American Society of Clinical Oncology 27(11): 1884-1892.

Quinn, J. A., M. E. Dolan, et al. (2001). "Phase II Trial of BCNU plus O6-benzylguanine for patients with recurrent or progressive malignant glioma (abstr # 251)." Proc Am Assoc Clin Oncol 20: 64a.

Quinn, J. A., S. X. Jiang, et al. (2009). "Phase II trial of Gliadel plus O6-benzylguanine in adults with recurrent glioblastoma multiforme." Clinical cancer research : an official journal of the American Association for Cancer Research 15(3): 1064-1068.

Quinn, J. A., S. X. Jiang, et al. (2009). "Phase II trial of temozolomide (TMZ) plus irinotecan (CPT-11) in adults with newly diagnosed glioblastoma multiforme before radiotherapy." J Neurooncol 95(3): 393-400.

Quinn, J. A., S. X. Jiang, et al. (2009). "Phase I trial of temozolomide plus O6-benzylguanine 5-day regimen with recurrent malignant glioma." Neuro-oncology 11(5): 556-561.

Quinn, J. A., D. A. Reardon, et al. (2003). "Phase II trial of temozolomide in patients with progressive low-grade glioma." J Clin Oncol 21(4): 646-651.

Reardon, D. A., A. Desjardins, et al. (2008). "The emerging role of anti-angiogenic therapy for malignant glioma." Current treatment options in oncology 9(1): 1-22.

Reardon, D. A., A. Gajjar, et al. (1998). "Bithalamic involvement predicts poor outcome among children with thalamic glial tumors." Pediatr Neurosurg 29(1): 29-35.

Reardon, D. A., J. A. Quinn, et al. (2004). "Phase 2 trial of BCNU plus irinotecan in adults with malignant glioma." Neuro Oncol 6(2): 134-144.

Reed, N. and D. H. Gutmann (2001). "Tumorigenesis in neurofibromatosis: new insights and potential therapies." Trends Mol Med 7(4): 157-162.

Rodriguez, F. J., B. W. Scheithauer, et al. (2008). "Ependymoma and intraparenchymal calcifying pseudoneoplasm of the neural axis: incidental collision or unique reactive phenomenon?" Acta neuropathologica 115(3): 363-366.

Romer, J. T., H. Kimura, et al. (2004). "Suppression of the Shh pathway using a small molecule inhibitor eliminates medulloblastoma in Ptc1(+/-)p53(-/-) mice." Cancer cell 6(3): 229-240.

Ron, E., B. Modan, et al. (1988). "Tumors of the brain and nervous system after radiotherapy in childhood." The New England journal of medicine 319(16): 1033-1039.

Rorke, L. B. (1983). "The cerebellar medulloblastoma and its relationship to primitive neuroectodermal tumors." J Neuropathol Exp Neurol 42(1): 1-15.

Rorke, L. B., R. J. Packer, et al. (1996). "Central nervous system atypical teratoid/rhabdoid tumors of infancy and childhood: definition of an entity." Journal of neurosurgery 85(1): 56-65.

Rosenblum, M. K., M. Matsutani, et al. (2000). CNS Germ cell tumors. Pathology & Genetics Tumors of the central nervous system. P. Kleihues and W. K. Cavenee. Lyons, France, IARC Press: 208-214.

Rubin, J. B. and D. H. Gutmann (2005). "Neurofibromatosis type 1 - a model for nervous system tumour formation?" Nature reviews. Cancer 5(7): 557-564.

Rudin, C. M., C. L. Hann, et al. (2009). "Treatment of medulloblastoma with hedgehog pathway inhibitor GDC-0449." The New England journal of medicine 361(12): 1173-1178.

Sampson, J. H., G. Akabani, et al. (2003). "Progress report of a Phase I study of the intracerebral microinfusion of a recombinant chimeric protein composed of transforming growth factor (TGF)-alpha and a mutated form of the Pseudomonas exotoxin termed PE-38 (TP-38) for the treatment of malignant brain tumors." J Neurooncol 65(1): 27-35.

Schwalbe, E. C., J. C. Lindsey, et al. (2011). "Rapid Diagnosis of Medulloblastoma Molecular Subgroups." Clin Cancer Res.

Scotto, K. W. and J. R. Bertino (2001). Chemotherapy suceptibility and resistance. The Moleercular Basis of Canc. J. Mendelsohn, P. M. Howley and M. A. Israel. Philadephia, W.B. Saunders: 387-400.

Shibamoto, Y., M. Takahashi, et al. (1997). "Prognosis of intracranial germinoma with syncytiotrophoblastic giant cells treated by radiation therapy." Int J Radiat Oncol Biol Phys 37(3): 505-510.

Singh, A. D., C. L. Shields, et al. (1999). "New insights into trilateral retinoblastoma." Cancer 86(1): 3-5.

Smith, M. A., B. Freidlin, et al. (1998). "Trends in reported incidence of primary malignant brain tumors in children in the United States." J Natl Cancer Inst 90(17): 1269-1277.

Stewart, D. J. (1994). "A critique of the role of the blood-brain barrier in the chemotherapy of human brain tumors." J Neurooncol 20(2): 121-139.

Tada, T., T. Takizawa, et al. (1999). "Treatment of intracranial nongerminomatous germ-cell tumor by high-dose chemotherapy and autologous stem-cell rescue." J Neurooncol 44(1): 71-76.

Taylor, R. E. (2004). "Review of radiotherapy dose and volume for intracranial ependymoma." Pediatric blood & cancer 42(5): 457-460.

Tekautz, T. M., C. E. Fuller, et al. (2005). "Atypical teratoid/rhabdoid tumors (ATRT): improved survival in children 3 years of age and older with radiation therapy and high-dose alkylator-based chemotherapy." Journal of clinical oncology : official journal of the American Society of Clinical Oncology 23(7): 1491-1499.

Tsikitis, M., Z. Zhang, et al. (2005). "Genetic ablation of Cyclin D1 abrogates genesis of rhabdoid tumors resulting from Ini1 loss." Proceedings of the National Academy of Sciences of the United States of America 102(34): 12129-12134.

Turner, C. D., S. Gururangan, et al. (2002). "Phase II study of irinotecan (CPT-11) in children with high-risk malignant brain tumors: the Duke experience." Neuro-oncol 4(2): 102-108.

Walter, A. W., R. K. Mulhern, et al. (1999). "Survival and neurodevelopmental outcome of young children with medulloblastoma at St Jude Children's Research Hospital." Journal of clinical oncology : official journal of the American Society of Clinical Oncology 17(12): 3720-3728.

Warren, K. E., A. A. Aikin, et al. (2005). "Phase I study of O6-benzylguanine and temozolomide administered daily for 5 days to pediatric patients with solid tumors." Journal of clinical oncology : official journal of the American Society of Clinical Oncology 23(30): 7646-7653.

Warren, K. E., S. Goldman, et al. (2011). "Phase I trial of lenalidomide in pediatric patients with recurrent, refractory, or progressive primary CNS tumors: Pediatric Brain Tumor Consortium study PBTC-018." Journal of clinical oncology : official journal of the American Society of Clinical Oncology 29(3): 324-329.

Warren, K. E., M. C. Patel, et al. (2001). "Phase I trial of lobradimil (RMP-7) and carboplatin in children with brain tumors." Cancer Chemother Pharmacol 48(4): 275-282.

Watson, G. A., R. P. Kadota, et al. (2001). "Multidisciplinary management of pediatric low-grade gliomas." Semin Radiat Oncol 11(2): 152-162.

Westphal, M., D. C. Hilt, et al. (2003). "A phase 3 trial of local chemotherapy with biodegradable carmustine (BCNU) wafers (Gliadel wafers) in patients with primary malignant glioma." Neuro-oncology 5(2): 79-88.

Wisoff, J. H., J. M. Boyett, et al. (1998). "Current neurosurgical management and the impact of the extent of resection in the treatment of malignant gliomas of childhood: a report of the Children's Cancer Group trial no. CCG-945." J Neurosurg 89(1): 52-59.

Woehrer, A., I. Slavc, et al. (2010). "Incidence of atypical teratoid/rhabdoid tumors in children: a population-based study by the Austrian Brain Tumor Registry, 1996-2006." Cancer 116(24): 5725-5732.

Wolden, S. L., I. J. Dunkel, et al. (2003). "Patterns of failure using a conformal radiation therapy tumor bed boost for medulloblastoma." J Clin Oncol 21(16): 3079-3083.

Yan, H., D. W. Parsons, et al. (2009). "IDH1 and IDH2 mutations in gliomas." The New England journal of medicine 360(8): 765-773.

Yu, J., H. Deshmukh, et al. (2009). "Alterations of BRAF and HIPK2 loci predominate in sporadic pilocytic astrocytoma." Neurology 73(19): 1526-1531.

6

Malignant Brain Tumors in Childhood

Giovanni Scarzello, Maria S. Buzzaccarini and Guido Sotti
Department of Radiotherapy, IOV - IRCCS, Padova
Italy

1. Introduction

Twenty percent of all neoplasms in children arise in the central nervous system (CNS) and the incidence of these tumors has increased in the last years. The World Health Organization (WHO) classification of CNS tumors is shown in Tab. 1 (1).

2. Etiology

Although most brain tumors are sporadic, a number of pediatric brain tumor presentations are associated with recognized genetic syndromes. About 15–20% of children with neurofibromatosis (NF1) present with CNS neoplasms, usually gliomas of the optic pathways or low-grade tumors of the diencephalon, cerebral hemispheres, or posterior fossa (2). Low-grade gliomas associated with NF1 may be less aggressive than similar gliomas in the general population. The indolent subependymal giant cell astrocytoma occurs in children with tuberous sclerosis. Childhood brain tumors are frequently noted in families with the Li–Fraumeni syndrome and children with the syndrome are also at high risk for secondary, treatment related tumors (5). Radiation-induced meningiomas have long been recognized.

3. Supratentorial brain tumors

3.1 Clinical presentation

Supratentorial tumors generally present with localizing neurologic symptoms; symptoms and signs may develop over extended time intervals and are often protean. Seizures are the most common symptom in cerebral hemispheric lesions, especially with tumors arising in the temporal lobe. Lateralizing neurologic signs occur in thalamic region tumors, often associated with symptoms of increased intracranial pressure. Also suprasellar tumors may occlude the foramen of Monro, raising elevated intracranial pressure. Visual field deficits and or decreased acuity and endocrine abnormalities like diminished growth hormone, cortisol or thyroid production, diabetes insipidus, delayed or precocious puberty, are often apparent with midline suprasellar lesions. Children with suprasellar tumors may show the diencephalic syndrome with hyperactivity and asthenia despite normal or high food intake (4). Pineal region tumors produce hydrocephalus by compressing the aqueduct of Sylvius; specific ocular signs like the Parinaud syndrome (decreased upward gaze, near-light dissociation of the papillary response and convergence nystagmus) are classically noted.

TUMORS OF NEUROEPITHELIAL TISSUE
- **Astrocytic tumors**
  - astrocytoma
  - anaplastic astrocytoma
  - glioblastoma
  - pilocytic astrocytoma
  - pleomorphic xanthoastrocytoma
  - subependymal giant cell astrocytoma
- **Oligodendroglial tumors**
  - oligodendroglioma
  - anaplastic oligodendroglioma
- **Ependymal tumors**
  - ependymoma
  - anaplastic ependymoma
  - myxopapillary ependymoma
- **Mixed gliomas**
  - oligodendroglioma
  - others
- **Choroids plexus tumors**
- **Neuronal tumors**
  - gangliocytoma
  - gaglioglioma
  - desmoplastic infantile neuroepithelioma
  - dysembryoplastic neuroepithelial tumor
  - central neurocytoma

PINEAL PARENCHYMAL TUMORS
  - pineocytoma
  - pineoblastoma

EMBRYONAL TUMORS
- **Medulloepithelioma**
- **Neuroblastoma**
- **Ependymoblastoma**
- **Primitive neuroectodermal tumors**
- **Medulloblastoma**
- **Cerebral (supratentorial), spinal PNET**

TUMORS OF MENINGOTHELIAL CELLS
- **Meningioma**
- **Malignant meningiomas**

TUMORS OF THE UNCERTAIN HISTOGENESIS
- **Hemangioblastoma**

GCTs
- **Germinoma**
- **Embryonal carcinoma**
- **Endodermal sinus tumor**
- **Choriocarcinoma**
- **Teratoma**
- **Mixed GCTs**

TUMORS OF THE SELLAR REGION
- **Pituitary adenoma**
- **Craniopharyngioma**

Table 1. Histopathologic Classification of CNS Tumors – WHO Classification 2007

3.2 Low-grade supratentorial astrocytomas

Low-grade astrocytomas (LGA) represent the most common category of pediatric brain tumors. The most frequent site of origin is the cerebellum, followed by the midline diencephalon and the cerebral hemispheres. In about 3% of cases LGA, mostly if located in the diencephalon, present with subarachnoid dissemination; an uncommon subgroup of diffuse LGA encroaches more than one lobe often with no clear mass: this diffuse pattern of growth is classified as gliomatosis cerebri (5).

Imaging commonly shows a isointense lesion on computed tomograpy and T1 MRI sequences and hyperintense on T2, with variable enhancement with gadolinium. Small or large cysts and calcifications may be present. LGA histological findings are low cellularity, little nuclear atypia, and few or no mytosis. Although the term "low grade" applies to all pediatric gliomas that are not anaplastic, the various histiotypes differ in the degree of infiltration, relative aggressiveness, and prognosis. Juvenile pilocytic astrocytomas (JPAs) and diffuse fibrillary astrocytomas (DFA) comprise the majority of pediatric low-grade gliomas. Less common LGAs include gemistocytic astrocytomas, pleomorphic xanthoastrocytomas, desmoplastic infantile astrocytomas, protoplasmic astrocytomas, and subependymal giant cell astrocytomas. Management depends on tumor location, patient age, presence of a genetic mutation, the goal of treatment is long term disease control or cure with function preservation. Outcome is largely favorable.

3.2.1 Therapy

3.2.1.1 Surgery

For resectable LGA surgery (S) is the first and sole intervention providing excellent control of disease. Low recurrence rates are reported after total resection: with a 5-year progression-free survival (PFS) ranging from 95 to 100% for JPAs and gangliogliomas to 80% for grade II DFA (6). Resection of tumors involving the dominant medial temporal lobe, motor strip region, or the Broca speech cortex may not be possible without inducing severe neurologic deficits. Partial resection may provide initial intervention for decompression and histopathologic diagnosis. LGA of the diencephalon are technically challenging because of the deep location and eloquent area.

3.2.1.2 Radiation Therapy

Radiation Therapy (RT) is an established, effective treatment for pediatric LGA, achieving tumor response and durable control in a significant proportion of cases (7). An analysis from Pollack et al. showed improved disease control at 10 years after irradiation following incomplete resection of cerebral hemispheric astrocytomas: 82% PFS with RT versus 42% after S alone. The same study showed no significant benefit in overall survival (OS)(8). A recent phase II prospective study published by Merchant et al. showed excellent event-free survival (EFS) (87% and 74% at 5 and 10 years, respectively) and OS over 90% at 10 years for children treated with three-dimensional (3D) conformal irradiation to the MRI-defined tumor volume (9). These results have been associated with excellent functional outcomes (10). The decreased volume of normal brain exposed to moderate or high radiation doses using conformal techniques with small margins may significantly decrease some of the serious radiation-induced side effects (11). There are no contemporary data suggesting a benefit of postoperative irradiation for completely resected LGA. For incompletely resected LGA, early administration of irradiation may not benefit the patient. Current indications for

RT after a near total resection (with imaging evidence of disease residual) include symptoms or signs that might improve with RT or post surgical progression in a location not amenable to safe, definitive second resection. Other factors considered are histological subtype or biology.

3.2.1.3 Chemotherapy

Chemotherapy (CT) has been used with increasing frequency for LGA as a strategy to delay or avoid RT; less data regarding CT response for progressive disease following irradiation are available. CT can provide disease control for months to years, more often achieving stable disease or partial response than complete remission; most tumors progress within 3-4 years, requiring RT at that time. The age below which CT is more appropriate is controversial and dependent on factors such as tumor size and location, presence of NF mutation, or developmental or neurocognitive delays. Packer et al. reported age to be the only significant prognostic factor, with 3-year PFS rate of 74% for children 5 year old versus 39% for older children (12). In COG, the age of 10 years has been chosen for trial eligibility in studies evaluating CT as initial treatment (13). Individual centers have used thresholds of 3 or 5 years of age. Favorable control rates and relative absence of serious toxicity have established carboplatin and vincristine as the "standard" first line CT in younger children (14). Temozolomide, an alkylating agent with modest responsiveness in recurrent LGA, is currently in trial with carboplatin-vincristine to try to prolong drug tolerance (15). The five-drug University of California at San Francisco (UCSF) regimen (6-thioguanine, procarbazine, dibromodulcitol, lomustine, and vincristine) has been reported to be similarly efficacious; a randomized trial comparing carboplatin-vincristine to this regimen has been completed in COG, suggesting equal or greater efficacy with the five-drug regimen (13). Bevacizumab in combination with irinotecan has been investigated for recurrent LGA with promising response rates for heavily pretreated patients (16). The decision to proceed with CT or RT relates to patient age and clinical presentation; factors beyond age alone include symptoms and signs, potential for additional neurocognitive deficits, the likelihood of durable benefit from respective chemotherapeutic regimens, and the radiation volume required in weighing relative potential toxicities. Although not proven to be problematic, there is no confirmation that the response rate and durability of disease control following RT are independent on prior failure on CT.

3.3 Optic pathway tumors

Optic pathway tumors (OPTs) represent 5% of childhood brain tumors and may involve one or more anatomic sections of the optic system: optic nerves, optic chiasm, optic tracts, optic radiations. They can be small and localized or extensive and infiltrative. Tumors involving the chiasm are difficult to distinguish from tumors originating in the hypothalamus, therefore they are commonly grouped with hypothalamic gliomas as one entity. OPTs occur predominantly in young children: 25% present before 18 months of age and 50% present before 5 years. Up to 25% of childhood OPTs occur in children with NF1 and 10-20% of children with NF1 are found to have OPTs on MRI. Clinical presentation is most often with diminished vision. In young children, increased intracranial pressure endocrinopathies and diencephalic syndrome may predominate. Histologically, more than 90% of OPTs are LGA, most often JPAs, with infrequent gangliogliomas or hamartomas; malignant gliomas are uncommon (17). While acknowledging the sometimes indolent nature of OPTs, serial observations in major pediatric neuro-oncology clinics indicate progression in 75-85% of children, typically within 2 years of initial presentation. Tumors confined to the optic nerves may behave in a more hamartomatous fashion. Children with NF1 have a more indolent course with lower rates of progression and longer latency intervals (17). Other signs of the neoplastic behavior of OPTs include extension to or invasion of the adjacent hypothalamus and posterior extension to the optic tracts and optic radiations. Infrequently, optic chiasmatic and hypothalamic tumors demonstrate diffuse leptomeningeal disease (18). Mortality within 10 years of diagnosis is uncommon, although ultimate disease-related mortality has been documented in up to 40% of cases (19). The rare but documented occurrence of spontaneous regression of OPTs (20) is also to be noted. Several series identify chiasmatic OPTs as optic pathway-hypothalamic gliomas, acknowledging the difficulty in identifying the origin of tumors that intimately involve both the chiasm and the hypothalamus (14). Although lesions extending to or originating in the hypothalamus may be somewhat more aggressive than lesions confined to the visual pathways, up to 50% of selected, asymptomatic children have been free of progression for 5 years or longer without therapeutic intervention. Preliminary data suggest adequate retrieval with secondary therapy at the time of progression during observation (17).

3.3.1 Therapy

3.3.1.1 Surgery

S has been the preferred treatment for unilateral tumors of the optic nerve (21,22), but care should be taken to avoid visual compromise or other surgical complications as alternative therapies are quite successful. Observation may be selected, especially if there is residual vision associated with a lesion confined to the intraorbital optic nerve. Alvord and Lofton (21) reported progression in 70% of children with untreated lesions within 6 years of diagnosis, although it was rarely associated with tumor-related mortality. Most series indicate more indolent behavior in children with neurofibromatosis (22). For lesions involving the optic chiasm, there are limited data suggesting a role for surgical resection. Decompression or limited resection may be successful in restoring vision. Typical chiasmatic lesions that involve components of the visual pathways beyond the optic chiasm and hypothalamic region may be managed without biopsy confirmation. Most of these tumors are LGA and often can be managed according to the clinical and imaging diagnosis. Globular tumors that involve the chiasm and hypothalamus are best biopsied if this can be performed safely; a small percentage of these lesions may be more aggressive malignant gliomas (23).

3.3.1.2 Radiation Therapy

Irradiation is indicated for significant visual or neurologic deficits at presentation or documented progression by clinical evaluation or neuroimaging after observation, S or CT (12,21,24). RT is highly effective for OPTs: 10-year PFS rates exceed 80% (25,31). Although OS at 10 years is unaffected by the initial therapeutic approach, PFS rates at 5 and 10 years are substantially higher after RT (26). Serial imaging studies document significant tumor response in more than 50% of children after irradiation (25). Transient post irradiation tumor enlargement, often in the setting of central cystic degeneration, has been well documented (19). Close observation and medical management rather than aggressive intervention for presumed tumor progression is advised, particularly for lesions that may appear to progress within 6–12 months after RT. Visual improvement has been reported in

25-35% of children after irradiation (19,27). Visual deterioration is reported in 10-20% of children after RT, largely related to cystic degeneration and consequent increased mass effect at the chiasm or unrecognized elevated intracranial pressure (19,26). Vision should be monitored closely during RT and in the months following completion. OPTs are associated with unique late radiation-related sequelae. The young age at diagnosis, central location, and often extensive anatomic involvement challenge the ability to deliver adequate RT while preserving neurocognitive function; the problem is further accentuated in children with NF1, itself associated with cognitive delays (25,28). There is also concern about late vascular events: the incidence of occlusive vasculopathy at the circle of Willis in children with brain tumors is highest among those with OPTs, especially in younger children (29). There is also a heightened concern regarding the risk of second malignancy in patients with NF1 (30). The Toronto group has uniquely reported a 10% incidence of second malignant neoplasms after irradiation for OPTs; of interest, a series from Children's Hospital of Los Angeles showed the same rate of anaplastic degeneration in JPA after surgery alone (31, 32).

3.3.1.3 Chemotherapy

Because of the radiation associated morbidities in young children with OPT, Packer et al. explored primary CT in children younger than 5 years. Initial experience with actinomycin D and vincristine resulted in stabilization in a majority of children and objective tumor reduction in approximately 25%. Although more than 60% of children needed RT by 5 years after diagnosis, the approach resulted in a substantial delay in RT, with a median time to progression of 3 years (33). Subsequent experience with an 18 month regimen of carboplatin and vincristine for LGA including those of the hypothalamic region and OPTs has shown a significant rate of objective tumor reduction, early progression in only 10%, and 3 year PFS that ranges from 75% for children younger than 5 years to 39% for those older than 5 years (12). Similar results have been reported with the UCSF five drug regimen (34). Early experience suggests favorable outcome with secondary RT after progression during or after CT; recent observations related to the timing of initiating RT suggest that long term disease control and function are not diminished with prolonged preirradiation intervals (12,24). Toxicity with carboplatin and vincristine has been limited, and early data suggest continued intellectual development during CT (35). There is a balance between duration of disease control, clearly superior with RT and less durable control with CT apparently without the serious morbidities associated with RT in the younger age group (17,26). In current practice, most children below 5-10 years receive CT as initial intervention, with some centers extending this to all prepubertal children. It is important not to avoid RT even in younger children when despite CT, progressive visual loss is apparent.

3.4 Oligodendroglioma

Oligodendrogliomas represent 1-2% of supratentorial tumors in children. The generally circumscribed tumors occur most often in the cerebral hemispheres. Treatment recommendations are based largely on adult experience with S and RT (36). Adults show excellent response to procarbazine, lomustine, and vincristine (PCV) or to temozolomide CT, particularly in anaplastic oligodendrogliomas with isochromosome 1p or p53 mutations (37). Given differences in biology, it is unclear whether chemosensitivity can be extrapolated to children. Gross total resection (GTR) is the treatment of choice for accessible lesions. GTR has been documented in 20-25% of all cases, apparently more often in children and adolescents (30). The OS rate at 10 years after total excision is reported to be about 60% (38). For incompletely resected oligodendrogliomas, a short-term benefit for RT has been documented reported 5 year OS rate of 25% after subtotal resection, compared with 62% with the addition of irradiation to doses greater than 50 Gy; by 10 years, the OS rates were 31% with RT and 25% without RT (39). Adjuvant RT is typically withheld for differentiated oligodendrogliomas in children, even with incomplete resection. Histologic grade has been cited as a prognostic indicator in oligodendrogliomas. Anaplastic oligodendrogliomas are managed similarly to other malignant supratentorial gliomas, although the outcome tends to be superior to those with anaplastic astrocytoma and glioblastoma. Limited CT has been associated with sufficient tumor reduction to permit delayed S in tumors initially unresectable (40).

3.5 Ganglioglioma

Gangliogliomas are uncommon neoplasms comprised of neuronal and glial elements, occurring primarily in children and young adults. Gangliogliomas present most often in the mesial aspect of the temporal lobes, with seizures as the dominant symptom (41,42). Pediatric tumors uncommonly present in the posterior fossa. The lesions are typically well circumscribed and resectable (41,43). Gangliogliomas are classically coded as WHO grade I, well differentiated histologically with no atypia or anaplasia (42). S alone is the standard initial intervention; 10 year DFS has been reported in 97% of pediatric cases after S (42). Malignant transformation at progression or recurrence is rare; almost 10% of cases show nuclear atypia or anaplastic components (grade II or III, respectively) (43). Malignant degeneration to glioblastoma (grade IV) is decidedly uncommon in children and adolescents (44). Prolonged PFS survival has been noted in small series with RT following incomplete resection or recurrence; the efficacy following malignant degeneration is less apparent (44).

3.6 Rare low-grade neoplasms

Neurocytomas are clinically indolent tumors that present as intraventricular lesions, usually in the lateral ventricles with attachment to the midline septum pellucidum; most are diagnosed in adolescents and young adults. Neurocytomas are composed of small neuronal cells thought to represent a benign neoplasm derived from cells midway in the maturation process of neuronal differentiation (41). These tumors are genetically distinct from the oligodendrogliomas and dysembryoplastic neuroepithelial tumors (DNETs), with which they can be confused both clinically and histologically (42). The lesion is generally resectable; prognosis has been related to the rate of proliferation (43). These tumors respond to RT; small series have suggested improved outcome in cases with less than total resection when followed by RT. DNETs are biologically indolent, often large cerebral cortical tumors typically presenting with a long standing seizure history (45). Symptoms typically arise in children younger than 12 years; the mean age at diagnosis is 14. The tumors may be considered hamartomatous, classically are well demarcated, and show no contrast on MRI; uncommonly, DNETs present as complex solid and cystic lesions with enhancement, calcification, and intralesional hemorrhage (46). These tumors may be followed, but S is needed for seizure control; although they appear to be responsive to RT, there is no documented role for postoperative therapy (45).

3.7 Malignant gliomas

Supratentorial malignant gliomas represent approximately 6% of brain tumors in children. Histologic grading divides high grade gliomas (HGG) into anaplastic astrocytoma, WHO

Grade III and glioblastoma, WHO Grade IV (1). Children have a higher proportion of anaplastic astrocytomas among the malignant gliomas and have longer survival intervals (47). Adult primary malignant gliomas appear to arise denovo and are associated with amplification of the epidermal growth factor receptor (EGFR) gene and PTEN; less common secondary malignant gliomas evolve from low grade tumors and typically have TP53 mutations (48). Supratentorial malignant gliomas arise primarily as cerebral hemispheric tumors; 20–30% present centrally in the thalamus or basal ganglia. Imaging characteristics are similar to those in adults, with often poorly marginated, peripherally enhancing lesions on MRI or computed tomography associated with surrounding white matter changes due to edema; the enhancing components correlate with the cellular, vascularized periphery of the tumor complex. The infiltrative characteristics of HGG necessitate some caution in aggressive S and high-dose local RT; interest in functional imaging for both stereotactic surgical planning and RT reflects the acknowledged heterogeneity of the tumors and invasiveness beyond areas identified by anatomic imaging (49). Even with acknowledged infiltration at a distance from the overt tumor, clinical data show both a direct relationship between the degree of resection and duration of tumor control as well as a pattern of failure that is overwhelmingly at the primary target volume even after high dose focal RT (50,51). Leptomeningeal dissemination had been reported in up to 15% of children at diagnosis; however, a large prospective CCG trial showed disease beyond the primary site only anecdotally (52). The diagnosis of HGG in children has often been challenging to the neuropathologist. Central review of pathology in the CCG-945 trial showed that 36% of cases entered, based on an institutional diagnosis of anaplastic astrocytomas or glioblastoma, were felt to have a discordant diagnosis, primarily LGA, based on the reviewers' interpretation (53).

3.7.1 Therapy

3.7.1.1 Surgery

Surgical resection often has been limited in extent by the poorly circumscribed nature of the tumor and the attendant lack of aggressive neurosurgical intent. The large CCG series indicated that more than GTR and near total resection was achieved in only 37% of cases: 49% of lesions arising in the superficial cerebral hemispheres, 45% of lesions arising in the cerebellum, and 8% of those arising in the central structures (50). There is a significant relationship between degree of resection and outcome. Five year PFS in the initially reported CCG-945 experience was 44% and 26% for anaplastic astrocytomas and glioblastoma, after more than 90% removal, compared with 22% and 4%, respectively, after less aggressive resection (50).

3.7.1.2 Radiation Therapy

RT is a primary component of initial management of pediatric malignant gliomas. Adult studies have documented the impact of adequate RT on OS, although survival beyond 2 years occurs almost entirely among those with anaplastic astrocytoma rather than glioblastoma. Treatment has evolved to local RT, with margins reflecting the known pattern of microscopic extension and functional imaging to guide evolving therapeutic approaches. A series of dose escalating trials have yet to demonstrate a convincing impact on disease control (51,56). Current trials use 3D conformal RT or IMRT to dosage levels, similar to those used in adults (51,57).

3.8 Embryonal CNS tumors: Primitive neuroectodermal tumors and pineoblastoma

Primitive neuroectodermal tumors (PNETs) are aggressive cerebral tumors occurring predominantly in young children comprising 2-3% of pediatric CNS neoplasms. The tumor consists of undifferentiated neuroepithelial cells with areas of divergent differentiation toward glial, neuronal, and mesenchymal lines (1). Embryonal tumors typically present as solid or partially cystic lesions. Although PNETs and cerebral neuroblastoma may present as well demarcated lesions, most embryonal tumors are generally invasive (58). Leptomeningeal dissemination is apparent at the time of diagnosis or at the time of initial tumor recurrence or progression in approximately one third of children; there is some controversy regarding the frequency of CSF failure in initially localized cerebral neuroblastoma, but most reports indicate CNS dissemination at a rate similar to that of the other embryonal tumor types (59). Medulloepithelioma is the most primitive embryonal tumor, histologically showing features of primitive medullary epithelium and primitive tubular structures; focal differentiation toward glial, neuronal, or mesenchymal lines is often present. Primitive polar spongioblastoma is a rare cerebral tumor thought to be derived from migrating glial precursor cells and characterized by immature unipolar glial cells. Ependymoblastoma is a poorly differentiated embryonal tumor with ependymal differentiation marked by multilayered rosettes similar to those seen in retinoblastoma (1). The tumor is felt to be a specific embryonal neoplasm, different from the differentiated and anaplastic ependymomas that occur both in the posterior fossa and supratentorially. Cerebral neuroblastoma ranges histologically from an undifferentiated tumor similar to the extra-CNS childhood neuroblastoma, often including unilayered Homer–Wright rosettes, to lesions demonstrating ganglionic differentiation (60). The tumor most often confused with medulloblastoma histologically and by contiguous anatomic location is the pineoblastoma. The tumor is believed to arise from pineal parenchymal cells, histologically signified by undifferentiated small round cells, usually including scattered Homer–Wright rosettes. (61).

3.8.1 Therapy

The basic principle of S is often limited by disease site and extent. The PNETs may be resectable in up to 50% of cases, especially when cystic (58,59). Pineoblastomas are generally approached for stereotactic biopsy or limited resection (61,62). Postoperative RT is indicated for the embryonal CNS tumors. Classic studies indicate disease control in fewer than 25% of cases with sPNET and pineoblastoma (58,63). A review of the SIOP/UKCCSG experience showed high rates of disease control with cranio spinal irradiation (CSI) for pineoblastomas with or without CT. The use of immediate postoperative RT and subsequent CT in CCG resulted in a 60% survival rate in children over 1.5-3 years with pineoblastomas (61). Overall results in other more recent series highlight interest in high-dose CT (e.g., high-dose methotrexate in the HIT regimens from the German studies or high-dose therapy with peripheral stem cell rescue) following irradiation (64).

3.9 Intracranial germ cell tumors

Intracranial GCTs are rare in North America and Europe, representing less than 2-4% of pediatric CNS neoplasms; in Japan and Taiwan they are reported to represent up to 11% of childhood brain tumors. The full range of germ cell histiotypes presents as primary CNS tumors: pure germinomas (60-70% of intracranial GCTs), "malignant" germ cell types (embryonal carcinomas, endodermal sinus tumors, and choriocarcinomas, collectively 15-

20% of CNS GCTs), and teratomas (benign, immature, and malignant types, 15–20%) (1). Malignant teratomas are admixtures of benign teratomatous lesions with one or more malignant germ cell lines such as embryonal carcinoma, endodermal sinus tumor, or choriocarcinoma or with malignant elements of rhabdomyosarcoma, neuroblastoma, or epithelial carcinoma (65,66,67). GCTs are conventionally categorized into two highly prognostic histological subgroups: pure germinomas and non germinomatous (or "malignant") germ cell tumors (NGGCTs). NGGCTs include GCTs with any malignant germ cell component and or any tumor that secretes AFP or high levels of β-HCG. Some international trials have classified these tumors simply as "secreting" and "non secreting" based on the high likelihood of secretion from malignant germ cell components and lack germinomas (68). Pure germinomas carry a much more favorable prognosis, and therefore are generally treated less aggressively than NGGCTs. CNS GCTs usually occur as midline third ventricular lesions. These tumors most often arise in the pineal region (50–60%) or from the infundibulum-pituitary stalk in the suprasellar region (30-35%). Less common locations for primary intracranial GCTs include the basal ganglia or thalamic nuclei (67,68). Involvement of multiple tumor sites around the third ventricle is common, most often the pineal and suprasellar regions concurrently; such tumors are referred to as "multiple midline germinomas" and appear to represent multicentric tumor development or subependymal infiltration around the ventricle rather than subarachnoid or CSF pathway metastasis. Up to 20% of intracranial germinomas present as multiple midline tumors, especially noted in adolescent males; this phenomenon is much more frequently encountered with pure germinomas, but has been reported with NGGCTs (69). Leptomeningeal spread through the cerebrospinal axis may be seen, but is much less common. Pineal germinomas occur with a higher prevalence in adolescent males. Suprasellar germinomas occur throughout the first two decades; there is no gender predilection for this location. Teratomas tend to occur in younger children, and other malignant histiotypes (e.g., embryonal carcinoma, endodermal sinus tumor) generally present in older children, adolescents, and young adults. A unique spectrum of neoplasms presents a broad differential diagnosis for tumors arising in the posterior third ventricular region. Approximately 80% of the pineal region tumors in children and adolescents are GCTs (60–70%) or pineal parenchymal tumors (10–20%). In very young children, the most common tumor type is the pineoblastoma. Less common histiotypes include glial tumors (astrocytomas, ependymomas) and arachnoid cysts. Pinealoblastomas are embryonal CNS tumors described earlier. Pineocytomas are "mature" parenchymal cell neoplasms, which are rare in children, clinically benign in adolescents but potentially malignant in younger children (70). The differential diagnosis for suprasellar tumors is also rather broad, including astrocytomas and craniopharyngiomas (together, more than 80% of lesions in this location) as well as GCTs. Pineal GCTs present most often with increased intracranial pressure caused by compression of the adjacent Sylvian aqueduct. Ocular signs are classically noted as the Parinaud syndrome: a triad of decreased upward gaze, abnormal pupillary responses described as near-light dissociation (limited constriction to light but retained pupillary response to accommodation; otherwise known as the Argyll–Robertson pupil), and convergence nystagmus (71). Findings occur as a result of pressure from the pineal tumor on the superior colliculus of the tectum. In suprasellar GCTs, the classic triad of presenting symptoms is diabetes insipidus, precocious or delayed puberty and visual deficits. Diabetes insipidus or other symptoms of suprasellar disease in conjunction with an apparently isolated pineal tumor are virtually diagnostic of a multiple midline germinoma and should be treated as such. Conversely, care should be taken in evaluating the pineal region with suprasellar tumors (72). Evaluation for GCT should include MRI of the brain with and without gadolinium with thin cuts through the suprasellar and pineal regions. A screening MRI of the spine should be obtained with axial images through any regions suspicious for disease. Lumbar puncture with CSF cytology and CSF AFP and β-HCG should be obtained with caution, especially in children with large pineal tumors or potentially persistent increased intracranial pressure. Serum AFP and β-HCG should also be measured. AFP is usually present in serum and CSF in embryonal carcinoma, endodermal sinus tumor, or malignant teratoma. β-HCG is elevated in a subset of germinomas (10–20% of pure germinomas show levels above 10 IU, up to 70–100 IU; levels above 100–200 IU are found in germinomas with syncytiotrophoblastic giant cells); significant elevation (typically more than 1000IU) is diagnostic of choriocarcinoma (67,73). If there is any detectable elevation of AFP above institutional norm (generally, serum 5–10 ng/dL; CSF 2–5 ng/dL), this is diagnostic of malignant germ cell histiotypes; the tumor is classified as an NGGCT. β-HCG elevation may be seen in pure germinomas; the appropriate cut-off for categorization as a NGGCT is controversial. The COG ultimately recognized values 75 to 100 IU/L; this may be a conservative number (74). Additional baseline studies should include a full evaluation of hypothalamic and pituitary function, ophthalmological examination, and baseline neuropsychological testing.

3.9.1 Therapy

Treatment of CNS GCTs is controversial, from the decision to establish histology to the role of S, radiation parameters, and CT. Although excellent disease control has been reported in series based on clinical and imaging diagnosis without histological confirmation, specific RT, CT, and S are best guided by a histologic diagnosis. At present, clinicians routinely recommend confirmation of pathology for all GCTs, regardless of location. When there is a significant elevation of tumor markers in serum or CSF, clinicians may consider the diagnosis of an NGGCT without a biopsy. Similarly, a classical imaging presentation with β-HCG above normal is sometimes considered pathognomonic of germinomas. Others advocate for histological verification in all settings, as some studies indicate important prognostic implications based on histological subtypes (67,75). Historically, the non operative approach for pineal region tumors had been to assume the relative dominance of germinoma, especially among adolescent males with pineal region tumors, and initiate local irradiation as a "histologic test." Prompt tumor reduction after 20–25 Gy was interpreted to be diagnostic of germinoma, and subsequent therapy used modified radiation parameters based on institutional use of local, cranial, or CSI fields (76). If a tumor showed limited early response to the "test" dosage, then S was entertained, or subsequent therapy was based on the presumption of a benign or malignant tumor. Major improvements in neurosurgical techniques have markedly decreased rates of morbidity and mortality and in modern practice, the "radiation dose test" is not a recommended approach. RT has long been the standard sole treatment or an essential element of treatment for pure germinomas; it is an important component of multimodality therapy for NGGCTs. Intracranial pure germinomas are quite chemoresponsive; the use of combined CT and limited-volume and or limited-dose irradiation has been an alternative approach in treating these tumors (77). The use of CT alone has been associated with unacceptable recurrence and mortality rates for GCTs (83). For NGGCTs, RT alone has achieved disease control in only 20–45% of tumors, and combined modality therapy, also including CT and potential surgical resection, is standard (75,76,78).

3.9.2 Surgery

The goal of surgical resection or biopsy is to provide accurate diagnosis, and in some cases, improve disease control. For patients with suspected GCT without elevation of tumor markers, biopsy is considered mandatory to confirm diagnosis of germinoma and to attempt to rule out malignant germ cell components. Contemporary surgical techniques permit stereotactic or open biopsy for both suprasellar and pineal region tumors with low rates of morbidity and mortality (79). Although it is clear that limited tissue sampling may lead to misdiagnosis for some patients, particularly in the setting of a mixed histology tumor, aggressive up front resection is not advocated by the majority of institutions in Europe and North America as higher rates of morbidity and mortality have been encountered; delayed S for persistent disease after CT is preferred (80). There is no known advantage to achieving a GTR for pure germinomas. However, a benefit of surgical resection for NGGCT has been suggested even if it is somewhat controversial (78,81,82). Some series have shown a trend toward improved control with more aggressive resection for malignant histiotypes. As stated above, others advocate initial CT with consideration of second-look S for tumors or components of tumors that do not respond. Often, teratoma components of these tumors do not respond to CT and may even grow, for these cases, surgical resection is therapeutic and provides local control. For patients with pineal region tumors that present with hydrocephalus, decompression of the ventricles is required, often urgently. The placement of a ventriculoperitoneal shunt or external ventricular drain can provide relief of hydrocephalus. Endoscopic third ventriculostomy is a particularly attractive, alternative method of treating hydrocephalus by diverting CSF flow and obtaining a biopsy under direct visualization. This procedure is more sensitive than MRI for detection of metastatic deposits

3.9.3 Radiation Therapy

For pure germinomas, RT has been the major curative modality. Long-term disease control rates range from 80% to more than 90–95% with the use of irradiation alone (76,83,84). There is ongoing controversy regarding the appropriate RT volume (local tumor with or without wider volumes that have included third ventricular, full ventricular, full cranial or CSI) and dose (40–50 Gy for primary RT). Whether primary RT is the best course of treatment, is often a complex decision based on tumor site and extent, the child's age, and the child's functional status at presentation, presenting a choice between RT alone or a combination of CT and reduced-dose, limited-volume irradiation (85). The recently closed COG trial, ACNS 0232, attempted to determine the better treatment; RT alone or CT and response based reduced volume and dose irradiation. Unfortunately, this trial closed due to poor accrual leaving this important question unanswered. For NGGCTs, combined CT and RT is the standard, again with some uncertainty regarding the appropriate radiation volume: local, whole ventricle, whole brain, or CSI (78,79). The use of stereotactic radiosurgery to boost local disease visible on imaging after and persistent after CT and fractionated RT is rational, but investigational for children with persistent NGGCT that cannot be safely removed by S (88).

3.9.4 Chemotherapy

Intracranial GCTs are chemosensitive, with excellent objective response rates documented for cyclophosphamide; carboplatin; cisplatin and etoposide; ifosfamide, carboplatin, and etoposide; cisplatin, etoposide, and bleomycin (73,81,86). Objective response rates approach 100% for germinomas (89,90). Several series using pre irradiation CT and limited-volume, "response-adjusted" attenuation of radiation doses has shown excellent disease control rates. Initially explored in the United States by Allen with the use of cyclophosphamide and, later, platinating agents, this treatment has resulted in a large proportion of complete or substantial responses, with long-term disease control after local irradiation to reduced dose levels of 24–36 Gy (78,86,89). Carboplatin, most often in combination with etoposide, has replaced cisplatin for germinomas because the drug is associated with fewer long-term sequelae (90). The major short-term morbidity has been difficulties handling fluid and electrolyte balance in children with suprasellar tumors, often associated with diabetes insipidus and/or salt-wasting syndromes. This has been associated with early mortality during CT. The aim of combined CT and RT has not been to improve disease control, but to potentially improve long-term functional outcomes by decreasing radiation doses and/or volumes (85,91). The recently abandoned Phase III COG study had randomized patients with local disease to whole ventricular RT followed by a boost to the primary tumor bed or pre irradiation CT (two cycles of carboplatin and etoposide) followed by involved field, reduced dose RT if complete response was documented; if not, two cycles of cisplatin and cyclophosphamide were administered. Radiation dose depended upon response at the completion of the additional CT. For patients with disseminated disease, CSI was required, doses depend upon response to CT. The use of CT alone for intracranial germinomas has been tested in the international protocols coordinated by Balmaceda and colleagues (74). This trial included pure germinomas and NGGCTs. The first drug regimen tested (carboplatin, etoposide, bleomycin, cyclophosphamide) achieved high initial response rates, but disease progression or recurrence occurred in 50% of patients (both pure germinomas and NGGCTs); unacceptable CT-related mortality approximated 10% (83). Failures occurred primarily in the primary site at the ventricular system, with 5% in the spine. Although Merchant et al. (94) reported systematic salvage following CT-alone failure with high-dose cyclophosphamide and craniospinal irradiation, the more aggressive combined therapy regimen is excessive in a significant cohort of children who would enjoy favorable outcome with less intensive initial RT. For NGGCTs, prognosis with irradiation alone is inadequate; overall long-term survival rates approximate 20–40%. The addition of platinum-based CT has markedly improved outcome, with short-term OS rates in excess of 70%. CT has become a standard component of therapy for these tumors prior to RT. CT on both the French Society of Pediatric Oncology (SFOP) and recently completed COG study used alternating cycles of carboplatin-etoposide and ifosphamide-etoposide (93). The regimen has been both efficacious and well tolerated. High-dose CT with stem cell rescue has shown promise for relapsed GCTs (94). For the subgroup of patients who do not experience a CR to all other modalities of treatment, this approach has been considered and was recommended for patients who did not undergo CR to CT and could not safely undergo a second look S.

3.10 Posterior fossa brain tumors

Nearly one half of all childhood brain tumors arise in the posterior fossa. The most common types are medulloblastoma, LGA of the cerebellum, brainstem gliomas, and ependymomas.

3.11 Medulloblastoma

Medulloblastoma (MB) is a primitive cerebellar tumor of neuroectodermal origin. The tumor is the most common malignant brain tumor in children and adolescents, accounting for 20% of pediatric brain tumors. The classic description defined MB an embryonal tumor of the cerebellum, derived from undifferentiated progenitor medulloblasts located in the cerebellar external granular layer. The WHO classification of CNS neoplasms identifies embryonal tumors as a subset of the neuroepithelial neoplasms that are particularly prominent among pediatric brain tumors (1). Histologically, MB is a densely cellular neoplasm composed predominantly of undifferentiated small, round, blue cells. Differentiation may be toward neuronal or glial lines in the more common "classic variant"(1,95). Differentiation along mesenchymal lines defines a variant called medullomyoblastoma. Approximately, 10% to 20% of MBs can be categorized as desmoplastic type, marked by relatively hypocellular areas of prominent nodularity in reticulin-free zones, occurring most often in the cerebellar hemispheres. Desmoplastic MB is associated with mutations within the sonic hedgehog (SHH)-patched (PTCH) pathway and overexpression of IGF-2 (96,97). There is considerable excitement about the SHH pathway as a target for newly developing molecular-targeted therapies (98). Anaplastic tumors are marked by nuclear pleomorphism and high mitotic rate; these tumors overlap with large cell MB and are marked by chromosomal loss 17p, MYC amplification, and poor prognosis (97). Over expression of ERBB2 may also be related to anaplastic large cell tumors and is a similarly negative prognosticator. The histologic grade of MB has only recently been linked to prognosis. Extensive nodularity has been correlated with favorable outcome; desmoplastic variant is similarly a marker of more favorable diseases (99). The degree of anaplasia has been associated with inferior survival rates (100). Tumors with extra neural metastasis, either at diagnosis or as a pattern of failure, are more often associated with markedly anaplastic histology. From the clinical genetics standpoint, MB is the CNS tumor most often associated with germ line mutations and familial diseases. The most frequent association is between Gorlin syndrome (nevoid basal cell carcinoma syndrome) and desmoplastic MB, both related to the tumor suppressor gene PTCH and the SHH receptor. In addition, mutations of the SHH-PTCH pathway are found in 10% to 20% of "sporadic" MB. TP53 mutations mark the Li-Fraumeni syndrome, associated with a small percentage of MB. Mutations of the APC gene define Turcot syndrome of colonic polyposis, also seen in conjunction with MB. Mutations of the WNT pathway, developmentally linked to proliferation of stem cells in the sub ventricular zone, were first noted in children with Turcot syndrome. The pathway is activated in 5% to 10% of sporadic MB with classic histopathology, manifest by accumulation of intranuclear β-catenin and associated with quite favorable prognosis; Wnt/Wg-active tumors are associated with iso -chromosome 16 (98,100). Notch 2 over expression has also been noted in MB, interesting as hypoxia appears to promote neural stem cell proliferation through Notch. Other molecular correlations important in understanding the current directions in MB include TrkC expression, directly proportional to survival and ErbB2 expression. The latter factor is biologically related to cerebellar granular cell proliferation, migration, and invasion; elevated levels of ErbB2 are associated with poor outcome. The median age at diagnosis is 5 to 6 years. Approximately 20% of MB present in infants younger than 2 years and 10% occur in young adults. Boys are affected more often than girls. Presenting symptoms are those classically associated with posterior fossa lesions in children: symptoms related to elevated intracranial pressure and ataxia. Elevated intracranial pressure results from the tumor obstructing CSF flow through the sylvian aqueduct and the fourth ventricle. Approximately 75% of MB present in the midline cerebellar vermis. The tumor characteristically grows into and fills the fourth ventricle. Infiltration around the fourth ventricle is common, often involving the brachium pontis and extending onto the ventricular floor. Nearly one in four tumors arises within the cerebellar hemispheres, more commonly with desmoplastic histology. On MRI, MB is well-defined, solid lesions with uniform or, less often, no homogeneous contrast enhancement. Correlation between MR spectroscopic findings and metastasis at diagnosis has been reported (101). By computed tomography, the tumor often is hyperdense, reflecting high cellularity. MB is the classic CNS tumor associated with CSF seeding or metastasis. The standard of care requires postoperative staging, based on imaging of the brain to assess degree of resection and potential subarachnoid metastasis, spinal MRI and lumbar CSF cytology. Subarachnoid dissemination has been reported at diagnosis in 20% to 35% of children (102). Neuraxis disease typically involves the spinal subarachnoid space; intracranial metastasis is less common. The Chang (103) clinical staging system was developed in the pre-CT era and is based on the size and invasiveness of the primary tumor at surgery ("T stage") and evidence of spread outside the posterior fossa ("M stage"). Progressive tumor size and invasion of the brainstem defined increasing local tumor burden and aggressive behavior, classified as T 1-4. With the advent of computed tomography and MRI, it became apparent that imaging identification of brainstem invasion is not as reliable as surgical observation. There are no modern data to substantiate a role for T stage as an independent parameter predicting outcome or defining therapy (104,105). Comparisons in otherwise early MB (defined as M0 with complete or near total resection) and in series addressing advanced MB have shown equivalent outcome among those with brainstem invasion (T3b) and those without such (T1-3a). M stage is based on subarachnoid metastasis, coding abnormal CSF cytology (M1) or imaging evidence of non contiguous tumor in the cranium (M2) or spine (M3). Extraneural disease is present in fewer than 2% of cases at presentation, coded as M4. M stage remains a highly significant prognostic factor; intensity of therapy in current protocols and outcome are strongly related to the presence or absence of metastatic disease (106). Current clinical trials and standard management in North America define clinical risk categories for MB as average risk (children older than 3 years with no metastatic disease after near total or total resection, with less than 1.5 cm^2 residual on early postoperative imaging) or high risk (overt metastatic disease based on CSF cytology or neuroimaging, or the presence of more than 1.5 cm^2 residual on early postoperative imaging; more recently, all children younger than 3 years of age typically have been classified as high risk. With appropriately aggressive surgical intent in most centers in the United States and Europe, more than 65% to 75% of children above 3 years of age are staged as average risk. Of the 25% to 35% staged as high risk, more than 85% present with metastatic disease at diagnosis: primarily M3 (60%), but also M1 (30%), and M2 (10%); significant residual tumor at the primary site is present in ≥15% of cases (101).

3.11.1 Therapy

3.11.1.1 Surgery

In 1930 Harvey Cushing demonstrated the inability of S alone to cure MB; only 1 of 61 patients survived 3 years after S with or without limited RT (107). Maximal judicious surgical resection underlies most contemporary series. GTR (no evidence of residual tumor seen at S and negative post-operative imaging) and near total resection (more than 90% resection estimated by the surgeon and less than 1.5 cm^2 residual on postoperative imaging) have resulted in superior outcome in comparison to subtotal or partial resection and biopsy only. Data from the Children's Cancer Group (CCG) indicate gross total or near total resection in approximately 90% of children (104). In an earlier CCG trial, 5-year EFS was 78% for children with M0 disease and less than 1.5 cm^2 residual, compared with 54% for those with larger residual volumes. For tumors adherent to or invading the brainstem, a report from St. Jude Children's Research Hospital showed no advantage to pursuing GTR compared with near total removal, with none of the cases exhibiting more than 1.5 cm^2 residual; morbidity appeared to be greater with the more aggressive surgical approach. With maximal safe resection a principle of therapy, the impact of minimal residual is difficult to discern; key is the distinct advantage of treatment on an average-risk regimen whenever possible, assuming such is a M0 disease (106). Operative mortality has been reduced to 2% or less in pediatric neurosurgical centers. However, aggressive S may be associated with significant morbidity (107,108). The posterior fossa syndrome has been described in 15% to 25% of children after posterior fossa craniotomy (109). The syndrome is signified by difficulty swallowing, truncal ataxia, mutism, and, less often, respiratory failure; recent imaging data suggest the etiology may be a cerebello cerebral diaschisis (110). The routine use of ventriculo-peritoneal shunts to reduce intracranial pressure before posterior fossa craniotomy resulted in significant improvement in morbidity and mortality, when introduced 40 years ago. Children with ventriculoperitoneal shunts typically become shunt dependent. Shunt failure or infection may complicate long-term survival, necessitating revision or replacement in nearly 25% of children measured 5 years after insertion. In many academic pediatric neurosurgical centers, it is a standard procedure to place a ventricular drain, as needed, at the time of S. The surgeon often can document reestablishment of CSF flow after fourth ventricular tumor resection. Later shunt insertion may be needed in 20% to 25% of children (111,112). A delayed shunt insertion approach provides physiologic CSF dynamics for the majority of children, avoiding potential late events related to a ventriculoperitoneal shunt.

3.11.1.2 Radiation Therapy

The efficacy of RT in MB was reported within a decade of Cushing's initial description of the tumor. Cutler et al. (113) reported the radiation responsiveness of MB and the value of preventive RT of the entire neuraxis based on Cushing's clinical series. The seminal report documenting cure of MB with CSI was published by Bloom et al. in 1969: they reported 32% survival at 5 years and 25% DFS at 10 years (114). Numerous reports have subsequently confirmed increasing rates of disease control with modern radiation techniques; at standard CSI dose levels, RT alone achieves durable disease control in 65% to 75% of patients with average-risk disease (115). Modifications of radiation volume, dosage, and fractionation have been explored. The outcome following postoperative irradiation alone in average-risk MB using conventional radiation parameters (POG-CCG trial, one arm of which used CSI to 36 Gy, posterior fossa boost to 54 Gy resulting in 65% 7 year EFS) has been used as a basis for non randomized comparisons in establishing current standards for combined modality therapy in North America. The result is systematic reduction in CSI dosage to 23.4 Gy; with well documented efficacy now in average-risk disease when combined with contemporary cisplatin based CT (116,117). Agreement on combined chemo radiation is based on disease control rates that appear to be superior to those achieved with irradiation alone for both average-risk and high-risk presentations, a randomized European trial demonstrating improved outcome with chemo radiation compared to contemporary RT alone and several studies suggesting improvement in the risk: benefit ratio based on dose-volume modeling and evolving clinical data (118,119,120,121).

3.11.1.3 Chemotherapy

Phase II trials have documented the chemo responsiveness of MB to alkylating agents: platinum compounds, etoposide, antimetabolites, and camptothecins (122,123). The trial documenting the efficacy of adjuvant CT was reported by CCG, combining the attenuated CSI dose in average risk patients that had shown only 55% EFS at 5 years in the POG-CCG trial referenced in the prior section with concurrent vincristine and post irradiation cisplatin, vincristine, and CCNU; the 79% PFS at 5 years confirmed earlier institutional experience to show among the best disease control rates then documented in this (124). The International Society for Pediatric Oncology (SIOP)-United Kingdom Children's Cancer Study Group (UKCCSG) PNET-3 trial showed improved EFS with limited pre irradiation CT and full-dose irradiation versus equivalent irradiation alone: 78% EFS at 5 years with pre irradiation vincristine, etoposide, carboplatin and cyclophosphamide compared to 65% with irradiation alone (118). A large randomized trial assessing reduced-dose CSI followed by cisplatin and vincristine with "standard" CCNU versus cyclophosphamide confirmed overall EFS more than 80% with no difference in disease control on either CT arm; early analysis suggests that a larger number of secondary neoplasm may be apparent in the cyclophosphamide arm (117). St. Jude reported a prospective trial using post irradiation cyclophosphamide, vincristine and cisplatin; 83% EFS was obtained without sometimes toxic vincristine during RT and with a marked reduction in oto toxicity attending post irradiation cisplatin when the latter was given with amifostine (125). The standard of care for children with average risk MB throughout North America has been accepted as reduced dose CSI (23.4 Gy) followed by CT including an alkylating agent, vincristine and cisplatin. For patients with high risk disease, studies through the 1990s typically showed 5-year EFS at the 40% to 50% level following full dose irradiation and CT (126,127). St. Jude's SJMB 96 study has shown 70% 5-year EFS following the same CT, preceded by full-dose CSI. Randomized trials have shown somewhat conflicting results regarding the sequence of postoperative therapy: POG showed 60% 5 year EFS in high-risk MB regardless of postoperative preirradiation CT (cyclophosphamide, vincristine, cisplatin) or the opposite sequence, both using full-dose CSI. The German HIT'91 trial showed superior results with post operative RT followed by CCNU, vincristine and cisplatin compared to postoperative ifosfamide, etoposide, high-dose methotrexate, cisplatin and cytosine arabinoside followed by irradiation: 83% 5-year EFS compared to 53%, respectively for M0 patients; no difference was noted in the M2–3 cohort, both at 40% EFS (127). CCG 9931 documented a 17% PD rate during a prolonged, 5 month preirradiation regimen, again showing only 43% EFS in high-risk disease (121). Similar trials have noted that outcome in average-risk patients receiving preirradiation CT correlates with response to CT; in the Milan trial, those with CR-PR to preirradiation CT enjoyed 94% PFS compared to 61% if only SD or PD attended CT (128). Several studies note that the time to initiating irradiation is related to disease control. For disease recurrent after RT with or without CT, numerous studies demonstrate chemo responsiveness to single agents, multiagent combinations, and high-dose therapy with hematologic stem cell rescue. Except in the infant setting, durable secondary disease control following initial CSI has only rarely been achieved despite aggressive, high-dose CT and further irradiation (129,130,131). Local irradiation can provide further control at the primary site (132). Trials of intrathecal CT in this setting are of interest, but to date with only limited phases I and II data (133).

3.12 Embryonal and malignant glial tumors in infants and young children

Children younger than 3 years account for 15% to 25% of pediatric CNS neoplasms (134,135). Symptoms in this age group usually include enlarged head, lethargy, and vomiting. Tumors are predominantly supratentorial; in comparison to older children, infant tumors are more often malignant and may be more frequently metastatic at diagnosis. The most common types include astroglial tumors primarily low grade; among infants less than 1 year old, up to 25% are high-grade malignant gliomas, embryonal neoplasms and ependymomas. Atypical teratoid rhabdoid tumors (ATRTs) occur predominantly in this age group (1,136,137). A significant proportion of intracranial teratomas and choroid plexus tumors present in young children below 12 to 18 months of age. Infantile desmoplastic neuroepithelial tumors also arise predominantly in the very young. These lesions often are quite large, are peripherally located, and appear aggressive histologically, but typically display rather "benign," low-grade behavior, rarely recurring after primary resection (1). OS rates for the embryonal brain tumors presenting in children younger than 3 to 4 years are lower than for older children (138,139). Tumor type, pattern of growth, and the therapeutic ratio for both S and RT are unfavorable when compared to older children. Operative morbidity and mortality rates are higher in infants; after RT, cognitive dysfunction, somatic alterations, endocrine deficits, and neurotoxicity are more pronounced than in older children 140). For malignant gliomas, there is actually suggestion that outcome exceeds that of older children and adults, based on apparent differences in biology and disease response to CT (141).

3.12.1 Therapy

For embryonal tumors with long-established chemosensitivity, a number of trials between 1985 and 2000 explored the use of prolonged primary postoperative CT using delayed, diminished, or no irradiation. Several large series documented a high rate of chemoresponsiveness to a "standard" four-drug regimen (including cyclophosphamide, cisplatin, vincristine, etoposide) or to systemic methotrexate; durable disease control without RT was limited to 25-35% of cases in most trials, typically in those with localized disease amenable to complete resection at diagnosis (135,140,142,143). Successive trials from the German POG tested progressively more intense systemic and intrathecal methotrexate with an alternating drug program incorporating the agents noted above. While overall PFS in the HIT SKK 87 trial (1987 to 1993) was 53% in the favorable resected, M0 cohort, the study showed youngsters with desmoplastic MB enjoyed nearly 90% PFS. The SKK 92 study (1992 to 1997) intensified methotrexate and noted overall 5 year PFS of 58%; among the resected M0 group, 5 year PFS was 82%, with 14 of 17 survivors treated with S and CT only, absent RT which was used only for residual progressive disease. Once again, the results with desmoplastic histology were exceptional: 85% PFS compared to 34% PFS in those with classic MB (144). The second direction was suggested by Khalifa and the French group, where primary CT showed only 29% PFS at 5 years even among the most favorable, resected M0 cohort. Notable was the OS rate of 73%, reflecting excellent "salvage" therapy with high-dose CT, busulfan-thiotepa, and local RT; among 39 patients treated, 5-year postsecondary treatment survival was 77% for those with M0 disease initially and at failure (143,145). Although the St. Jude group had also documented excellent salvage with CSI alone, the functional consequences of more limited RT in this age group seem self evident (140,142). Both POG and the Pediatric Brain Tumor Consortium (PBTC) initiated trials in the late 1990s testing CT with planned, localized irradiation after the initial 4 months of CT. Results are yet in analysis, recognizing that among the M0 group that proceeded to consolidative local RT on PBTC 001, 5-year PFS is 85% and OS, 95%. All infant trials to date have shown poor outcome for the 20% of patients presenting with neuraxis dissemination, OS rates rarely exceeding 10% to 25% (143,145). Although CSI is curative in a significant proportion of children, the consequences of CSI at effective dose levels are not considered acceptable (141). Alternative use of aggressive, high-dose CT alone has been fraught with otherwise unseen toxicity, including toxic deaths and EFS for favorable presentations approximating 50%; outcome in the M+ cohort has been essentially zero. Separate from MB is the immature, highly aggressive ATRT (1,146). ATRTs occur predominantly in young children, presenting in the posterior fossa; those occurring in children older than 3 years are more often supra-tentorial lesions. The lesions are histologically distinctive, and diagnosis by light microscopy and immuno-histochemistry is often definitive. The tumor is associated with monosomy of chromosome 22, a finding in common with extraneural primary rhabdoid tumors. Genetically, the tumor is associated with loss of the tumor suppressor gene hSNF5/INI1 in more than 75% of cases; absence of INI1 by FISH is diagnostic (139,146,147). Up to 15% to 25% of cases show leptomeningeal dissemination at diagnosis (148). Although ATRTs often respond to CT (especially carboplatin-containing regimens), the disease course has been marked by rapid recurrence and neuraxis dissemination. There is an increasing evidence that the outcome is related to post operative RT; recent trials incorporate early local RT for children as young as 12 to 18 months old, ideally limiting postoperative CT to 4 to 6 weeks (137,139,146,148). For children older than 3 years of age, use of post -operative CSI followed by CT has resulted in 78% 2-year EFS compared to 11% for younger children in whom irradiation was delayed or avoided (148).

3.12.2 Surgery

As in older children, complete resection is often the primary predictor of disease control; for infant MB, the differences in outcome strongly favor attempted GTR in every major series regardless of the type and intensity of postoperative management. In the initial Baby POG study, OS for MB was 40%, compared with 60% for the one third of children who had undergone GTR and 69% for those with GTR and localized disease (135). In the latest published GHOP trial, PFS among all M0 cases falls from 82% to 50% based on the absence or presence of residual tumor post S, respectively (144). Delayed definitive S has been utilized for sizable MB or supratentorial PNETs in this age group. After initial CT, tumors may be reduced in size and vascularity, resulting in more successful tumor resection. Choroid plexus tumors are often malignant carcinomas in this age group. The tumors typically arise in the lateral ventricles; histology can be uncertain in predicting benign or malignant behavior, with carcinomas marked largely by brain invasiveness and atypia. Complete resection alone appears to be adequate, with few recurrent tumors following imaging confirmed removal even without added CT or RT (149).

3.12.3 Radiation Therapy

Evolving combinations of systematic or selected consolidative RT, RT for disease progression, or multimodality salvage regimens incorporating low or high-dose RT have resulted in RT as a component of therapy for nearly half of all surviving children in this age group. Important in the context of current strategies is identification of those cases most likely to benefit from local irradiation, with consensus developing toward noting those with classic histology and localized MB or those with incompletely resected M0 desmoplastic MB. Using planned RT, typically within the first 4 months of postoperative CT, is key to avoiding the scenario of requiring more aggressive irradiation and CT for those who progress during or after more prolonged CT. Although salvage CSI has been successful in controlling more than 40% of recurrent MB, the ultimate 40% to 60% disease control was balanced by a median IQ of only 62 at 7 years (149). The latter finding has dampened enthusiasm for salvage CSI, at least at dosage levels greater than 24 Gy, in this age group.

3.12.4 Chemotherapy

The initial van Eys study of primary mechlorethamine vincristine, procarbazine, and prednisone (MOPP) CT at M.D. Anderson Cancer Center showed long term survival in 8 of 11 infants with MB; 6 had not received RT (150). In the first POG trial with initial postoperative CT, the regimen included cycles of cyclophosphamide with vincristine and cisplatin with etoposide; response rates varied between MB, 48% partial and complete response rate among those with imaging residual, and malignant gliomas, 60% (110). PFS and OS rates at 5 years were 32% and 40% for MB, 43% and 50% for malignant gliomas, and 0% and 0% for pineoblastomas; overall 5 year survival was 27% for supratentorial PNETs (107). As in subsequent infant trials, failures beyond 2 years have been uncommon except with ependymomas (140, 142,145,146). Most of the subsequent infant studies have used variations of the four drug regimens noted in the first POG trial; more intensive regimens have shown benefit in specific subsets of infant malignant tumors (143). The Head Start series of intensive CT have evolved to similar four drug induction with second S for residual local tumor, followed by myeloablative doses of thiotepa, etoposide, and carboplatin. In the selected M0 resected medulloblastoma cohort, EFS at 5 years was 52%; OS of 70% those requiring irradiation for disease progression; toxicity has remained a problem with this approach.

3.13 Ependymomas

Intracranial ependymomas represent 5% to 8% of intracranial neoplasms in children. More than 90% of pediatric ependymomas occur as intracranial tumors; primary spinal cord tumors are relatively uncommon in children, where ependymomas represent 25% of primary spinal tumors. Two-thirds ependymomas in children present as posterior fossa lesions, arising along the inner surface of the fourth ventricle or at the cerebellopontine angle (CPA). It is quite common for such tumors to grow into the foramina of Luschka, on either side of the brainstem, toward and to the CPA (151,152). Presentation in the CPA is noted less commonly, occurring particularly in very young children. Fourth ventricular tumors also extend caudally beyond foramen magnum and into the upper cervical spine; extension is either from caudal growth from foramen of Luschka or, more commonly, through the foramen of Magendie and then posteriorly from the cervicomedullary junction caudally (153). Growth below the foramen magnum marks nearly 50% of fourth ventricular lesions. Supratentorial ependymomas account for one third of childhood presentations, occurring predominantly as extra ventricular cerebral hemispheric tumors; growth is commonly adjacent to the third or lateral ventricular regions (153). Ependymomas consist histologically of polygonal cells with large vesicular nuclei and cytoplasmic granules. Characteristic are ependymal rosettes, formed by tumor cells oriented radially around a central lumen; cells also have a tendency to orient themselves around blood vessels, forming perivascular pseudorosettes (1,154). Molecular genetic analyses highlight the origin of ependymomas from populations of neural progenitor cells that are genetically distinct in the supratentorial, posterior fossa, and spinal regions anatomically related patterns of gene expression and regions of chromosomal loss or gain mark the three sites independently (154).

The WHO classification defines ependymomas as grade 1 (subependymomas or myxopapillary spinal ependymomas), grade 2 (classical ependymomas, including cellular, papillary, clear cell, and tancytic types), and grade 3 (anaplastic) (1,154). Subependymomas are benign neoplasms most often arising under the fourth ventricle, but also similarly adjacent to the lateral ventricles. Myxopapillary tumors are indolent lesions occurring primarily in young adults, specifically in the region of the cauda equina. Cellular tumors occur in extraventricular regions with a relatively low mitotic rate. Papillary ependymomas present along the ventricular surfaces. Clear cell tumors mimic oligodendrogliomas histologically, occurring primarily as supratentorial lesions; there is a suggestion that this variant is somewhat aggressive. Tancytic tumors grow as fascicles, usually within the spinal cord. Anaplastic ependymomas are marked by high mitotic rate, microvascular proliferation, and pseudopalisading necrosis. Ependymoblastoma are extremely rare, highly malignant primitive embryonal tumors occurring in infants as supratentorial lesions with features of an ependymal neoplasm; they are not considered in the classification of ependymomas, but rather as embryonal tumors. There have been conflicting reports regarding the correlation between tumor grade and survival. Some prominent neuropathologists in the 1980s reported no correlation between anaplasia or grade and clinical behavior (155). More recent series identify histology as one of the dominant features related to disease control after aggressive S and RT (156). Merchant et al. (157) reviewed the St. Jude historical experience, noting 3 year PFS of 84% among the 70% of children with differentiated ependymomas and 28% for the 30% of cases with anaplastic features. Late follow-up of Merchant's expanded series confirms the impact of tumor grade on outcome. Multi-institutional reviews reflecting independent experience at 11 major US centers and that within the former POG document histopathology as a significant factor, with higher rates of 5-year EFS associated with differentiated histology but no statistical difference in OS for those with anaplastic tumors; the latter report includes a review of 1444 cases in the English literature between 1900 and 2005 substantiating such findings (158). Earlier data suggested a correlation between anaplasia and the frequency of neuraxis dissemination, particularly among fourth ventricular lesions. Merchant's recent report detailing the largest prospective trial similarly documents a significant correlation between anaplastic histology and a higher rate of distant failure (159). Chromosomal abnormalities are present in approximately 50% of tumors, most commonly loss of the long arm of chromosome 22 or 6 orgain in chromosome 1q. Alterations in the Wnt/β-catenin signaling pathway have been related to tumorigenesis in anaplastic ependymomas (160). The p53 pathway appears to be intact in ependymomas, although p53 induced G1 growth arrest is apparent in ependymomas, potentially implicated in radiation resistance (161). The tumors show expression of the ErbB receptors. Ependymomas are somewhat more common in boys, although young children show equal sex distribution or even a slight female predominance. The median age at diagnosis is 4 to 5 years; one third occur in children younger than 3 years, with typically inferior likelihood of disease control (151, 152,157,162). Ependymomas represent a somewhat higher proportion of CNS tumors in infants and young children.

Symptoms usually are non specific and related to fourth ventricular obstruction with headaches, vomiting and ataxia. Children with disease involving the CPA often show torticollis or cranial nerve signs. MRI often shows a non homogeneously enhancing lesion, diagnostic when there is characteristic involvement through the foramen of Luschka. Computed tomography often shows stippled calcification.

3.13.1 Therapy

3.13.1.1 Surgery

Extent of resection is the dominant factor influencing outcome. Fourth ventricular lesions usually are adherent along the brainstem, especially at the level of the obex, where surgical damage can result in significant cardiorespiratory compromise. Total or near total resection has classically been realized in 50% to 75% of cases (151,156,162,163,164). Current image guided neurosurgical techniques and recognition of the importance of GTR have allowed major referral centers to achieve GTR in 80% to 90% of instances, sometimes requiring a second procedure to complete S before adjuvant RT (157). Even in very young children, complete or near complete resection is often feasible prior to initiating further therapy. The relationship between extent of resection and disease control has been apparent for several decades, with EFS averaging 50% to 75% after GTR compared with 30% to 45% with incomplete removal (165,166). With optimal postoperative RT in the prospective St. Jude trial, degree of resection is the single most significant correlate with outcome: 7-year EFS falls from 77% after GTR to 34% with near total or subtotal resection. Even in cases with metastatic disease at diagnosis, the impact of GTR on both 5-year EFS and OS is impressive, with 35% and 59% reported in a retrospective multinstitutional review. Total resection is associated with a low rate of operative mortality, 2.5% or less, and morbidity, 10% to 25% incidence of new neurologic deficits (167,168). Postoperative cranial nerve deficits are common, including components of the posterior fossa syndrome (164). The proximity of vital centers makes GTR in the fourth ventricle rather challenging, particularly for those arising in or extending to the CPA (164,166). Total resection of supratentorial ependymomas is more readily achieved (184). The St. Jude experience with GTR in 96% of tumors originating in the CPA is marked by a 30% major complication rate, including need for tracheostomy, gastrostomy feeding tube, or major cranial nerve palsies. The rationale, continued improvement in neurologic function over time, and overall functional status of often young children has encouraged the neurosurgical team to continue aggressive resection for primary presentations, second S before irradiation, or for local recurrence (175). In young children with moderate disease residual, the option of initial CT with delayed S prior to RT has been noted for some time and is still under exploration (167,168).

3.13.1.2 Radiation Therapy

RT has been a routine component of therapy for ependymomas since the 1950s. The favorable results summarized above, following GTR, are based on the addition of postoperative RT in almost all instances (151,163,164). Earlier, two classic retrospective series confirmed the contribution of RT: Pollack et al. (162) recorded overall 5-year survival of 45% with surgery and irradiation, compared with 13% with Surgery alone, while Rousseau et al. (163) noted 63% survival at 5 years after RT and 23% without. Although there are limited data from Epstein's New York University experience suggesting disease control for differentiated supratentorial ependymomas following S alone, there are very little data documenting favorable disease control rates absent irradiation for posterior fossa presentations, patients with anaplastic histology, or those with any degree of residual disease (166). The prospective Italian Association for Pediatric Hematology and Oncology protocol reports inferior outcome when RT is deferred following S alone, with both inferior disease control and greater morbidity attendant to requisite second S. The excellent results with complete resection and postoperative RT, even in children as young as 12 to 18 months of age, are best demonstrated by Merchant's series from St. Jude, where assiduously contoured target volumes for 3D CRT to relatively high-dose levels resulted in 74% EFS at 5 years, with 87% local tumor control and 85% OS; the rate of local failure is 16% at 7 years (157). The series shows little decrement in outcome at 7 years, recognizing that longer term data reporting results from Children's Hospital of Philadelphia (CHOP), University of Pennsylvania, and Washington University, St. Louis, both show a 10% or greater decline in EFS and OS between 5 and 10 years postirradiation (169). The coordination of aggressive surgical resection and prompt postoperative RT, even in the younger age cohort, resulted in an excellent rate of tumor control and OS with noted but relatively low rates of acute and subacute morbidities from S and RT; prospective data suggest relatively limited functional morbidities to date (170). Disease control rates and local tumor control are equivalent in cohorts younger or older than 3 years in the St. Jude data, based largely on S and RT (157). The recently completed COG trial ACNS0121 studied children more than 12 months of age with postoperative RT for those with complete or near total resection except supratentorial differentiated ependymomas, the latter to be observed after confirmed GTR; children with significant local residual had the option of initial CT followed by second look S prior to RT. There is a modest literature regarding retreatment for ependymomas recurrent following prior S and RT, with or without CT. Resection and full dose local reirradiation to 50 to 54 Gy resulted in secondary disease control for 10 of 13 children following local recurrence; among 12 children with metastatic recurrence retreated with CSI, the 4 year secondary EFS was 53% (170). Tolerance has been surprisingly good, as reported in more eclectic series with stereotactic radiosurgery used for reirradiation in children and adults (171).

3.13.1.3 Chemotherapy

Ependymomas are only modestly chemosensitive tumors, with objective responses most apparent after exposure to cisplatin and oral etoposide (152,157,172). The only prospective, randomized trial that tested adjuvant CT (CCNU, vincristine, prednisone) after S and irradiation was completed by CCG in the early 1980's (173). The trial was small, but there was no suggestion of improved disease control with CT; a subsequent randomized trial of adjuvant CCNU-vincristine-prednisone versus the "8-in-1" regimen showed no improvement in either arm of the trial; the group concluded that local tumor control was the dominant issue, inadequately addressed systemically. Needle reported a limited institution pilot study in children 3 to 14 year old where moderately aggressive carboplatin-vincristine alternating with ifosfamide-etoposide resulted in a 74% 5 year PFS rate, noting half the cohort had incomplete resection; the data reflect a combination intentionally derived from infant protocols, and it is in the latter setting that further assessment of dose intensive CT is ongoing. Gilbertson's documentation of ERBB2 and ERBB4 coexpression in more then 75% of ependymomas specimens has prompted studies in the PBTC testing lapatinib, a molecular targeting agent active in preclinical models against ERBB expressing xenografts (174). Preliminary reports have not been encouraging with this approach, but trials of molecular agents are ongoing. Infant studies may be interpreted positively in documenting that approximately 20% to 25% of children with ependymomas can be controlled with S and CT, absent RT; the more recent UKCCSG/SIOP study alone shows radiation free EFS at 5 years of 42% (157,158,175). The CCG 9921 experience resulted in 5 year EFS of 32% with OS of 59% (142). The multidrug regimens have included the traditional four drug combination (cisplatin, etoposide, vincristine, and cyclophosphamide) or, more recently, the UKCCSG/SIOP dose intensive regime including sequential carboplatin and vincristine, high-dose methotrexate and vincristine, cyclophosphamide, and cisplatin (157,158). The St. Jude experience with a carboplatin based regimen showed 33% 5 year PFS and 62% OS in a series utilizing post CT irradiation with any imaging evidence of residual (141). The impact of RT on disease control in young children had been suggested in the first POG infant brain tumor study: children less than 3 year old received RT after 1 year of CT and those younger than 2 years were scheduled to receive irradiation after 2 years of CT. Long-term disease control was significantly higher in the older cohort, interpreted as likely to be related to earlier RT (157). Part of the rationale for continuing primary CT in this age group is the potential ability for post CT S and RT to achieve ultimate disease control: the 5 year OS in the SFOP series was 59% despite the 22% rate of PFS. Timmermann et al. concluded that the 27% EFS at 3 years following HIT SKK 87 and 92 CT (high-dose methotrexate based, both systemic and intrathecal) is inadequate, resulting in local failures in 75% of cases prior to irradiation and a 3 year OS rate of 56% (176).

3.14 Brainstem glioma

The brainstem is the connecting structure that joins the long tracts from the cerebral hemispheres and midline diencephalic nuclei with the cerebellar tracts. Brainstem tumors are a heterogeneous group of tumors that share common astrocytic histologies but evidence divergent neoplastic behavior and degrees of differentiation, related to the anatomic region of involvement. Brainstem tumors are classified by the anatomic area involved and the macroscopic appearance or pattern of growth: focal lesions are tumors that are discrete or distinctly marginated on imaging, without apparent infiltration beyond the primary lesion, relatively limited in volume, and histology which is low grade, usually JPA, less often fibrillary astrocytoma (177,178). Focal tumors occur most often in the tectal plate and adjacent to pontine nuclei, sharing low grade histology with the largely exophytic tumors arising dorsally exophytic at the ponto medullary junction or in other locations of the brainstem (179). The more common diffusely infiltrating brainstem gliomas (DIBSG) arise in the pons, diffusely expanding the pons and extending rostrally to the cerebral peduncles of the midbrain and sometimes through the internal capsule of the thalamic region, or growing caudally to the medulla or upper spinal cord, less often through the peduncles into the cerebellum. DIBSG account for 75% to 85% of brainstem neoplasms in children and adolescents; focal and exophytic tumors represent 15% to 25% of cases (177,178,180,181). The duration of symptoms correlates with the type of brainstem glioma. Children with DIBSG report a brief history of neurologic symptoms, typically measured in weeks and certainly less than 6 months. Neurologic signs associated with the pontine DIBSGs include cranial nerve deficits, long tract signs, and ataxia; dyspraxia and dysphagia are also rather common (180,181). Elevated intracranial pressure secondary to obstructive hydrocephalus is often present in midbrain tumors or in the expansile dorsally exophytic tumors that fill the fourth ventricle, but noted in fewer than 15% of children with pontine DIBSGs. The focal brainstem tumors are often associated with prolonged, more limited symptoms, findings confined to deficits in one or two cranial nerves alone, ataxia, or dyspraxia, typically with minor long tract signs and a history measured in months or years (177,179,181,182). MRI is the definitive test for diagnosis and delineation of tumor extent and type. The typical diffusely infiltrating pontine glioma is homogeneous and hypointense on T1 imaging but readily appreciated on T2 sequence. DIBSGs expand the pons, often showing exophytic growth in the ventral, dorsal, and/or lateral directions as infiltrating lesions with indistinct margins; gadolinium enhancement is usually absent or minimal. Diffusion tensor imaging and tractography often show sparing of the dorsal columns of the pons with infiltration splaying the longitudinal tracts. Focal brainstem tumors by definition show distinct margins, typically enhancing briskly. 18FDG PET is hypermetabolic in DIBSG; imaging histologic correlations show hyperactivity only among grade 4 or glioblastoma cases; anaplastic astrocytomas were isometabolic with normal brain or hypometabolic, while low-grade fibrillary gliomas were isometabolic (183). As a group, brainstem tumors constitute approximately 10% of intracranial tumors in children. The peak incidence occurs between the ages of 5 and 9 years; boys are affected more commonly than girls. The most common presenting symptomsfor DIBSGs include diplopia, lateralizing motor weakness, and difficulty with speech, swallowing, and walking. Neurologic signs include ataxia, cranial nerve palsies and long tract signs. Tumors of the midbrain and medulla may be diffuse or focal; even diffuse tumors typically show much less infiltration and expansion of the brainstem than seen with the pontine gliomas. Focal intrinsic tumors do occur in the pons, often as localized tumors of a cranial nerve nucleus or along the cerebellopontine peduncle. Biopsy of the classic, diffusely infiltrating pontine glioma is generally unnecessary (178,181,182,184). Following trials in the 1980s of systematic open biopsy that yielded some of the basic knowledge correlating imaging and histopathology, biopsy related neurologic compromise has led most US and European centers to biopsy only the 15% to 20% of atypical brainstem tumors, often demonstrating JPA or fibrillary astrocytoma (183). Stereotactic guidance has resulted in a rather safe approach to the brainstem tumors, with series from Paris, Germany, and Brussels showing current histopathology and clinic imaging correlations while reporting only minor, typically transient new neurologic deficits inapproximately 10% of instances (183,185). The more recent biopsy series shows rather divergent histopathology, clearly dependent on the selection criteria for biopsy: 22 of 24 children showed anaplastic astrocytoma or glioblastoma, with 1 PNET and 1 JPA reported from Hospital Necker-Enfants, compared to 10 of 20 in a more selected series from Brussels, the remainder showing fibrillary astrocytoma, JPA, PNET, or germ cell tumor (185). There is no consistent correlation between histology and outcome; all diffusely infiltrating pontine tumors show extremely poor duration of response to RT and median survival of less than 1 year (182, 186). Brainstem tumors have recently been shown to express ERBB1, with the degree of overexpression or less common amplification proportional to increasing histologic grade (187). The finding suggests that ErbB orEGFR inhibitors may be worth studying in these tumors, allowing selected therapeutic interventions. A protocol considered by the PBTC would select patients for temozolomide based on MGMT expression and erlotinib if EGFR is positive. A small subset of DIBSG may show CNS dissemination. Gururangan et al. described neuraxis metastasis in 17% of 96 patients at a median of 15 months after diagnosis, presenting as parenchymal dissemination, leptomeningeal metastasis, or subependymal spread (188). The dorsally exophytic "benign" brainstem tumor characteristically fills the fourth ventricle, presenting with symptoms and signs of elevated intracranial pressure. In most cases, the tumor enhances briskly with gadolinium. The origin from the floor of the fourth ventricle may be suggested by MRI but is usually apparent only at the time of S. These tumors are almost always JPA; the prognosis has been quite favorable (184,189). Focal tumors of the pons are uncommon. One specific presentation includes isolated facial nerve palsy or similar, limited neurologic dysfunction associated with a small, enhancing intrapontine lesion. Such tumors are JPAs and enjoy a favorable prognosis (190). Tumors of the midbrain may involve the tegmentum or the tectal plate. Tegmental tumors usually are fibrillary astrocytomas. The tumors may involve the tegmentum focally or may infiltrate through much of the midbrain. Lesions may show uniform enhancement or little contrast enhancement. Presenting signs include extra ocular muscle palsy or long track involvement. Biopsy is preferred, especially for lesions contiguous with the pineal region. Tectal plate tumors usually are quite small and well demarcated, confined to the tectal plate. MRI shows the focal nature of tectal lesions, most often signified by brisk enhancement; biopsy generally confirms JPA. These tumors are typically indolent; observation alone is usually the treatment of choice (179,180). If the tumor is anatomically confined to the tectum and stable over an initial 3 to 6 month period of observation, biopsy may be deferred unless there is evidence of tumor progression necessitating therapy (180,190). When lesions are atypical, larger than 10 cc in volume, or when there is some question whether the lesion originated in the adjacent pineal region, biopsy may be needed at diagnosis. If it is confirmed as a LGA, observation is appropriate.

3.15 Therapy

3.15.1 Surgery

The role of S in classic pontine gliomas is limited. Interest in biopsy in the current era is largely to define the biology of the more common DIBSG and to document diagnosis for the atypical brainstem tumors, both intrinsic and exophytic (191,192). For dorsally exophytic tumors, judicious incomplete resection will establish the diagnosis and reduce the obstructing mass in the fourth ventricular region. Although there is no documented advantage to aggressive S, it may be advantageous to remove the bulk of the lesion posteriorly, establishing CSF flow and reducing the bulk of tumor when it can be reasonably separated from the underlying margin of normal, functioning brainstem. Aggressive S as a primary intervention is often associated with unnecessary morbidity. Partial resection alone is associated with 50% to 70% EFS at 5 to 10 years (189). Small focal lesions intrinsic to the pons may be biopsied if safely approachable; one cannot insist on biopsy if the differential diagnosis is limited and the biopsy-associated morbidity is high. Lesions in the tegmentum should be biopsied, although the potential morbidity of stereotactic biopsy is recognized because of the proximity of the central veins. Occasional resection has been reported for midbrain tumors (192). Tumors of the lower medulla or cervicomedullary region are similar to low grade astrocytomas of the spinal cord. Biopsy and attempted GTR have been reported; results after S alone have been impressive but limited to a small number of neurosurgical centers. Histology usually is LGA; malignant gliomas have been reported (191).

3.15.2 Radiation Therapy

Children with diffusely infiltrating pontine gliomas often respond impressively to RT. Up to 70% show improvement in neurologic symptoms and signs over the course of irradiation;

objective reduction in tumor on MRI is apparent within 8 to 12 weeks of initiating RT. Unfortunately, signs of progressive disease are apparent systematically within 6 to 12 months (193). Clinical response has also been noted in tegmental midbrain lesions and tumors of the medulla, where RT is more likely to achieve long term disease control. For tectal plate or dorsally exophytic pontomedullary astrocytomas, RT is typically deferred until signs of disease progression are apparent on imaging (189). Once progression has been documented on serial imaging, there has been almost uniform disease control measured out to more than 5 years after local irradiation. Intrinsic focal pontine lesions often require RT at diagnosis to control attendant neurologic signs. With the availability of precision volume techniques, the risk benefit ratio may favor earlier RT in localized, low grade brainstem lesions (194).

3.15.3 Chemotherapy

Despite documented transient response, there is little evidence of efficacy for CT in brainstem tumors. An earlier prospective, randomized trial of CCNU, vincristine, and prednisone showed no benefit in these tumors despite purported efficacy in supratentorial high grade gliomas (195). Adjuvant studies with concurrent or sequential CT or, more recently, trials incorporating molecular targeting agents have failed to alter the PFS or OS data in this disease (196,197). Despite efficacy in adults with hemispheric malignant gliomas, temozolomide has shown no advantage in DIBSG in children (198). Preirradiation CT regimens have shown some responsiveness, but early disease progression during CT and a lack of objective benefit in postRT intervals to progression have largely dampened enthusiasm for this approach, although a limited recent French trial testing preRT BCNU, cisplatin, and high-dose methotrexate continues to generate interest (199). Cross-study analyses of serial POG brainstem glioma trials actually suggested a detrimental effect when cisplatinum was added to high dose hyperfractionated RT (200). Trials of non cytotoxic radiosensitizers have also been conducted in phases I and II settings for DIBSG; more recent experience with motexafin gadolinium has revealed little benefit (201). Demonstration that large molecules can be perfused directly through the brainstem using an intraaxial catheter for convection enhanced delivery raises the possibility of direct infusion of biologic agents for brainstem gliomas, a concept now being addressed in a phase I trial at the U.S. National Institutes of Health (202). For focal, LGA, the use of CT before RT is an extrapolation from diencephalic low grade tumors, which may be rational in selected settings (203). For the majority of children, even those younger than 4 years, symptomatic or progressive dorsally exophytic or focal pontine lesions can be treated effectively with focal radiation techniques. It is difficult to anticipate any significant advantage in delaying definitive therapy with intervening CT.

3.16 Cerebellar astrocytomas

Cerebellar astrocytomas (CA) make up 10% to 15% of childhood brain tumors and 25% of posterior fossa neoplasms. These tumors are typically low grade, well circumscribed, and slowly growing with prominent cyst formation (204,205). The classic cystic CA presents as a unilocular cyst with a single prominent mural nodule. The cerebellum is one of the most common sites of origin for LGA in children, JPAs comprise 80% to 95% of cases and DFA account for 5% to 15% (206). DFAs tend to be less circumscribed, more infiltrative and expansile, with a less favorable prognosis relative to JPA; the diffuse tumors arise specified, or as oligoastrocytomas. Malignant gliomas are quite uncommon in the childhood cerebellum. The median age at diagnosis is 5 to 6 years, with 20% of cases younger than 3 years; astrocytomas of this location are rarely found in infants (206,207). Presenting symptoms often are confined to those associated with elevated intracranial pressure, with less frequent altered cerebellar function; cranial nerve deficits are uncommon. The majority of tumors arise in the cerebellar hemispheres; approximately one third are primary vermis lesions. Most tumors are confined to the cerebellum; a minority extend to the cerebellopontine peduncle or the posterior aspect of the brainstem. The most characteristic appearance on computed tomography or MRI is a large, well circumscribed tumor with prominent cysts. The nodular or solid portion of the tumor characteristically enhances briskly; the cyst wall may or may not demonstrate contrast enhancement. The nodular and cystic components are considered part of the tumor; both components should be addressed at the time of S (206,207). Cerebellar JPAs have uncommonly been associated with multifocal CNS involvement, representing either neuraxis dissemination or concurrent multifocal presentation (208).

3.16.1 Therapy

3.16.1.1 Surgery

S is the treatment of choice for CA and the amount of resection has been found to be the most important prognostic factor for outcome. For classic cystic CA, GTR has been reported in 70% to 90% of cases (209). PFS for these children is in excess of 90%. Even in the setting of documented should residual, many tumors remain indolent. After imaging confirmed GTR, recurrence is uncommon, noted at 5% to 10% in major series (206,207,208). After incomplete resection, disease progression has been reported in 30% to 60% of cases at 5 years or more, long term survival remains above 65% (205,206,209). Infiltrative tumors and DFA are less likely to be amenable to GTR and are associated with a higher rate of disease progression or recurrence. Despite the indolent nature of these tumors, the median time to recurrence is about 2 years (205,206). Children who experience tumor recurrence amenable to resection may benefit from a second S.

3.16.1.2 Radiation Therapy

There is no established role for RT in the primary management of CA amenable to GTR and prognostic factors that may predict relapse after initial S alone be considered. Most series indicate greater risk of later disease progression in recurrent tumors, infiltrative tumors, astrocytomas that cannot be completely resected, and tumors with diffuse fibrillary histology or more aggressive histologic subtypes (206,207,208,209). Indications for RT include progression of incompletely resected tumors not amenable to second S and incomplete resection following recurrence. This is an uncommon situation for JPA, but is seen more frequently in tumors with diffuse fibrillary histology. Given recent data showing the efficacy of CT in delaying disease progression, CT may be the preferred initial adjuvant treatment for these more aggressive presentations in very young children (210). There are no data substantiating improvement in disease control with postoperative RT following a complete resection (207,209,211). Lesions with an infiltrative pattern involving the peduncle or brainstem may require early RT when symptomatic or progressive. The treatment of high-grade CA generally includes multiple modalities and postoperative RT is recognized as the standard of care. CSF dissemination is a recognized pattern of failure; CSI is typically considered only when overt CNS metastasis is documented (206,208,211).

3.16.1.3 Chemotherapy

Because most LGA located in the cerebellum are amenable to S and do not require adjuvant therapy, it is relatively rare to use CT for this specific tumor site. Multiple chemotherapeutic agents have been shown to delay progression (210,212). The most commonly administered regimen is the combination of carboplatin and vincristine.

4. References

[1] Louis DN, Ohgaki H, Wiestler OD, et al. WHO Classification of Tumours of the Central Nervous System. 4th ed. World Health Organization; 2007.

[2] Lewis RA, Gerson LP, Axelson KA, et al. von Recklinghausen neurofibromatosis. II. Incidence of optic gliomata. Ophthalmology. 1984;91:929–935.

[3] Li FP, Fraumeni JF Jr. Soft-tissue sarcomas, breast cancer, and other neoplasms. A familial syndrome? Ann Intern Med. 1969;71:747–752.

[4] Relling MV, Rubnitz JE, Rivera GK, et al. High incidence of secondary brain tumours after radiotherapy and antimetabolites. Lancet. 1999;354:34–39.

[5] Perry A. Pathology of low-grade gliomas: an update of emerging concepts. Neuro-Oncol. 2003;5:168–178.

[6] Wisoff JH, Sanford RA, Heier LA, et al. Primary neurosurgery for pediatric low-grade astrocytomas: a prospective multi-institutional study. Neurosurgery. 2009.

[7] Shaw EG, Wisoff JH. Prospective clinical trials of intracranial low-grade glioma in adults and children. Neuro-Oncol. 2003;5:153–160.

[8] Pollack IF, Claassen D, al-Shboul Q, et al. Low-grade gliomas of the cerebral hemispheres in children: an analysis of 71 cases. JNeurosurg. 1995;82:536–547.

[9] Merchant TE, Kun LE, Wu S, et al. Phase II trial of conformal radiation therapy for pediatric low-grade glioma. J Clin Oncol .2009;27:3598–3604.

[10] Merchant TE, Conklin HM, Wu S, et al. Late effects of conformal radiation therapy for pediatric patients with low-grade glioma: prospective evaluation of cognitive, endocrine, and hearing deficits. J Clin Oncol. 2009;27:3691–3697.

[11] Marcus KJ, Goumnerova L, Billett AL, et al. Stereotactic radiotherapy for localized low-grade gliomas in children: final results of a prospective trial. Int J Radiat Oncol Biol Phys. 2005;61:374–379.

[12] Packer RJ, Ater J, Allen J, et al. Carboplatin and vincristine chemotherapy for children with newly diagnosed progressivelow-grade gliomas. J Neurosurg . 1997;86:747–754.

[13] Chemotherapy for progressive low grade astrocytoma in children less than 10 years old: a Phase III Intergroup COG Study. Internet; 2009.

[14] Packer RJ. Chemotherapy: low-grade gliomas of the hypothalamus and thalamus. Pediatr Neurosurg. 2000;32:259–263.

[15] Khaw SL, Coleman LT, Downie PA, et al. Temozolomide in pediatric low-grade glioma. Pediatr Blood Cancer. 2007;49:808–811.

[16] Packer RJ, Jakacki R, Horn M, et al. Objective response of multiply recurrent low-grade gliomas to bevacizumab and irinotecan. Pediatr Blood Cancer. 2009;52:791–795.

[17] Janss AJ, Grundy R, Cnaan A, et al. Optic pathway and hypothalamic/chiasmatic gliomas in children younger than age 5 years with a 6 year follow-up. Cancer . 1995;75:1051–1059.

[18] Pollack IF, Hurtt M, Pang D, et al. Dissemination of low grade intracranial astrocytomas in children. Cancer. 1994;73:2869–2878.
[19] Tao ML, Barnes PD, Billett AL, et al. Childhood optic chiasm gliomas: radiographic response following radiotherapy and long-term clinical outcome. Int J Radiat Oncol Biol Phys . 1997;39:579–587.
[20] Schmandt SM, Packer RJ, Vezina LG, et al. Spontaneous regression of low-grade astrocytomas in childhood. Pediatr Neurosurg.2000;32:132–136.
[21] Alvord EC Jr, Lofton S. Gliomas of the optic nerve or chiasm. Outcome by patients' age, tumor site, and treatment. J Neurosurg .1988;68:85–98.
[22] Hoffman HJ, Humphreys RP, Drake JM, et al. Optic pathway/hypothalamic gliomas: a dilemma in management. Pediatr Neurosurg. 1993;19:186–195.
[23] Medlock MD, Scott RM. Optic chiasm astrocytomas of childhood. Surgical management. Pediatr Neurosurg. 1997;27:129–136.
[24] Listernick R, Louis DN, Packer RJ, et al. Optic pathway gliomas in children with neurofibromatosis 1: consensus statement from the NF1 Optic Pathway Glioma Task Force. Ann Neurol. 1997;41:143–149.
[25] Bataini JP, Delanian S, Ponvert D. Chiasmal gliomas: results of irradiation management in 57 patients and review of literature. Int J Radiat Oncol Biol Phys. 1991;21: 615–623.
[26] Jenkin D, Angyalfi S, Becker L, et al. Optic glioma in children: surveillance, resection, or irradiation? Int J Radiat Oncol Biol Phys. 1993;25:215–225.
[27] Bataini JP, Delanian S, Ponvert D. Chiasmal gliomas: results of irradiation management in 57 patients and review of literature. IntJ Radiat Oncol Biol Phys. 1991;21: 615–623.
[28] Packer RJ. Chemotherapy: low-grade gliomas of the hypothalamusand thalamus. Pediatr Neurosurg. 2000;32:259–263.
[29] Rudoltz MS, Regine WF, Langston JW, et al. Multiple causes ofcerebrovascular events in children with tumors of the parasellarregion. J Neurooncol . 1998;37:251–261.
[30] Sharif S, Ferner R, Birch JM, et al. Second primary tumors in neurofibromatosis patients treated for optic glioma: substantial risks after radiotherapy. J Clin Oncol. 2006;24:2570–2575.
[31] Krieger MD, Gonzalez-Gomez I, Levy ML, et al. Recurrence patterns and anaplastic change in a long-term study of pilocytic astrocytomas. Pediatr Neurosurg. 1997;27:1–11.
[32] Dirks PB, Jay V, Becker LE, et al. Development of anaplastic changes in low-grade astrocytomas of childhood. Neurosurgery. 1994;34:68–78.
[33] Packer RJ, Sutton LN, Bilaniuk LT, et al. Treatment of chiasmatic/hypothalamic gliomas of childhood with chemotherapy: an update. Ann Neurol. 1988;23:79–85.
[34] Prados MD, Edwards MS, Rabbitt J, et al. Treatment of pediatric low-grade gliomas with a nitrosourea-based multiagent chemotherapy regimen. J Neuro-Oncol. 1997;32:235–241.
[35] Friedman HS, Krischer JP, Burger P, et al. Treatment of children with progressive or recurrent brain tumors with carboplatin or iproplatin: a Pediatric Oncology Group randomized phase IIstudy. J Clin Oncol 1992;10:249–256.
[36] Razack N, Baumgartner J, Bruner J. Pediatric oligodendrogliomas. Pediatr Neurosurg. 1998;28:121–129.
[37] Ino Y, Betensky RA, Zlatescu MC, et al. Molecular subtypes of anaplastic oligodendroglioma: implications for patient management at diagnosis. Clin Cancer Res. 2001;7:839–845.

[38] Shaw EG, Scheithauer BW, O'Fallon JR, et al. Oligodendrogliomas: the Mayo Clinic experience. J Neurosurg. 1992;76:428-434.
[39] Shaw EG, Scheithauer BW, O'Fallon JR. Management of supratentorial low-grade gliomas. Oncology. 1993;7:97-104,107.
[40] Gajjar A, Heideman RL, Kovnar EH, et al. Response of pediatric low grade gliomas to chemotherapy. Pediatr Neurosurg.1993;19:113-118.
[41] Leenstra JL, Rodriguez FJ, Frechette CM, et al. Central neurocytoma: management recommendations based on a 35-year experience. Int J Radiat Oncol Biol Phys. 2007;67:1145-1154
[42] Fujisawa H, Marukawa K, Hasegawa M, et al. Genetic differences between neurocytoma and dysembryoplastic neuroepithelial tumor and oligodendroglial tumors. J Neurosurg.2002;97:1350-1355.
[43] Yasargil MG, von Ammon K, von Deimling A, et al. Central neurocytoma: histopathological variants and therapeutic approaches. J Neurosurg. 1992;76:32-37.
[44] Kim DG, Paek SH, Kim IH, et al. Central neurocytoma: the role of radiation therapy and long term outcome. Cancer.1997;79:1995-2002.
[45] Daumas-Duport C, Scheithauer BW, Chodkiewicz JP, et al.Dysembryoplastic neuroepithelial tumor: a surgically curable tumor of young patients with intractable partial seizures. Reportof thirtynine cases. Neurosurgery. 1988;23:545-556.
[46] Daumas-Duport C. Dysembryoplastic neuroepithelial tumours. Brain Pathology. 1993;3:283-295
[47] Broniscer A, Gajjar A. Supratentorial high-grade astrocytoma and diffuse brainstem glioma: two challenges for the pediatric oncologist. Oncologist. 2004;9:197-206.
[48] Louis DN, Holland EC, Cairncross JG. Glioma classification: a molecular reappraisal. Am J Pathol. 2001;159:779-786.
[49] Heideman RL, Kuttesch J Jr, Gajjar AJ, et al. Supratentorial malignant gliomas in childhood: a single institution perspective. Cancer. 1997;80:497-504.
[50] Nagashima G, Suzuki R, Hokaku H, et al. Graphic analysis of microscopic tumor cell infiltration, proliferative potential, and vascular endothelial growth factor expression in an autopsy brain with glioblastoma. Surg Neurol. 1999;51:292-299.
[51] Pirotte BJ, Levivier M, Goldman S, et al. Positron emission tomography-guided volumetric resection of supratentorial high-grade gliomas: a survival analysis in 66 consecutive patients. Neurosurgery. 2009;64:471-481.
[52] Wisoff JH, Boyett JM, Berger MS, et al. Current neurosurgicalmanagement and the impact of the extent of resection in the treatment of malignant gliomas of childhood: a report of theChildren's Cancer Group trial no. CCG-945. J Neurosurg.1998;89:52-59.
[53] Chan JL, Lee SW, Fraass BA, et al. Survival and failure patterns of high-grade gliomas after three-dimensional conformal radiotherapy. J Clin Oncol. 2002;20:1635-1642.
[54] Wagner S, Benesch M, Berthold F, et al. Secondary disseminationin children with high-grade malignant gliomas and diffuse intrinsic pontine gliomas. Br J Cancer. 2006;95:991-997.
[55] Narayana A, Yamada J, Berry S, et al. Intensity-modulated radiotherapy in high-grade gliomas: clinical and dosimetric results. IntJ Radiat Oncol Biol Phys. 2006;64:892-897.
[56] Park I, Tamai G, Lee MC, et al. Patterns of recurrence analysis in newly diagnosed glioblastoma multiforme after three-dimensional conformal radiation therapy with

respect to preradiation therapy magnetic resonance spectroscopic findings. Int J Radiat Oncol Biol Phys. 2007;69:381–389.
[57] Lee IH, Piert M, Gomez-Hassan D, et al. Association of 11C-methionine PET uptake with site of failure after concurrent temozolomide and radiation for primary glioblastoma multiforme. Int J Radiat Oncol Biol Phys. 2009;73: 479–485.
[58] Pigott TJ, Punt JA, Lowe JS, et al. The clinical, radiological and histopathological features of cerebral primitive neuroectodermaltumours. Br J Neurosurg. 1990;4:287–297.
[59] Albright AL, Wisoff JH, Zeltzer P, et al. Prognostic factors in chil-dren with supratentorial (non pineal) primitive neuroectodermaltumors. A neurosurgical perspective from the Children's CancerGroup. Pediatr Neurosurg. 1995;22:1–7.
[60] Rubinstein LJ. Embryonal central neuroepithelial tumors and their differentiating potential. A cytogenetic view of a complex neuro-oncological problem. J Neurosurg. 1985;62: 795–805.
[61] Jakacki RI, Zeltzer PM, Boyett JM, et al. Survival and prognosticfactors following radiation and/or chemotherapy for primitive neuroectodermal tumors of the pineal region in infants and children: a report of the Children's Cancer Group. J Clin Oncol.1995;13:1377–1383.
[62] Pizer BL, Weston CL, Robinson KJ, et al. Analysis of patients with supratentorial primitive neuro-ectodermal tumours entered intothe SIOP/UKCCSG PNET 3 study. Eur J Cancer. 2006;42:1120–1128.
[63] Gaffney CC, Sloane JP, Bradley NJ, et al. Primitive neuroectodermal tumours of the cerebrum. Pathology and treatment. J Neurooncol. 1985;3:23–33.
[64] Chintagumpala M, Hassall T, Palmer S, et al. A pilot study of risk-adapted radiotherapy and chemotherapy in patients with supratentorial PNET. Neuro-Oncol. 2009;11:33–40.
[65] Burger PC, Scheithauer BW, Vogel FS. Surgical Pathology of theNervous System and its Coverings. 4th ed. New York: Churchill Livingstone; 2002.
[66] McLendon RE, Rosenblum MC, Bigner DD. Russell & Rubinstein's Pathology of Tumors of the Nervous System (Contemporary Neurology). 7th ed. London: A Hodder Arnold; 2006.
[67] Glenn OA, Barkovich AJ. Intracranial germ cell tumors: a compre-hensive review of proposed embryologic derivation. Pediatr Neurosurg. 1996;24:242–251.
[68] Sawamura Y, Ikeda J, Shirato H, et al. Germ cell tumours of thecentral nervous system: treatment consideration based on 111cases and their long-term clinical outcomes. Eur J Cancer.1998;34:104–110.
[69] Cunliffe CH, Fischer I, Karajannis M, et al. Synchronous mixedgerm cell tumor of the pineal gland and suprasellar region with apredominant angiomatous component: a diagnostic challenge. J Neurooncol. 2009;93:269–274.
[70] Schild SE, Scheithauer BW, Schomberg PJ, et al. Pineal parenchymal tumors. Clinical, pathologic, and therapeutic aspects. Cancer.1993;72:870–880.
[71] Erlich SS, Apuzzo ML. The pineal gland: anatomy, physiology, and clinical significance. J Neurosurg. 1985;63:321–341.
[72] Maghnie M, Cosi G, Genovese E, et al. Central diabetes insipidusin children and young adults. N Engl J Med. 2000; 343:998–1007.
[73] MacDonald SM, Desai N, Heller G, et al. MRI changes in the "normal" pineal gland following chemotherapy for suprasellar germ celltumors. Pediatr Hematol Oncol. 2008;25:5–15.

[74] Balmaceda C, Heller G, Rosenblum M, et al. Chemotherapy without irradiation a novel approach for newly diagnosed CNS germcell tumors: results of an international cooperative trial. The First International Central Nervous System Germ Cell Tumor Study. J Clin Oncol. 1996;14:2908-2915.
[75] Finlay J, da Silva NS, Lavey R, et al. The management of patients with primary central nervous system (CNS) germinoma: current controversies requiring resolution. Pediatr Blood Cancer.2008;51:313-316.
[76] Matsutani M, Sano K, Takakura K, et al. Primary intracranial germcell tumors: a clinical analysis of 153 histologically verified cases. J Neurosurg. 1997;86:446-455.
[77] Dearnaley DP, A'Hern RP, Whittaker S, et al. Pineal and CNS germcell tumors: Royal Marsden Hospital experience 1962-1987. Int JRadiat Oncol Biol Phys. 1990;18:773-781.
[78] Kretschmar C, Kleinberg L, Greenberg M, et al. Preradiation chemotherapy with response-based radiation therapy in childrenwith central nervous system germ cell tumors: a report from theChildren's Oncology Group. Pediatr Blood Cancer. 2007;48:285-291.
[79] Calaminus G, Bamberg M, Baranzelli MC, et al. Intracranial germcell tumors: a comprehensive update of the European data. Neuropediatrics. 1994;25:26-32.
[80] Regis J, Bouillot P, Rouby-Volot F, et al. Pineal region tumors andthe role of stereotactic biopsy: review of the mortality, morbidity,and diagnostic rates in 370 cases. Neurosurgery. 1996;39:907-912.
[81] Calaminus G, Bamberg M, Harms D, et al. AFP/beta-HCG secretingCNS germ cell tumors: long-term outcome with respect to initialsymptoms and primary tumor resection. Results of the cooperativetrial MAKEI 89. Neuropediatrics. 2005;36:71-77.
[82] Allen JC, Kim JH, Packer RJ. Neoadjuvant chemotherapy for newly diagnosed germ-cell tumors of the central nervous system. J Neurosurg. 1987;67:65-70.
[83] Robertson PL, DaRosso RC, Allen JC. Improved prognosis of in-tracranial non-germinoma germ cell tumors with multimodalitytherapy. J Neurooncol. 1997;32:71-80.
[84] Shibamoto Y, Takahashi M, Sasai K. Prognosis of intracranial germinoma with syncytiotrophoblastic giant cells treated by radiation therapy. Int J Radiat Oncol Biol Phys. 1997;37:505-510.
[85] Haas-Kogan DA, Missett BT, Wara WM, et al. Radiation therapy for intracranial germ cell tumors. Int J Radiat Oncol Biol Phys.2003;56:511-518.
[86] Paulino AC. Induction chemotherapy and involved-field radiotherapy for intracranial germinoma. J Clin Oncol. 2002;20:2911-2912.
[87] Sawamura Y, Shirato H, Ikeda J, et al. Induction chemotherapy followed by reduced volume radiation therapy for newly diagnosed central nervous system germinoma. J Neurosurg.1998;88:66-72.
[88] Lafay-Cousin L, Millar BA, Mabbott D, et al. Limited field radiation for bifocal germinoma. Int J Radiat Oncol Biol Phys.2006;65:486-492.
[89] Kondziolka D, Hadjipanayis CG, Flickinger JC, et al. The role ofradiosurgery for the treatment of pineal parenchymal tumors. Neurosurgery. 2002;51:880-889.
[90] Kitamura K, Shirato H, Sawamura Y, et al. Preirradiation evaluation and technical assessment of involved-field radiotherapy using computed tomographic (CT) simulation and neoadjuvant chemotherapy for intracranial germinoma. Int J Radiat Oncol BiolPhys. 1999;43:783-788.

[91] Paulino AC, Wen BC, Mohideen MN. Controversies in the management of intracranial germinomas. Oncology .1999;13:513–521.
[92] Merchant TE, Davis BJ, Sheldon JM, et al. Radiation therapy forrelapsed CNS germinoma after primary chemotherapy. J ClinOncol. 1998;16:204–209.
[93] A phase II study to assess the ability of neoadjuvant chemotherapy and second look surgery to eliminate all measurable diseaseprior to radiotherapy for NGGCT. Internet; 2009.
[94] Modak S, Gardner S, Dunkel IJ, et al. Thiotepa-based high-dosechemotherapy with autologous stem-cell rescue in patients with recurrent or progressive CNS germ cell tumors. J Clin Oncol.2004;22:1934–1943.
[95] Burger PC, Grahmann FC, Bliestle A, et al. Differentiation in the medulloblastoma. A histological and immunohistochemical study. Acta Neuropathol. 1987;73:115–123.
[96] Rubin JB, Rowitch DH. Medulloblastoma: a problem of developmental biology. Cancer Cell. 2002;2:7–8.
[97] Gilbertson RJ. Medulloblastoma: signalling a change in treatment. Lancet Oncol. 2004;5:209–218.
[98] de Bont JM, Packer RJ, Michiels EM, et al. Biological background ofpediatric medulloblastoma and ependymoma: a review from a trans-lational research perspective. Neuro Oncol. 2008;10:1040–1060.
[99] Berman DM, Karhadkar SS, Hallahan AR, et al. Medulloblastoma growth inhibition by hedgehog pathway blockade. Science. 2002;297:1559–1561.
[100] Brown HG, Kepner JL, Perlman EJ, et al. "Large cell-anaplastic"medulloblastomas: a Pediatric Oncology Group study. J Neuropathol Exp Neurol. 2000;59:857–865.
[101] Pomeroy SL, Tamayo P, Gaasenbeek M, et al. Prediction of central nervous system embryonal tumour outcome based on gene expression. Nature. 2002;415:436–442.
[102] Kortmann RD, Kuhl J, Timmermann B, et al. Postoperative neoadjuvant chemotherapy before radiotherapy as compared to immediate radiotherapy followed by maintenance chemotherapy in thetreatment of medulloblastoma in childhood: results of the Germanprospective randomized trial HIT'91. Int J Radiat Oncol Biol Phys. 2000;46:269–279.
[103] Chang CH, Housepian EM, Herbert C Jr. An operative staging system and a megavoltage radiotherapeutic technic for cerebellar medulloblastomas. Radiology. 1969;93:1351–1359.
[104] Zeltzer PM, Boyett JM, Finlay JL, et al. Metastasis stage, adjuvant treatment and residual tumor are prognostic factors for medulloblastoma in children: conclusions from the Children's Cancer Group 921 randomized phase III study. J Clin Oncol. 1999;17:832–845.
[105] Bailey CC, Gnekow A, Wellek S, et al. Prospective randomised trial ofchemotherapy given before radiotherapy in childhood medulloblastoma. International Society of Paediatric Oncology (SIOP) and the(German) Society of Paediatric Oncology (GPO): SIOP II. Med Pediatr Oncol. 1995;25:166–178.
[106] Packer RJ, Rood BR, MacDonald TJ. Medulloblastoma: present concepts of stratification into risk groups. Pediatr Neurosurg. 2003;39:60–67.
[107] Cushing H. Experiences with the cerebellar medulloblastomas: a critical review. Acta Pathol Microbiol Scand. 1930; 1:1–86.
[108] Douglas JG, Barker JL, Ellenbogen RG, et al. Concurrent chemotherapy and reduced dose cranial spinal irradiation followed by conformal posterior fossa tumor bed boost for average-risk medulloblastoma: efficacy and patterns of failure. Int J Radiat Oncol Biol Phys. 2004;58:1161–1164.

[109] Miller NG, Reddick WE, Kocak M, et al. Cerebellocerebral diaschisis is the likely mechanism of postsurgical posterior fossa syndrome in pediatric patients with midline cerebellar tumors. Am J Neuroradiol. 2010;31;288–294.

[110] Miller NG, Reddick WE, Kocak M, et al. Cerebellocerebral diaschisis is the likely mechanism of postsurgical posterior fossa syndrome in pediatric patients with midline cerebellar tumors. Am J Neuroradiol. 2010;31;288–294.

[111] Oyharcabal-Bourden V, Kalifa C, Gentet JC, et al. Standard risk medulloblastoma treated by adjuvant chemotherapy followed by reduced dose craniospinal radiation therapy: a French Society ofPediatric Oncology Study. J Clin Oncol. 2005;23:4726–4734.

[112] Grill J, Lellouch-Tubiana A, Elouahdani S, et al. Preoperativechemotherapy in children with high-risk medulloblastomas: a feasibility study. J Neurosurg. 2005;103:312–318.

[113] Cutler EC, Sosman MC, Vaughan WW. Place of radiation in treatment of cerebellar medulloblastoma: report of 20 cases. Am J Roentgenol Radium Ther Nucl Med. 1936;35:429–453.

[114] Bloom HJG, Glees J, Bell J. The treatment and prognosis of medulloblastoma in children. AJR Am J Roentgenol. 1969; 105:43–62.

[115] Carrie C, Grill J, Figarella-Branger D, et al. Online quality control,hyperfractionated radiotherapy alone and reduced boost volume forstandard risk medulloblastoma: long-term results of MSFOP 98. J Clin Oncol. 2009;27: 1879–1883.

[116] Merchant TE, Kun LE, Krasin MJ, et al. Multi institution prospective trial of reduced dose craniospinal irradiation (23.4 Gy) followed by conformal posterior fossa (36 Gy) and primary site irradiation (55.8 Gy) and dose-intensive chemotherapy for average-risk medulloblastoma. Int J Radiat Oncol Biol Phys. 2008;70:782–787.

[117] Packer RJ, Gajjar A, Vezina G, et al. Phase III study of cranio spinalradiation therapy followed by adjuvant chemotherapy for newly di-agnosed average-risk medulloblastoma. JClin Oncol. 2006;24:4202–4208.

[118] Taylor RE, Bailey CC, Robinson KJ, et al. Impact of radiotherapy parameters on outcome in the International Society of PaediatricOncology-United Kingdom Children's Cancer Study Group PNET-3 study of preradiotherapy chemotherapy for M0–M1 medulloblastoma. Int J Radiat Oncol Biol Phys. 2004;58:1184–1193.

[119] Mulhern RK, Merchant TE, Gajjar A, et al. Late neurocognitive sequelae in survivors of brain tumours in childhood. Lancet Oncol. 2004;5:399–408.

[120] Merchant TE, Kiehna EN, Li C, et al. Modeling radiation dosimetry to predict cognitive outcomes in pediatric patients with CNS embryonal tumors including medulloblastoma. Int J Radiat Oncol BiolPhys. 2006;65:210–221.

[121] Allen J, Donahue B, Mehta M, et al. A phase II study of preradiotherapy chemotherapy followed by hyperfractionated radiotherapy for newly diagnosed high-risk medulloblastoma-primitiveneuroectodermal tumor: a report from the Children's OncologyGroup (CCG 9931). Int J Radiat Oncol Biol Phys. 2009;74:1006–1011.

[122] Heideman RL, Kovnar EH, Kellie SJ, et al. Preirradiation chemotherapy with carboplatin and etoposide in newly diagnosed embryonal pediatric CNS tumors. J Clin Oncol. 1995;13:2247–2254.

[123] Stewart CF, Iacono LC, Chintagumpala M, et al. Results of a phaseII upfront window of pharmacokinetically guided topotecan inhigh-risk medulloblastoma and supratentorial primitive neuroectodermal tumor. J Clin Oncol. 2004;22: 3357–3365.

[124] Packer RJ, Goldwein J, Nicholson HS, et al. Treatment of childrenwith medulloblastomas with reduced-dose craniospinal radiationtherapy and adjuvant chemotherapy: a Children's Cancer GroupStudy. J Clin Oncol. 1999;17:2127–2136.
[125] Fouladi M, Chintagumpala M, Ashley D, et al. Amifostine protectsagainst cisplatin-induced ototoxicity in children with average-risk medulloblastoma. J Clin Oncol. 2008; 26: 3749–3755.
[126] Taylor RE, Bailey CC, Robinson KJ, et al. Outcome for patients withmetastatic (M2-3) medulloblastoma treated with SIOP-UKCCSGPNET-3 chemotherapy. Eur J Cancer. 2005; 41:727–734.
[127] von HK, Hinkes B, Gerber NU, et al. Long-term outcome and clinical prognostic factors in children with medulloblastoma treated inthe prospective randomised multicentre trial HIT'91. Eur J Cancer. 2009;45:1209–1217.
[128] Gandola L, Massimino M, Cefalo G, et al. Hyperfractionated accelerated radiotherapy in the Milan strategy for metastatic medulloblastoma. J Clin Oncol. 2009;27:566–571.
[129] Shih CS, Hale GA, Gronewold L, et al. High-dose chemotherapy with autologous stem cell rescue for children with recurrent malignant brain tumors. Cancer. 2008; 112: 1345–1353.
[130] Massimino M, Gandola L, Spreafico F, et al. No salvage using high-dose chemotherapy plus-minus reirradiation for relapsing previously irradiated medulloblastoma. Int J Radiat Oncol Biol Phys. 2009;73:1358–1363.
[131] Gururangan S, Krauser J, Watral MA, et al. Efficacy of high-dosechemotherapy or standard salvage therapy in patients with recurrent medulloblastoma. Neuro Oncol. 2008;10:745–751.aaaaaaaaa
[132] Saran F, Baumert BG, Creak AL, et al. Hypofractionated stereotactic radiotherapy in the management of recurrent or residual medulloblastoma-PNET. Pediatr Blood Cancer. 2008;50:554–560.
[133] Kramer K, Humm JL, Souweidane MM, et al. Phase I study of targeted radioimmunotherapy for leptomeningeal cancers using intra-Ommaya 131-I-3F8. J Clin Oncol. 2007;25:5465–5470.
[134] Childhood Brain Tumor Consortium. Supplement Report: Primary Brain Tumors in the United States, 2004. Hinsdale, IL: Central Brain Tumor Registry of the United States, 2008.
[135] Larouche V, Huang A, Bartels U, et al. Tumors of the central nervous system in the first year of life. Pediatr Blood Cancer. 2007;49:1074–1082.
[136] Meyers SP, Khademian ZP, Biegel JA, et al. Primary intracranial atypical teratoid-rhabdoid tumors of infancy and childhood: MRI features and patient outcomes. AJNR Am J Neuroradiol. 2006;27:962–971.
[137] Packer RJ, Biegel JA, Blaney S, et al. Atypical teratoid-rhabdoid tumor of the central nervous system: report on workshop. J Pediatr Hematol Oncol. 2002;24:337–342.
[138] Cohen BH, Packer RJ, Siegel KR, et al. Brain tumors in children under 2 years: treatment, survival and long-term prognosis. Pediatr Neurosurg. 1993;19:171–179.
[139] Tekautz TM, Fuller CE, Blaney S, et al. Atypical teratoid- rhabdoid tumors (ATRT): improved survival in children 3 years of age and older with radiation therapy and high-dose alkylator-based chemotherapy. J Clin Oncol. 2005;23: 1491–1499.
[140] Walter AW, Mulhern RK, Gajjar A, et al. Survival and neurodevelopmental outcome of young children with medulloblastoma at St. Jude Children's Research Hospital. J Clin Oncol. 1999;17:3720–3728.

[141] Sanders RP, Kocak M, Burger PC, et al. High-grade astrocytoma in very young children. Pediatr Blood Cancer. 2007; 49:888–893.
[142] Fouladi M, Gururangan S, Moghrabi A, et al. Carboplatin-based primary chemotherapy for infants and young children with CNS tumors. Cancer. 2009;115:3243–3253.
[143] Geyer JR, Sposto R, Jennings M, et al. Multiagent chemotherapyand deferred radiotherapy in infants with malignant brain tumors: a report from the Children's Cancer Group. J Clin Oncol. 2005;23:7621–7231.
[144] Grill J, Sainte-Rose C, Jouvet A, et al. Treatment of medulloblastoma with postoperative chemotherapy alone: an SFOP prospective trial in young children. Lancet Oncol. 2005;6:573–580.
[145] Rutkowski S, Bode U, Deinlein F, et al. Treatment of early childhood medulloblastoma by postoperative chemotherapy alone. N Engl J Med. 2005;352:978–986.
[146] Ridola V, Grill J, Doz F, et al. High-dose chemotherapy with autologous stem cell rescue followed by posterior fossa irradiation for local medulloblastoma recurrence or progression after conventional chemotherapy. Cancer. 2007;110: 156–163.
[147] Squire SE, Chan MD, Marcus KJ. Atypical teratoid-rhabdoid tumor: the controversy behind radiation therapy. J Neurooncol. 2007;81:97–111.
[148] Biegel JA, Kalpana G, Knudsen ES, et al. The role of INI1 and theSWI/SNF complex in the development of rhabdoid tumors: meet-ing summary from the workshop on childhood atypical teratoid-rhabdoid tumors. Cancer Res. 2002; 62:323–328.
[149] Chi SN, Zimmerman MA, Yao X, et al. Intensive multimodality treatment for children with newly diagnosed CNS atypical teratoid rhabdoid tumor. J Clin Oncol. 2009;27: 385–389.
[150] Krishnan S, Brown PD, Scheithauer BW, et al. Choroid plexus papillomas: a single institutional experience.J Neurooncol. 2004;68:49–55.
[151] Ater JL, van Eys J, Woo SY, et al. MOPP chemotherapy without ir-radiation as primary postsurgical therapy for brain tumors in infants and young children. J Neurooncol. 1997;32:243–252.
[152] Nazar GB, Hoffman HJ, Becker LE, et al. Infratentorial ependymomas in childhood: prognostic factors and treatment. J Neurosurg. 1990;72:408–417.
[153] Veelen-Vincent ML, Pierre-Kahn A, Kalifa C, et al. Ependymoma in childhood: prognostic factors, extent of surgery, and adjuvant therapy. J Neurosurg. 2002;97:827–835.
[154] Yuh EL, Barkovich AJ, Gupta N. Imaging of ependymomas: MRI and CT. Childs Nerv Syst. 2009;25:1203–1213.
[155] Taylor MD, Poppleton H, Fuller C, et al. Radial glia cells are candidate stem cells of ependymoma. Cancer Cell. 2005;8: 323–335.
[156] Ross GW, Rubinstein LJ. Lack of histopathological correlation ofmalignant ependymomas with postoperative survival. J Neurosurg. 1989;70:31–36.
[157] Merchant TE, Jenkins JJ, Burger PC, et al. Influence of tumor grade on time to progression after irradiation for localized ependymoma in children. Int J Radiat Oncol Biol Phys. 2002;53:52–57.
[158] Merchant TE, Li C, Xiong X, et al. Conformal radiotherapy after surgery for paediatric ependymoma: a prospective study. Lancet Oncol. 2009;10:258–266.
[159] Tihan T, Zhou T, Holmes E, et al. The prognostic value of histological grading of posterior fossa ependymomas in children: a Children's Oncology Group study and a review of prognostic factors. Mod Pathol. 2008;21:165–177.

[160] Palm T, Figarella-Branger D, Chapon F, et al. Expression profiling of ependymomas unravels localization and tumor grade specific tumorigenesis. Cancer. 2009;115:3955-3968.
[161] Gaspar N, Grill J, Geoerger B, et al. p53 Pathway dysfunction in primary childhood ependymomas. Pediatr Blood Cancer. 2006;46:604-613.
[162] Pollack IF, Gerszten PC, Martinez AJ, et al. Intracranial ependymomas of childhood: long-term outcome and prognostic factors. Neurosurgery 1995;37:655-666.
[163] Rousseau P, Habrand JL, Sarrazin D, et al. Treatment of intracranial ependymomas of children: review of a 15-year experience. Int J Radiat Oncol Biol Phys. 1994;28:381-386.
[164] Shim KW, Kim DS, Choi JU. The history of ependymoma management. Childs Nerv Syst. 2009;25:1167-1183.
[165] Zacharoulis S, Ji L, Pollack IF, et al. Metastatic ependymoma: a multiinstitutional retrospective analysis of prognostic factors. Pediatr Blood Cancer. 2008;50:231-235.
[166] Hukin J, Epstein F, Lefton D, et al. Treatment of intracranial ependymoma by surgery alone. Pediatr Neurosurg. 1998; 29:40-45.
[167] Duffner PK, Krischer JP, Sanford RA, et al. Prognostic factors in infants and very young children with intracranial ependymomas. Pediatr Neurosurg. 1998;28:215-222.
[168] Grundy RG, Wilne SA, Weston CL, et al. Primary postoperative chemotherapy without radiotherapy for intracranial ependymoma in children: the UKCCSG/SIOP prospective study. Lancet Oncol. 2007;8:696-705.
[169] Mansur DB, Perry A, Rajaram V, et al. Postoperative radiation therapy for grade II and III intracranial ependymoma. Int J Radiat Oncol Biol Phys. 2005;61:387-391.
[170] Merchant TE, Kiehna EN, Li C, et al. Radiation dosimetry predicts IQ after conformal radiation therapy in pediatric patients with localized ependymoma. Int J Radiat Oncol Biol Phys. 2005;63:1546-1554.
[171] Merchant TE, Boop FA, Kun LE, et al. A retrospective study of surgery and reirradiation for recurrent ependymoma. Int J Radiat Oncol Biol Phys. 2008;71:87-97.
[172] Robertson PL, Zeltzer PM, Boyett JM, et al. Survival and prognosticfactors following radiation therapy and chemotherapy for ependymomas in children: a report of the Children's Cancer Group. J Neurosurg. 1998;88:695-703.
[173] Evans AE, Anderson JR, Lefkowitz-Boudreaux IB, et al. Adjuvant chemotherapy of childhood posterior fossa ependymoma: cranio-spinal irradiation with or without adjuvant CCNU, vincristine, and prednisone: a Children's Cancer Group study. Med Pediatr Oncol. 1996;27:8-14.
[174] Gilbertson RJ, Bentley L, Hernan R, et al. ERBB receptor signaling promotes ependymoma cell proliferation and represents a potential novel therapeutic target for this disease. Clin Cancer Res. 2002;8:3054-3064.
[175] Bouffet E, Tabori U, Bartels U. Paediatric ependymomas: should we avoid radiotherapy? Lancet Oncol. 2007;8:665-666.
[176] Timmermann B, Kortmann RD, Kuhl J, et al. Role of radiotherapy in anaplastic ependymoma in children under age of 3 years: results of the prospective German brain tumor trials HIT-SKK 87 and 92. Radiother Oncol. 2005;77:278-285.
[177] Barkovich AJ, Krischer J, Kun LE, et al. Brain stem gliomas: a classification system based on magnetic resonance imaging. Pediatr Neurosurg. 1990;16:73-83.
[178] Albright AL, Price RA, Guthkelch AN. Brain stem gliomas of children. A clinicopathological study. Cancer. 1983;52: 2313-2319.

[179] Ternier J, Wray A, Puget S, et al. Tectal plate lesions in children. J Neurosurg. 2006;104:369–376.

[180] Freeman CR, Farmer JP. Pediatric brain stem gliomas: a review. Int J Radiat Oncol Biol Phys. 1998;40:265–271.

[181] Donaldson SS, Laningham F, Fisher PG. Advances toward an understanding of brainstem gliomas. J Clin Oncol. 2006; 24:1266–1272.

[182] Freeman CR, Bourgouin PM, Sanford RA, et al. Long term survivorsof childhood brain stem gliomas treated with hyperfractionated radiotherapy. Clinical characteristics and treatment related toxicities. The Pediatric Oncology Group. Cancer. 1996;77:555–562.

[183] Schumacher M, Schulte-Monting J, Stoeter P, et al. Magnetic resonance imaging compared with biopsy in the diagnosis of brainstem diseases of childhood: a multicenter review. J Neurosurg. 2007;106:111–119.

[184] Pierre-Kahn A, Hirsch JF, Vinchon M, et al. Surgical management of brain-stem tumors in children: results and statistical analysis of 75 cases. J Neurosurg. 1993;79:845–852.

[185] Roujeau T, Machado G, Garnett MR, et al. Stereotactic biopsy of diffuse pontine lesions in children. J Neurosurg. 2007;107:1–4.

[186] Shrieve DC, Wara WM, Edwards MS, et al. Hyperfractionated radiation therapy for gliomas of the brainstem in children and in adults. Int J Radiat Oncol Biol Phys. 1992;24: 599–610.

[187] Gilbertson RJ, Hill DA, Hernan R, et al. ERBB1 is amplified and over-expressed in high-grade diffusely infiltrative pediatric brain stem glioma. Clin Cancer Res. 2003;9:3620–3624.

[188] Gururangan S, McLaughlin CA, Brashears J, et al. Incidence and patterns of neuraxis metastases in children with diffuse pontine glioma. J Neurooncol. 2006;77:207–212.

[189] Pollack IF, Hoffman HJ, Humphreys RP, et al. The long-term outcome after surgical treatment of dorsally exophytic brainstem gliomas. J Neurosurg. 1993;78:859–863.

[190] Farmer JP, Montes JL, Freeman CR, et al. Brainstem gliomas. A 10-year institutional review. Pediatr Neurosurg. 2001;34:206–214.

[191] Epstein F, McCleary EL. Intrinsic brainstem tumors of childhood: surgical indications. J Neurosurg. 1986;64:11–15.

[192] Lesniak MS, Klem JM, Weingart J, et al. Surgical outcome follow ing resection of contrast-enhanced pediatric brainstem gliomas. Pediatr Neurosurg. 2003;39:314–322.

[193] Freeman CR, Krischer JP, Sanford RA, et al. Final results of a studyof escalating doses of hyperfractionated radiotherapy in brain stem tumors in children: a Pediatric Oncology Group study. Int J Radiat Oncol Biol Phys. 1993;27:197–206.

[194] Combs SE, Steck I, Schulz-Ertner D, et al. Long-term outcome of high precision radiotherapy in patients with brain stem gliomas: results from a difficult to treat patient population using fractionated stereotactic radiotherapy. Radiother Oncol. 2009;91:60–66.

[195] Jenkin RD, Boesel C, Ertel I, et al. Brainstem tumors in childhood: a prospective randomized trial of irradiation with and without adjuvant CCNU, VCR, and prednisone. A report of the Children's Cancer Study Group. J Neurosurg. 1987;66:227–233.

[196] Allen J, Siffert J, Donahue B, et al. A phase I/II study of carboplatin combined with hyperfractionated radiotherapy for brainstem gliomas. Cancer. 1999;86:1064–1069.

[197] Korones DN, Fisher PG, Kretschmar C, et al. Treatment of childrenwith diffuse intrinsic brain stem glioma with radiotherapy, vincristineand oral VP-16: a Children's Oncology Group phase II study. Pediatr Blood Cancer. 2008;50:227-230.
[198] Broniscer A, Iacono L, Chintagumpala M, et al. Role of temozolomide after radiotherapy for newly diagnosed diffuse brainstem glioma in children: results of a multi institutional study (SJHG-98). Cancer. 2005;103:133-139.
[199] Frappaz D, Schell M, Thiesse P, et al. Preradiation chemotherapymay improve survival in pediatric diffuse intrinsic brainstem gliomas: final results of BSG 98 prospective trial. Neuro Oncol. 2008;10:599-607.
[200] Freeman CR, Kepner J, Kun LE, et al. A detrimental effect of acombined chemotherapy radiotherapy approach in children with diffuse intrinsic brain stem gliomas? Int J Radiat Oncol Biol Phys. 2000;47:561-564.
[201] Bradley KA, Pollack IF, Reid JM, et al. Motexafin gadolinium and involved field radiation therapy for intrinsic pontine glioma ofchildhood: a Children's Oncology Group phase I study. Neurooncol. 2008;10:752-758.
[202] Lonser RR, Walbridge S, Garmestani K, et al. Successful and safe perfusion of the primate brainstem: in vivo magnetic resonanceimaging of macromolecular distribution during infusion. JNeurosurg. 2002;97:905-913.
[203] Allen JC, Siffert J. Contemporary chemotherapy issues for children with brainstem gliomas. Pediatr Neurosurg. 1996;24:98-102.
[204] Ilgren EB, Stiller CA. Cerebellar astrocytomas. Clinical characteristics and prognostic indices. J Neurooncol. 1987; 4:293-308.
[205] Schneider JH Jr, Raffel C, McComb JG. Benign cerebellar astrocytomas of childhood. Neurosurgery. 1992;30:58-62.
[206] Pencalet P, Maixner W, Sainte-Rose C, et al. Benign cerebellar astrocytomas in children. J Neurosurg. 1999;90:265-273.
[207] Sgouros S, Fineron PW, Hockley AD. Cerebellar astrocytoma ofchildhood: long-term follow-up. Childs Nerv Syst. 1995;11:89-96.
[208] Prados M, Mamelak AN. Metastasizing low grade gliomas in chil-dren. Redefining an old disease. Cancer. 1994;73: 2671-2673.
[209] Garcia DM, Marks JE, Latifi HR, et al. Childhood cerebellar astrocytomas: is there a role for postoperative irradiation? Int J RadiatOncol Biol Phys. 1990;18:815-818.
[210] Packer RJ, Ater J, Allen J, et al. Carboplatin and vincristine chemotherapy for children with newly diagnosed progressive low-grade gliomas. J Neurosurg. 1997;86:747-754.
[211] Larson DA, Wara WM, Edwards MS. Management of childhood cerebellar astrocytoma. Int J Radiat Oncol Biol Phys. 1990;18:971-973.
[212] Packer RJ, Jakacki R, Horn M, et al. Objective response of multiplyrecurrent low-grade gliomas to bevacizumab and irinotecan. Pediatr Blood Cancer. 2009;52:791-795.

Part 5

Role of Neuroimaging in CNS Tumors

7

Preoperative Estimation and Resection of Gliomas Using Positron Emission Tomography/Computed Tomography Neuronavigation

Yang Shuyuan[1,2], Zhang Chuan[1], Yue Shuyuan[1], Cai Li[3], Gao Shuo[3] and Zhu Tao[1]
[1]*Department of Neurosurgery, Tianjin Medical University General Hospital*
[2]*Tianjin Neurological Institute; Key Laboratory of Post-trauma Neur12o-repair and Regeneration in* Variations and Regeneration of Nervous System
[3]*PET-CT Center, Tianjin Medical University General Hospital*
P.R. China

1. Introduction

Gliomas are the most common primary neoplasm of the brain, and their treatment presents a number of challenging diagnostic and therapeutic problems for neuro-oncologists. The outcomes for patients with glioma can be quite variable, and there is no consensus regarding the best treatment. To this point, the most widely accepted treatment has been surgical excision, followed by radiotherapy and chemotherapy. Gliomas, however, tend to be diffuse, with ill-defined borders, particularly in grade II and a part of grade III tumors, making them difficult to distinguish from normal or edematous brain tissue during the excision. The percentage of gliomas that are completely removed through surgical intervention is disappointingly now, and this generally leads to a poor prognosis. However, cases where the glioma has been completely removed show a significant improvement in long-term prognosis compared to cases where the glioma was only partially removed. Although complete excision might be an unrealistic goal at this time, these findings suggest that even just increasing the amount of tumor excised has potential prolonging patient survival.

In glioma surgery, precise histological diagnosis during the initial operation is crucial since treatment strategies and prognosis can differ greatly depending on the histological grade. Gliomas diffusely infiltrate neighboring brain structures and are characterized by regional variations of histological malignancy [1]. Therefore, detection of the highly malignant region and delineation of the extent of the tumor are critical during preoperative evaluation.

Recently, positron emission tomography (PET) has been used for evaluation of glioma metabolism. The representative radiolabeled tracers are 18F-fluorodeoxyglucose (FDG) and 11C-methionine (MET). Methionine is an endogenous, essential amino acid and enters tumor cells via the L-amino acid transporter to meet the demands of accelerated protein and RNA synthesis. MET is widely used because less of the amino acid tracer is taken up by healthy brain tissue, which results in greater contrast between tumor and normal brain tissue than what can be seen with FDG PET [2]. MET PET has been reported to delineate both benign and malignant gliomas more accurately than computed tomography (CT) or magnetic resonance imaging (MRI) [3, 4], and has been used in the diagnosis and follow-up of glioma patients [5-6]. On the other hand, malignant tumors are well known to have higher rates of glucose utilization and glycolysis, which would argue for the use of FDG PET. Several reports have demonstrated that FDG uptake in gliomas is highly correlated with the degree of malignancy [7-12]. FDG PET is ill-suited for the detection of gliomas, however, because the rate of glucose utilization of normal brain cortex is relatively high [13-15], so that when a hypermetabolic lesion is near the cortical or subcortical gray matter, it is often difficult to differentiate between tumor and normal tissue [16]. In addition, FDG uptake is known to be non-specific: high FDG accumulation has been observed in inflammatory cells and granulation tissue as well as in viable cancer cells [17-18].

Neuronavigation can precisely locate intracranial lesions and track these targets dynamically, facilitating a more complete removal of the tumor. A comprehensive survey showed neuronavigation-guided surgery of 52 primary glioblastomas achieved complete tumor resection in 31% of cases, versus 19% in a series of conventional operations [19]. These data demonstrate that neuronavigation can increase resection of glioblastoma without prolonging operating time, and increase survival time. However, computed tomography (CT) and magnetic resonance (MR) imaging cannot show the border of glioma accurately because of the tumor biological characteristics. PET shows the metabolic characteristics of tissue, which has a unique advantage in the operation of glioma using neuronavigation.

2. Method and clinical data

2.1 Patients

From May 2004 to May 2010, a total of 71 patients with gliomas received PET/CT with FDG and MET. There were 44 males and 27 females, all between the ages of 6 to 72 years old (mean 41.7±17.2). The most common presenting symptoms included headache, nausea, vomiting, seizures, hemiparesis/aphasis, and cognitive dysfunction, etc. All patients were treated surgically, and diagnosis was confirmed by pathology.

2.2 MRI and CT

All patients underwent brain CT, plain MRI, and enhanced MRI scans.

MRI studies were performed using a 1.5-tesla MRI system (1.5T Signa Twin-speed, infinity with Excite I; GE Medical Systems, Milwaukee, Wisconsin, U.S.A.), or a 3.0-tesla MRI system (Signa Excite HD 3.0T; GE Medical Systems) within 1 month before PET/CT imaging. The conventional imaging protocol consisted of fluid-attenuated inversion recovery sequence T1-weighted imaging (repetition time [TR] 2025 msec, echo time [TE] 8.4 msec, inversion time 750 msec, slice thickness 6.0 mm, slice gap 1.5 mm, field of view 24x18 cm, matrix 320x224, number of excitations [NEX] 2), fast-recovery fast spin-echo sequence T2-weighted imaging (TR 4000 msec, TE 110 msec, slice thickness 3.0 mm, no slice gap, field of view 24x24 cm, matrix 512x512, NEX 2), spin-echo echo-planar imaging sequence diffusion-weighted imaging (TR 10,000 msec, TE 80.1 msec, slice thickness 3.0 mm, no slice gap 1.5 mm, field of view 24x24 cm, matrix 128x128, NEX 1), and spin-echo sequence T1-weighted imaging (TR 500 msec, TE 8.4 msec, flip angle 75, slice thickness 3.0 mm, no slice gap, field of view 24x24 cm, matrix 256x150, NEX 1) 2 minutes after injection of gadolinium-diethylenetriaminepenta-acetic acid (0.1 mmol/kg). We used non-contrast-enhanced transaxial T1-weighted images (T1WI) and T2-weighted images (T2WI) for image fusion.

2.3 PET/CT

18F-fluorodeoxyglucose (FDG) and 11C-methionine (MET) were produced in a MINItrace cyclotron, with TRACERlab MXFDG and TRACERlab FXc synthesizer (GE Medical Systems, Milwaukee, Wisconsin, U.S.A.). PET/CT was performed using a Discovery LS PET/CT unit (GE Medical Systems, Milwaukee, Wisconsin, U.S.A.). Patients fasted for at least 6 hours prior to the PET/CT examination. A dose of 222-370 MBq (6-10 mCi) FDG and/or 555-740 MBq (15-20 mCi) MET was injected intravenously within 1 minute. Static emission scanning was performed at least 40 minutes after FDG injection or at least 20 minutes after MET injection. PET was performed in three-dimensional (3D) mode (field of view 15 cm, slice thickness 5.0 mm, slice gap 4.25 mm, matrix 128x128). The lamellar CT protocol was slice thickness 2.5 mm, slice gap 0, and matrix 512x512. Six reference markers were fixed to the scalp around the tumor before the PET/CT investigation.

2.4 PET\CT diagnosis

Visual analysis: PET/CT scans of the glimoa were referenced to MRI images of the lesion, and the uptake of imaging reagents was classified. Uptake lower than or close to white matter uptake was defined as low metabolism; uptake higher than white matter uptake but significantly lower than gray matter uptake was defined as moderate metabolism; and uptake near, equal to or higher than gray matter uptake was defined as high metabolism. In addition to reagent concentration within the lesion, the analysis also included reagent distribution, lesion shape, uniform or not and whether the boundary clearly.

Semi-quantitative analysis: the center region with highest reagent concentration was marked, avoiding necrotic cystic areas, to outline regions of interest (ROI). Tumor standard uptake values (SUV) were derived, and the ratios of the tumor-to-contralateral white matter (T/WM) and tumor-to-contralateral gray cortex (T/GM) were calculated.

2.5 PET-assisted neuronavigation glioma surgery

Intraoperative neuronavigation was performed using a VectorVision®2 system (Brain LAB AG, Heimstetten, Germany). PET, CT, and MRI data were input into the project graphic workstation, the markers were identified, and the 3D images were rebuilt. The 3D PET image was then coregistered automatically with the 3D MRI or CT image using the registration program of the project system, and the fused image adjusted manually.

Patients were anesthetized, and their heads were fixed in a Mayfield head frame. The operative project data were input into the neuronavigation workstation, and the markers were registered with an error of ±1.5 mm. The tumor resection was then carried out, directed by the neuronavigation system. The extent of the operative target was confirmed using the neuronavigation system.

3. Pathologic examination

3.1 HE staining

Sections taken from each operation specimen were fixed with formalin, embedded in paraffin, and stained with hematoxylin and eosin. The histological diagnosis was determined by an experienced neuropathologist according to the WHO classification of tumors of the central nervous system.

3.2 Ki-67 LI

Proliferative activity was measured by obtaining the Ki-67 proliferation index by histochemical staining of pathological specimens. Paraffin-embedded tumor specimens were recut into 3–4 μm serial sections. Immunohistochemical staining was carried out on sections using monoclonal murine antibody MIB-1, an antibody to Ki-67 (1/100 dilution; DAKO Corp.). MIB-1 recognizes the Ki-67 antigen, a 345- and 395-kDa nuclear protein common to proliferating human cells (21). Sections were then incubated in secondary antibody for 30 min at 25°C, incubated with streptavidin peroxidase, and then washed in phosphate-buffered saline. 3,3-Diaminobenzidine tetrahydrochloride was used as a substitute substrate-chromogen solution, and sections were counterstained with Meyer's haematoxylin. For negative controls, tissue sections were incubated with mouse IgG instead of anti-Ki-67 nuclear antigen antibody. After cell staining, fields were selected randomly for cell counting. Serial sections were reviewed by an experienced neuropathologist. A minimum of 1,000 cells were counted per tissue section. All cells with nuclei staining of any intensity were defined as positive. The Ki-67 score (%) (Ki-67 LI) was defined as the percentage of cells that stained positively for Ki-67 nuclear antigen. The proliferative activity score, quantified as the percentage of MIB-1 stained nuclei per total nuclei in the sample, was estimated from a representative slide selected by the neuropathologist.

4. Results

4.1 Patient and tumor characteristics

12 cases had resections guided by PET-neuronavigation, including 2 cases of fibrous astrocytoma, 2 cases of mixed oligodendro -astrocytoma, 3 cases of anaplastic astrocytoma, 1 case of anaplastic oligodendroglioma, 1 case of anaplastic oligodendro -astrocytoma and 3 cases of glioblastoma. For heterogeneous areas of MET and FDG metabolism, specimens from the hot spots of MET and FDG uptake were resected separately with navigation, and sent to pathology.

4.2 PET visual analysis

FDG PET examination: 38 of the patients in the study had high-grade gliomas (grade III, or IV). Visual analysis revealed high metabolic lesions with clear boundary in 36 of the 38 cases. FDG distribution within the lesion area was uneven; cystic and necrotic areas were defect for reagent, and the edematous area around the tumor showed reduced metabolism. In the remaining 3 high-grade cases (1 medulloblastoma and 2 anaplastic astrocytomas) visual analysis revealed moderate metabolism. 33 of the patients in the study had low-grade gliomas (grade I, or II). In 31 of the 33 cases, visual analysis revealed either moderate or low metabolic lesions, and FDG distribution was relatively homogeneous. However, when the tumor was located within the gray/white matter junction, the high metabolism of surrounding normal gray matter often made it difficult to distinguish the lesion boundaries. The remaining 2 low-grade cases (both oligodendrogliomas) displayed high metabolism. FDG PET visualization results were concordant with pathological grading in 66 of the 71 cases (coincidence rate= 93%).

MET PET examination: Visual analysis revealed high metabolism in 66 of the 71 cases. Visual analysis of the remaining 5 cases (all grade II fibrous astrocytomas) revealed low metabolism. However, compared with FDG, MET uptake in normal brain tissue has very low background, which can provide a better contrast to scope the tumor border, and helpful to detect the low-grade glioma. In some cases, FDG and MET were inconsistent at the concentrated area.

Characteristic	No. of cases
Age (yrs)	
6-72 (average 41.7±17.2)	71
Sex	
Female	44
Male	27
WHO classification	
Grade I	8
pilocytic astrocytoma	3
dysembryoplastic neuroepithelial tumor	3
subependymal giant cellular astrocytoma	1
ganglion cellular glioma	1
Grade II	25
Astrocytoma	12
Oligodendroglioma	5
Oligodendro - astrocytoma	8
Grade III	21
Anaplastic astrocytoma	14
Anaplastic oligodendroglioma	3
Anaplastic oligoastrocytoma	4
Grade IV	17
Glioblastoma	14
medulloblastoma	2
PNET	1

Table 1. Patients and tumor characteristics

4.3 PET semi-quantitative analysis and Ki-67 LI

PET semi-quantitative analysis: the centre region with highest reagent concentration was marked, avoiding necrotic cystic area, to outline regions of interest (ROI), derived tumor standard uptake value (SUV); then calculate the ratios of the tumor / contralateral white

matter (T / WM) and tumor / contralateral gray cortex (T / GM). PET semi-quantitative indicators and Ki-67 LI results were shown in Table 2. Analysis of variance (One-Way ANOVA) for FDG: the results showed statistically significant differences between groups (F_{SUV} = 9.371, $F_{T/WM}$ = 9.907, $F_{T/GM}$ = 17.867, both P <0.01), between low-grade (grade I and II) gliomas and high-grade (grade III and IV) (P <0.01), between III and IV grade (T/GM FDG, P = II 0.029). However, various indicators did not show manifest difference between grade I and (P> 0.05). MET results displayed only T/GM MET in statistically significant difference between groups (FT/GM = 3.026, P = 0.048), and between II and IV grade (P = 0.011). The remaining indicators were no significant differences (P> 0.05).
Correlation analysis showed that: FDG and MET PET in three semi-quantitative indexes were positively correlated, SUV, T/WM and T/GM of the correlation coefficient r values were 0.608, 0.708, and 0.716 (all P <0.001) . T/GM FDG and T/GM MET was positively correlated with Ki-67 LI, r were 0.610, 0.729 (all P <0.001).

Tumor Grade	n	SUV_{FDG}	T/WM_{FDG}	T/GM_{FDG}	SUV_{MET}	T/WM_{MET}	T/GM_{MET}	Ki-67 LI
WHO I	8	4.38±4.36	1.43±0.54	0.45±0.14	3.94±1.57	4.18±1.6	1.98±0.93	2.95±0.75
WHO II	25	5.02±2.68	1.57±0.62	0.58±0.21	3.58±3.29	4.13±2.28	1.91±1.07	5.35±3.98
WHO III	21	11.69±7.77	2.84±0.81	1.11±0.47	5.11±2.42	5.29±3.12	2.84±1.24	10.41±7.70
WHO IV	17	13.59±4.80	3.86±1.76	1.54±0.47	5.39±2.11	6.29±1.5	3.51±1.2	25.35±1.82

Table 2. PET semi-quantitative index and Ki-67 LI.

4.4 PET and CT, MRI

For the typical grade IV glioblastoma, MRI showed the mass as hypointense on the T1-weighted images, and hyperintense on the T2-weighted images, with irregular ring enhancement accompanied by necrosis or cystic tissue. But in three of the glioblastoma cases, CT and MRI scans revealed the tumor located in the corticomedullary junction area, invading the cortex, with some slightly enhanced spots in the lesion, and peripheral edema surrounding the tumor with no clear boundary. FDG and MET PET showed irregular areas of high concentration with clear borders (especially MET). The most concentrated area of distribution inconsistent between FDG and MET in some cases, but the tumor boundary was roughly same. Under the guidance of neuronavigation, tumor samples were taken at the most concentrated FDG and MET areas respectively (Fig. 1). Pathological findings revealed: tumor cells densely located at the MET concentrated area with obvious atypical nuclei and highly proliferative vascular endothelial cell, as the typical glioblastoma grade IV character. Patholodical findings for the FDG area revealed less tightly packed cells, with no obvious vascular endothelial cell proliferation, which was the junction between tumor and normal brain tissue (Fig. 2-4).

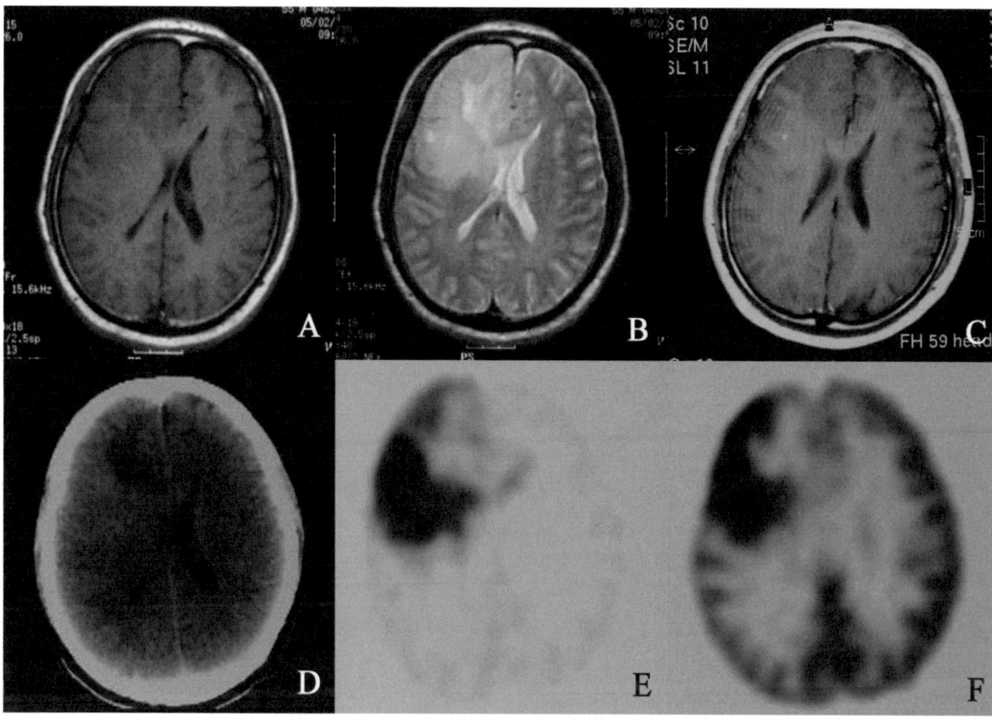

Fig. 1. A 55-year-old man with a diffuse lesion in the right frontal lobe. A-C: T1-weighted (A) and T2-weighted (B) magnetic resonance (MR) images, and T1-weighted MR image with contrast medium (C), showing a mass in the right frontal lobe with unclear margin as slightly hypointense on the T1- weighted and hyperintense on the T2-weighted images, with some slightly enhanced spots in the lesion. D: Computed tomography scan, showing the lesion as equal or slightly increased density, with an unclear border, in and below the right frontal lobe cortex. E: 11C-methionine positron emission tomography (PET) scan, showing an irregular area of high uptake with a clear border in the right frontal lobe. The area of highest MET uptake was in the posterior part of the lesion. F: 18F-fluorodeoxyglucose PET scan, showing an irregular area of high uptake which was relatively well defined in the frontal lobe. The highest FDG uptake area was in front of the MET hot area.

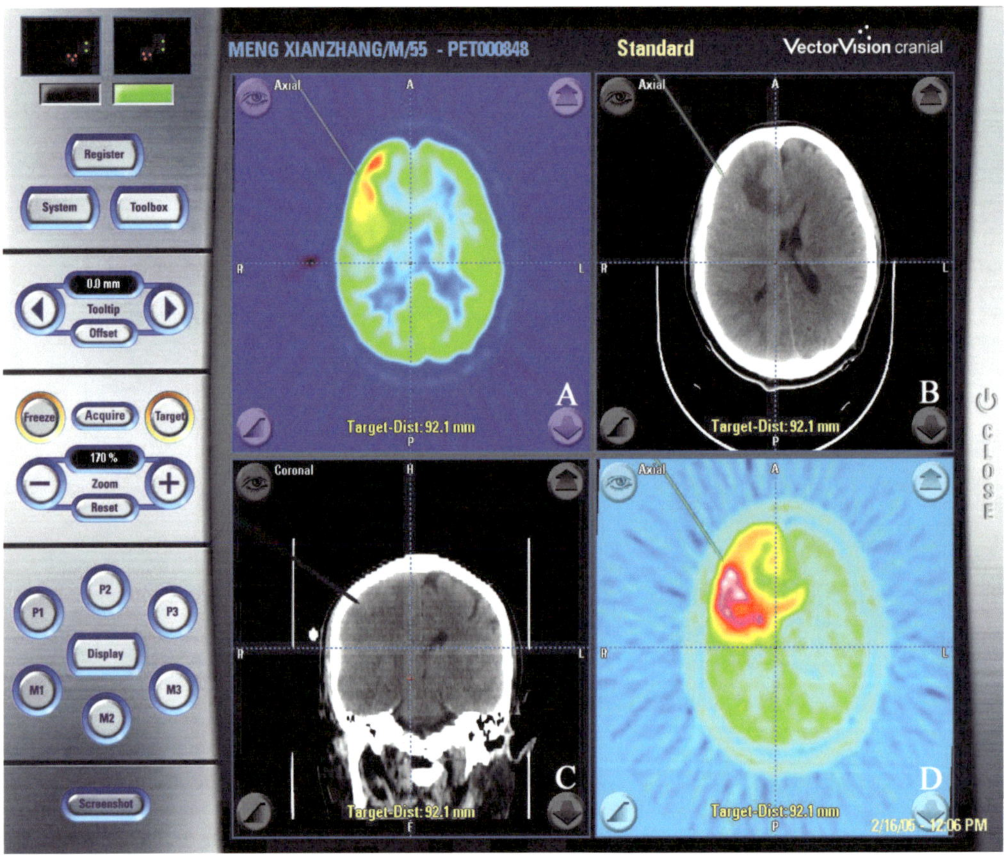

Fig. 2. Positron emission tomography (PET) neuronavigation system monitoring images captured during the operation. A: 18F-fluorodeoxyglucose PET scan; B, C: CT scans; D: 11C-methionine PET scan. CT provided the anatomic background. PET provided more distinct information of the tumor.

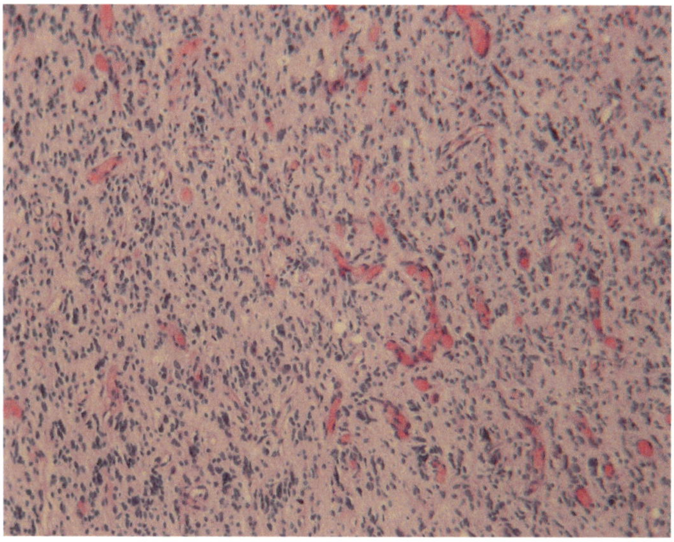

Fig. 3. Photomicrograph of the specimen resected from the hot spot demonstrated by 11C-methionine positron emission tomography showing glioblastoma, World Health Organization grade 4. Nucleus deformation, and cell and vessel proliferation were prominent. Hematoxylin and eosin stain, x100.

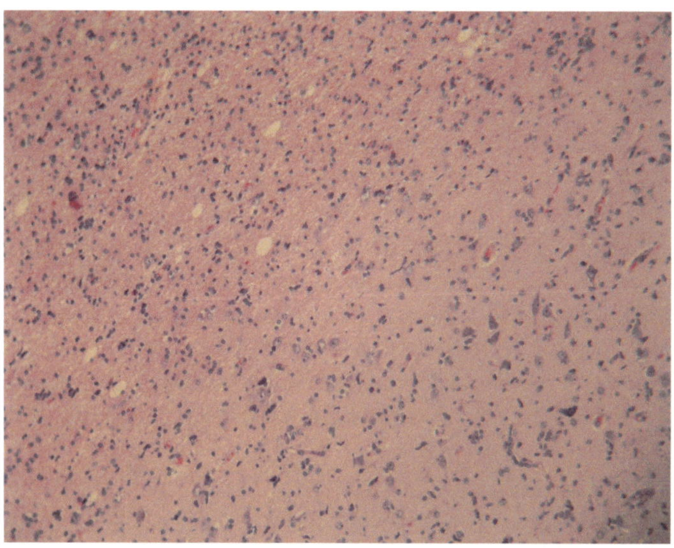

Fig. 4. Photomicrograph of the specimen resected from the hot spot demonstrated by [18F]fluorodeoxyglucose positron emission tomography showing the margin of the tumor. Nucleus deformation, and cell and vessel proliferation were similar to that of astrocytoma grade II. Hematoxylin and eosin stain, x100.

For gliomas grade II and III, MRI showed the tumor as an irregular hypointensity or an irregular hyperintensity surrounded by edema with ill-defined boundaries on the T1-weighted and T2-weighted images respectively. The lesion displayed mild enhancement or no enhancement. PET imaging, especially, MET distribution was more helpful in illustrating the tumor boundaries. Oligodendrogliomas and Oligodendroastrocytoma in particular showed the high MET concentrations (Figure 5).

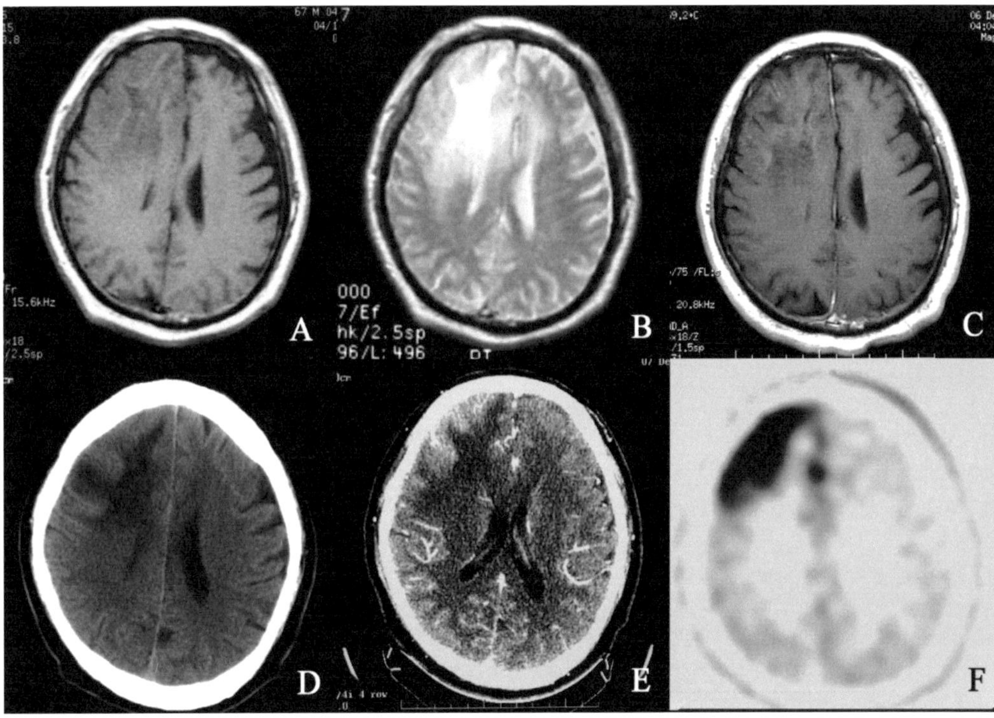

Fig. 5. A 65-year-old man with a diffuse lesion in the right frontal lobe. A-C: T1-weighted magnetic resonance images (A, B), and with contrast medium (C), showing a mass with unclear margins in the right frontal lobe, appearing as slightly hypointense on the T1-weighted and hyperintense on the T2-weighted images without obvious enhancement. D, E: Computed tomography scan (D) and with contrast medium (E) , showing the irregular lesion as uniform density with an unclear border and slight enhancement deep within the right frontal lobe cortex. F: 11C-methionine positron emission tomography scan, showing an irregular high uptake area in and below the right frontal lobe cortex with a clear margin.

4.5 PET neuronavigation surgery

In 4 cases of grade II gliomas, visual inspection of the surface of the brain was normal except for some localized slight gyral broadening, such that tumor location could not be determined by gross visualization. Tumor boundaries could not be clearly determined with CT and MRI scans. PET scans (especially MET), however, allowed for satisfactory delineation of the tumor boundaries. Because of this, the resections were performed using MET PET/CT neuronavigation. During the resection, the tumor tissue appeared approximately normal in color, with a slightly tenacious texture, and moderate bleeding.

After complete resection, the cross section and periphery of the tumor were checked. The cut surface appeared much like normal brain, with no necrosis or capsule (Figure 6).

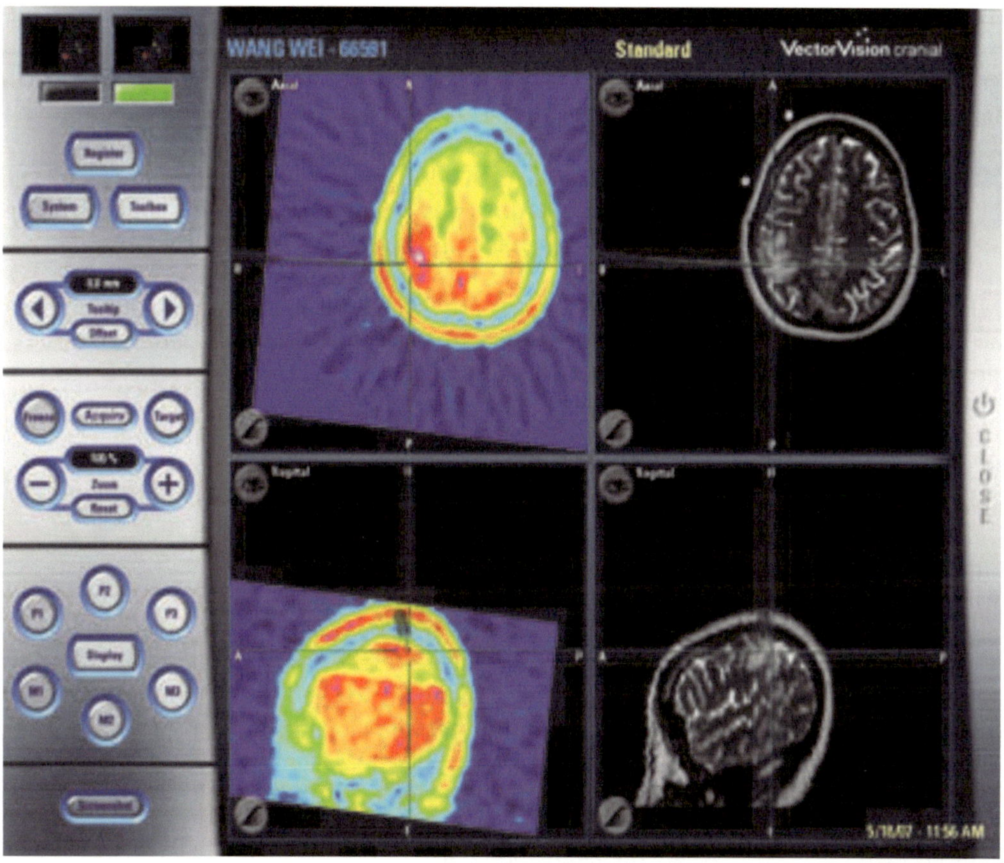

Fig. 6. Positron emission tomography (PET) neuronavigation system monitoring images captured during the operation. A 56-year-old woman with a diffuse lesion in the right frontoparital lobe. The pathological diagnosis of the tumor is Oligodendroglioma.

Grade III and IV gliomas were characterized by abnormal color, texture and blood supply, and were all resected under the guidance of PET-assisted navigation. The specimens taken from different tracer concentrated areas were sent to pathology. Postoperative imaging demonstrated complete resection of the suspected tumor area (Figure 4).

5. Discussion

5.1 The value of PET assessment for preoperative glioma

In 1982, Di Chiro confirmed by FDG PET that a tumor's malignancy level is closely related to the tissue's glucose utilization [20]. FDG PET is widely utilized to detect malignant tumors. Increased glucose uptake is usually associated with higher malignancy and aggressiveness. In glimoas, due to high uptake in cortex and basal ganglia, and low uptake in white matter, FDG uptake showed a close relationship with histological grade or prognosis [7-12]. Patronas et al. reported that FDG uptake is a more accurate reflection of tumor grade than contrast enhancement [21], and Goldman et al. [10] proved that FDG uptake in gliomas correlated regionally with presence of anaplasia by means of FDG PET-guided stereotactic biopsy. Although FDG PET is the gold-standard detection tool for regional malignancy in gliomas, it is not perfect. In terms of delineating tumor boundaries precisely, FDG PET is obviously inferior to MET PET [2]. MET increased uptake in tumor mainly reflects the increase in amino acid trafficking activity, and indirectly represents the increase in protein synthesis. MET, however, proved better than FDG in distinguishing tumor boundaries, as the lower uptake in normal brain tissue allows for better contrast between normal and tumor tissue. In addition, fusion of MET with MRI or CT images allowed for better detection of low-grade tumors close to the cortex, smaller tumors, and tumor boundaries. Therefore, combined use of FDG and MET is reasonable in detecting regional malignancy and in delineating the extent of viable tumor tissue for preoperative evaluation of glioma surgery [22-24]. This study also found that the most concentrated area for each tracer was sometimes inconsistent in the high-grade gliomas. Comparison with pathology reports showed that MET uptake in tumor cells was more specific. [25]

Metabolic characteristics of different types of gliomas were diverse. Our and other studies found that oligodendrogliomas and oligodendroastrocytoma displayed high uptake of both MET and FDG. Oligodendrogliomas showed particularly high uptake, with MET uptake close to the level seen in anaplastic astrocytomas, and pathologically the tumor cells were highly condensed. Previous studies have demonstrated that pilocytic astrocytomas may have higher FDG and MET uptake [26]. In our study, 2 cases of pilocytic astrocytoma showed high metabolism of MET, even higher than that seen in grade II astrocytomas, but low FDG metabolism, histopathology revealed extensive capillaries. One case of subependymal giant cell astrocytoma with tuberous sclerosis showed moderate FDG uptake, and significantly elevated MET uptake, close to levels seen in glioblastomas. Pathology on this case revealed large tumor cells surrounded by a large number of expanded blood vessels. Therefore, the MET uptake of gliomas (especially low-grade gliomas) may be dependent not only on proliferative activities but also on other factors such as cerebral blood volume [27], amount of microvessels [18, 28], and cell density [29].

SUV is the most common semi-quantitative indicator, but it may be affected by many factors, such as age, blood glucose level, and medication. As such, it may not be well suited as a means for comparison across repeated examinations, and amongst different individuals.

Using the uptake ratios between the lesion and normal tissue can overcome the shortcomings. Our results show that the T/GM is of the best indicator for grading gliomas, and that FDG is better than MET in estimating a tumor's pathological character.

Recent studies have confirmed that MET uptake is closely related to the proliferation of brain tumors. During the early exponential growth phase, tumor cells can show a high degree of MET concentration. Whereas at the plateau phase MET uptake is much lower. So the level of MET uptake could be regarded as a sign of tumor cell proliferation, but it is controversial whether FDG uptake is related to cell proliferation. Our study demonstrated that uptake levels of FDG and MET in gliomas were associated with Ki-67 LI. Ki-67 LI which revealed the tumor proliferation was a prognostic indicator for cancer patients, and PET which revealed the tumor metabolic activity can also help evaluate the tumor proliferation and prognosis [30-32] .

5.2 PET comparing with MRI and CT

MRI and CT can display the brain organization structure clearly, and as such these are the main non-surgical methods used to initially diagnose gliomas. Currently MRI is the first choice for diagnosing tumor pathological grade and for determining the location and extent of the tumor. The malignant part of tumor is most often located in or near the area of blood-brain barrier breakdown, in which case it would appear as an area of enhancement on an MRI with medium contrast. However, T1- and T2-weighted MRI are often insufficient to definitively determine the relationship between tumor and normal or edematous tissue. This is the case with many grade II gliomas, and sometimes is seen even in grade III and IV gliomas. Furthermore, if the tumor is not located near the blood-brain barrier breakdown or the barrier has not broken down, it is near impossible to distinguish between healthy and tumor tissue, nor can the regional heterogeneity of the tumor be shown. Clinical studies have shown that gliomas often extend beyond the contrast-enhanced margin and that approximately 80% of tumor relapses occur within a 2-cm margin around the original enhanced lesion [33]. Therefore, neuronavigation using only MR imaging cannot be relied upon to outline the target completely.

In addition to CT and MR imaging, metabolic imaging with PET has been considered. PET can be used to estimate the grade and malignancy of the glioma before operation, evaluate the prognosis and the outcome of radiotherapy and chemotherapy, and show the tumor extent and heterogeneity [30, 34]. Clinical studies using radiolabeled amino acid PET, such as MET, have demonstrated superior delineation of the glioma mass compared with MRI. The use of PET over MRI allowed for differentiation between tumor and edematous tissue, and recognition of different areas of proliferation in different parts of the tumor. Confirmation of the target of stereotactic biopsy and radiotherapy by PET provides high sensitivity and specificity [35-38].

5.3 PET optimizing neuronavigation surgery

Invasive growth of gliomas showed no obvious boundaries, especially in gradeII and III. Visualization of the border between tumor tissue and normal brain tissue is extremely difficult, and complete resections are very rare when using conventional surgical method. The use of neuronavigation imaging data to demarcate the glioma boundaries, however, facilitates the implementation of total tumor resection.

Because of excellent tissue resolution, MRI (especially enhanced MRI) is often used as the input for neuronavigation during glioma resections. However, for grade II glioma, some grade III, and a few glioblastoma grade IV, MRI scans were not able to determine lesion boundaries or distinguishand it from the surrounding edema. In the absence of apparent BBB damage, enhanced MRI was not able to show full the tumor extent, or the proliferation of heterogeneity within the tumor. In addition, the enhanced MRI may not show the real extent of the tumor invasion, so in some cases, MRI alone could not determine the surgical target. Our study revealed 9 cases in which high-grade gliomas showed mild or no enhancement on MRI, but high uptakes of FDG and MET on PET images.PET imaging, in particular, MET PET can clearly display the boundaries of glioma, the distinction between the tumor and surrounding edema, and the proliferation of different tumor areas [32, 34]. The data to determine the target for the application of PET stereotactic biopsy and stereotactic radiation therapy, confirm its high sensitivity and specificity [36-38]. The new PET/CT technique has significantly improved the precision of PET and combines the advantages of structural and functional imaging [39]. Combined with a neuronavigation system, PET could provide more comprehensive and precise imaging data to help more completely remove the tumor [40]. The project graphic workstation of our VectorVision®2 neuronavigation system could fuse the PET and MR or CT images.

We used the PET neuronavigation system to guide the surgery in twelve patients with glioma which had been difficult to confirm by routine CT and MR imaging. In particular, the actual tumor margin was undefined, and tumor and edema were not distinguished. In contrast, PET clearly identified the extent and invasiveness of the tumors, and provided the reliable data needed for neuronavigation-guided excision. In our study, grade II gliomas could not be distinguished from the normal brain tissue by visual inspection, and the boundary was not visible in the resected specimen. These operations were then continued using PET neuronavigation guidance. The degree of proliferation in different parts of some high grade gliomas could not be distinguished using MRI. In contrast, PET demonstrated distinctly both the tumor extent and the degree of proliferation in the various areas by the different uptakes of FDG and MET. Histological examination of the specimens showed that PET neuronavigation provided reliable distinction between normal brain tissue and glioma, the uptake of PET tracers can indicate the degree of proliferation. MET was more effective for this purpose than FDG [41].

6. Conclusion

PET imaging can fully reflect the tumor metabolic status, useful to preoperative assessment of brain glioma, and provide a new assistant for navigation of glioma surgery, especially when conventional imaging is difficult to determine the degree of malignancy and the extent of glioma. In addition, under the navigation, samples taken from different metabolic region, are profound to study on the biological characteristics of glioma.

7. References

[1] Paulus W, Peiffer J. Intratumoral histologic heterogeneity of gliomas. A quantitative study. Cancer 64:442–447, 1989

[2] Singhal T, Narayanan TK, Jain V, Mukherjee J, Mantil J. 11C-L-methionine positron emission tomography in the clinical management of cerebral gliomas. Mol Imaging Biol 10:1–18, 2008

[3] Pirotte B, Goldman S, Dewitte O, Massager N, Wikler D, Lefranc F, Ben Taib NO, Rorive S, David P, Brotchi J, Levivier M. Integrated positron emission tomography and magnetic resonance imaging-guided resection of brain tumors: a report of 103 cnsecutive procedures. J Neurosurg 104:238–253, 2006

[4] Tovi M, Lilja A, Bergstrom M, Ericsson A, Bergstrom K, Hartman M. Delineation of gliomas with magnetic resonance imaging using Gd-DTPA in comparison with computed tomography and positron emission tomography. Acta Radiol 31:417–429, 1990

[5] Braun V, Dempf S, Weller R, Reske SN, Schachenmayr W, Richter HP. Cranial neuronavigation with direct integration of (11)C methionine positron emission tomography (PET) data–results of a pilot study in 32 surgical cases. Acta Neurochir (Wien) 144:777–782 discussion 782, 2002

[6] Kracht LW, Miletic H, Busch S, Jacobs AH, Voges J, Hoevels M, Klein JC, Herholz K, Heiss WD. Delineation of brain tumor extent with [11C]L-methionine positron emission tomography: local comparison with stereotactic histopathology. Clin Cancer Res 10:7163–7170, 2004

[7] Kaschten B, Stevenaert A, Sadzot B, Deprez M, Degueldre C, Del Fiore G, Luxen A, Reznik M. Preoperative evaluation of 54 gliomas by PET with fluorine-18-fluorodeoxyglucose and/or carbon-11-methionine. J Nucl Med 39:778–785, 1998

[8] Alavi JB, Alavi A, Chawluk J, Kushner M, Powe J, Hickey W, Reivich M. Positron emission tomography in patients with glioma. A predictor of prognosis. Cancer 62:1074–1078, 1988

[9] Borbely K, Nyary I, Toth M, Ericson K, Gulyas B. Optimization of semi-quantification in metabolic PET studies with 18F-fluorodeoxyglucose and 11C-methionine in the determination of malignancy of gliomas. J Neurol Sci 246:85–94, 2006

[10] Goldman S, Levivier M, Pirotte B, Brucher JM, Wikler D, Damhaut P, Stanus E, Brotchi J, Hildebrand J. Regional glucose metabolism and histopathology of gliomas. A study based on positron emission tomography-guided stereotactic biopsy. Cancer 78:1098–1106, 1996

[11] Ogawa T, Inugami A, Hatazawa J, Kanno I, Murakami M, Yasui N, Mineura K, Uemura K. Clinical positron emission tomography for brain tumors: comparison of fludeoxyglucose F18 and L-methyl-11C-methionine. AJNR Am J Neuroradiol 17:345–353, 1996

[12] Padma MV, Said S, Jacobs M, Hwang DR, Dunigan K, Satter M, Christian B, Ruppert J, Bernstein T, Kraus G, Mantil JC. Prediction of pathology and survival by FDG PET in gliomas. J Neurooncol 64:227–237, 2003

[13] Benard F, Romsa J, Hustinx R. Imaging gliomas with positron emission tomography and single-photon emission computed tomography. Semin Nucl Med 33:148–162, 2003

[14] Chen W. Clinical applications of PET in brain tumors. J Nucl Med 48:1468–1481, 2007

[15] Kubota K. From tumor biology to clinical Pet: a review of positron emission tomography (PET) in oncology. Ann Nucl Med 15:471–486, 2001

[16] Delbeke D, Meyerowitz C, Lapidus RL, Maciunas RJ, Jennings MT, Moots PL, Kessler RM. Optimal cutoff levels of F-18 fluorodeoxyglucose uptake in the differentiation of low-grade from high-grade brain tumors with PET. Radiology 195:47–52, 1995

[17] Kato T, Shinoda J, Oka N, Miwa K, Nakayama N, Yano H, Maruyama T, Muragaki Y, Iwama T. Analysis of 11Cmethionine uptake in low-grade gliomas and correlation with proliferative activity. AJNR Am J Neuroradiol 29:1867–1871, 2008

[18] Nojiri T, Nariai T, Aoyagi M, Senda M, Ishii K, Ishiwata K, Ohno K. Contributions of biological tumor parameters to the incorporation rate of L: -[methyl-(11)C] methionine into astrocytomas and oligodendrogliomas. J Neurooncol 93:233–241, 2009

[19] Wirtz CR, Albert FK, Schwaderer M, Heuer C, Staubert A, Tronnier VM, Knauth M, Kunze S: The benefit of neuronavigation for neurosurgery analyzed by its impact on glioblastoma surgery. Neurol Res 22: 354-360, 2000

[20] Di Chiro G, DelaPaz RL, Brooks RA, et al. Glucose utilization of cerebral gliomas measured by [18F] fluorodeoxyglucose and positron emission tomography. Neurology 32:1323~1329, 1982

[21] Patronas NJ, Brooks RA, DeLaPaz RL, Smith BH, Kornblith PL, Di Chiro G. Glycolytic rate (PET) and contrast enhancement (CT) in human cerebral gliomas. AJNR Am J Neuroradiol 4:533–535, 1983

[22] Goldman S, Levivier M, Pirotte B, Brucher JM, Wikler D, Damhaut P, Dethy S, Brotchi J, Hildebrand J. Regional methionine and glucose uptake in high-grade gliomas: a comparative study on PETguided stereotactic biopsy. J Nucl Med 38:1459–1462, 1997

[23] Bergstrom M, Collins VP, Ehrin E, Ericson K, Eriksson L, Greitz T, Halldin C, von Holst H, Langstrom B, Lilja A et al. Discrepancies in brain tumor extent as shown by computed tomography and positron emission tomography using [68 Ga]EDTA, [11C]glucose, and [11C]methionine. J Comput Assist Tomogr 7:1062–1066, 1983

[24] Mosskin M, Ericson K, Hindmarsh T, von Holst H, Collins VP, Bergstrom M, Eriksson L, Johnstrom P. Positron emission tomography compared with magnetic resonance imaging and computed tomography in supratentorial gliomas using multiple stereotactic biopsies as reference. Acta Radiol 30:225–232, 1989

[25] Giammarile F, Cinotti LE, Jouvet A, Ramackers JM, Saint Pierre G, Thiesse P, Jouanneau E, Guyotat J, Pelissou-Guyotat I, Setiey A, Honnorat J, Le Bars D, Frappaz D. High and low grade oligodendrogliomas (ODG): correlation of amino-acid and glucose uptakes using PET and histological classifications. J Neurooncol 68:263–274, 2004

[26] Utriainen M, Metsahonkala L, Salmi TT, et al. Metabolic characterization of childhood brain tumors: comparison of 18F-fluorodeoxyglucose and 11C-methionine positron emission tomography. Cancer 95: 1376~1386, 2002

[27] Sadeghi N, Salmon I, Decaestecker C, Levivier M, Metens T, Wikler D, Denolin V, Rorive S, Massager N, Baleriaux D, Goldman S. Stereotactic comparison among cerebral blood volume, methionine uptake, and histopathology in brain glioma. AJNR Am J Neuroradiol 28:455–461, 2007

[28] Kracht LW, Friese M, Herholz K, Schroeder R, Bauer B, Jacobs A, Heiss WD. Methyl-[11C]- l-methionine uptake as measured by positron emission tomography correlates to microvessel density in patients with glioma. Eur J Nucl Med Mol Imaging 30:868–873, 2003

[29] Okita Y, Kinoshita M, Goto T, Kagawa N, Kishima H, Shimosegawa E, Hatazawa J, Hashimoto N, Yoshimine T. (11)Cmethionine uptake correlates with tumor cell density rather than with microvessel density in glioma: a stereotactic image-histology comparison. Neuroimage 49:2977–2982, 2010

[30] Schaller B. Usefulness of positron emission tomography in diagnosis and treatment follow-up of brain tumors. Neurobiol Dis 15:437-448, 2004

[31] Wei Chen. Clinical applications of PET in brain tumors. J Nucl Med 48:1468-1481, 2007

[32] Wong TZ, van der Westhuizen GJ, Coleman RE. Positron emission tomography imaging of brain tumors. Neuroimaging Clin N Am 12(4):615-626, 2002

[33] Gorska-Chrzastek M, Grzelak P, Bienkiewicz M, Tybor K, Zakrzewska E, Mikolajczak R, Stefanczyk L, Kusmierek J: Assessment of clinical usefulness of 131I alpha-methyl-tyrosine and fused SPECT/MRI imaging for diagnostics of recurrent cerebral gliomas. Nucl Med Rev Cent East Eur 7:135-141,2004

[34] Chung JK, Kim YK, Kim SK, Lee YJ, Paek S, Yeo JS, Jeong JM, Lee DS, Jung HW, Lee MC: Usefulness of 11C-methionine PET in the evaluation of brain lesions that are hypo- or isometabolic on 18F-FDG PET. Eur J Nucl Med Mol Imaging 29:176-182, 2002

[35] Floeth FW, Pauleit D, Wittsack HJ, Langen KJ, Reifenberger G, Hamacher K, Messing-Junger M, Zilles K, Weber F, Stummer W, Steiger HJ, Woebker G, Muller HW, Coenen H, Stabel M: Multimodal metabolic imaging of cerebral gliomas: positron emission tomography with [18F]fluoroethyl-L-tyrosine and magnetic resonance spectroscopy. J Neurosurg 102:318-327, 2005

[36] Hara T, Kondo T, Hara T, Kosaka N: Use of 18F-choline and 11C-choline as contrast agents in positron emission tomography imaging-guided stereotactic biopsy sampling of gliomas. J Neurosurg 99:474-479, 2003

[37] Lee JK, Liu RS, Shiang HR, Pan DH: Usefulness of semiquantitative FDG-PET in the prediction of brain tumor treatment response to gamma knife radiosurgery. J Comput Assist Tomogr 27:525-529, 2003

[38] Levivier M, Massager N, Wikler D, Lorenzoni J, Ruiz S, Devriendt D, David P, Desmedt F, Simon S, Van Houtte P, Brotchi J, Goldman S: Use of stereotactic PET images in dosimetry planning of radiosurgery for brain tumors: clinical experience and proposed classification. J Nucl Med 45:1146-1154, 2004

[39] von Schulthess GK. Positron emission tomography versus positron emission tomography/computed tomography: from "unclear" to "new-clear" medicine. Mol Imaging Biol 6:183-187, 2004

[40] Nakajo K, Tatsumi M, Inoue A, Isohashi K, Higuchi I, Kato H, Imaizumi M, Enomoto T, Shimosegawa E, Kimura T, Hatazawa J: Diagnostic performance of fluorodeoxyglucose positron emission tomography/magnetic resonance imaging fusion images of gynecological malignant tumors: comparison with positron emission tomography/computed tomography. Jpn J Radiol 28(2):95-100, 2010
[41] Yang S, Zhang C, Zhu T, Cai L, Gao S, Yue S, Wei W: Resection of gliomas using positron emission tomography/computed tomography neuronavigation. Neurol Med Chir (Tokyo) 47:397-401, 2007

8

The Brain Adjacent to Tumor (BAT)

Davide Schiffer, Laura Annovazzi, Valentina Caldera and Marta Mellai
Research Centre Policlinico di Monza/Consorzio di Neuroscienze,
University of Pavia, Vercelli,
Italy

1. Introduction

Gliomas represent the classical intra-axial tumors of the brain and glioblastoma multiforme (GBM) is the most frequent and malignant glioma. It is an extremely aggressive tumor with a high invasive potential. After treatments, it invariably resumes proliferation and its recurrences occur most often within 2 cm from the resection margins (Hochberg & Pruitt, 1980; Wallner et al., 1989; Oppitz et al., 1999). The dispersion of glioma cells in the surrounding normal brain puts them out of reach of surgery, radio- and chemotherapy, because outside of the limits of surgical resection and of the irradiated volume, established in order to avoid damages to the normal brain. The BAT, therefore, is the place where tumor cells migrate and invade and where a series of biological, pathological and molecular events occur as far as the interaction between host and tumor is concerned. Migrating cells from the tumor, reacting astroglia and microglial cells, elements of the immunological response or belonging to the monocytic phagocyting system reaching the tumor from the blood flow, and cells from gliogenetic zones of the brain make the BAT a melting pot of interactions among cells and factors. It has special importance also from the neuroimaging point of view for the recognition of the tumor limits and of peritumoral edema, which may have, at the same time, a prognostic significance (Ramakrishna et al., 2010). With MRI, beside the peripheral increase of T2 signal, uptake of gadolinium, hypodensities corresponding to vasogenic edema, necrotic cyst formation, other features can be shown by special technical procedures. The correlation, therefore, between neuroimaging and histopathology and molecular biology in the BAT is of the greatest interest.

2. Cell migration and invasion

The process of tumor cell invasion of the brain recognizes some fundamental steps (Nakada et al., 2007): cell detachment from the tumor mass; their attachment to the degraded extra-cellular matrix (ECM) and cell migration. Each of these steps is regulated by a series of molecular events with different gene expression profiles associated with motility, cytoskeleton modifications, transduction molecules, surface receptors and components of ECM (Table 1).

How GBM acquires an invasive phenotype is still discussed. It is known that carcinoma invasion is driven by an "epithelial to mesenchymal transition" (EMT) (Kalluri & Weinberg, 2009), which is activated by the helix-loop-helix protein TWIST1. Recently, a mesenchymal change in GBM has been recognized (Phillips et al., 2006; Tso et al., 2006; Carro et al., 2010), associated with a more aggressive phenotype. TWIST1 is up-regulated in GBM cell lines *in vitro* (Elias et al., 2005) and it promotes cell invasion through mesenchymal molecular and cellular changes which can be demonstrated by Affymetrix gene expression array. It mediates cell-cell adhesion, the interaction with the substrate, migration and cytoskeleton modifications, activating specific gene expression profiles of invasion and without involving the cadherin switch (Mikheeva et al., 2010). In the rim of GBM, there is an increase of the Na^+/H^+ exchanger regulatory factor1 (NHERF-1), which sustains glioma invasion and migration and, if inhibited, migration ceases and apoptosis increases and cells become more sensitive to Temozolomide (Kislin et al., 2009). Genes for matrix degrading are up-regulated both *in vivo* and *in vitro* in cells with ΔEGFR (Lal et al., 2002). Also Neuropilin-1, a receptor for semaphorin3A, is required for GBM cell migration. GBM cells secrete Sema3A endogenously, and RNA interference mediated down-regulation of Sema3A inhibits migration and alters cell morphology that is dependent on Rac1 activity. Sema3A depletion also reduces cell dispersal, which is recovered by supplying Sema3A exogenously (Bagci et al., 2009). Migrating glioma cells show a downregulation of the major histocompatibility complex (MHC) (Zagzag et al., 2005).

Detachment from the original site	CD44, NCAM,α- and β-Catenin, F-Actin, N-Cadherin, Hyaluronic acid
Attachment to ECM	Tenascin-C, Integrins, FAK, ILK
Degradation of ECM	ADAM, MMP, uPA, β-Cathepsin
Migration	EGF - EGFR, c-met - HGF

Table 1. Invasion phases with some relevant molecular steps.

Motility of glioma cells has been demonstrated both *in vivo* and *in vitro* (Pilkington, 1994); it increases with malignancy (Chicoine & Silbergeld, 1995) and it is at the basis of glioma spreading. The growth of gliomas is generally attributed to cell proliferation which conditions invasiveness, but not enough attention has been paid to cell motility.

2.1 Mechanisms of migration and invasion

GBM cells have been demonstrated to migrate individually with a mesenchymal mode of motility (Friedl & Wolf, 2003; Caspani et al., 2006; Beadle et al., 2008): a polarized extension of leading edge membrane processes in the direction of migration takes place. A complex interaction with the environment is realized, as it will be said below, with the creation of a track by the leader cell, followed by other cells. The cells travel mainly along white matter tracts and blood vessels (Zhong et al., 2010). Neoplastic glial cell motility is dependent upon dynamic remodeling of the actin cytoskeleton and vimentin characterizes developing and poorly differentiated glial cells, as nestin is typical of developing neuroectodermal cells. Cytoskeleton remodeling implies redistribution of many components, polarization and extension of active membrane processes with lamellipodia and filipodia (Lefranc et al., 2005). Co-expression of nestin and vimentin serves as a marker of enhanced motility and invasion in gliomas and GFAP has the opposite meaning (Bolteus et al., 2001). The ECM components, i. e. laminin, fibronectin, collagen IV, Tenascin-C and vitronectin interact with invading glioma cells as permissive substrates (Tysnes & Mahesparan, 2001) and many of them are upregulated in high-grade gliomas (Gladson, 1999). On the subject, different experimental tumor models are available.

CD44, a transmembrane glycoprotein functioning as an adhesion molecule, plays a role in cell detachment from the tumor mass. It is the principal receptor of hyaluronan and inhibits adhesion of glioma cells to fibronectin, laminin, vitronectin and collagen I. It is present in glioblastomas (Fig. 1) and shows numerous isoforms derived from alternative splicing the functions of which are still unclear. Cleaved by ADAM (a disintegrin and a metalloproteinase) it promotes cell migration, but if it is blocked invasion is reduced (Bolteus et al., 2001). In the same fraction of the process, neural cell adhesion molecules (NCAM) can act as a paracrine inhibitor of glioma cell locomotion, whereas other molecules such as cadherins that are calcium-dependent transmembrane cell adhesion glycoproteins mediating cell-cell β-adhesion, play a role as well (Perego et al., 2002).

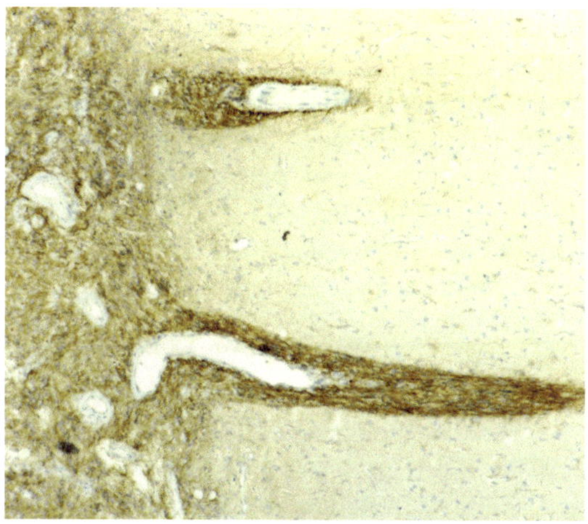

Fig. 1. CD44 positive invading cells, DAB, x100.

ECM proteins have a great importance in cell migration and ECM can be remodeled by glioma cells which produce their own matrix. Tenascin-C is highly concentrated around hyperplastic vessels in gliomas (Zagzag et al., 1995) and enhances migration of endothelial cells and phosphorylation of the focal adhesion kinase (FAK) that interacts with integrin-β1 mediating tenascin C signaling (Plopper et al., 1995). It is over-expressed in invasive gliomas (Mariani et al., 2001). The interest for tenascin recently increased, because specific anti-tenascin antibodies labeled with I^{131} have been used for therapy (Bigner et al., 1995; Goetz et al., 2003).

The proteins of the matrix must be disrupted by proteases or protease-activators such as the zinc-dependent enzymes metalloproteinases (MMPs), classified as collagenases, gelatinases and stromelysin and secreted as proenzymes, which are in balance with their inhibitors or tissue inhibitors of metalloproteinases (TIMPs). Several studies demonstrated the expression of these genes in brain tumors (Pagenstecher et al., 2001) and MMPs have been shown to potentiate tumor cells to migrate along white matter tracts (Belien et al., 1999) or activating other growth factors (McCawley & Matrisian, 2001a, 2001b) and to support gliomas to develop angiogenesis (Forsyth et al., 1999). GBM cell invasiveness and MMP2 expression are suppressed *in vitro* by PAX6 (Mayes et al., 2006). ADAM family has similar effects (Yong et al., 2001; Bauvois, 2004) and it seems to play a role in tumor invasion (Wildeboer et al., 2006).

Urokinase-type plasminogen activator (uPA) binds to its receptor converting plasminogen to plasmin that degrades fibrin, laminin, fibronectin amd proteoglycan. Among cysteine proteinases, cathepsin B must be reminded. Cell adhesion to ECM is favored by integrins, composed by transmembrane glycoprotein units of which β1 is the critical one. Integrins variously occur on glioma cells both in cell lines and biopsies and can be considered as the rungs of a ladder on which cells attach (Tysnes & Mahesparan, 2001). Upregulation of many integrins has been found in glioma cells, compared with normal brain and astrocytes, with α3β1, αvβ1, αvβ3 and αvβ5 playing major roles in migration of tumor astrocytes (Rutka et al., 1999). The *αvβ3* complex can recognize several ligands, such as laminin, fibronectin, vitronectin and Tenascin-C and it can play a role in the angiogenesis activating VEGFR-2. A particular importance has been recently given to lectins, which are carbohydrate-binding proteins, and in particular to selectins and galectins (Lefranc et al., 2005).

Cell migration and invasion are regulated by many factors, first of all EGFR. *In vitro*, cells with strong expression of EGFR are more stimulated to migrate than those with lower expression (Tysnes et al., 1997). Cells with highly amplified EGFR are found at the invading edge of the tumor rather than at the solid tumor centres (Okada et al., 2003), Another very important factor in the regulation of tumor glial cell motility is PTEN: its phosphatase-independent domains reduce the invasive potential of glioma cells, distinctly of the PKB/Akt pathway (Maier et al., 1999). PTEN/Akt/PI3-K/mTOR pathway regulates also the switch between migration and apoptosis and in this context the role played by NF*k*B must not be forgotten. There is a complicated integrin-mediated signaling to which kinases such as FAK and ILK belong. FAK seems to be necessary for integrin-mediated motility (Sieg et al., 2000) and it is in the focus of a very complicated circuit (Günther et al., 2003). Integrins play also a role in cell growth and proliferation. Other factors involved in controlling cell motility are the scatter factor/hepatocyte growth factor (SF/HGF) (Lamszus et al., 1999) and TGF-β1 (Merzak et al., 1995). The regulation of the entire process of cell invasion is really not so simple (Demuth & Berens, 2004) and integrin receptors and focal adhesions, the FAK/Src signaling, the actin function and GTPase in mesenchymal migration have been the most studied steps (Zhong et al., 2010).

A series of novel molecules have been proposed influencing glioma invasion (Nakada et al., 2007). Among extracellular secreted proteins there are: IGFBP (insulin-like-growth-factor-binding protein), Cyr61 (cystein-rich 61/connective tissue growth factor), angiopoietin 2, YKI40, Autotaxin. Among membrane-type proteins Fn14/TWEAK, member of TNF super-family, EphB2/ephrin-B3, of the receptor protein tyrosine kinases, CD155, member of the immunoglobulin family of cell adhesion molecules, have been listed together with intracellular proteins (Nakada et al., 2007)

New synthetic low-molecular weight inhibitors are unceasingly investigated against specific molecular targets of glioma invasion, but one aspect of the process must be kept in mind. There is an inverse correlation between cell motility and cell proliferation (Dalrymple et al., 1994; Giese et al., 1996; Schiffer et al., 1997; Mariani et al., 2001). If migrating cells lower their proliferation rate, they become resistant to treatments and decrease their ability to undergo apoptosis, maybe through activation of PI3/Akt pathway (Joy et al., 2003). From the therapeutic point of view it is important that glioma invasion and angiogenesis share common mechanisms (Lakka et al., 2005).

3. Pathological findings

The study of glioma diffusion is very important from the diagnostic and therapeutic point of view and biomathematical models have been recently developed for a better understanding

(Swanson et al., 2003). It has been calculated that the velocity of tumor expansion is linear with time and varies from about 4 mm/year for low-grade gliomas to 3 mm /month for high grade gliomas. In tumor spheroids, tumor cells diffuse experimentally in the three dimensions following a mathematical model (Stein et al., 2007). Other models are useful in assessing different biological properties of GBM (Eikenberry et al., 2009).

After surgical resection of GBM, recurrence originates from residual invasive cells that in 96% of patients arise from the resection margin, 2-3 cm from the resection cavity (Burger et al., 1983), close to highly cellular tumor (Giese et al., 2003). It has been shown that patients with absence of tumor cells in the adjacent normal nervous tissue had better survival than those with tumor cells (Mangiola et al., 2008). A complete study has been carried out on residual tissue after removal of the tumor and it has been demonstrated that residual cells are distinct from the cells found in routinely resected GBM tissue. They vary in content of stem/progenitor cells, proliferative and invasive capacity, marker and molecular target profiles, and sensitivity to *in vitro* drug and irradiation challenges. Thus, one may speculate that residual cells represent distinct, malignant GBM subentities (Glas et al., 2010).

It is long debated whether infiltrated tissue can be recognized by MRI, not only when adjacent to tumor, but also at a distance. It has been observed that low grade gliomas, which locate preferentially in the insula and the supplementary motor area, spread along distinct sub-cortical fasciculi (Mandonnet et al., 2006). Analyzing different peri-tumor areas with different MRI methods, it has been shown that fractional anisotropy and not apparent diffusion coefficient can be used for evaluating glioma cell invasion. An attempt to classify different peritumoral tissues by a voxel-wise analytical solution using serial diffusion MRI has been made (Ellingson et al., 2011).

Neuropathology is long since discussing infiltrating and invading cells in the BAT and also at a distance from the tumor (Schiffer, 2006). The main problem is how to recognize them, being nuclear anomalies often not sufficient signs. Today, Nestin expression (Kitai et al., 2010) and mainly IDH1-2 mutations (Capper et al., 2010) are convincingly useful in this matter. Critical contributions during the last decades outlined how gliomas spread in the brain and a systematic study has been carried out in one hundred autopsy cases of glioblastomas and astrocytomas (Table 2) (Schiffer, 1986). The knowledge of the spreading modalities of gliomas is particularly useful when a tumor type must be recognized in small surgical samples by its spreading modalities, when these are the only tumor signs present in the sample. Even more difficult is to assess whether a tissue sample contains or not glioma cells.

Gliomas may spread in the homolateral hemisphere and/or to the contralateral hemisphere, mainly along the long axis of short and long fibre bundles. Typical is the diffusion to the contralateral hemisphere through corpus callosum and lamina terminalis. Fibre bundles may also represent an obstacle to diffusion, when they are reached by tumor cells along their short axis. Each tumor location has preferential pathways: fronto-parietal tumors may spare the temporal lobe and the opposite occurs with occipital tumors. Temporal tumors may spread toward hypothalamus and low midline structures or the temporal stem. Interestingly, glioblastomas with evident astrocytic areas, very likely remnants of a previous astrocytoma, spread more frequently to the same hemisphere, whereas glioblastomas, very likely of primary origin, spread through corpus callosum. The Table 2 shows the spreading modalities of a series of glioblastomas.

Anatomical structures	%	Tumor type
Homolateral diffusion	44	1 >3 > 2
Contralateral diffusion	56	3 > 2 > 1
Sub-arachnoidal diffusion	25	2 > 3 > 1
Sub-pial diffusion	9	2 > 1 > 3
Corpus callosum	35	3 > 2 > 1
Septum pellucidum - fornix	18	3 > 2 > 1
Infiltration > 2 cm from tumor edge	22	2 > 3 > 1
Seeding on ventricular walls	6	3 > 2
Multicentric growth	8	2 > 3 > 1
Necrotic tumor with no regrowth	10	1 0 0

Table 2. Spreading modalities of glioblastoma. 1 = tumors with evident astrocytic character; 2 = tumors with diffuse anaplastic aspect; 3 = tumors with a mixed character.

The cerebral cortex may be invaded from tumors located in the white matter, either with or without a perineuronal satellitosis, or from the sub-pial infiltration of a tumor that has invaded from the opposite gyrus, or from cells coming down from sub-arachnoidal seedings along penetrating vessels. Basal ganglia are invaded by local tumors that invade also corpus callosum, or by adjacent tumors. Frequently they reach the temporal stem or the hypothalamus. Septum pellucidum is often passed through by tumor cells which establish a traffic between hypothalamus and basal cortical structures and corpus callosum.
Sub-arachnoidal seeding is frequent (Nishio et al., 1982; Rosenblum, 1995), sometimes as small clusters of tumor cells, visible at naked eyes. Anterior basal, posterior cerebellar and lateral cisterns are involved and even sagittal scissura can be involved when the gyrus cynguli is invaded. When tumor cells invade the underlying cortex, this shows a remarkably intense gliosis. Also spreading in the ventricular system is frequent: tumor cells collect on the ventricular surface and adhere to it where ependymal cells are lacking on an area of pilocytic gliosis.

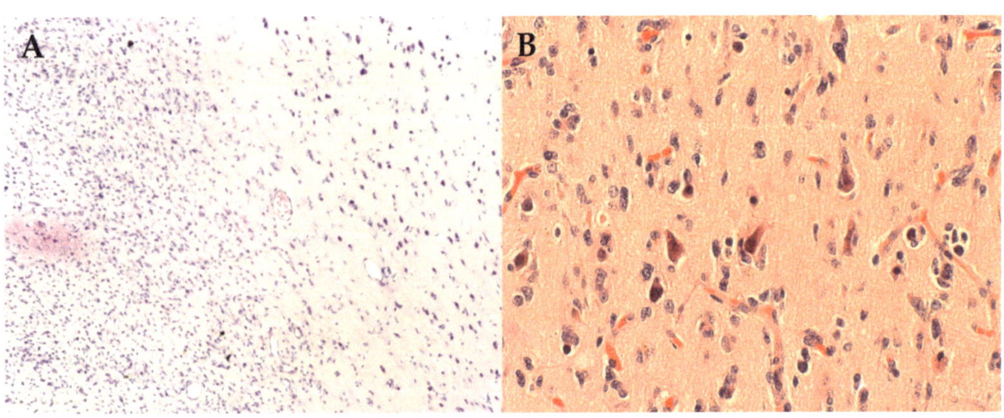

Fig. 2. A - Sharp edge toward normal brain, H&E, x 100; B - Infiltrated cortex with dying neurons, H&E, x 200.

The most important aspect of tumor spreading is the existence of a gradient of tumor cell density towards normal tissue and it could be really interesting to know how far from the tumor edge neoplastic cells can be found and recognized (Fig. 4A, B, C). This datum could be of paramount importance either during intervention, in the attempt of not leaving behind tumor cells, or for establishing post-surgical irradiation modalities: classically a 2 cm distance from the tumor edge is considered a limit of safety (Burger et al., 1988). Sometimes, an infiltrated cortex represents the whole sample removed at the intervention or the sample does not contain the typical signs of the maximum grade of malignancy: necroses, vascular proliferations or high cell proliferation. In these cases, one should be based on the knowledge of what kind of relationships exist among the different tumor features. For example, between cell invasion and cell proliferation. There are *in vitro* evidences suggesting that the two events may be antithetic (Pilkington, 1992; Merzak et al., 1995) and examples of infiltrating, but non-proliferating tumor cells are known (Dalrymple et al., 1994; Schiffer, 1997).

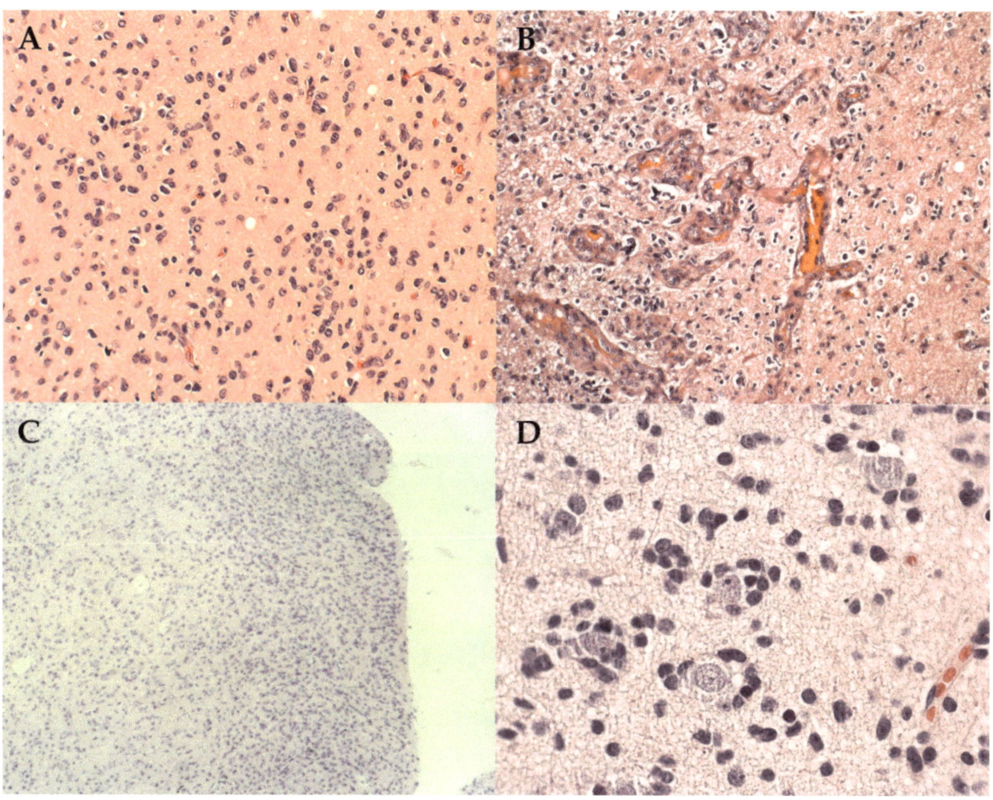

Fig. 3. A – Deeply infiltrated cortex, H&E, x 200; B - Neoformed vessels at the tumor edge, H&E, x 100; C – Invading cells accumulated in the molecular layer, H&E, x 100; D - Perineuronal satellitosis, H&E, x 200.

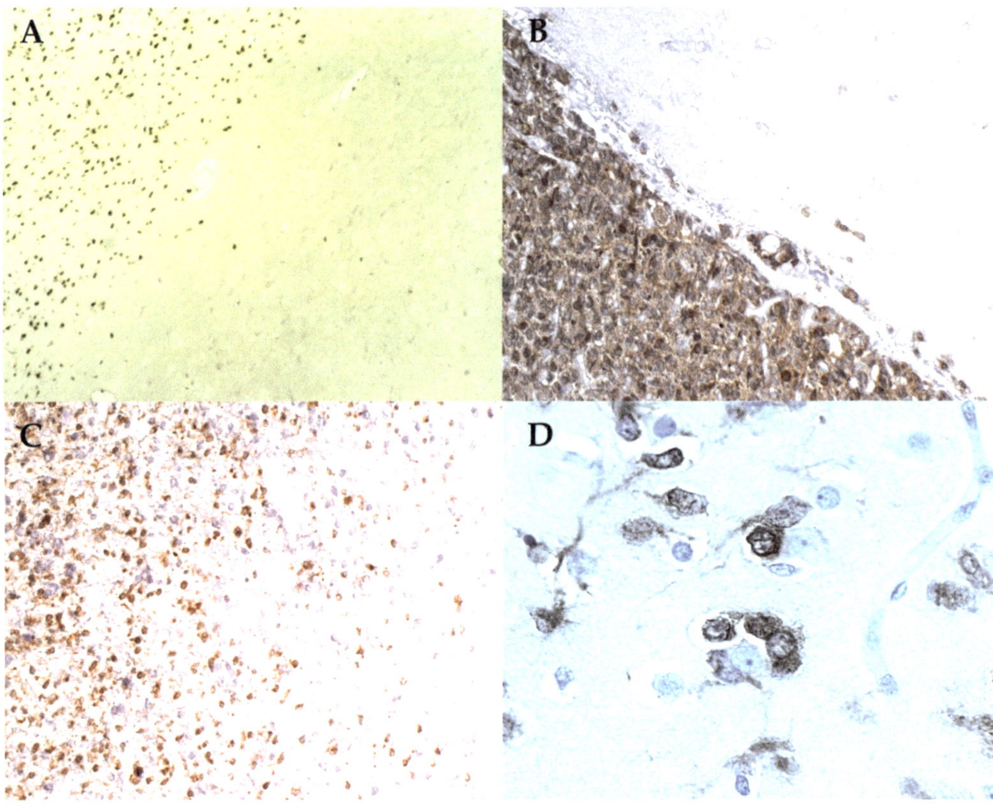

Fig. 4. A - The proliferation ceases at the sharp tumor edge, Ki.67/MIB.1, x 100; B - Sharp tumor edge, IDH1^{R132H} mutation, x 200; C – Gradient of proliferating cells, Ki.67/MIB.1, x 100; D - Positive perineuronal satellites, IDH1^{R132H} mutation, x 400.

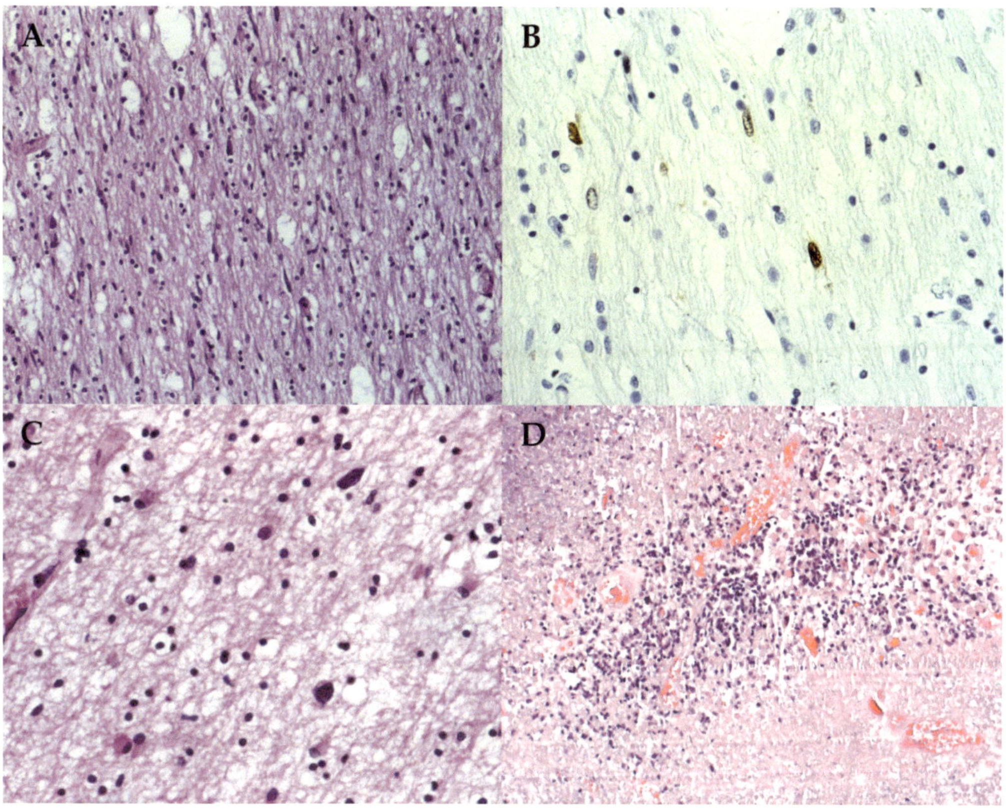

Fig. 5. A - Infiltrated white matter, H&E, x 200; B - PCNA-positive nuclei in the corpus callosum, H&E, x 200; C - Deformed nuclei in the BAT, H&E, x 200; D – Island of viable tumor cells in a radionecrosis, H&E, x 100.

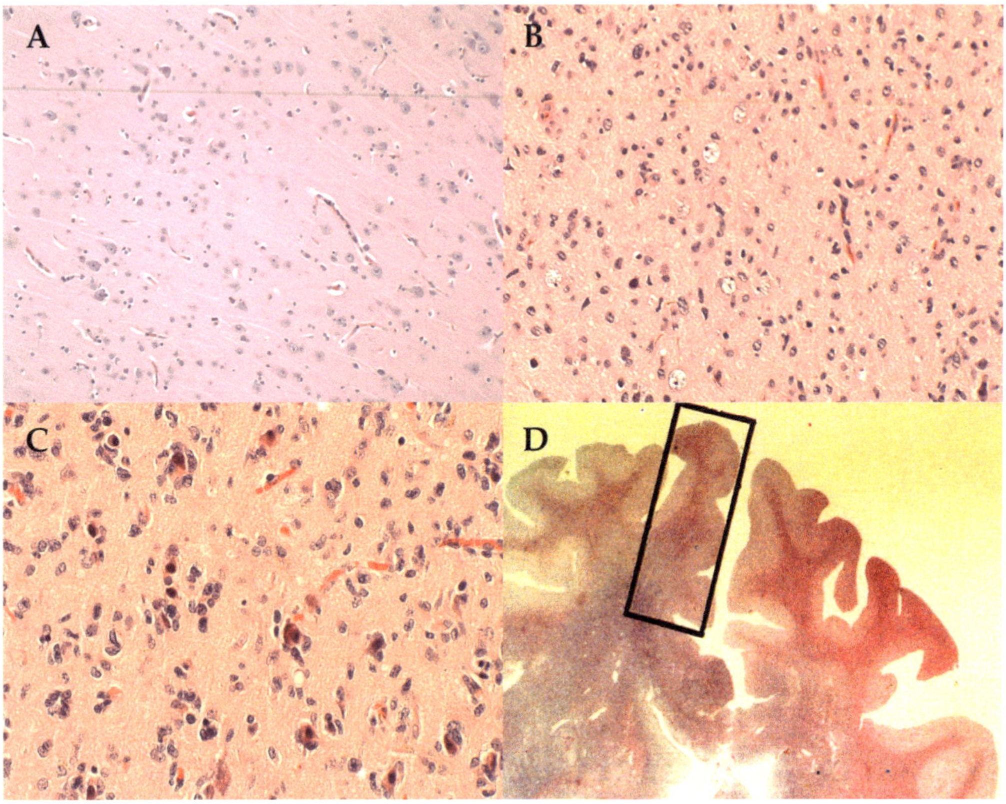

Fig. 6. A - Normal cortex, H&E, x 100; B - Invaded cortex, H&E, x 200; C – id. with sclerotic neurons, H&E, x 200; D – Gradient of tumor cells in a gyrus, H&E.

1. Normal white matter	96±10
2. Tumor peripheral area	213±36
3. Infiltrated area	171±13
4. Apparently normal area	148±8
5. Edematous infiltrated area	55±8

Table 3. Cell Count in the gradient of Fig. 6D (mean number of nuclei per μm^2).

Between the solid tumor and the cortex there is a cell density gradient (Fig. 2A, 2B, 3A) more frequently than between solid tumor and the white matter where the border is usually sharp. There is also a gradient for mitoses and nuclei stained for proliferation markers, such as Ki.67/MIB.1 (Fig. 4A). Sharp borders (Fig. 4B) and cell gradient are, therefore, antithetic. It frequently happens to recognize in completely normal long fibre bundles tumor cells by Ki.67/MIB.1 or PCNA or IDH1-2 mutations (Fig. 5A, 5B). Perineuronal satellitosis is another invasion modality (Fig. 3D, 4D).

The occurrence of isolated tumor cells can be ascertained by these methods (Burger et al., 1986; Schiffer et al., 1997), or by stereotactic procedures (Kelly et al., 1987) or by systematic topographic studies (Burger et al., 1988; Burger & Kleihues, 1989). Tumor cell occurrence in the final part of the cell gradient, where it is more difficult to recognize them, can also be deduced from cell counting showing a higher number of cells than normal (Fig. 6D, Table 3) (Schiffer et al., 1997). Not infrequently, the antitheticity between cell proliferation and migration can be verified in the infiltrated cortex where tumor cells migrating to the cortical surface show a very low MIB.1 LI (Labeling Index), whereas this increases again when the cells terminate migration and accumulate under the pia membrane in the outer cortical layer (Fig. 3C) (Schiffer et al., 1997). *In vitro*, the two properties may appear as mutually exclusive: cells expressing A2B5, i.e. gangliosides, which are highly expressed during development in migratory cells (Small et al., 1987), are not labeled by BrdU or PCNA (Pilkington, 1992, 1994). Isolated tumor cells and solid tumor cells seem to be under a different genetic control (Liotta & Stetler-Stevenson, 1991) and this is very important, because radiotherapy and certain forms of chemotherapy are likely to be scarcely effective on poorly proliferating cells. On the contrary, the proliferation rate of subarachnoidal seedings and of the cells invading the cortex is very high.

Interesting are the re-growth modalities of malignant gliomas after radio-therapy (Schiffer et al., 1982). They are not discussed in this chapter and radionecrosis is just mentioned, but the finding of abnormal, pleomorphic nuclei around the tumor after irradiation (Fig. 5C) or the occurrence of nests of viable tumor cells in a radionecrosis (Fig. 5D) around tumor must be reminded.

4. Migration of neural stem cells (NSCs) toward gliomas

Targeting brain tumor stem cells (BTSCs) for therapy is a new goal today and conversely it has been found that NSCs can target tumors (Shah et al., 2005). NSCs exhibit tumor-homing capability: immortalized murine NSCs, implanted into glioma-bearing rodents, distributed within and around tumors, even migrating to the contralateral hemisphere (Aboody et al., 2000). Genetically engineered NSCs with their tropism for gliomas may have an adverse effect on the latter (Ehtesham et al., 2002; Shah et al., 2003; Kim et al., 2005; Uhl et al., 2005), especially if they are also transduced with herpes simplex virus-thymidine kinase (*HSVtk*) gene and followed by the administration of systemic ganciclovir (Li et al., 2006; Rath et al., 2009; Tyler et al., 2009). Human NSCs implanted in rat brains containing a C6 glioma migrated in the direction of the expanding tumor (Jeon et al., 2008). The same properties are shown by mesenchymal stem cells, injected either into carotid arteries or intracerebrally (Nakamura et al., 2004; Nakamizo et al., 2005) and by hematopoietic progenitor cells (Tabatabai et al., 2005).

Endogeneous progenitor cells have been observed to migrate from the sub-ventricular zone (SVZ) toward a murine experimental glioblastoma (Glass et al., 2005). The migrated nestin-positive cells were positive for Ki-67/MIB.1 and 35% of them for musashi-1 (Pirzkall et al., 2002). Chemokines, angiogenic cytokines and glioma-produced ECM can play a role in the NSC tropism (Xu et al., 2007). It is possible to take advantage of the natural capacity of chemokines to initiate migratory responses, and to use this ability to enhance tumor-inhibitory neural progenitor cells to target an intracranially growing glioma (Honeth et al., 2006). The therapeutic possibilities offered by NSCs are continuously increasing. For example, they can be engineered as sources of secreted therapeutics, exploiting their mobility toward nervous system lesions. They could function as minipumps (Chen et al., 2007).

Rat embryonic progenitor cells transplanted at a distance from a glioma grown in the striatum migrate and co-localize with it. They modify their phenotype, express vimentin and reduce the volume of the tumor, demonstrating that a cross-talk exists between them and the tumor (Staflin et al., 2007). It has been shown that hypoxia is a key factor in determining NSC tropism to glioma and that this is mediated by stromal-derived factor.1 and its receptor (SDF-1/CXCR4), urokinase-type plasminogen activator and its receptor (uPA/uPAR) and VEGF/VEGFR2 (Zhao et al., 2008). It could be interesting to try to enhance motility of adult NSCs towards central nervous system injury or disease and to take into account that EGFR could play a role, because of its participation to malignant transformation (Ayuso-Sacido et al., 2006). It has also been recognized that a limitation exists to the possibility of migration of neural precursors from SVZ to an induced cortical glioblastoma in mice. The limitation is given by age and the proliferation potential of SVZ: adult mice supply fewer cells than younger mice, depending on the expression of D-type Cyclins as Cyclin D1 is lost during aging and only Cyclin D2 remains (Walzlein et al., 2008).
Recently, novel treatment strategies using NSCs have been proposed, for example the suicide gene therapy using converting enzyme (Barresi et al., 2003) and others and new ones will emerge from further studies of NSCs and BTSCs (Oh & Lim, 2009). Just a warning: is it possible that tumors grow from transplanted NSCs (Amariglio et al., 2009)?

5. Microglia/macrophages

It is a common knowledge that malignant gliomas are rich in microglia/macrophages. They are classified as ramified or resident microglia, ameboid or activated microglia, macrophages and perivascular microglia (Fig. 7A) (Graeber & Streit, 1990); therefore, they are both intrinsic to the CNS and blood-borne recently arrived, because of the local production of chemoattractans (Frei et al., 1992). They are increased either in the centre or in the periphery of the tumors (Roggendorf et al., 1996) and it has been calculated that up to one third of cells in glioma biopsies are represented by macrophages (Morimura et al., 1990; Roggendorf et al., 1996). Undoubtedly, they proliferate in response to tumor growth and have a cytotoxic defense function (Sutter et al., 1991), as well as the capacity for antigen presentation (Flugel et al., 2001), but they can also promote tumor infiltration and proliferation as well (Huettner et al., 1997; Graeber et al., 2002).
Macrophages (Fig. 7B) have long been recognized as critical components of immunity against tumors, because, when appropriately stimulated, they can attack tumor cells by contact interaction or secreting cytotoxic and cytostatic factors (Burke et al., 2002). However, they can also contribute to tumor development, secreting growth factors such as angiogenic factors, proteinases, which degrade the matrix, and immunosuppressor factors (Bingle et al., 2002). Their dual function is exerted mainly through TNF which demonstrates both an anti-cancer (Lejeune et al., 1998) and a pro-cancer activity (Orosz et al., 1993). However, it has also been shown that TNF can reduce glioma growth and prolong survival (Villeneuve et al., 2005).
Together with fibroblasts, pericytes, neutrophils, mastcells, lymphocytes, dendritic cells and endothelial cells, macrophages belong to the category of stromal cells which interact with the tumor, as said before, *via* cell-cell or by cytokine- or chemokine-mediated signaling. Tumor cells may influence stromal cells to produce growth factors such as VEGF, TNFα, TGFβ, IL1 or chemokines CCL2, CXCL8, CXCL12 that promote angiogenesis and tumor growth and, conversely, tumor cells are stimulated to produce chemokines influencing

angiogenesis and growth. There is an autocrine and a paracrine tumor growth stimulation (Somasundaram & Herlyn, 2009). The enrichment of stromal cells, especially microglia/macrophages, in the BAT strongly influences immunoregulation and tumor growth on the one side and represents a defense from the tumor on the other side. The observation that there is a positive relationship between microglia/macrophages and tumor initiating cells in the two opposite directions is relevant to the problem (Yi et al., 2011). The possibility to follow the concept that microglia can be exploited in tumor therapy remains today "in its infancy" (Graeber et al., 2002) and it must be interpreted also in a negative sense: the demonstration that microglia/macrophages promote glioma progression means that their inhibition can be a useful therapeutic tool (Zhai et al., 2011).

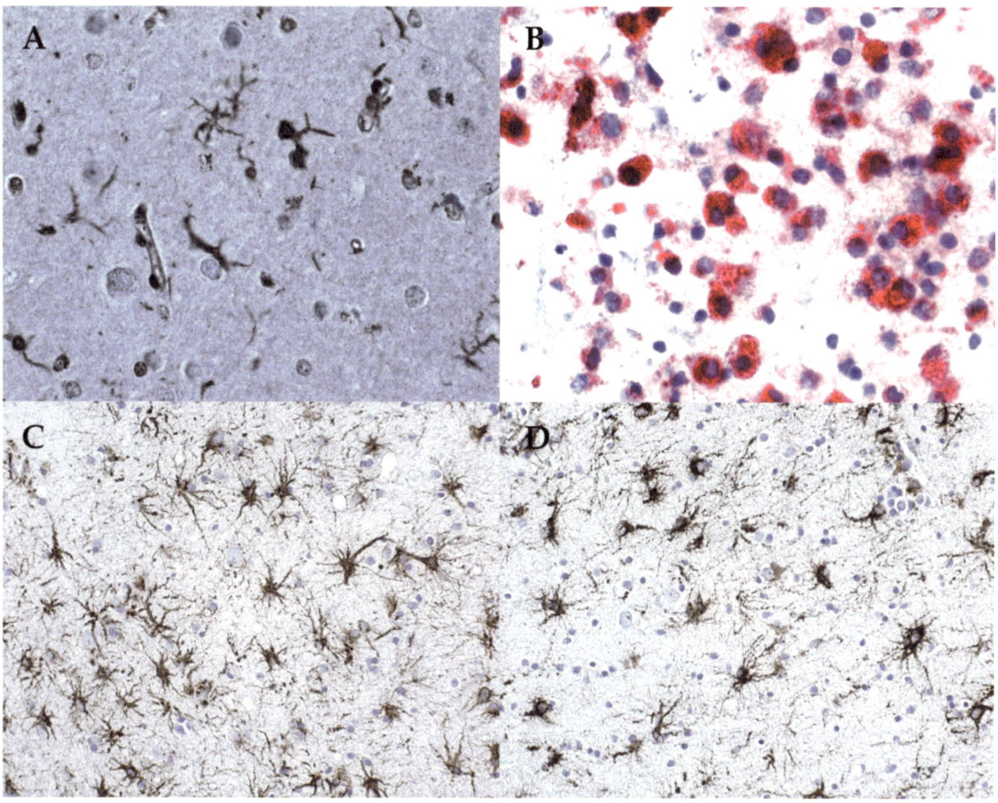

Fig. 7. A - Microglia cells in the cortex around the tumor, CD68, DAB, x 400; B - Macrophages in the BAT, CD68, DAB, x 400; C - Reactive astrocytes in the BAT, GFAP, DAB, x 400; D - Reactive astrocytes in a moderately infiltrated BAT, GFAP, DAB, x 400.

6. Reactive astrocytes

Astrocytes respond rapidly and dramatically to CNS injuries through hypertrophy and then hyperplasia. The first sign of a CNS injury is a progressive development of their cytoplasm to reach a gemistocytic aspect, followed by the production of processes which become in time longer and thicker to form isomorphic or anisomorphic gliosis. The best known hallmark of reactive astrocytes is up-regulation of intermediate filament (IF) proteins, in

particular GFAP, that is one among the 65 IF proteins identified in humans (Hermann & Aebi, 2004). In normal astrocytes, GFAP is the major IF protein, being the expression of Vimentin variable and low (Pixley & De Vellis, 1984). The cells show fine processes extending from the thicker ones. In reactive conditions, a hypertrophy of cellular processes with up-regulation of GFAP and Vimentin expression and re-expression of Nestin occur and a number of genes are involved with the cell functions (Hernandez et al., 2002). There are analogies between glial reaction and physiological maturation of astrocytes during embryogenesis. In initial phases, the fine processes originate directly from the cell soma and then from the thick and long processes (Bushong et al., 2004). Nestin and Vimentin would be the main IF of immature, whereas GFAP and Vimentin of the mature astrocytes (Clarke et al., 1994; Eliasson et al., 1999). In the post-natal brain, GFAP and Vimentin would replace Nestin (Wei et al., 2002). In normal rat brain, Nestin occurs in few astrocytes of the brain stem, whereas in reactive astrocytes it has been observed everywhere: in hippocampus by lesions with kainic acid (Clarke et al., 1994), in hemispheres in experimental ischemia (Duggal et al., 1997) and in trauma where Nestin expression increases in time with GFAP (Sahin Kaya et al., 1999). A complicated and not yet completely solved problem remains that of hyperplasia. It can be realized through an increased number of regional astroglia cells in response to a *noxa*, or by proliferation and migration of sub-ependymal cells (Takamiya et al., 1988; Schiffer et al., 1993; Frisén et al., 1995; Holmin et al., 1997). It was shown that subsets of reactive astrocytes can recapitulate stem cell/progenitor features after damage (Buffo et al., 2010), i.e. some astrocytes acquire stem cell properties after injury and hence may provide a promising cell type to initiate repair after brain injury (Buffo et al., 2008).
Peritumoral reactive gliosis (Fig. 7C, 7D) has a particular importance because of three main characteristics: reactive astrocytes divide by mitosis as tumor cells do; progressively they lose Nestin and increase GFAP expression, as during development and they may exert regionally a series of metabolic and molecular influences (Schiffer, 1997). The most important point is that reactive astrocytes may be included in the advancing tumor in which they become progressively no more recognizable from tumor cells. The question is whether they disappear suffocated by the high density of tumor cells, or if they remain, unrecognizable from tumor cells, contribute to the pleomorphic aspect of gliomas or they are transformed into tumor cells (Tamagno & Schiffer, 2006). The precise origin of reactive astrocytes is still a matter of debate, i.e. whether they are mostly migrated progenitor cells from the sub-ventricular zone (Clarke et al., 1994; Frisén et al., 1995; Lin et al., 1995; Sahin Kaya et al., 1999) or originating from regional astrocytes (Duggal et al., 1997; Li et al., 1999). There is no evidence that tumors can develop from the proliferating reactive glia; however, they might originate from radial glia, which has the capability to proliferate and into which differentiated astrocytes can regress under certain stimuli (Magavi et al., 2000).

7. Autocrine glutamate signalling

Glutamate can promote glioma cell invasion. Glioma cells lack functional EAAT transporters (Ye et al., 1999) and, therefore, glutamate is released rather than taken up (Ye et al., 1999). Glutamate promotes tumor growth, besides causing neuronal excitotoxicity on the neurons surrounding tumor and, therefore, being responsible for the epileptic seizures frequently associated in the symptomatology of gliomas (Sontheimer, 2003). Glutamate release is caused by the cellular cystine uptake *via* x_C^- which is a heterodimeric protein complex made by a catalytic light chain xCT and a regulatory heavy chain 4F2hc localizing the transporter into the membrane (Sato et al., 1999). It imports cystine for the synthesis of glutathione with exchange of glutamate (McBean & Flynn, 2001). It has been demonstrated that glioma cells *in vitro* are stimulated to migrate in response to glutamate (Lyons et al., 2007). The role played by glutamate in the BAT is frequently emphasized, but it does not seem to be adequately considered.

8. Peritumoral edema and infiltration zone

The main problem for invasive gliomas is how far from the tumor border invasive cells can be found. Theoretically, as already said, a zone of two centimetres has been calculated as the limit of target volume for radiotherapy. Even though from the pathological point of view it is a common experience that cells can go farther, the limit expresses the maximum distance from the tumor border seen by MRI compatible with the preservation of the normal nervous tissue with radiotherapy and the minimum for including the most part of invasive cells in the radiation field. In this way the diffusion of tumor cells in the BAT overlaps with peritumoral edema, making it difficult for MRI to distinguish the invasive zone. In low grade gliomas and in secondary GBM such a distinction could be made, even not in the entire BAT, by detection of IDH1-2 mutations in the surgical samples, with the exception of primary GBM (Capper et al., 2010; Mellai et al., 2011).

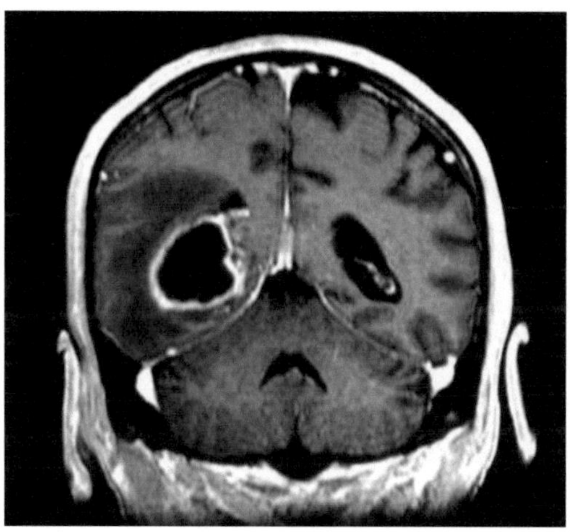

Fig. 8. MRI, T1, peritumoral edema (From the courtesy of Dr. Consuelo Valentini, Dept. Radiology, CTO Hospital, Turin).

For neuroimaging, the coexistence of invasive cells and edema in the BAT (Fig. 8) represents a real problem, because there is not a precise answer to the question whether conventional MRI can distinguish between edema due to reactively altered vital brain tissue from edema plus invasive cells. Using more sophisticated MRI with 1.5 Tesla, it seems that this can be possible. In experimental tumors transplanted into the mice, superimposing immunohistochemistry to MRI it has been observed that in edema districts around the tumor reactive astrocytes, activated microglia, increased expression of aquaporin-4 and invasive tumor cells can be found (Engelhorn et al., 2009). The working concept that brain blood barrier (BBB) is preserved in the BAT to the point that attempts have been made for crossing it to allow chemotherapeutics drugs to reach invasive cells (Madsen & Hirschberg,

2010), is not completely true. In some experiences, BBB after experiments with dexamethasone is considered in the BAT as partially disrupted (Straathof et al., 1998).

Very interesting are the observations on the expression of Aquaporin (AQP4) that is the highest in peritumoral tissue where it correlates with edema, whereas in the tumor it correlates with HIF.1α, VEGF and the grade of malignancy (Mou et al., 2010). In the daily experience of radiologists, radiotherapists and neurosurgeons, the border zone between tumor infiltration and normal brain tissue represents a crucial point, because it is difficult to define the margin for the purposes of treatment planning: to leave small areas of tumor infiltration out of the treatment volume or to include too much normal nervous tissue in it. That is to say to increase the risk of recurrence or that of nervous tissue toxicity (Pirzkall et al., 2004). It must not to be forgotten that volume is a factor of toxicity beside dose and time (Marks et al., 1981) and that small-volume radiotherapy decreases neuropsychological sequelae in comparison with large volume-radiotherapy (Hochberg & Pruitt, 1980; Maire et al., 1987).

It has been demonstrated that tumor cells can be revealed > 3 cm distant from the contrast-enhancing margin of the tumor (Matsukado et al., 1961; Burger et al., 1988) and relapses occur within 2 cm from the original tumor (Hochberg & Pruitt, 1980; Wallner et al., 1989; Oppitz et al., 1999). Therefore, tumor cell invasion is realized inside the area of edema.

With conventional MRI, the detection of tumor infiltration is even more difficult when this is very low and recently attempts are being made with more specific MRI procedures. Magnetic resonance spectroscopy imaging (MRSI), that so much information produced on glioma grading (Law et al., 2003; Nelson, 2003), demonstrated that infiltration could be detected along white matter fibre tracts (Pirzkall et al., 2001, 2002). It is known that with MRSI metabolic changes can be investigated in brain lesions. In gliomas, for example, there is an increase of choline-containing compounds and a decrease of N-acetyl-aspartate (NAA) signal (Pirzkall et al., 2001). Creatine is used to calculate the ratios. It has been demonstrated that MRSI is a valuable tool for assessing residual tumor after surgery (Pirzkall et al., 2004); however, tNAA seems to be more suitable to detect low tumor cell infiltration (Stadlbauer et al., 2007). The problem of detecting tumor cell infiltration in peritumoral edema started to be solved in neuroimaging, even though it cannot be said that it has been completely solved. It parallels that of distinguishing recurrent tumor from radiation injury that can be accomplished by multivoxel 3D Oritin MR spectroscopy (^{1}H-MRS) (Zeng et al., 2007).

9. Conclusions

Different cell types can be found in the BAT, but they do not exhaust all its phenotypic features. Other events may occur in the peritumoral tissue and one of them, calcifications, may have repercussions on neuroimaging of tumors. Calcifications may be found either at a distance from the tumor or in the infiltration zone, because reached by the advancing tumor with time. Another event is the occurrence of teleangectatic vessels just outside the zone of solid tumor or in the healthy tissue and successively included in the invading tumor.

The aspect of the greatest interest is that the existence itself of a BAT as before depicted and its thickness are not a constant finding around malignant gliomas. Sometime it happens that the tumor confines with the normal tissue in a sharp way and there is no tumor cell gradient. This is not infrequent when the tumor meets a white matter bundles perpendicularly. Conversely, when it proceeds from the deep white matter to the cortex along ascending and descending fibres the cell gradient can be very wide, to the point that it can be difficult to establish, without an accurate cell count (Schiffer, 2006), where the tumor ends. This is a real challenge for neuroimaging, because theorethically tumor cells can be found at any distance from the tumor and the safety margins are more conventional than real. Just think to the passage through the corpus callosum, septum pellucidum, commissures, and seeding in the subarachnoidal spaces. The occurrence of tumor cells far from the tumor, can be a problem relevant to gliomagenesis and the relationship between brain and glioma origin (Schiffer et al., 2006, 2010), falling, therefore, outside the present chapter.

Another crucial point is that the cell composition of the BAT can be manifold with an inconstant proportion among them in the different zones of the front between tumor and the healthy tissue. For example, the quota of macrophages/microglia may greatly vary, as well as that of reactive astrocytes, depending also on the treatments received from the tumor. For example, in tumors after radiotherapy large areas of packed macrophages can be found around the tumor, not identifiable directly with radionecrosis (Schiffer et al., 1980). On the contribution of migrating stem cells from the SVZ there is no available information on human pathology. Their participation to the BAT is just deduced from experimental neuro-oncology and it is an hypothesis to be taken into account. That of BAT is a working concept that will be fruitful in the future, together with the advancement of neuroimaging.

10. References

Aboody, K.S., Brown, A., Rainov, N.G., Bower, K.A., Liu, S., Yang, W., Small, J.E., Herrlinger, U., Ourednik, V., Black, P.M., Breakefield, X.O., & Snyder, E.Y. (2000). Neural stem cells display extensive tropism for pathology in adult brain: evidence from intracranial gliomas. *Proceedings of the National Academy of Sciences of the United States of America,* Vol.97, No.23, pp. 12846-12851, ISSN 0027-8424

Amariglio, N., Hirshberg, A., Scheithauer, B.W., Cohen, Y., Loewenthal, R., Trankhtenbrot, L., Paz, N., Koren-Michowitz, M., Waldman, D., Leider-Trejo, L., Toren, A., Constantini, S., & Rehcavi, G. (2009). Donor-derived brain tumor following neural stem cell transplantation in an ataxia-teleangectasia patient. *PLoS Medicine,* Vol.6, No.2, pp. e1000029, ISSN 1549-1676

Ayuso-Sacido, A., Graham, C., Greenfield, J.P., & Boockvar, J.A. (2006). The duality of epidermal growth factor receptor (EGFR) signalling and neural stem cell phenotype: cell enhancer or cell transformer? *Current Stem Cell Research & Therapy,* Vol.1, No.3, pp. 387-394, ISSN 1574-888X

Bagci, T., Wu, J.K., Pfannl, R., Ilag, L.L., & Jay, D.G. (2009). Autocrine semaphorin 3A signaling promotes glioblastoma dispersal. *Oncogene,* Vol. 28, No. 40, pp. 3537-3550, ISSN 0950-9232

Barresi, V., Belluardo, N., Sipione, S., Mudò, G., Cattaneo, E., & Condorelli, D.F. (2003). Transplantation of prodrug-converting neural progenitor cells for brain tumor therapy. *Cancer Gene Therapy,* Vol.10, No.5, pp. 396-402, ISSN 0929-1903

Bauvois, B. (2004). Transmembrane proteases in cell growth and invasion: new contributors to angiogenesis? *Oncogene,* Vol.23, No.2, pp. 317-329, ISSN 0950-9232

Beadle, C., Assanah, M.C., Monzo, P., Vallee, R., Rosenfeld, S.S., & Canoll, P. (2008). The role of myosin II in glioma invasion of the brain. *Molecular Biology of the Cell,* Vol.19, No.8, pp. 3357-3368, ISSN 1059-1524

Beliën, A.T., Paganetti, P.A., & Schwab, M.E. (1999). Membrane-type 1 matrix metalloprotease (MT1-MMP) enables invasive migration of glioma cells in central nervous system white matter. *Journal of Cell Biology,* Vol.144, No.2, pp. 373-384. ISSN 0021-9525

Bigner, D.D., Brown, M., Coleman, R.E., Friedman, A.H., Friedman, H.S., McLendon, R.E., Bigner, S.H., Zhao, X.G., Wikstrand, C.J., & Pegram, C.N. (1995). Phase I studies of treatment of malignant gliomas and neoplastic meningitis with 131I-radiolabeled monoclonal antibodies anti-tenascin 81C6 and anti-chondroitin proteoglycan sulfate Me1-14 F (ab')2--a preliminary report. *Journal of Neuro-Oncology,* Vol.24, No.1, pp. 109-22, ISSN 0167-594X

Bingle, L., Brown, N.J., & Lewis, C.E. (2002). The role of tumour-associated macrophages in tumour progression: implications for new anticancer therapies. *Journal of Pathology,* Vol.196, No.3, pp. 254-265, ISSN: 0022-3417

Bolteus, A.J., Berens, M.E., & Pilkington, G.J. (2001). Migration and invasion in brain neoplasms. *Current Neurology and Neuroscience Reports,* Vol.1, No.3, pp. 225-32, ISSN 1528-4042

Buffo, A., Rite, I., Tripathi, P., Lepier, A., Colak, D., Horn, A.P., Mori, T., & Götz, M. (2008). Origin and progeny of reactive gliosis: A source of multipotent cells in the injured brain. *Proceedings of the National Academy of Sciences of the United States of America,* Vol.105, No.9, pp. 3581-3586, ISSN 0027-8424

Buffo, A., Rolando, C., & Ceruti, S. (2010). Astrocytes in the damaged brain: molecular and cellular insights into their reactive response and healing potential. *Biochemical Pharmacology,* Vol.79, No.2, pp. 77-89, ISSN 0006-2952

Burger, P.C., Dubois, P.J., Schold, S.C. Jr, Smith, K.R. Jr, Odom, G.L., Crafts, D.C., & Giangaspero, F. (1983). Computerized tomographic and pathologic studies of the untreated, quiescent, and recurrent glioblastoma multiforme. *Journal of Neurosurgery,* Vol.58, No.2, pp. 159-169, ISSN 0022-3085

Burger, P.C., Shibata, T., & Kleihues, P. (1986). The use of the monoclonal antibody Ki-67 in the identification of proliferating cells: application to surgical neuropathology. *American Journal of Surgical Pathology,* Vol.10, No.9, pp. 611-617, ISSN 0147-5185

Burger, P.C., Heinz, E.R., Shibata, T., & Kleihues, P. (1988). Topographic anatomy and CT correlations in the untreated glioblastoma multiforme. *Journal of Neurosurgery,* Vol.68, No.5, pp. 698-704, ISSN 0022-3085

Burger, P.C., & Kleihues, P. (1989). Cytologic composition of the untreated glioblastoma with implications for evaluation of needle biopsies. *Cancer,* Vol.63, No.10, pp. 2014-2023, ISSN 1097-0142

Burke, B., Tang, N., Corke, K.P., Tazzyman, D., Ameri, K., Wells, M., & Lewis, CE. (2002). Expression of HIF-1alpha by human macrophages: implications for the use of macrophages in hypoxia-regulated cancer gene therapy. *The Journal of Pathology,* Vol.196, No.2, pp. 204-212, ISSN 0022-3417

Bushong, E.A., Martone, M.E., & Ellisman, M.H. (2004). Maturation of astrocyte morphology and the establishment of astrocyte domains during postnatal hippocampal development. *International Journal of Developmental Neuroscience,* Vol.22, No.2, pp. 73-86, ISSN 0736-5748

Capper, D., Weissert, S., Balss, J., Habel, A., Meyer, J., Jäger, D., Ackermann, U., Tessmer, C., Korshunov, A., Zentgraf, H., Hartmann, C., & von Deimling, A. (2010).

Characterization of R132H mutation-specific IDH1 antibody binding in brain tumors. *Brain Pathology,* Vol.20, No.1, pp. 245-254, ISSN 1015-6305

Carro, M.S., Lim, W.K., Alvarez, M.J., Bollo, R.J., Zhao, X., Snyder, E.Y., Sulman, E.P., Anne, S.L., Doetsch, F., Colman, H., Lasorella, A., Aldape, K., Califano, A., & Iavarone, A. (2010). The transcriptional network for mesenchymal transformation of brain tumours. *Nature,* Vol.463, No.7279, pp. 318-325, ISSN 0028-0836

Caspani, E.M., Echevarria, D., Rottner, K., & Small, J.V. (2006). Live imaging of glioblastoma cells in brain tissue shows requirement of actin bundles for migration. *Neuron Glia Biology,* Vol.2, No.2, pp. 105-114, ISSN 1741-0533

Chen, H.I., Bakshi, A., Royo, N.C., Magge, S.N. & Watson, D.J. (2007). Neural stem cells as biological minipumps: a faster route to cell therapy for the CNS? *Current Stem Cell Research & Therapy,* Vol.2, No.1, pp. 13-22, ISSN 1574-888X

Chicoine, M.R., & Silbergeld, D.L. (1995). The in vitro motility of human gliomas increases with increasing grade of malignancy. *Cancer,* Vol.75, No.12, pp. 2904-2909, ISSN 1097-0142

Clarke, S.R., Shetty, A.K., Bradley, J.L., & Turner, D.A. (1994). Reactive astrocytes express the embryonic intermediate neurofilament nestin. *Neuroreport,* Vol.5, No.15, pp. 1885-1888, ISSN 0959-4965

Dalrymple, S.J., Parisi, J.E., Roche, P.C., Ziesmer, S.C., Scheithauer, B.W., & Kelly, P.J. (1994). Changes in proliferating cell nuclear antigen expression in glioblastoma multiforme cells along a stereotactic biopsy trajectory. *Neurosurgery,* Vol.35, No.6, pp. 1036-1045, ISSN 0148-396X

Demuth, T., & Berens, M.E. (2004). Molecular mechanisms of glioma cell migration and invasion. *Journal of Neuro-Oncology,* Vol.70, No.2, pp. 217-228, ISSN 0167-594X

Duggal, N., Schmidt-Kastner, R., & Hakim, A.M. (1997). Nestin expression in reactive astrocytes following focal cerebral ischemia in rats. *Brain Research,* Vol.768, No.1-2, pp. 1-9, ISSN 0006-8993

Ehtesham, M., Kabos, P., Kabosoya, A., Neuman, T., Black, K.L. & Yu, J.S. (2002). The use of interleukin 12-secreting neural stem cells for the treatment of intracranial glioma. *Cancer Research,* Vol.62, No.20, pp. 5657-5663, ISSN 0008-5472

Eikenberry, S.E., Sankar, T., Preul, M.C., Kostelich, E.J., Thalhauser, C.J., & Kuang, Y. (2009). Virtual glioblastoma: growth, migration and treatment in a three-dimensional mathematical model. *Cell proliferation,* Vol.42, No.4, pp. 511-528, ISSN 0960-7722

Elias, M.C., Tozer, K.R., Silber, J.R., Mikheeva, S., Deng, M., Morrison, R.S., Manning, T.C., Silbergeld, D.L., Glackin, C.A., Reh, T.A., & Rostomily, R.C. (2005). TWIST is expressed in human gliomas and promotes invasion. *Neoplasia,* Vol.7, No.9, pp. 824-837, ISSN 1522-8002

Eliasson, C., Sahlgren, C., Berthold, C.H., Stakeberg, J., Celis, J.E., Betsholtz, C., Eriksson, J.E., & Pekny, M. (1999). Intermediate filament protein partnership in astrocytes. *Journal of Biological Chemistry,* Vol.274, No.34, pp. 23996-24006, ISSN 0021-9258

Ellingson, B.M., Laviolette, P.S., Rand, S.D., Malkin, M.G., Connelly, J.M., Mueller, W.M., Prost, R.W., & Schmainda, K.M. (2011). Spatially quantifying microscopic tumor invasion and proliferation using a voxel-wise solution to a glioma growth model and serial diffusion MRI. *Magnetic Resonance in Medicine,* Vol.65, No.4, pp. 1131-1143, ISSN 0740-3194

Engelhorn, T., Savaskan, N.E., Schwarz, M.A., Kreutzer, J., Meyer, E.P., Hahnen, E., Ganslandt, O., Dörfler, A., Nimsky, C., Buchfelder, M., & Eyüpoglu, I.Y. (2009).

Cellular characterization of the peritumoral edema zone in malignant brain tumors. *Cancer Science,* Vol.100, No.10, pp. 1856-1862, ISSN 1347-9032

Flügel, A., Bradl, M., Kreutzberg, G.W., & Graeber, M.B. (2001). Transformation of donor-derived bone marrow precursors into host microglia during autoimmune CNS inflammation and during the retrograde response to axotomy. *Journal of Neuroscience Research,* Vol.66, No.1, pp. 74-82, ISSN 0360-4012

Forsyth, P.A., Wong, H., Laing, T.D., Rewcastle, N.B., Morris, D.G., Muzik, H., Leco, K.J., Johnston, R.N., Brasher, P.M., Sutherland, G., & Edwards, D.R. (1999). Gelatinase-A (MMP-2), gelatinase-B (MMP-9) and membrane type matrix metalloproteinase-1 (MT1-MMP) are involved in different aspects of the pathophysiology of malignant gliomas. *British Journal of Cancer,* Vol.79, No.11-12, pp. 1828-1835, ISSN 0007-0920

Frei, K., Piani, D., Malipiero, U.V., Van Meir, E., de Tribolet, N., & Fontana, A. (1992). Granulocyte-macrophage colony-stimulating factor (GM-CSF) production by glioblastoma cells. Despite the presence of inducing signals GM-CSF is not expressed in vivo. *The Journal of Immunology,* Vol.148, No.10, pp. 3140-3146, ISSN 0022-1767

Friedl, P., & Wolf, K. (2003). Tumour-cell invasion and migration: diversity and escape mechanisms. *Nature Reviews Cancer,* Vol.3, No.5, pp.362-374, ISSN 1474-175X

Frisén, J., Johansson, C.B., Török, C., Risling, M., & Lendahl, U. (1995). Rapid, widespread, and longlasting induction of nestin contributes to the generation of glial scar tissue after CNS injury. *Journal of Cell Biology,* Vol.131, No.2, pp. 453-464, ISSN 0021-9525

Giese, A., & Westphal, M. (1996). Glioma invasion in the central nervous system. *Neurosurgery,* Vol.39, No.2, pp. 235-252, ISSN 0148-396X

Giese, A., Bjerkvig, R., Berens, M.E., & Westphal, M. (2003). Cost of migration: invasion of malignant gliomas and implications for treatment. J Clin Oncol. Vol.21, No.8, pp. 1624-1636, ISSN 0732-183X.

Gladson, C.L. (1999). The extracellular matrix of gliomas: modulation of cell function. *Journal of Neuropathology & Experimental Neurology,* Vol.58, No.10, pp. 1029-1040, ISSN 0022-3069

Glas, M., Rath, B.H., Simon, M., Reinartz, R., Schramme, A., Trageser, D., Eisenreich, R., Leinhaas, A., Keller, M., Schildhaus, H.U., Garbe, S., Steinfarz, B., Pietsch, T., Steindler, D.A., Schramm, J., Herrlinger, U., Brüstle, O., & Scheffler, B. (2010). Residual tumor cells are unique cellular targets in glioblastoma. *Annals of Neurology,* Vol.68, No.2, pp. 264-269, ISSN 0364-5134

Glass, R., Synowitz, M., Kronenberg, G., Walzlein, J.H., Markovic, D.S., Wang, L.P., Gast, D., Kiwit, J., Kempermann, G. & Kettenmann, H. (2005). Glioblastoma-induced attraction of endogeneous neural precursor cells is associated with improved survival. *The Journal of Neuroscience,* Vol.25, No.10, pp. 2637-2646, ISSN 0270-6474

Goetz, C., Riva, P., Poepperl, G., Gildehaus, F.J., Hischa, A., Tatsch, K., & Reulen, H.J. (2003). Locoregional radioimmunotherapy in selected patients with malignant glioma: experiences, side effects and survival times. *Journal of Neuro-Oncology,* Vol.62, No.3, pp. 321-328, ISSN 0167-594X

Graeber, M.B., & Streit, W.J. (1990). Microglia: immune network in the CNS. *Brain Pathology,* Vol.1, No.1, pp. 2-5, ISSN 1015-6305

Graeber, M.B., Scheithauer, B.W., & Kreutzberg, G.W. (2002). Microglia in brain tumors. *Glia,* Vol.40, No.2, pp. 252-259, ISSN 1098-1136

Günther, W., Skaftnesmo, K.O., Arnold, H., & Terzis, A.J. (2003). Molecular approaches to brain tumour invasion. *Acta Neurochirurgica,* Vol.145, No.12, pp. 1029-1036, ISSN 0001-6268

Hernandez, M.R., Agapova, O.A., Yang, P., Salvador-Silva, M., Ricard, C.S., & Aoi, S. (2002). Differential gene expression in astrocytes from human normal and glaucomatous optic nerve head analyzed by cDNA microarray. *Glia,* Vol.38, No.1, pp. 45-64, ISSN 1098-1136

Herrmann, H., & Aebi, U. (2004). Intermediate filaments: molecular structure, assembly mechanism, and integration into functionally distinct intracellular Scaffolds. *Annual Review of Biochemistry,* Vol.73, pp. 749-789, ISSN 0066-4154

Hochberg, F.H., & Pruitt, A. (1980). Assumptions in the radiotherapy of glioblastoma. *Neurology,* Vol.30, No.9, pp. 907-911, ISSN 0028-3878

Holmin, S., Almqvist, P., Lendahl, U., & Mathiesen, T. (1997). Adult nestin-expressing subependymal cells differentiate to astrocytes in response to brain injury. *European Journal of Neuroscience,* Vol.9, No.1, pp. 65-75, ISSN 0953-816X

Honeth, G., Staflin, K., Kalliomäki, S., Lindvall, M. & Kjellman, C. (2006). Chemokine-directed migration of tumor-inhibitory neural progenitor cells towards an intracranially growing glioma. *Experimental Cell Research,* Vol.312, No.8, pp. 1265-1276, ISSN 0014-4827

Huettner, C., Czub, S., Kerkau, S., Roggendorf, W., & Tonn, J.C. (1997). Interleukin 10 is expressed in human gliomas in vivo and increases glioma cell proliferation and motility in vitro. *Anticancer Research,* Vol.17, No.5A, pp. 3217-3224, ISSN 0250-7005

Jeon, J.Y., An, J.H., Kim, S.U., Park, H.G. & Lee, M.A. (2008). Migration of human neural stem cells toward an intracranial glioma. *Experimental and Molecular Medicine,* Vol40, No.1, pp. 84-91, ISSN, 1226-3613

Joy, A.M., Beaudry, C.E., Tran, N.L., Ponce, F.A., Holz, D.R., Demuth, T., & Berens, M.E. (2003). Migrating glioma cells activate the PI3-K pathway and display decreased susceptibility to apoptosis. *Journal of Cell Science,* Vol.116, No.Pt21, pp. 4409-4417, ISSN 0021-9533

Kalluri, R., & Weinberg, R.A. (2009). The basics of epithelial-mesenchymal transition. *The Journal of Clinical Investigation,* Vol. 119, No. 6, pp. 1420-1428. Erratum in: *The Journal of Clinical Investigation,* (2010), Vol.120, No.5, p. 1786, ISSN 0021-9738

Kelly, P.J., Daumas-Duport, C., Scheithauer, B.W., Kall, B.A., & Kispert, D.B. (1987). Stereotactic histologic correlations of computed tomography- and magnetic resonance imaging-defined abnormalities in patients with glial neoplasms. *Mayo Clinic Proceedings,* Vol.62, No.6, pp. 450-459, ISSN 0025-6196

Kim, S.K., Cargioli, T.G., Machluf, M., Yang, W., Sun, Y., Al-Hashem, R., Kim, S.U., Black, P.M. & Carroll, R.S. (2005). PEX-producing human neural stem cells inhibit tumor growth in a mouse glioma model. *Clinical Cancer Research,* Vol.11, No.16, pp. 5965-5970, ISSN 1078-0432

Kislin, K.L., McDonough, W.S., Eschbacher, J.M., Armstrong, B.A., & Berens, M.E. (2009). NHERF-1: modulator of glioblastoma cell migration and invasion. *Neoplasia,* Vol.11, No.4, pp. 377-387, ISSN 1522-8002

Kitai, R., Horita, R., Sato, K., Yoshida, K., Arishima, H., Higashino, Y., Hashimoto, N., Takeuchi, H., Kubota, T., & Kikuta, K. (2010). Nestin expression in astrocytic tumors delineates tumor infiltration. *Brain Tumor Pathology,* Vol.27, No.1, pp. 17-21, ISSN 1433-7398

Lal, A., Glazer, C.A., Martinson, H.M., Friedman, H.S., Archer, G.E., Sampson, J.H., & Riggins, G.J. (2002). Mutant epidermal growth factor receptor up-regulates molecular effectors of tumor invasion. *Cancer Research,* Vol.62, No.12, pp. 3335-3339, ISSN 0008-5472

Lakka, S.S., Gondi, C.S., & Rao, J.S. (2005). Proteases and glioma angiogenesis. *Brain Pathology,* Vol.15, No.4, pp. 327-341, ISSN 1015-6305

Lamszus, K., Laterra, J., Westphal, M., & Rosen, E.M. (1999). Scatter factor/hepatocyte growth factor (SF/HGF) content and function in human gliomas. *International Journal of Developmental Neuroscience,* Vol.17, No.5-6, pp. 517-530, ISSN 0736-5748

Law, M., Yang, S., Wang, H., Babb, J.S., Johnson, G., Cha, S., Knopp, E.A., & Zagzag, D. (2003). Glioma grading: sensitivity, specificity, and predictive values of perfusion MR imaging and proton MR spectroscopic imaging compared with conventional MR imaging. *American Journal of Neuroradiology,* Vol.24, No.10, pp. 1989-1998 ISSN 0195-6108

Lefranc, F., Brotchi, J., & Kiss, R. (2005). Possible future issues in the treatment of glioblastomas: special emphasis on cell migration and the resistance of migrating glioblastoma cells to apoptosis. *Journal of Clinical Oncology,* Vol.23, No.10, pp. 2411-2422, ISSN 0732-183X

Lejeune, F.J., Rüegg, C., & Liénard, D. (1998). Clinical applications of TNF-alpha in cancer. *Current Opinion in Immunology,* Vol.10, No.5, pp. 573-580, ISSN 0952-7915

Li, Y., & Chopp, M. (1999). Temporal profile of nestin expression after focal cerebral ischemia in adult rat. *Brain Research,* Vol.838, No.1-2, pp. 1-10, ISSN 0006-8993

Li, Z.B., Zeng Z.J., Chen, Q., Luo, S.Q., & Hu, W.X. (2006). Recombinant AAV-mediated HSVtk gene transfer with direct intratumoral injections and Tet-On regulation for implanted human breast cancer. *BMC Cancer,* Vol.6, p. 66, ISSN 1471-2407

Lin, R.C., Matesic, D.F., Marvin, M., McKay, R.D., & Brüstle, O. (1995). Re-expression of the intermediate filament nestin in reactive astrocytes. *Neurobiology of Disease,* Vol.2, No.2, pp. 79-85, ISSN 0969-9961

Liotta, L.A., & Stetler-Stevenson, W.G. (1991). Tumor invasion and metastasis: an imbalance of positive and negative regulation. *Cancer Research,* Vol.51, No.18 Suppl, pp. 5054s-5059s, ISSN 0008-5472

Lyons, S.A., Chung, W.J., Weaver, A.K., Ogunrinu, T., & Sontheimer, H. (2007). Autocrine glutamate signaling promotes glioma cell invasion. *Cancer Research,* Vol.67, No.19, pp. 9463-9471, ISSN 0008-5472

Madsen, S.J., & Hirschberg, H. (2010). Site-specific opening of the blood-brain barrier. *Journal of Biophotonics,* Vol.3, No.5-6, pp. 356-367, ISSN 1864-063X

Magavi, S., Leavitt, B.R., & Macklis, J.D. (2000). Induction of neurogenesis in the neocortex of adult mice. *Nature,* Vol.405, No.6789, pp. 951-955, ISSN 0028-0836

Maier, D., Jones, G., Li, X., Schönthal, A.H., Gratzl, O., Van Meir, E.G., & Merlo, A. (1999). The PTEN lipid phosphatase domain is not required to inhibit invasion of glioma cells. *Cancer Research,* Vol.59, No.21, pp. 5479-5482, ISSN 0008-5472

Maire, J.P., Coudin, B., Guérin, J., & Caudry, M. (1987). Neuropsychologic impairment in adults with brain tumors. *American Journal of Clinical Oncology,* Vol.10, No.2, pp. 156-162, ISSN 0277-3732

Mandonnet, E., Capelle, L., & Duffau, H. (2006). Extension of paralimbic low grade gliomas: toward an anatomical classification based on white matter invasion patterns. *Journal of Neuro-Oncology,* Vol.78, No.2, pp. 179-185, ISSN 0167-594X

Mangiola, A., De Bonis, P., Maira, G., Calducci, M., Sica, G., Lama, G., Lauriola, L., & Anile, C. (2008). Invasive tumor cells and prognosis in a selected population of patients with glioblastoma multiforme. *Cancer,* Vol.113, No.4, pp. 841-846, ISSN 0008-543X

Mariani, L., Beaudry, C., McDonough, W.S., Hoelzinger, D.B., Demuth, T., Ross, K.R., Berens, T., Coons, S.W., Watts, G., Trent, J.M., Wei, J.S., Giese, A., & Berens, M.E. (2001). Glioma cell motility is associated with reduced transcription of proapoptotic and proliferation genes: a cDNA microarray analysis. *Journal of Neuro-Oncology,* Vol.53, No.2, pp. 161-176, ISSN 0167-594X

Marks, J.E., Baglan, R.J., Prassad, S.C., & Blank, W.F. (1981). Cerebral radionecrosis: incidence and risk in relation to dose, time, fractionation and volume. *International Journal of Radiation Oncology, Biology, Physics,* Vol.7, No.2, pp. 243-252, ISSN 0360-3016

Matsukado, Y., Maccarty, C.S., & Kernohan, J.W. (1961). The growth of glioblastoma multiforme (astrocytomas, grades 3 and 4) in neurosurgical practice. *Journal of Neurosurgery,* Vol.18, pp. 636-644, ISSN 0022-3085

Mayes, D.A., Hu, Y., Teng, Y., Siegel, E., Wu, X., Panda, K., Tan, F., Yung, W.K., & Zhou, Y.H. (2006). PAX6 suppresses the invasiveness of glioblastoma cells and the expression of the matrix metalloproteinase-2 gene. *Cancer Research,* Vol.66, No.20, pp. 9809-9817, ISSN 0008-5472

McBean, G.J., & Flynn, J. (2001). Molecular mechanisms of cystine transport. *Biochemical Society Transactions,* Vol.29, No.Pt6, pp. 717-722, ISSN 0300-5127

McCawley, L.J., & Matrisian, L.M. (2001a). Matrix metalloproteinases: they're not just for matrix anymore! *Current Opinion in Cell Biology,* Vol.13, No.5, pp. 534-540, ISSN 0955-0674

McCawley, L.J., & Matrisian, L.M. (2001b). Tumor progression: defining the soil round the tumor seed. *Current Biology,* Vol.11, No.1, pp. R25-27, ISSN 0960-9822

Mellai, M., Piazzi, A., Caldera, V., Monzeglio, O., Lanotte, M., Valente G., & Schiffer, D. (2011). *IDH1* and *IDH2* mutations, immunohistochemistry and associations in a series of brain tumors. *Journal of Neuro-Oncology,* published online: 04 June 2011

Merzak, A., Koochekpour, S., Dkhissi, F., Raynal, S., Lawrence, D., & Pilkington, G.J. (1995). Synergism between growth factors in the control of glioma cell proliferation, migration and invasion in vitro. *International Journal of Oncology,* Vol.6, pp. 1079-1085, ISSN 1019-6439

Mikheeva, S.A., Mikheev, A.M., Petit, A., Beyer, R., Oxford, R.G., Khorasani, L., Maxwell, J.P., Glackin, C.A., Wakimoto, H., González-Herrero, I., Sánchez-García, I., Silber, J.R., Horner, P.J., & Rostomily, R.C. (2010). TWIST1 promotes invasion through mesenchymal change in human glioblastoma. *Molecular Cancer,* Vol.9: 194, ISSN 1476-4598

Morimura, T., Neuchrist, C., Kitz, K., Budka, H., Scheiner, O., Kraft, D., & Lassmann, H. (1990). Monocyte subpopulations in human gliomas: expression of Fc and complement receptors and correlation with tumor proliferation. *Acta Neuropathologica,* Vol.80, No.3, pp. 287-294, ISSN 0001-6322

Mou, K., Chen, M., Mao, Q., Wang, P., Ni, R., Xia, X., & Liu, Y. (2010). AQP-4 in peritumoral edematous tissue is correlated with the degree of glioma and with expression of VEGF and HIF-alpha. *Journal of Neuro-Oncology,* Vol.100, No.3, pp. 375-383, ISSN 0167-594X

Nakada, M., Nakada, S., Demuth, T., Tran, N.L., Hoelzinger, D.B., & Berens, M.E. (2007). Molecular targets of glioma invasion. *Cellular and Molecular Life Sciences,* Vol.64, No.4, pp. 458-478, ISSN 1420-682X

Nakamizo, A., Marini, F., Amano, T. & Khan, A. (2005). Human bone-marrow derived mesenchymal stem cells in the treatment of gliomas. *Cancer Research,* Vol.65, No.8, pp. 3307-3318, ISSN 0008-5472

Nakamura, K., Ito Y., Kawano, Y., Kurozumi, K., Kobune, M., Tsuda, H., Bizen, A., Honmou, O., Niitsu, Y. & Hamada, H. (2004). Antitumor effect of genetically engineered mesenchymal stem cells in a rat model. *Gene Therapy,* Vol.11, No.14, pp. 1155-1164, ISSN 0969-7128

Nelson, S.J. (2003). Multivoxel magnetic resonance spectroscopy of brain tumors. *Molecular Cancer Therapeutics,* Vol.2, No.5, pp. 497-507, ISSN 1535-7163

Nishio, S., Korosue, K., Tateishi, J., Fukui, M., & Kitamura, K. (1982). Ventricular and subarachnoid seeding of intracranial tumors of neuroectodermal origin--a study of 26 consecutive autopsy cases with reference to focal ependymal defect. *Clinical Neuropathology,* Vol.1, No.2, pp. 83-91, ISSN 0722-5091

Oh, M.C. & Lim, D.A. (2009). Novel treatment strategies for malignant gliomas using neural stem cells. *Neurotherapeutics,* Vol.6, No.3 pp. 458-463, ISSN 1933-7213

Okada, Y., Hurwitz, E.E., Esposito, J.M., Brower, M.A., Nutt, C.L., & Louis, D.N. (2003). Selection pressures of TP53 mutation and microenvironmental location influence epidermal growth factor receptor gene amplification in human glioblastomas. *Cancer Research,* Vol.63, No.2, pp. 413-416, ISSN 0008-5472

Oppitz, U., Maessen, D., Zunterer, H., Richter, S., & Flentje, M. (1999). 3D-recurrence-patterns of glioblastomas after CT-planned postoperative irradiation. *Radiotherapy and Oncology,* Vol.53, No.1, pp. 53-57, ISSN 0167-8140

Orosz, P., Echtenacher, B., Falk, W., Rüschoff, J., Weber, D., & Männel, D.N. (1993). Enhancement of experimental metastasis by tumor necrosis factor. *The Journal of Experimental Medicine,* Vol.177, No.5, pp. 1391-1398, ISSN 0022-1007

Pagenstecher, A., Wussler, E.M., Opdenakker, G., Volk, B. & Campbell, I.L. (2001). Distinct expression patterns and levels of enzymatic activity of matrix metalloproteinases and their inhibitors in primary brain tumors. *Journal of Neuropathology and Experimental Neurology,* Vol.60, No.6, pp. 598-612, ISSN 0022-3069

Perego, C., Vanoni, C., Massari, S., Raimondi, A., Pola, S., Cattaneo, M.G., Francolini, M., Vicentini, L.M., & Pietrini, G. (2002). Invasive behaviour of glioblastoma cell lines is associated with altered organisation of the cadherin-catenin adhesion system. *Journal of Cell Science,* Vol.115, No.Pt16, pp. 3331-3340, ISSN 0021-9533

Phillips, H.S., Kharbanda, S., Chen, R., Forrest, W.F., Soriano, R.H., Wu, T.D., Misra, A., Nigro, J.M., Colman, H., Soroceanu, L., Williams, P.M., Modrusan, Z., Feuerstein, B.G. & Aldape, K. (2006). Molecular subclasses of high-grade glioma predict prognosis, delineate a pattern of disease progression, and resemble stages in neurogenesis. *Cancer Cell,* Vol.9, No.3, pp. 157-173, ISSN 1535-6108

Pilkington, G.J. (1992). Glioma heterogeneity in vitro: the significance of growth factors and gangliosides. *Neuropathology and Applied Neurobiology,* Vol.18, No.5, pp. 434-442, ISSN 0305-1846

Pilkington, G.J. (1994). Tumour cell migration in the central nervous system. *Brain Pathology,* Vol.4, No.2, pp. 157-166, ISSN 1015-6305

Pirzkall, A., McKnight, T.R., Graves, E.E., Carol, M.P., Sneed, P.K., Wara, W.W., Nelson, S.J., Verhey, L.J., & Larson, D.A. (2001). MR-spectroscopy guided target delineation for high-grade gliomas. *International Journal of Radiation Oncology, Biology, Physics,* Vol.50, No.4, pp. 915-928, ISSN 0360-3016

Pirzkall, A., Nelson, S.J., McKnight, T.R., Takahashi, M.M., Li, X., Graves, E.E., Verhey, L.J., Wara, W.W., Larson, D.A., & Sneed, P.K. (2002). Metabolic imaging of low-grade gliomas with three-dimensional magnetic resonance spectroscopy. *International Journal of Radiation Oncology, Biology, Physics,* Vol.53, No.5, pp. 1254-1264, ISSN 0360-3016

Pirzkall, A., Li X., Oh, J., Chang, S., Berger, M.S., Larson, D.A., Verhey, L.J., Dillon, W.P., & Nelson, S.J. (2004). 3D MRSI for resected high-grade gliomas before RT: tumor extent according to metabolic activity in relation to MRI. *International Journal of Radiation Oncology, Biology, Physics,* Vol.59, No.1, pp. 126-137, ISSN 0360-3016

Pixley, S.K., & De Vellis, J. (1984). Transition between immature radial glia and mature astrocytes studied with a monoclonal antibody to vimentin. *Brain Research,* Vol.317, No.2, pp. 201-209, ISSN 0006-8993

Plopper, G.E., McNamee, H.P., Dike, L.E., Bojanowski, K., & Ingber, D.E. (1995). Convergence of integrin and growth factor receptor signaling pathways within the focal adhesion complex. *Molecular Biology of the Cell,* Vol.6, No.10, pp. 1349-1365, ISSN 1059-1524

Ramakrishna, R., Barber, J., Kennedy, G., Rizvi, A., Goodkin, R., Winn, R.H., Ojemann, G.A., Berger, M.S., Spence, A.M., & Rostomily, R.C. (2010). Imaging features of invasion and preoperative and postoperative tumor burden in previously untreated glioblastoma: Correlation with survival. *Surgical neurology international,* Vol.1, pii 40, ISSN 2152-7806

Rath, P., Shi, H., Maruniak, J.A., Litofsky, N.S., Maria, B.L. & Kirk, M.D. (2009). Stem cells as vectors to deliver HSV/tk gene therapy for malignant gliomas. *Current Stem Cell Research & Therapy,* Vol.4, No.1, pp. 44-49, ISSN 1574-888X

Roggendorf, W., Strupp, S., & Paulus, W. (1996). Distribution and characterization of microglia/macrophages in human brain tumors. *Acta Neuropathologica,* Vol. 92, No. 3, pp. 288-293, ISSN 0001-6322

Rosenblum, M.L. (1995). Factors influencing tumor cell traffic in the central nervous system. *Surgical Neurology,* Vol.43, No.6, p. 595, ISSN 0090-3019

Rutka, J.T., Muller, M., Hubbard, S.L., Forsdike, J., Dirks, P.B., Jung, S., Tsugu, A., Ivanchuk, S., Costello, P., Mondal, S., Ackerley, C., & Becker, L.E. (1999). Astrocytoma adhesion to extracellular matrix: functional significance of integrin and focal adhesion kinase expression. *Journal of Neuropathology and Experimental Neurology,* Vol.58, No.2, pp. 198-209, ISSN 0022-3069

Sahin Kaya, S., Mahmood, A., Li Y., Yavuz, E., & Chopp, M. (1999). Expression of nestin after traumatic brain injury in rat brain. *Brain Research,* Vol.84, No.1-2, pp.153-157, ISSN 0006-8993

Sato, H., Tamba, M., Ishii, T., & Bannai, S. (1999). Cloning and expression of a plasma membrane cystine/glutamate exchange transporter composed of two distinct proteins. *The Journal of Biological Chemistry,* Vol.274, No.17, pp. 11455-11458, ISSN 0021-9258

Schiffer, D., Giordana, M.T., Paoletti, P., Soffietti, R., & Tarenzi, L. (1980). Pathology of human malignant gliomas after radiation and chemotherapy. *Acta Neurochirurgica,* Vol.53, No.3-4, pp. 205-216, ISSN 0001-6268

Schiffer, D., Giordana, M.T., Soffietti, R., & Sciolla, R. (1982). Histological observations on the regrowth of malignant gliomas after radiotherapy and chemotherapy. *Acta Neuropathologica,* Vol.58, No.4, pp. 291-299, ISSN 0001-6322

Schiffer, D. (1986). Neuropathology and imaging: the ways in which gliomas spreads and varies in its histological aspects, In: *Biology of brain tumors,* M.D. Walker and D.G.T. Thomas, (Ed.), pp. 286-290, Nijhoff, Boston.

Schiffer, D., Giordana, M.T., Cavalla, P., Vigliani, M.C., & Attanasio, A. (1993). Immunohistochemistry of glial reaction after injury in the rat: double stainings and markers of cell proliferation. *International Journal of Developmental Neuroscience,* Vol.11, No.2, pp. 269-280, ISSN 0736-5748

Schiffer, D., Cavalla, P., Dutto, A., & Borsotti, L. (1997). Cell proliferation and invasion in malignant gliomas. *Anticancer Research,* Vol.17, No.1A, pp. 61-69, ISSN 0250-7005

Schiffer, D. (1997). *Brain Tumors. Biology, pathology and clinical references,* (2nd edn), Springer, Berlin-Heidelberg- New York.

Schiffer, D. (2006). *Brain tumor pathology: Current diagnostic hotspots and pitfalls,* Springer, ISBN 10 1-4020-3997-2, Dordrecht, The Netherlands.

Schiffer, D., Annovazzi, L., Caldera, V., & Mellai, M. (2010). On the origin and growth of gliomas. *Anticancer Research,* Vol.30, No.6, pp. 1977-1998, ISSN 0250-7005

Shah, A.C., Benos, D., Gillespie, G.Y. & Markert, JM. (2003).Oncolytic viruses: clinical applications as vectors for the treatment of malignant gliomas. *Journal of Neuro-Oncology,* Vol.65, No.3, pp. 203-226, ISSN 0167-594X

Shah, K., Bureau, E., Kim, D.E., Yang, K., Tang, Y., Weissleder, R. & Breakefield, X.O. (2005). Glioma therapy and real-time imaging of neural precursor cell migration and tumor regression. *Annals of Neurology,* Vol.57, No.1, pp. 34-41, ISSN 0364-5134

Sieg, D.J., Hauck, C.R., Ilic, D., Klingbeil, C.K., Schaefer, E., Damsky, C.H., & Schlaepfer, D.D. (2000). FAK integrates growth-factor and integrin signals to promote cell migration. *Nature Cell Biology,* Vol.2, No.5, pp. 249-256, ISSN 1465-7392

Small, R.K., Riddle, P., & Noble, M. (1987). Evidence for migration of oligodendrocyte--type-2 astrocyte progenitor cells into the developing rat optic nerve. *Nature,* Vol.328, No.6126, pp. 155-157, ISSN 0028-0836

Somasundaram, R., & Herlyn, D. (2009). Chemokines and the microenvironment in neuroectodermal tumor-host interaction. *Seminars in Cancer Biology,* Vol.19, No.2, pp. 92-96, ISSN 1044-579X

Sontheimer, H. (2003). Malignant gliomas: perverting glutamate and ion homeostasis for selective advantage. *Trends in Neurosciences,* Vol.26, No.10, pp. 543-549, ISSN 0166-2236

Stadlbauer, A., Nimsky, C., Buslei, R., Pinker, K., Gruber, S., Hammen, T., Buchfelder, M., & Ganslandt, O. (2007). Proton magnetic resonance spectroscopic imaging in the border zone of gliomas: correlation of metabolic and histological changes at low tumor infiltration--initial results. *Investigative Radiology,* Vol.42, No.4, pp. 218-223, ISSN 0020-9996

Staflin, K., Lindvall, M., Zuchner, T. & Lundberg, C. (2007). Instructive cross-talk between neural progenitor cells and gliomas. *Journal of Neuroscience Research,* Vol.85, No.10, pp. 2147-2159, ISSN 0360-4012

Stein, A.M., Demuth, T., Mobley, D., Berens, M., & Sander, L.M. (2007). A mathematical model of glioblastoma tumor spheroid invasion in a three-dimensional in vitro experiment. *Biophysical Journal,* Vol.92, No.1, pp. 356-365, ISSN 0006-3495

Straathof, C.S., van den Bent, M.J., Ma J., Schmitz, P.I., Kros, J.M., Stoter, G., Vecht, C.J., & Schellens, J.H. (1998). The effect of dexamethasone on the uptake of cisplatin in 9L glioma and the area of brain around tumor. *Journal of Neuro-Oncology,* Vol.37, No. 1, pp. 1-8, ISSN 0167-594X

Sutter, A., Hekmat, A., & Luckenbach, G.A. (1991). Antibody-mediated tumor cytotoxicity of microglia. *Pathobiology,* Vol.59, No.4, pp. 254-258, ISSN 1015-2008

Swanson, K.R., Bridge, C., Murray, J.D., & Alvord, E.C. Jr. (2003). Virtual and real brain tumors: using mathematical modeling to quantify glioma growth and invasion. *Journal of the Neurological Sciences,* Vol.216, No.1, pp. 1-10, ISSN 0022-510X

Tabatabai, G., Bähr, O., Möhle, R., Eyüpoglu, I.Y., Boehmler, A.M., Wischhusen, J., Rieger, J., Blümcke, I., Weller, M. & Wick, W. (2005). Lessons from the bone marrow how malignant glioma cells attract adult hematopoietic progenitor cells. *Brain,* Vol.128, No.Pt9, pp. 2200-2211, ISSN 0006-8950

Takamiya, Y., Kohsaka, S., Toya, S., Otani, M., & Tsukada, Y. (1988). Immunohistochemical studies on the proliferation of reactive astrocytes and the expression of cytoskeletal proteins following brain injury in rats. *Brain Research,* Vol.466, No.2, pp. 201-210, ISSN 0006-8993

Tamagno, I., & Schiffer, D. (2006). Nestin expression in reactive astrocytes of human pathology. *Journal of Neuro-Oncology,* Vol.80, No.3, pp. 227-233, ISSN 0167-594X

Tso, C.L., Shintaku, P., Chen, J., Liu, Q., Liu, J., Chen, Z., Yoshimoto, K., Mischel, P.S., Cloughesy, T.F., Liau, L.M. & Nelson, SF. (2006). Primary glioblastomas express mesenchymal stem-like properties. *Molecular Cancer Research,* Vol.4, No.9, pp. 607-619, ISSN 1541-7786

Tyler, M.A., Ulasov, I.V., Sonabend, A.M., Nandi, S., Han, Y., Marler, S., Roth, J. & Lesniak, M.S. (2009). Neural stem cells target intracranial glioma to deliver an oncolytic adenovirus in vivo. *Gene Therapy,* Vol.16, No.2, pp. 262-278, ISSN 0969-7128

Tysnes, B.B., Haugland, H.K., & Bjerkvig, R. (1997). Epidermal growth factor and laminin receptors contribute to migratory and invasive properties of gliomas. *Invasion and Metastasis,* Vol.17, No.5, pp. 270-280, ISSN 0251-1789

Tysnes, B.B., & Mahesparan, R. (2001). Biological mechanisms of glioma invasion and potential therapeutic targets. *Journal of Neuro-Oncology,* Vol.53, No.2, pp. 129-147, ISSN 0167-594X

Uhl, M., Weiler, M., Wick, W., Jacobs, A.H., Weller, M. & Herrlinger, U. (2005). Migratory neural stem cells for improved thymidine kinase-based gene therapy for malignant gliomas. *Biochemical and Biophysical Research Communications,* Vol.328, No.1, pp. 125-129, ISSN 0006-291X

Villeneuve, J., Tremblay, P., & Vallières, L. (2005). Tumor necrosis factor reduces brain tumor growth by enhancing macrophage recruitment and microcyst formation. *Cancer Research,* Vol.65, No.9, pp. 3928-3936, ISSN 0008-5472

Wallner, K.E., Galicich, J.H., Krol, G., Arbit, E., & Malkin, M.G. (1989). Patterns of failure following treatment for glioblastoma multiforme and anaplastic astrocytoma. *International Journal of Radiation Oncology, Biology, Physics,* Vol.16, No.6, pp. 1405-1409, ISSN 0360-3016

Walzlein, J.H., Synowitz, M., Engels, B., Markovic, D.S., Gabrusiewicz, K., Nikolaev, E., Yoshikawa, K., Kaminska, B., Kempermann, G., Uckert, W., Kaczmarek, L., Kettenmann, H. & Glass, R. (2008). The antitumorigenic response of neural precursors depends on subventricular proliferation and age. *Stem Cells,* Vol.26, No.11, pp. 2945-2954, ISSN 0250-6793

Wei, L.C., Shi, M., Chen, L.W., Cao, R., Zhang, P., & Chan, Y.S. (2002). Nestin-containing cells express glial fibrillary acidic protein in the proliferative regions of central nervous system of postnatal developing and adult mice. *Brain Research. Developmental Brain Research,* Vol.139, No.1, pp. 9-17, ISSN 0165-3806

Wildeboer, D., Naus, S., Amy Sang, Q.X., Bartsch, J.W., & Pagenstecher, A. (2006). Metalloproteinase disintegrins ADAM8 and ADAM19 are highly regulated in human primary brain tumors and their expression levels and activities are associated with invasiveness. *Journal of Neuropathology and Experimental Neurology,* Vol.65, No.5, pp. 516-527, ISSN 0022-3069

Xu, F. & Zhu, J.H. (2007). Stem cells tropism for malignant gliomas. *Neuroscience Bulletin,* Vol.23, No.6, pp. 363-369, ISSN 1673-7067

Ye, Z.C., Rothstein, J.D., & Sontheimer, H. (1999). Compromised glutamate transport in human glioma cells: reduction-mislocalization of sodium-dependent glutamate transporters and enhanced activity of cystine-glutamate exchange. *Journal of Neuroscience,* Vol. 19, No. 24, pp. 10767-10777, ISSN 0270-6474

Yi, L., Xiao, H., Xu, M., Ye, X., Hu, J., Li, F., Li, M., Luo, C., Yu, S., Bian, X., & Feng, H. (2011). Glioma-initiating cells: A predominant role in microglia/macrophages tropism to glioma. *Journal of Neuroimmunology,* Vol.232, No.1-2, pp. 75-82, ISSN 0165-5728

Yong, V.W., Power, C., Forsyth, P., & Edwards, D.R. (2001). Metalloproteinases in biology and pathology of the nervous system. *Nature reviews. Neuroscience,* Vol.2, No.7, pp. 502-511, ISSN 1471-003X

Zagzag, D., Friedlander, D.R., Miller, D.C., Dosik, J., Cangiarella, J., Kostianovsky, M., Cohen, H., Grumet, M., & Greco, M.A. (1995). Tenascin expression in astrocytomas correlates with angiogenesis. *Cancer Research,* Vol.55, No.4, pp. 907-914, ISSN 0008-5472

Zagzag, D., Salnikow, K., Chiriboga, L., Yee, H., Lan, L., Ali, M.A., Garcia, R., Demaria, S., & Newcomb, E.W. (2005). Downregulation of major histocompatibility complex antigens in invading glioma cells: stealth invasion of the brain. *Laboratory Investigation,* Vol.85, No.3, pp. 328-341, ISSN 0023-6837

Zeng, Q.S., Li, C.F., Zhang, K., Liu, H., Kang, X.S., & Zhen, J.H. (2007). Multivoxel 3D proton MR spectroscopy in the distinction of recurrent glioma from radiation injury. *Journal of Neuro-Oncology,* Vol.84, No.1, pp. 63-69, ISSN 0167-594X

Zhai, H., Heppner, F.L., & Tsirka, S.E. (2011). Microglia/macrophages promote glioma progression. *Glia,* Vol.59, No.3, pp. 472-485, ISSN 1098-1136

Zhao, D., Najbauer, J., Garcia, E., Metz, M.Z., Gutova, M., Glackin, C.A., Kim, S.U. & Aboody, K.S. (2008). Neural stem cell tropism to glioma: critical role of tumor hypoxia. *Molecular Cancer Research,* Vol.6, No.12, pp. 1819-1829, ISSN 1541-7786

Zhong, J., Paul, A., Kellie, S.J., & O'Neill, G.M. (2010). Mesenchymal migration as a therapeutic target in glioblastoma. *Journal of Oncology,* Vol.2010, 430142, ISSN 1687-8469

Part 6

Neurosurgery in CNS Tumors

Insular Tumours

Francesco Signorelli[1], Giuseppe Barbagallo[2], Rodolfo Maduri[1], Claudio Schonauer[3], Jacques Guyotat[4] and Kost Elisevich[5]
[1]*Dept. of Neurosurgery, University "Magna Græcia", Catanzaro*
[2]*Dept. of Neurosurgery, University of Catania*
[3]*Dept. of Neurosurgery, La Schiana Hospital, Napoli*
[4]*Dept. of Neurosurgery, Hôpital Neurologique et Neurochirurgical "P. Wertheimer", Lyon*
[5]*Dept. Of Neurosurgery, Henry Ford Hospital, Detroit,*
[1,2,3]*Italy*
[4]*France*
[5]*United States of America*

1. Introduction

Tumours affecting the insular structure and perisylvian opercula are frequently managed conservatively regardless of their nature and clinical evolution, even if impending infiltration of nearby eloquent areas will further promote dysfunction. Our experience and those of others [Duffau et al., 2005; Hentschel & Lang, 2005; Sanai et al., 2010; Lang et al., 2001; Signorelli et al., 2010] has demonstrated that wide surgical resection of these lesions is nonetheless feasible since tumour burden often displaces more than it incorporates eloquent sites [Duffau et al., 2009; Hentschel & Lang, 2005; Sanai et al., 2010; Signorelli et al., 2010] and other sites will often compensate for the lost function of infiltrated tissues. However, accurate anatomic and functional knowledge of the sylvian fissure and structures located nearby is essential to perform any surgical act in this area, in order to decrease the risk of postoperative permanent deficits. The aim of our chapter is to provide the reader with an updated review of insular anatomy and function, of clinical presentation and diagnosis of insular gliomas and point out technical details helpful in guiding surgery through this region.

2. Surgical anatomy and functions of the insula

The insula of Reil, composed of anterior and posterior lobules divided by a central sulcus, is an anatomically and functionally complex structure, situated at the bottom of the sylvian fissure and involved in complex anatomicofunctional relations. It is pyramid-shaped and its perimeter is defined by anterior, superior and inferior periinsular sulci. The limen insulae represents its medial threshold. It is a white matter structure extending from the anterior perforated substance to the insular pole along the sylvian stem and situated in parallel with the lateral olfactory stria [Türe et al., 1999]. Deep to the central portion of the insula, in a lateral-to-medial direction, lie the extreme capsule, claustrum, external capsule and putamen with its subjacent globus pallidus. Superiorly, at the level of the periinsular sulcus, is the corticospinal tract; anteroinferiorly, the uncinate fasciculus; and, posteriorly, along the same sulcus, the arcuate fasciculus. The blood supply of the insula is derived from the second (M2) segment of the middle cerebral artery (MCA) through its short and medium-sized perforating vessels. Long perforators overlying the posterior lobule are larger in diameter and may supply the corona radiata, particularly, the corticospinal and thalamocortical fibers [Hentschel & Lang, 2005]. Most of the lenticulostriate branches originate around the MCA bifurcation and arise in a nearly even distribution from before and after the bifurcation although the number arising from M1 increases commensurate with its length [Tanriover et al., 2004]. The mean distance from the insular apex to the lateralmost lenticulostriate artery, the length of M1 notwithstanding, is less than 1.5 cm [Tanriover et al., 2004]. The periinsular sulcus marks the transition from M2 to M3 whereas the convexity surface of the opercula demarcates the M4 segment of the MCA. As a paralimbic structure, the insula is located at the crossroad of allo- and neocortex. It is adjacent to perisylvian essential language areas, the primary auditory area, both the primary motor (PMA) and sensory (PSA) areas of the lower face in addition to their associated subcortical pathways. The insula subserves several functions including olfaction, taste, reciprocal visual-vestibular inhibition and the integration of sensory input with autonomic and emotional responses. It is, in fact, considered an accessory sensorimotor area, involved in motor planning and the planning and initiation of speech articulation [Naidich et al., 2004]. Sympathetic control of cardiovascular tone and pain perception suggest a further integrative role for the insula in association with proximate limbic structures. In fact, the insula is thought to be critically involved in the biobehavioural dysfunction characteristic of schizophrenia [Makris et al., 2006] and sleep regulation [Murphy et al., 2009].

3. Clinical presentation and diagnosis of insular gliomas

The clinical presentation of gliomas is somewhat associated with grade. Insular low grade gliomas (LGGs) present with epilepsy in 58% of cases with little or no neurological impairment [Duffau et al., 2005]. On the other hand, high grade gliomas (HGGs) frequently cause surrounding vasogenic edema with tissue infiltration, resulting in local and hemispheric mass effect and sensorimotor and/or language deficits. Moreover, neuropsychological assessment often reveals a cognitive decline, most likely ensuing from regional edema, seizures or the adverse effects of antiepileptic drugs (AEDs) [Klein et al., 2003; Meyers & Hess, 2002]. The semiology of insular epilepsy reflects the heterogeneity of the region's functional anatomy [Ryvlin et al., 2006]. It may mimic temporal lobe epilepsy [Barba et al., 2007; Isnard et al., 2004; Penfield & Faulk, 1955] or nocturnal hypermotor epilepsy of frontal lobe origin [Dobesberger et al., 2008; Ryvlin et al., 2006]. Other common ictal features are those of a simple partial epilepsy with respiratory, viscerosensitive or oroalimentary symptoms [Guénot & Isnard, 2008; Ostrowsky et al., 2000;]. Spread to the suprasylvian opercular cortex may produce facial paresthesia or laryngeal constriction, gustatory illusions and hypersalivation with postictal facial paresis [Isnard et al., 2004; Prats et al., 1999]. Infrasylvian opercular ictal spread, on the other hand, may produce auditory hallucinations or a sensory aphasia [Bancaud, 1987]. Further spread of activity over the central convexity gives rise to contralateral hemisensory or hemimotor manifestations.

Magnetic resonance imaging (MRI) with T2-weighted and Fluid-Attenuated Inversion Recovery (FLAIR) images best delineates the extent of tumour infiltration, which can be limited to the insular lobe (Yasargil type 3a) or reach the perisylvian opercula (type 3b) and other paralimbic areas, namely the orbitofrontal and temporopolar regions (type 5), with or without involvement of core limbic structures [Yasargil et al., 1992] (fig. 1). Functional MRI [Roux et al., 2008; Signorelli et al., 2003;), magnetoencephalography [Mäkelä et al., 2006] and positron emission tomography [Sobottka et al., 2002] help define the neighbouring cortical distribution of language, auditory, sensory and motor function. Moreover, diffusion tensor imaging (DTI) and, in particular, tractography helps delineate the major interconnecting tracts surrounding the insula [Makris et al., 2006]. Merging 3-D cortical and subcortical anatomical pictures with individual functional maps provides highly relevant information for surgical planning. Ultimately, such information is supplemented by intraoperative cortical and subcortical stimulation as the final measure to optimize tumour removal while preserving local function [Duffau et al., 2006; Signorelli et al., 2010].

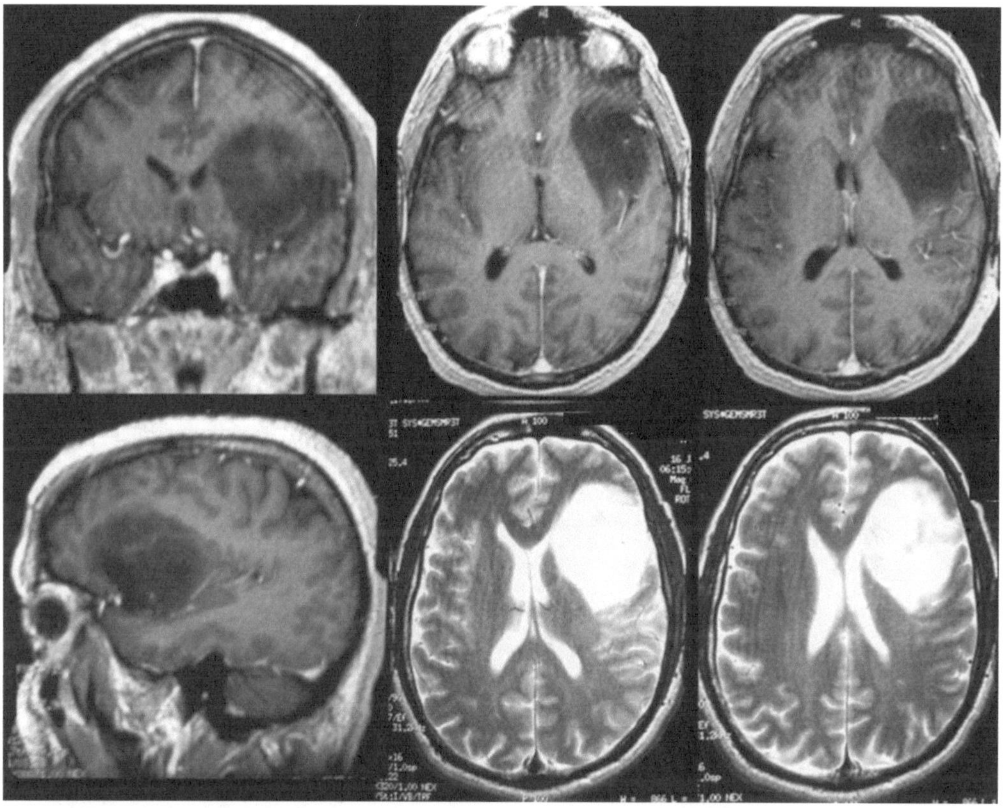

Fig. 1. Preoperative gadolinium enhanced T1- and T2-weighted MRI of a LGG infiltrating, left insular region, frontal and temporal operculum and fronto-orbital and temporopolar areas (5A of Yasargil classification). The tumour extends above the superior insular sulcus into the corona radiata.

4. Surgical procedure

Patients are positioned with a rest pad under the ipsilateral shoulder with the head turned 60° contralaterally, in order to allow the frontal and temporal lobes to separate when released so as to expose the sylvian fissure and avoid retraction. Moreover, this positioning provides a better orientation for the surgical perspective toward the posterior insular lobule, which is hidden by both the pre- and postcentral gyri [Hentschel & Lang, 2005]. We routinely apply cortico-subcortical electrical stimulation mapping (ESM) in order to locate and preserve eloquent sites and perform a tumour resection the limits of which are both anatomical and functional. An asleep-awake-asleep technique is used when operating on the dominant hemisphere. Neuronavigation is also useful for defining tumour boundaries and anatomic relationships with neural and vascular structures. The craniotomy is planned to include the whole perisylvian area from the pars orbitalis of the third frontal gyrus to the postcentral sulcus, the widest sulcus opening into the sylvian fissure and which, in general, delimits the posterosuperior corner of the insula (fig. 2).

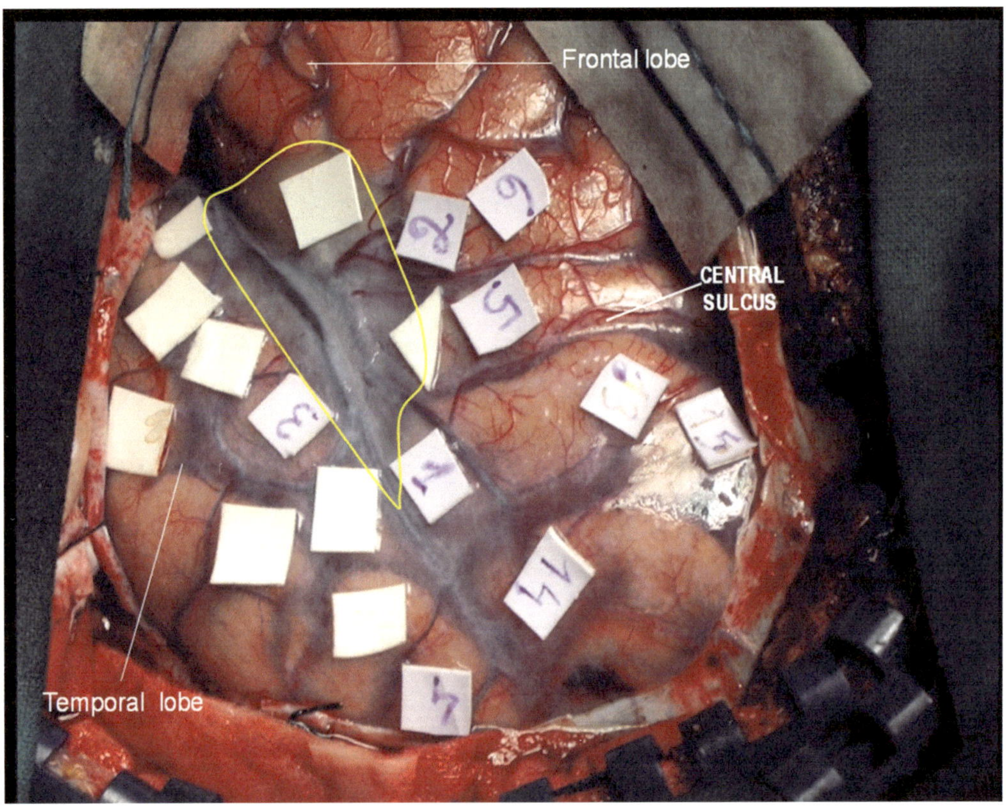

Fig. 2. Patient depicted in fig. 1. Craniotomy exposing widely the sylvian fissure, from pars orbitalis of F3 to the postcentral sulcus. Numbered tags indicate language sites (6, 2 speech arrest; 1, 3, 4 paraphasias; 13, 14, 15 anomia) and the primary motor area of the face (5).It is noteworthy that the functional sites are displaced at the periphery of the opercular tumoural infiltration (outlined in yellow).

Following ESM aimed at confirming the location of cortical language and sensorimotor areas, the superficial part of the lesion, which often infiltrates one or more of the frontal, parietal and temporal opercula, is removed so as to gain safe access into the depth of the sylvian fissure (fig. 3).

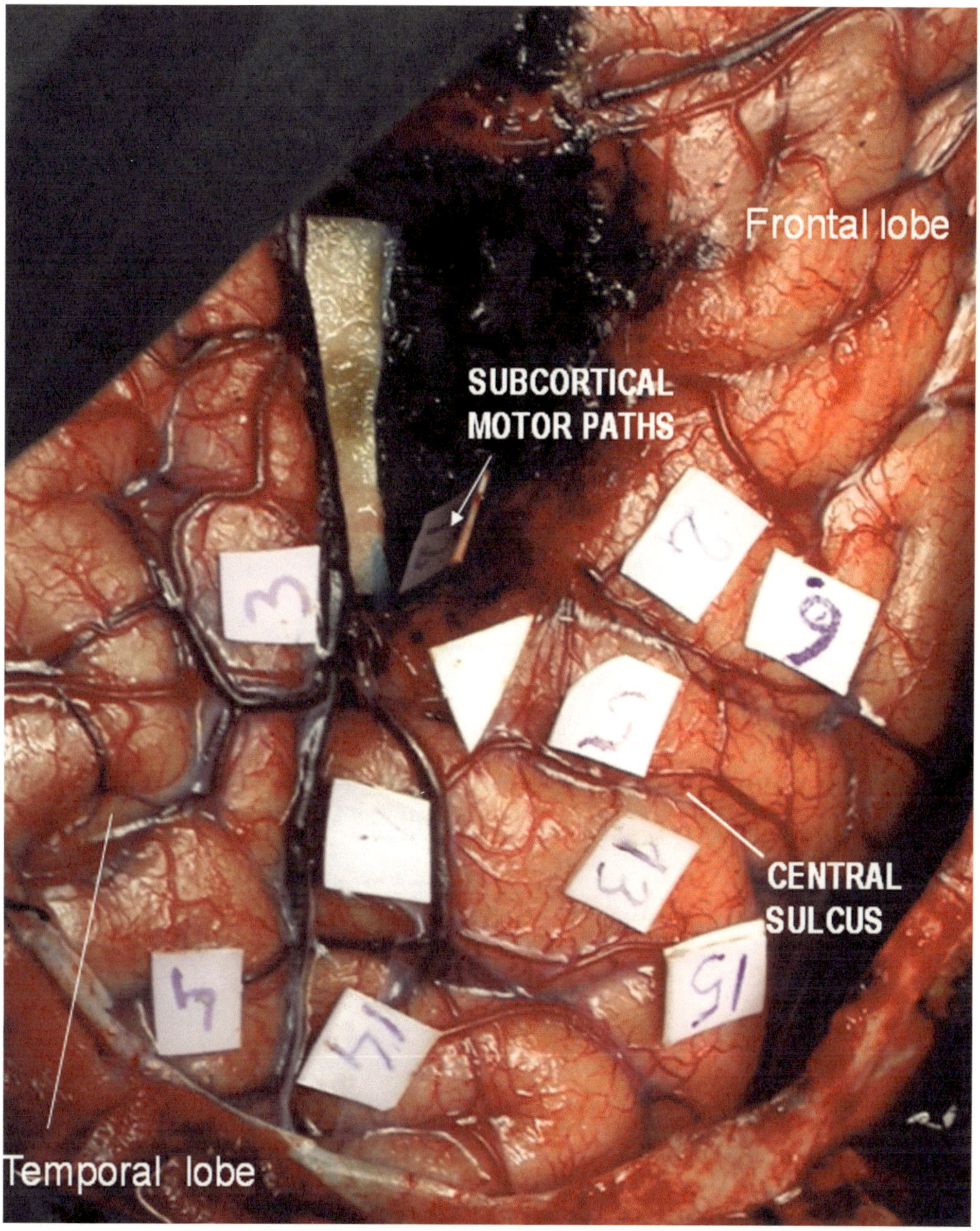

Fig. 3. After opercular resection, it is possible to reach the insular surface without retraction. Subcortical stimulation located motor pathwaysin the corona radiata, defining the posterior limit of tumoural resection in depth.

In most cases, the tumour displaces M2 branches centrifugally, indicating to the surgeon the site on the insular surface where the tumor is most proximate. Further use of ESM is required to search for possible language representation over the dominant insular cortex (fig. 4). The removal of insular gyri, when not harbouring language areas, is conducted medially to the putamen which is generally visible under the microscope as a gray, compact tissue that underlies a thin barrier of white matter [Yasargil et al., 1992]. Subcortical stimulation is used repeatedly beginning at a distance of two cm lateral to the posterior limb of the internal capsule, as measured by neuronavigational methods, in order to identify and preserve subcortical motor pathways. It is especially useful when extending tumour resection above the superior insular sulcus, where pyramidal fibers coursing through the corona radiata are found to be more superficial and where anatomic landmarks are lacking. Resection below the lenticular nucleus, at the level of the inferior limiting sulcus, may likewise interfere with sublenticular fibers of the posterior limb of the internal capsule. These are arranged in an anteroposterior direction to include the auditory and optic radiations [Rhoton, 2007]. Of utmost importance is the recognition of the vascular anatomy. Avulsion of the short branches of the MCA may injure the parent vessel with serious consequences. The long perforators, supplying the corona radiata, must be respected also to avoid ischemic injury of the white matter (Lang et al., 2001). In the area of the limen insulae, the lenticulostriate arteries originate commonly from the medial or superior aspect of the MCA, five mm or less around its bifurcation Their injury could lead to ischemic damage of the internal capsule. Electrical stimulation of the short and long gyri may result in speech arrest, particularly, in cases where a LGG has infiltrated the classic language area in the perisylvian opercula (fig. 4).

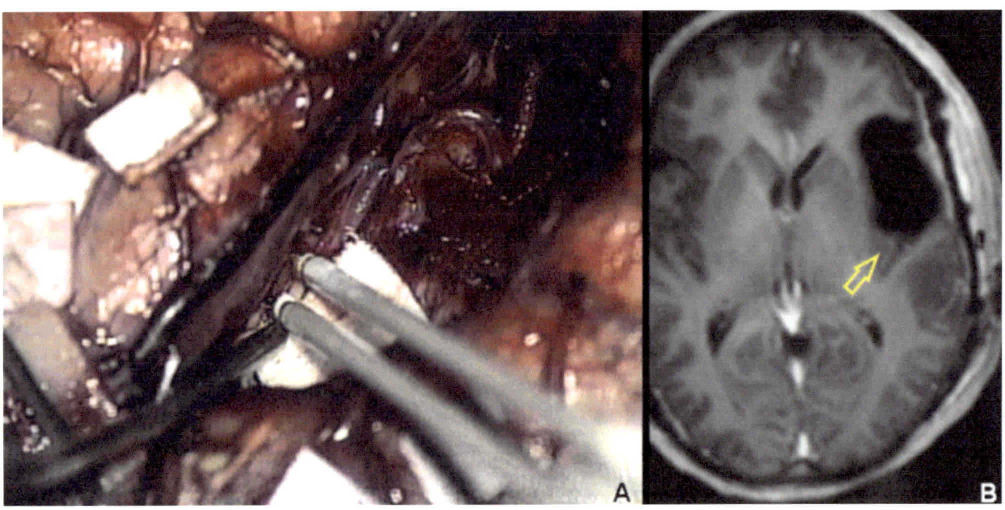

Fig. 4. A) The bipolar probe stimulates the cortical surface of posterior insular lobe. In this patient, patient, depicted in previous figures, insular cortical stimulation elicited speech arrest, which put a halt to tumoural resection. B) A postoperative (one month) T1-weighted Gd-enhanced MRI the tumoural residue is clearly seen at the level of the posterior insular lobe, where ESM elicited speech arrest (yellow arrow).

Seizures induced by ESM may be aborted by cooling the cortical surface with ice cold saline. The insular cortical areas where stimulation may evoke abdominal sensations or phenomena such as nausea, borborygmi, belching or chewing and/or tongue movements without speech arrest are not considered eloquent sites and may be removed when infiltrated by tumour. Stimulation of the uncinate fasciculus during removal of an infiltrated limen insulae is typically uneventful. On the other hand, stimulation of the white matter at the anterolateral border of the frontal horn of the left lateral ventricle will trigger speech arrest by depolarization of the subcallosal fasciculus and put a halt to resection (fig. 5). The posterosuperior limit of tumour resection is typically defined by identifying motor fibers in the corona radiata using ESM applied above the insular superior limiting sulcus (fig. 5). Most patients show immediate postoperative neurological aggravation which generally lasts no longer than one to two months emphasizing the proximity of eloquent structures.

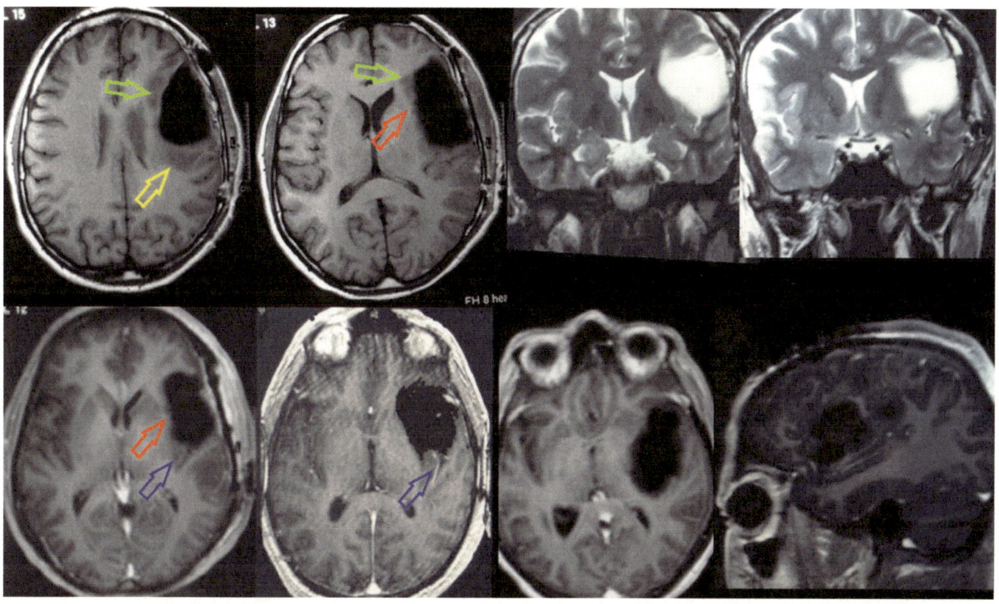

Fig. 5. One month Postoperative (one month) T1-weighted Gd-enhanced and T2-weighted MRI of the same patient previously illustrated, showing a subtotal tumour removal. Tumour remains at the level of the subcallosal fasciculus (green arrow), where stimulation elicited speech arrest with preserved repetition, at the level of the inferior occipitofrontal fasciculus (IOF, red arrow) in the anterior portion of capsula extrema, where stimulation elicited semantic paraphasias, into the corona radiata where subcortical motor pathways run (yellow arrow) and at the posterior insular lobe, where stimulation triggered speech arrest and dysarthria (blue arrow).

5. Discussion

Several well-designed controlled studies indicate that the degree of surgical resection of brain gliomas affects survival and the quality of life of patients [Pignatti et al., 2002; Stupp et al., 2005]. Significant cytoreduction is effective not just in reducing the mass effect of the lesion but it is more likely to remove the contingent of neoplastic cells that may manifest more aggressive behaviour through proliferation and invasiveness [Sanai et al., 2010]. Aggressive tumour removal is also more likely to mitigate a lesion-associated epilepsy [Sanai et al., 2010]. A significant percentage of LGGs, up to 25% in one series [Duffau & Capelle, 2004], invade the insula, raising doubt regarding their resectability. Surgical pursuit of such tumours is recommended to forestall clinical impairment, improve survival and lengthen the recurrence-free period [Duffau et al., 2009; Sanai et al., 2010]. Since the first report by Yasargil (Yasargil et al., 1992), few authors have dealt with the surgical treatment of tumours infiltrating the insula [Duffau et al., 2005; Hentschel & Lang, 2005; Lang et al., 2001; Sanai et al., 2010; Zentner et al., 1996]. A number of authors have emphasized the importance of functional mapping because of the eloquent nature of both insular and periinsular structures [Signorelli et al., 2003; Sobottka et al., 2002]. The use of sensory and/or motor evoked potentials [Zentner et al., 1996] or ESM [Duffau et al., 2005, 2006, 2009; Sanai et al., 2010; Signorelli et al., 2010] provide additional intraoperative landmarks by which to safely resect insular masses. Dominant hemisphere cortical language localization is advisable although language interference from direct stimulation of the insular cortex has seldom been reported [Duffau et al., 2005; Hentschel & Lang, 2005]. In our experience, insular tumours infiltrating the opercular region of the dominant hemisphere are responsible for functional reshaping of language areas with relocation onto the insular cortex. The insula is a secondary functional area that has the potential to take charge of lost function brought about by tumour infiltration of primary eloquent sites. Patients may present without a phasic deficit in language in such circumstances. Thus, testing language function in such patients harboring a dominant-sided insular LGG may reduce the risk of postoperative permanent impairment, which comes about in 14% of subjects when no language mapping is performed [Zentner et al., 1996].

6. Conclusion

Insular gliomas represent a surgical challenge because of the diverse functional importance of the insula and surrounding brain. Its accessibility within the convoluted perisylvian structure adds to this challenge. Newly acquired knowledge of structural and dynamic functional organization of the insula provide the surgeon the opportunity to plan and execute effective surgical resection of gliomas, once deemed inoperable, with acceptable risk. It follows that optimization of tumour removal coupled with an ultimate return of function improves the quality of life and survival.

7. References

Bancaud, J. (n.d.). Clinical symptomatology of epileptic seizures of temporal origin. *Revue neurologique*, Vol.43, No.5, (n.d. 1987), pp.392-400, ISSN 0035-3787

Barba, C.; Barbati, G.; Minotti, L.; Hoffman, D. & Kahane, P. (2006). Ictal clinical and scalp-EEG findings differentiating temporal lobe epilepsies from temporal 'plus' epilepsies. *Brain*, Vol.130, No.7, (May 2007), pp.1957-1967, ISSN 1460-2156

Dobesberger, J.; Ortler, M.; Unterberger, I.; Walser, G.; Falkenstetter, T.; Bodner, T.; Benke, T.; Bale, R.; Fiegele, T.; Donnemiller, E.; Gotwald, T. & Trinka E. (2007). Successful surgical treatment ofinsular epilepsy with nocturnal hypermotor seizures. *Epilepsia*, Vol.49, No.1, (October 2008), pp.159-162, ISSN 1528-1167

Duffau, H. & Capelle, L. (2004). Preferential brain locations of low-grade gliomas. *Cancer*, Vol.100, No.12, (April 2004), pp.2622-2626, ISSN 1097-0142

Duffau, H.; Taillandier, L.; Gatignol, P. & Capelle, L. (2005). The insular lobe and brain plasticity: Lessons from tumor surgery. *Clinical Neurology and Neurosurgery*, Vol.108, No.6, (September 2005), pp.543-548, ISSN 0303-8467

Duffau, H,; Moritz-Gasser, S. & Gatignol, P. (2009). Functional outcome after language mapping for insular for World Health Organization Grade II gliomas in the dominant hemisphere with 24 patients. *Neurosurgical Focus*, Vol.27, No.2, (August 2009), pp. 1-10, ISSN 1092-0684

Guénot, M. & Isnard, J. (2008). Epilepsy and insula. *Neurochirurgie*, Vol.54, No.3, (May 2008), pp.374-381, ISSN 0028-3770

Hentschel, SJ. & Lang, FF. (2005). Surgical resection of intrinsic insular tumors. *Neurosurgery*, Vol.57, No.1, (July 2005), pp.176-183, ISSN 1524-4040

Isnard, J.; Guénot, M.; Sindou, M. & Mauguière, F. (2004). Clinical manifestations of insular lobe seizures: a stereo-electroencephalographic study. *Epilepsia*, Vol.45, No.9, (April 2004), pp.1079-1090, ISSN 1528-1167

Klein, M.; Engelberts, NH.; van der Ploeg, HM.; Kasteleijn-Nolst Trenité, DG.; Aaronson, NK.; Taphoorn, MJ.; Baaijen, H.; Vandertop, WP.; Muller, M.; Postma, TJ. & Heimans, JJ. (n.d.). Epilepsy in low-grade gliomas: the impact on cognitive function and quality of life. *Annals of Neurology*, Vol.54, No.4, (September 2003), pp.514-520, ISSN 0364-5134

Lang, FF.; Olansen, NE.; DeMonte, F.; Gokaslan, ZL; Holland, EC.; Kalhorn, C. & Sawaya R. (2000). Surgical resection of intrinsic insular tumors: Complication avoidance. *Journal of Neurosurgery*, Vol.95, No.4, (October 2001), pp.638-650, ISSN 0022-3085

Mäkelä, JP.; Forss, N.; Jääskeläinen, J.; Kirveskari, E.; Korvenoja, A. & Paetau, R. (2005). Magnetoencefalography in neurosurgery. *Neurosurgery*, Vol.59, No.3, (June 2006), pp.493-510, ISSN 0022-3085

Makris, N.; Goldstein, J.; Kennedy, D.; Hodge, S.; Caviness, V.; Faraone, S.; Tsuang, M.& Seidman, L. (2005). Decreased volume of left and total anterior insular lobule in schizophrenia. *Schizophrenia Research*, Vol.83, No.2, (June 2006), pp.155-171, ISSN 0920-9964

Meyers, C. & Hess, KR. (2003). Multifaceted endpoints in brain tumor clinical trials: cognitive deterioration precedes MRI progression. (2002). *Neuro-oncology*, Vol.5, No.2, (December 2002), pp.89-95, ISSN 1523-5866

Murphy, M.; Riedner, BA.; Huber, R.; Massimini, M.; Ferrarelli, F; & Tononi, G. Source modelling sleep slow waves. (2008). *Proceedings of the national academy of sciences of the United States of America*, Vol.106, No.5, pp.1608-1613, ISSN 0027-8424

Naidich, TP.; Kang, E.; Fatterpekar, GM.; Delman, BN.; Gultekin, SH.; Wolfe, D.; Ortiz, O.; Yousry, I.; Weisman, M. & Yousry, TA. (2003). The insula: anatomic study and MR imaging display at 1.5T. *American Journal of Neuroradiology*, Vol.25, No.2, (February 2004), pp.222-232, ISSN 0195-6108

Ostrowsky, K.; Isnard, J.; Ryvlin, P.; Guénot, M.; Fischer, C. & Mauguière, F. (2000). Functional mapping of the insular cortex: clinical implication in temporal lobe epilepsy. *Epilepsia*, Vol.41, No.6, (June 2000), pp.681-686, ISSN 0013-9580

Penfield, W. & Faulk, ME Jr. (1955). The insula: further observations on its function. *Brain*, Vol.78, No.4 , (n.d.), pp.445-470, ISSN 0006-8950

Pignatti, F.; van den Bent, M.; Curran, D.; Debruyne, C.; Sylvester, R.; Therasse, P.; Afra, D.; Cornu, P.; Bolla, M.; Vecht, C. & Karim, AB. (2001). Prognostic factors for survival in adult patients with cerebral low-grade glioma. *Journal of Clinical Oncology*, Vol.20, No.8, (April 2002), pp.2076-2084, ISSN 1527-7755

Prats, JM.; Garaizar, C.; Garcia-Nieto ML & Madoz, P. (1999). Opercular epileptic syndrome: an unusual form of benign partial epilepsy in childhood. *Revista de Neurología,* Vol.29, No.4, (August 1999), p. 375-380. ISSN: 0210-0010

Rhoton, A.L. Jr. The cerebrum. Anatomy. (2002). *Neurosurgery,* Vol.61, No.1, (July 2007), pp.37-118, ISSN 0022-3085

Roux, FE.; Boukhatem, L.; Draper, L.; Sacko, O. & Démonet, J.F. (2008). Cortical calculation localization using electrostimulation. *Journal of neurosurgery,* (December 2008), Vol.110, No.6, pp.1291-1299, ISSN 0022-3085

Ryvlin, P.; Minotti, L.; Demarquay, G.; Hirsch, E.; Arzimanoglou, A.; Hoffman, D.; Guénot, M.; Picard, F.; Rheims, S. & Kahane, P. (2005). Nocturnal hypermotor seizures, suggesting frontal lobe epilepsy, can originate in the insula. *Epilepsia,* (April 2006), Vol.47, No.4, pp.755-765, ISSN 0013-9580

Sanai, N.; Polley, M.Y. & Berger, M.S. (2009). Insular glioma resection: assessment of patient morbidity, survival, and tumor progression. *Journal of neurosurgery,* (January 2010), Vol.112, No.1, pp.1-9, ISSN 0022-3085

Signorelli, F.; Guyotat, J.; Schneider, F.; Isnard, J. & Bret PH. (2010). Technical refinements for validating functional MRI-based neuronavigation data by electrical stimulation during cortical language mapping. *Minimally Invasive Neurosurgery,* Vol.46, No. , (October 2003), pp.265-268, ISSN 0946-7211

Signorelli, F.; Guyotat, J; Elisevich, K. & Barbagallo, GM. (2009). Review of current microsurgical management of insular gliomas. *Acta Neurochirurgica,* Vol.152, No.1, (January 2010), pp.19-26, ISSN 0942-0940

Sobottka, SB.; Bredow, J.; Beutgien-Baumann, B.; Reiss, G.; Schackert, G. & Steinmeier, R. Comparison of functional brain PET images and intraoperative brain mapping data using image-guided surgery. (2001). *Computer Aided Surgery,* Vol.7, No.6, (April 2002), pp. 317-325, ISSN 1092-9088

Tanriover, N.; Rhoton, A.L. Jr.; Kawashima, M.; Ulm, AJ. & Yasuda, A. (2004). Microsurgical anatomy of the insula and the sylvian fissure. *Journal of Neurosurgery,* Vol.100, No.5, (May 2004), pp.891-922, ISSN 0022-3085

Türe, U.; Yaşargil, MG; Al-Mefty, O. & Yasargil, DCH. (n.d.) Arteries of the insula. *Journal of Neurosurgery,* (April 2000), Vol.92, No.4, pp.676-687, ISSN 0022-3085

Yasargil, MG.; von Ammon, K.; Cavazos, E.; Doczi, T.; Reeves, JD. & Roth, P. (1992). Tumors of the limbic and paralimbic systems. *Acta Neurochirurgica,* Vol.116, No.2-4, (March 1992), pp.147-149, ISSN 0001-6268

Zentner, J.; Meyer, B.; Stangl, A. & Schramm, J. (1996). Intrinsic tumors of the insula: a prospective surgical study of 30 patients. *Journal of Neurosurgery,* Vol.85, No.2, (August 1996), pp.263-271, ISSN 0022-3085

Part 7

Radiation Therapy in CNS Tumors

10

Regional Chemotherapy and Brachytherapy for Malignant Glioma – Clinical Experience and Serial Experiments

Li Anmin, Fu Xiangping, Zhao Ming, Zhang Zhiwen,
Yi Linhua, Xue Jinghui and Zhang Yipeng
Department of Neurosurgery, First Affiliated Hospital of Chinese PLA General Hospital, China

1. Introduction

Malignant glioma (MG) is the most common type of malignant tumors derived from neuroepithelial tissue, and accounts for 46% of brain tumors. It has an incidence of 30-100/million and ranks third in adult mortality and second in child mortality in all cancer patients. Compared with malignant tumors from other tissues and organs, MG has much lower treatment success rates. Despite global efforts over the past thirty years, there has been no major breakthrough in treatment and patient survival has not significantly improved. The median survival time after diagnosis is eight months in patients receiving surgery alone and 11 months in patients receiving surgery plus adjuvant radiotherapy/chemotherapy. Conventional treatments for MG include surgical resection, adjuvant whole brain radiotherapy (WBRT), and systemic chemotherapy. Limitations of these treatments include:

1. Surgical resection: MG is highly invasive. As a result, total resection is typically not achieved in surgery. The operation may also activate residual tumor cells from the G0 phase to the proliferation phase, resulting in tumor recurrence of malignancy.
2. Post-operative WBRT. The effective dose for MG (73-80 Gy) is higher than the maximum tolerated dose for brain tissue (60 Gy). The therapeutic effects at a dose of 60 Gy are mediated primarily by radioactive ions that stimulate endotheliocytosis in the microvascular bed of the tumor. The endotheliocytosis results in embolism and decreased blood supply to tumor.
3. Post-operative chemotherapy. Upon systemic treatment, only ~20% of chemotherapeutic agents reach the brain. The blood brain barrier (BBB) around the post-operative tumor cavity also prevents the chemotherapeutic agents from reaching the site of action.

The weak immunogenicity of the glioma membrane and the heterogeneity of the cells have limited the application of immunotherapy. The unique biological properties and lack of effective clinical treatment creates a challenge for clinical practice and basic experimental research [1,2].

The growth of MG tends to be localized. Such a feature may represent an opportunity to develop novel treatment for MG [3]. Specifically, we propose that localized tumor should be treated with regional therapy.

Over 18 years of clinical research (Apr 1991 to Dec 2008), the authors developed new regional treatments. These new treatments incorporated three therapeutic concepts: emphasizing the "first strike" to the tumor, maintaining a high quality of life for the patients, and devising individual treatment plans for patients.

Clinical research provided satisfactory and promising outcomes for regional therapy. In addition, in vivo and in vitro experimental results showed that the implementation of regional treatment methods could control residual tumor growth and invasive behaviors. Data accumulated with 10-year follow-up in 379 patients confirmed that the new regional treatments improved the survival as well as the quality of life in patients with MG.

2. New regional therapies for MG

The authors introduced the idea that localized tumors should be treated with regional therapy and developed seven new methods for such regional therapy. With these new methods, we achieved 16.6% 3-year survival rate in MG patients. Strikingly, the tumor disappeared in 6.3% of the cases. The seven new methods can be classified as regional chemotherapy or brachytherapy.

i. Regional chemotherapy

1. Intra-tumoral interstitial chemotherapy
2. Selective/super-selective interventional chemotherapy via the cerebral artery
3. High-dose chemotherapy supported by autologous stem cells

ii. Brachytherapy

1. Intra-tumoral brachytherapy
2. Immunologically targeted radiotherapy via ^{131}I labeled McAb
3. Tumor interstitial brachytherapy
4. Brachytherapy for MG located in the brain stem or spinal cord

3. Intra-tumoral interstitial chemotherapy

Regional chemotherapy was explored for decades in the world [4-7]. In 1991, the authors used a patented chemotherapy reservoir (Li Anmin I reservoir, Fig.1-A) for postoperative intra-tumor interstitial chemotherapy. From Jan 2001 to Dec 2008, 151 of 379 patients received this chemotherapy.

3.1 Methods

After MG resection, the chemotherapy reservoir was implanted into the residual tumor cavity (Fig.1-B). Chemotherapeutic agents were injected into the extracranial capsule and then into the residual tumor cavity via the reservoir tube. The chemotherapeutic agents used for this treatment (BCNU, VM, and ACNU) have low molecular weight, and could permeate the residual tumor cavity wall and tumor cell membrane. Doses for these agents were 25 mg for BCNU, 50 mg for VM26, and 25-50 mg for ACNU. The injection began at 7 d after the operation and continued daily for 4 d. When tumor growth was under control (Fig. 2), the interval between the injections was increased to 30-40 d. The entire treatment lasted for 2 yr.

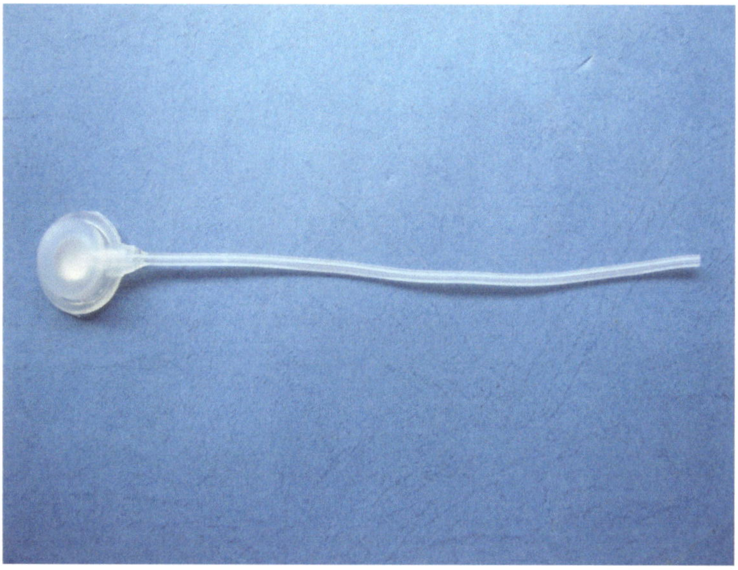

Fig. 1-A. Photo of Chemotherapeutic Reservoir (Li Anmin Type I Reservoir)

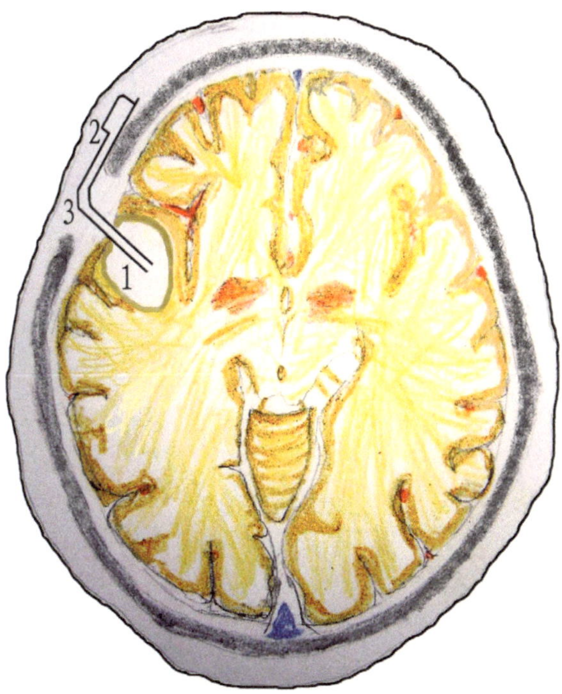

Fig. 1-B. The sketch of interstitially intratumoral chemotherapy postoperatively:
1. Residual tumor cavity, 2. Valve of the reservoir, 3. Tube of the reservoir

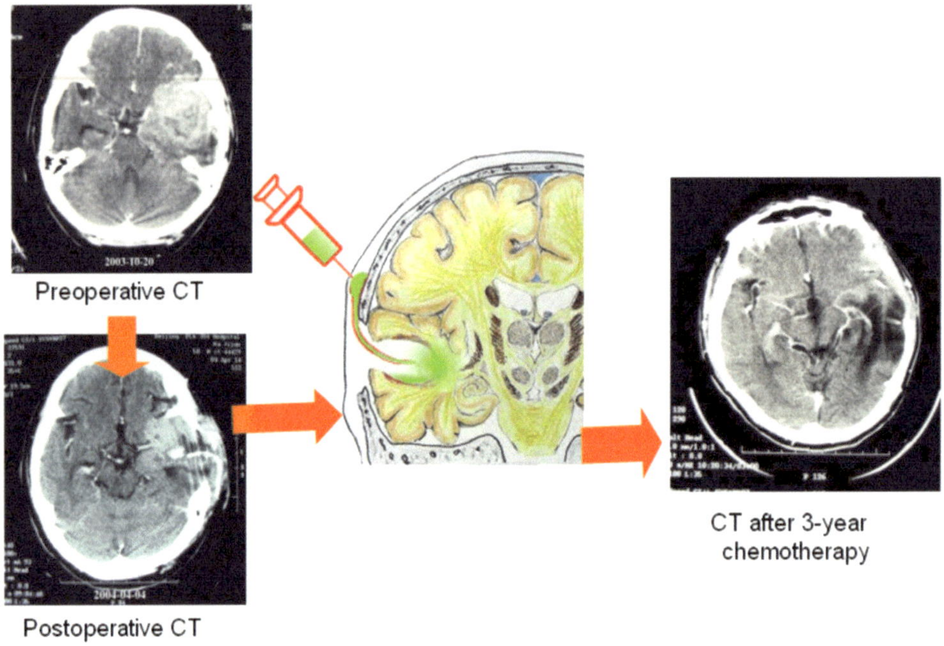

Fig. 2. The sketch of interstitially intratumoral chemotherapy

3.2 Side effects

There was no general toxicity during or after drug injection. Headache (typically tolerable was observed in some patients receiving VM26 or BCNU. Seizure developed in 2.7% of the patients receiving VM26 or BCNU. ACNU did not cause discomfort in any patient (Table 1).

The Li Anmin I reservoir has several advantages over Ommaya reservoir. First, the extracranial capsule of the new reservoir has a steel or titanium basement plate, which prevents it from being pierced during the drug injection. Second, the tube of the new reservoir extends from the side of the external capsule rather than from the bottom as in the Ommaya reservoir[8,9]. This new configuration facilitates fixation and reduces the capsule volume.

Overall, hawse has achieved positive therapeutic outcomes with tolerable adverse effects with this method. As a result, it is now widely adopted in China.

	BCNU	VM26	ACNU
Inhibitive efficiency	++	+	+++
Effective radius	cm	>3 cm	<3 cm
Necrosis feature	Coagulation necrosis	Liquefaction necrosis	Coagulation necrosis
Local effect	++	+++	++
Toxicity	++	+++	+

Table 1. Three chemotherapeutic agents used in intra-tumoral interstitial chemotherapy.

4. Selective/super-selective interventional chemotherapy via the cerebral artery

In early 1990s in China, interventional therapy via the cerebral artery was primarily a tool for the diagnosis and treatment of cerebrovascular diseases. In 1993, the authors presented the first use of interventional chemotherapy via cerebral artery for the treatment of MG.0

4.1 Methods

There are three major methods currently used by the authors in the cerebral interventional chemotherapy (Fig. 3): intervention by common carotid artery, intervention by femoral-internal carotid (supraclinoid)/vertebrobasilar artery (selective chemotherapy), and intervention by femoral-tumor feeding artery (super-selective chemotherapy).

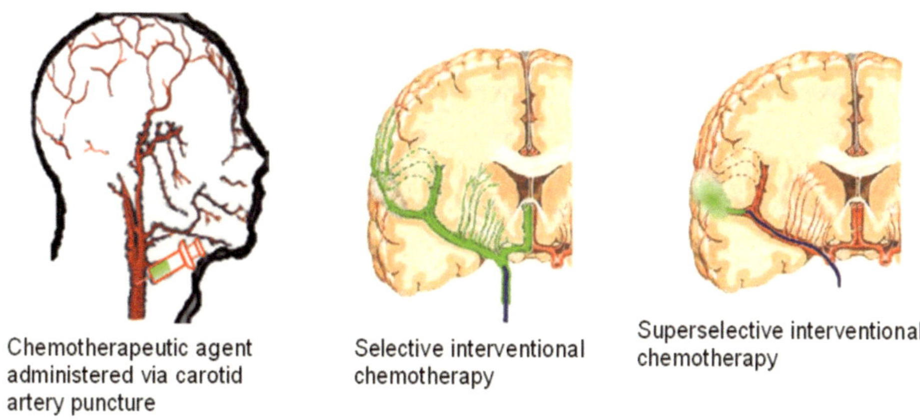

Fig. 3. The sketch of interventional chemotherapy via cerebral artery

4.2 Side effects

From Apr 1991 to Dec 2008, 677 patients received this therapy, and 4916 operations were performed. The side effects for interventional chemotherapy included three cases of vision reduction, perhaps due to embolism of retinal arteriole by chemotherapeutic micro-lipoparticles, one case of hemiplegia caused by breaking off of the plaque in the bifurcation and embolized of ICA during the punctuation of CCA. Leucopenia and thrombocytopenia developed in 92 cases (24.4%), but recovered within four weeks of withdrawal in most cases. In seven cases, white blood cell count was too low to continue the chemotherapy. Spontaneous hemorrhagic tendency (the thrombocytopenia after chemotherapy had no effective treatment to promote the recovery of bone marrow function) occurred in two cases. Myelofibrosis was observed in one case.

Cerebral artery interventional chemotherapy significantly reduced the adverse effects of chemotherapeutic agents and elevated the intratumoral local drug concentration by more than 15-fold (Fig. 4). From 2001 to 2008, 283 of 379 cases were treated with interventional chemotherapy, and 158 cases (56.0%) had favorable outcomes. This method has been adopted widely (Fig. 5).

Typical case:

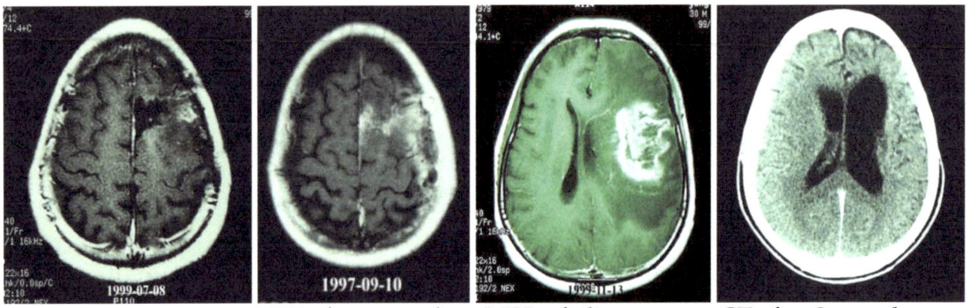

MRI after first surgery | MRI after second surgery | MRI of glioma recurrence | CT after 8-month chemotherapy

Fig. 5. The male patient was 30 years old with recurrent glioblastoma multiform, treated with interventional chemotherapy

5. High dose chemotherapy supported by Autologous Peripheral Blood Bone Marrow Stem Cell (APBBMSC)

Based on the dose-effect curve of chemotherapeutic agents, the authors used high-dose chemotherapy (twice the normal dose) to treat MG. In 2003, we introduced APBBMSC-supported high-dose chemotherapy for MG. Beginning at five days before chemotherapy, 300 μg of granulocyte colony stimulating factor (G-CSF) was injected daily to stimulate APBBMSCs. The APBBMSCs were isolated from peripheral blood and concentrated in a 60 mL suspension. The cell concentration was adjusted to 1.0×10^9 cells/mL with Tc-199 cell culture solution blended with buffer solution (60% Tc-199, 20% dimethyl sulfoxide, 20% autologous plasma). APBBMSC was stored in liquid nitrogen. After the high-dose chemotherapy, frozen APBBMSCs were thawed rapidly at 4ºC and administered intravenously at 48-72 h post-chemotherapy (Fig. 6).

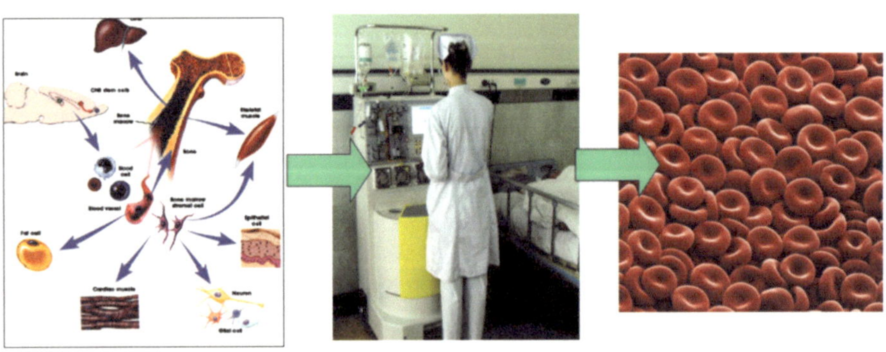

To activate bone marrow hemopoietic stem cells into peripheral circulation | The hemopoietic stem cells were collected and condensed. | The bone marrow stem cells were infused intravenously.

Fig. 6. The procedure of chemotherapy supported by autotransplantation of peripheral blood bone marrow stem cells.

Following this treatment, the WBC count decreased for 3-7 d, reaching the lowest values at 5-10 d, and increased to >1.0 × 10^9 cells/L in 6-10 d. The PLT levels typically returned to >50.0 × 10^9/L in 12-15 d. In the 74 patients receiving only conventional chemotherapy, WBC count reduced to <1.0 × 10^9/L and PLT levels reduced to <20.0 × 10^9/L. The low levels remained for 16-31 days before returning to normal.
In this series, the overall effective rate was 55.6% (total number of patients: 27; 2 CR cases, 13 PR cases, 10 MR cases, 1 NC case, and 1 PD case; Fig. 7).

Typical case:

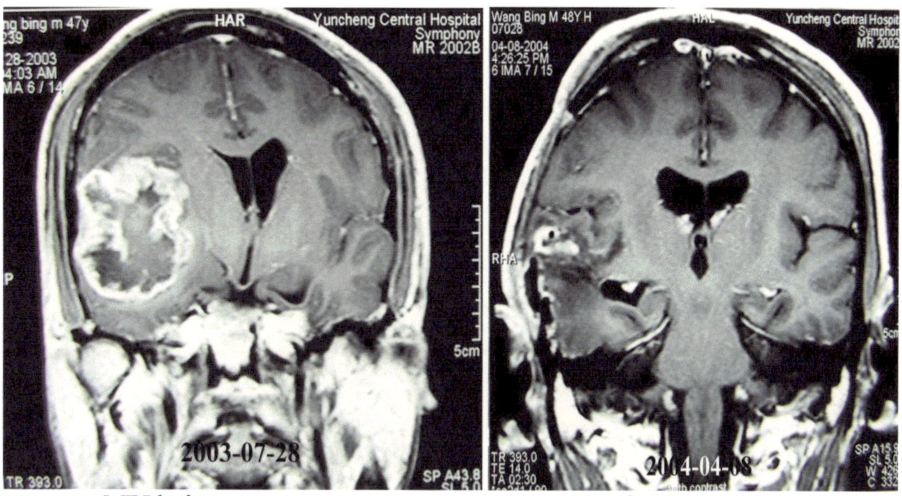

MRI before treatment MRI after 21-month treatment

Fig. 7. The male patient was 49 years old with recurrent GBM, treated with chemotherapy supported by autotransplantation of peripheral blood bone marrow stem cells, superselectively intervetional chemotherapy and targeted immunoradiotherapy with monoclonal antibody labelled ^{131}I.

This study indicated that APBBMSC-supported high-dose chemotherapy offers the advantage of rapid recovery of bone marrow after high-dose chemotherapy. Compared with bone marrow transplants following chemotherapy, APBBMSC-supported high-dose chemotherapy is easy to perform and could achieve rapid recovery of hematopoietic function with limited side effects [10].

6. Intra-tumoral brachytherapy

In 1993, the authors developed a radiotherapy reservoir (Li Anmin II reservoir, Fig. 8-A) to perform postoperative intra-tumoral brachytherapy for MG. This treatment was used in 172 of the 379 patients.

6.1 Methods

After surgical removal of the tumor, a brachytherapy reservoir was implanted into the residual tumor cavity, and the valve of the reservoir was embedded subcutaneously (Fig. 8-B). Radioactive isotopes (^{125}I or ^{131}I) were injected through the reservoir valve into the reservoir. The reservoir formed an oval-shaped radioactive envelope (Fig. 9), and produced localized, long-term, high-dosage irradiation to the residual cavity and the surrounding region for two half lives (^{125}I $t_{1/2}$=120 days and ^{131}I $t_{1/2}$=16 days).

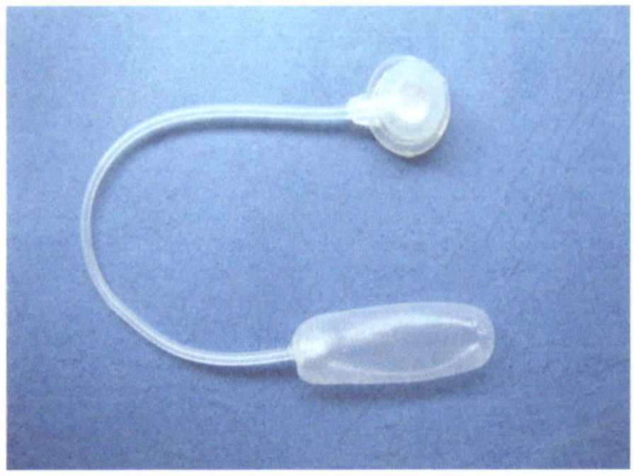

Fig. 8-A. Photo of Radiotherapeutic Reservoir (LiAnmin Type II reservoir)

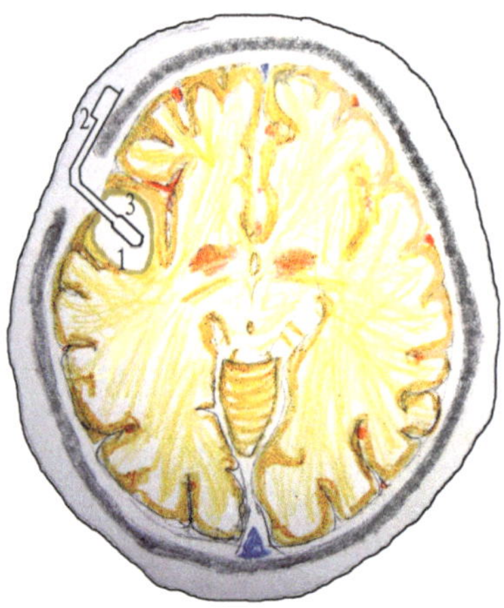

Fig. 8-B. The sketch of intratumoral brachytherapy: 1.Residual tumor cavity, 2. Valve of the reservoir, 3. Sack of the reservoir

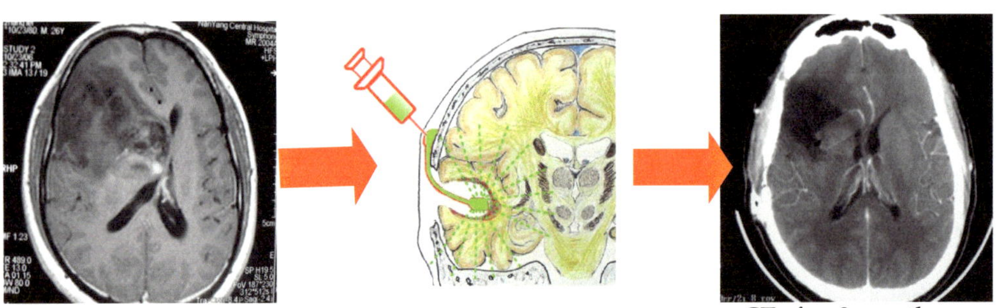

MRI before treatment | The sketch of treatment | CT after 9-month treatment

Fig. 9. The sketch of intratumoral brachytherapy

The isotopes emited high-energetic particles to damage the ultra micro-structure of DNA in MG cells. Simultaneously, hyperplasia of vascular endotheliocytes was induced, reducing blood supply to the tumor.

According to the radiometric determination from the water and wax model, brachytherapy produced a 3- to 5-fold larger absorption than routine extracranial irradiation of 10-20 cGy/h. These results are in accordance with Gutin's report. To measure the radioactivity absorbed in the remnant tumor, we used an radioactivity detector (NE Company UK Ionex 2500/3) and a finger-shaped ionization chamber. Calculation using the formula $Or = 51.2 \times C \sum \times (niEi\ \psi I) cGy/d$ resulted in 30.4-91.3 cGy/h or 730-3190 cGy/d absorption by remnant tumor.

The extent of brain edema in normal brain tissue was lower than that after routine radiotherapy. Light and electron microscopy of brain tissue samples from a patient treated by intra-tumoral brachytherapy revealed that there was no tumor growth within 3 cm of the implanted radioactive source and that tumor cells 4 cm from the source were inactive.

This treatment offers several advantages over routine radiotherapy. First, the isotope was much closer to the residual tumor cells (Fig. 10). As a result, efficacy was improved; toxicity was reduced. Second, the isotope was sealed within the reservoir without leakage into the body. Third, survival time and quality of life improved in this treatment compared to the control group. The survival time increased with increasing radioactive dose. Finally, according to tumor proliferation during treatment, when patients need additional treatment, the reservoir can be refilled with the radioactive isotope through the subcutaneous valve.

Typical case:

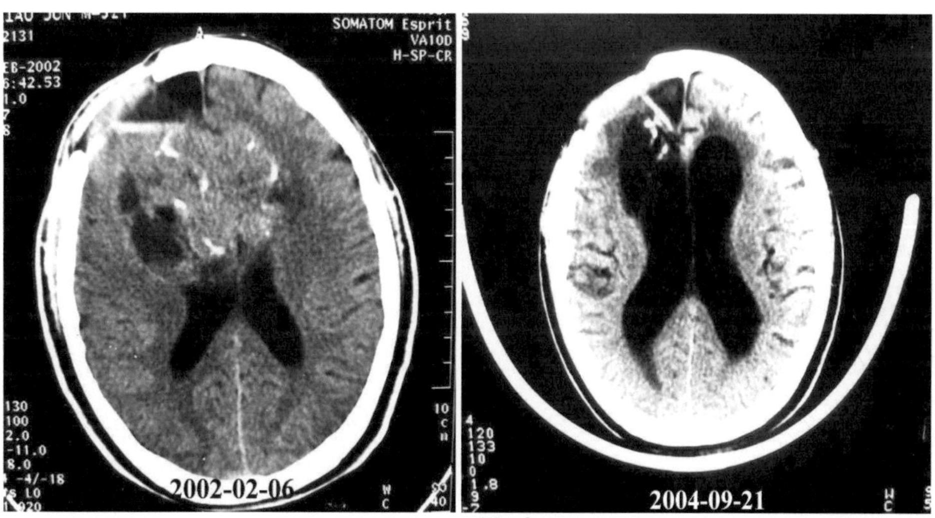

Postoperative CT scan before treatment

CT after 2-year treatment. The patient is still alive.

Fig. 10. The male patient was 57 years old with recurrent glioblastoma multiform, treated with intra-tumoral brachytherapy and intratumorally interstitial chemotherapy.

7. Intratumoral interstitial brachytherapy

Beginning in 2002, the authors performed interstitial brachytherapy in patients with tumors in central or functionally important locations. The Li Anmin I reservoir was implanted stereotactically (Fig. 11-A). 1.5 mL of 30 mCi ^{131}I solution was injected into the tumor site postoperatively at a constant speed (0.25 mL/h). Tumor cells were eliminated by short-distance radiation during the regeneration of interstitial fluid (Figs. 11-B and 12).

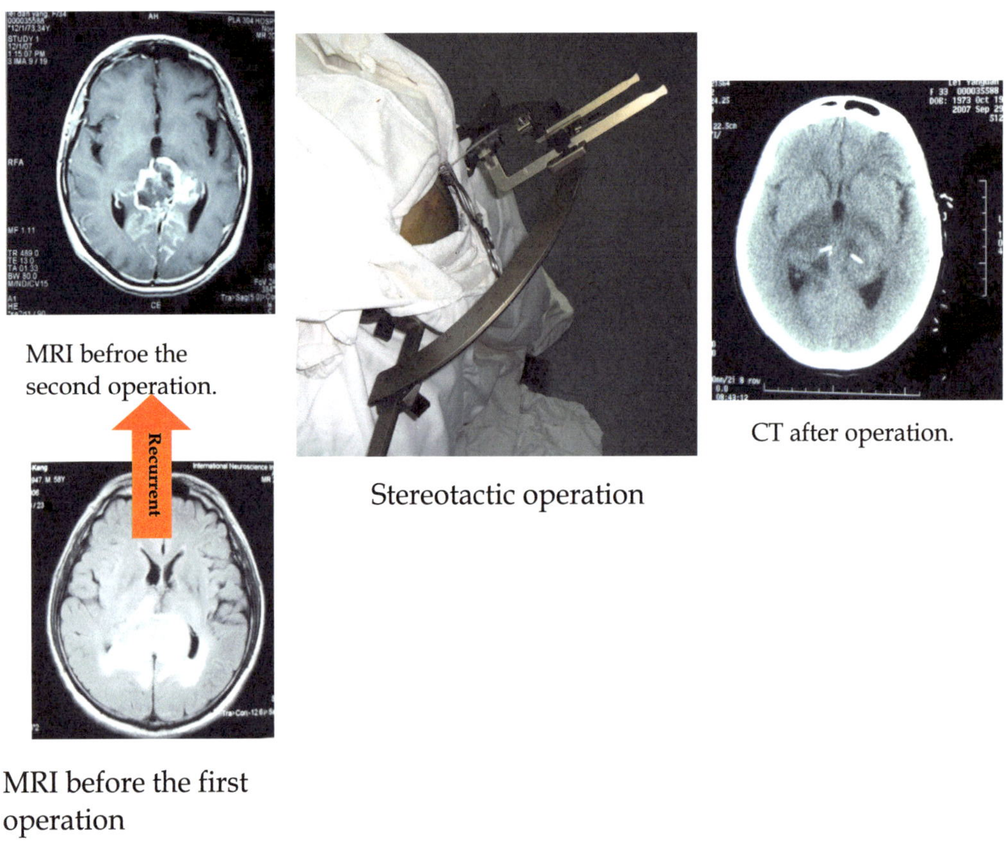

Fig. 11-A. The sketch of procedure of Intratumoral interstitial brachytherapy

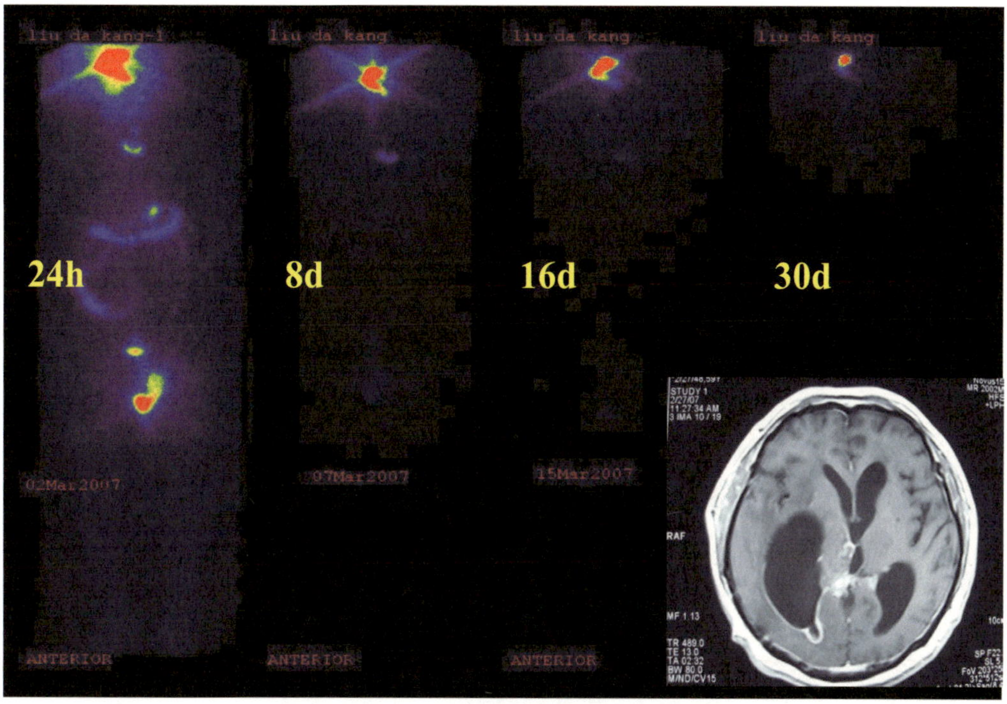

Fig. 11-B. CT and ECT at 24h, 8d, 16d and 30d after intratumoral interstitial brachytherapy.

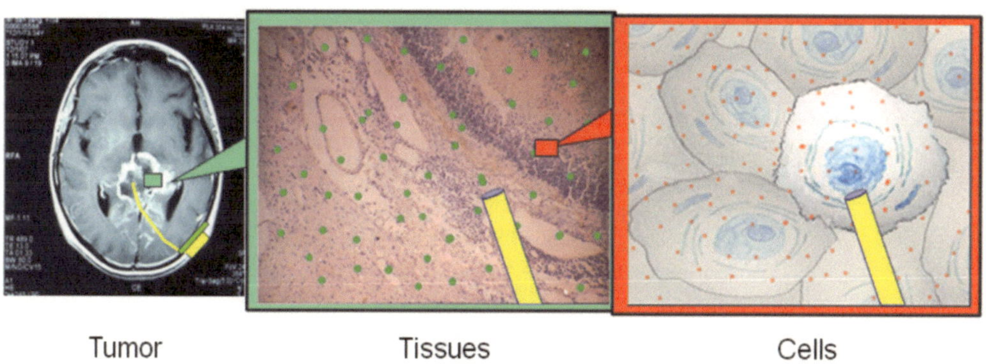

Fig. 12. The sketch of three structure levels of intratumoral interstitial brachytherapy for brain tumor.

This therapy involves three primary mechanisms (Fig. 13). First, a high-energy liquid radioactive source was placed at the interface of tumor and normal brain tissues, preventing the tumor from invading deep structures. Second, the liquid isotope flowed out of the reservoir into the interstitial fluid, irradiating tumor cells during the regeneration of the interstitial fluid. Finally, the liquid radioactive agents within the reservoir tube formed a radioactive column inside the tumor, subjecting it to continuous radiation for >16 d (2 half lives of ^{131}I). The ^{131}I fluid can be refilled to prolong the radioactive exposure.

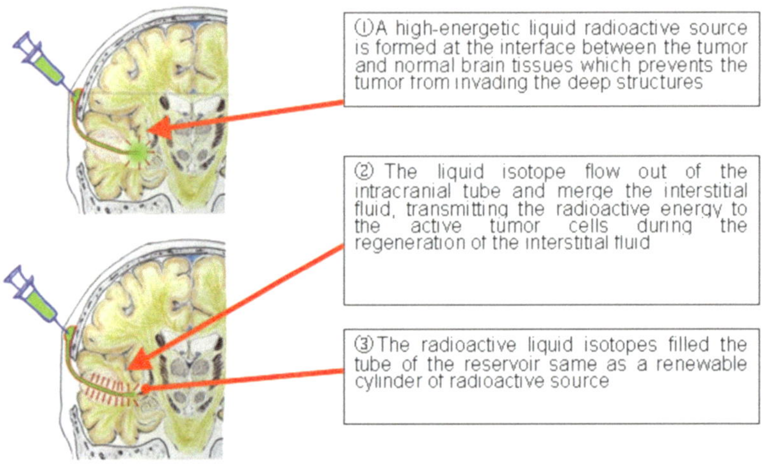

Fig. 13. The sketch of intratumoral interstitial brachytherapy

Based on long-term follow-up from Jan 2006 to Jul 2008, 33 patients who received the therapy had a prolonged survival time and a significantly improved quality of life (Fig. 14).

Typical case:

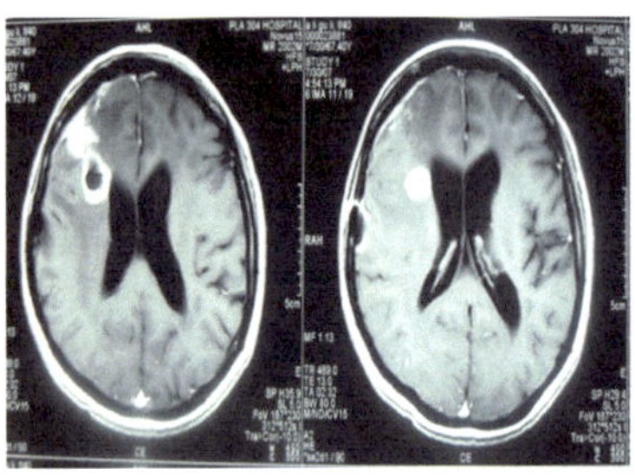

MRI of Recurrent glioma

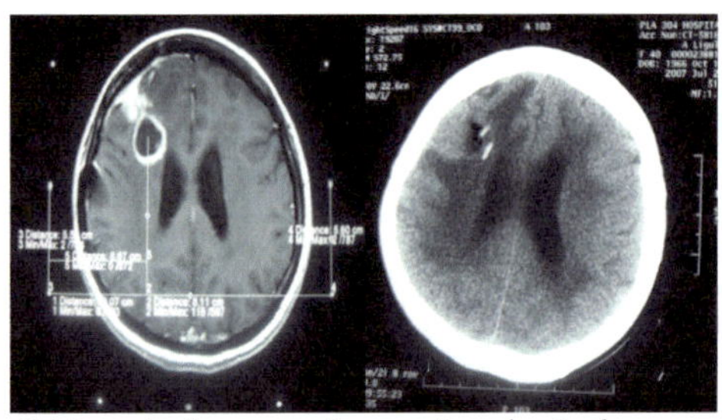

LiAnmin I reservoir was implanted stereotactically.
Postoprational CT showed the position of intratumoral tube.

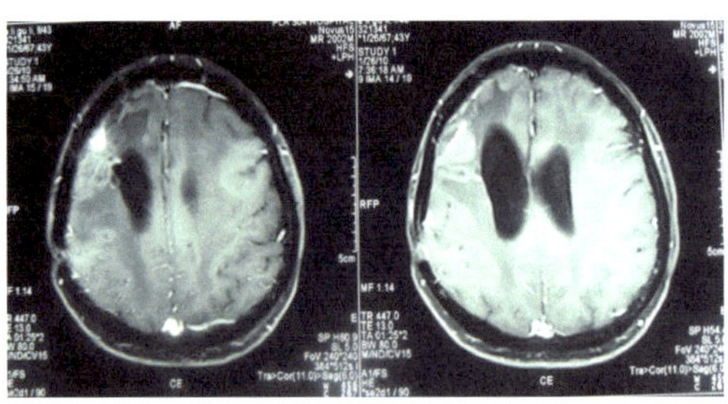

2.5 years after intratumoral interstitial brachytherapy

Fig. 14. Female, 42 years old, recurrent anaplastic astrocytoma

Treatment:

1. Intratumoral interstitial brachytherapy.
2. Selective/superselective interventional chemotherapy via cerebral artery

7.1 Complications and prevention

Hypothyroidism is a common complication in patients receiving long-term, cumulative exposure to micro-doses of ^{131}I, but could be prevented by iodine treatment prior to and during the exposure.

8. Immunologically targeted radiotherapy via monoclonal antibodies (McAb) loaded with ^{131}I

Immunologically targeted radiotherapy was designed for targeted brachytherapy [11]. Due to the weak immunogenicity and heterogeneity of glioma cells, an anti-nucleus McAb loaded with ^{131}I works better than an anti-membrane antibody. The chimeric McAb binds specifically to histones inside the dying tumor cells to destroy the adjacent tumor cells with high-dose local irradiation (Fig. 15).

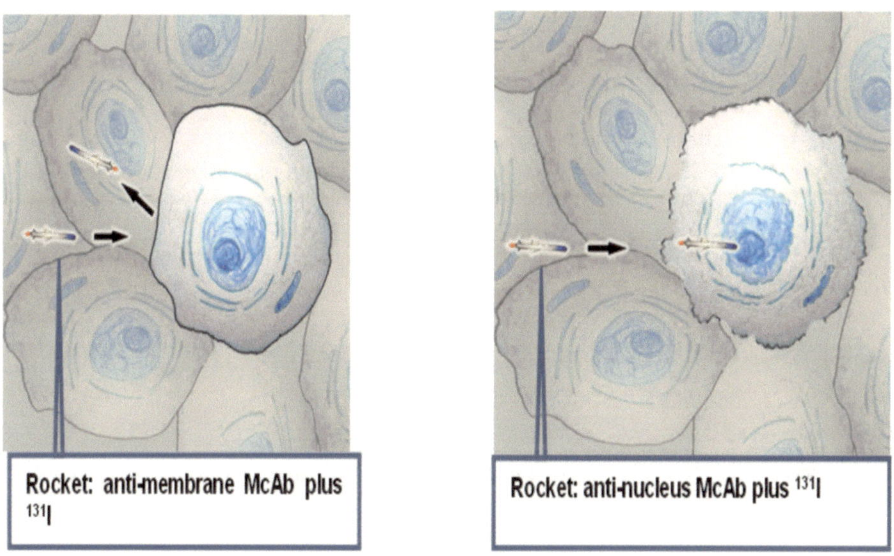

Illustration of Immunologically targeted radiotherapy via anti-membrane McAb the anti-membrane antibody couldn't recognize the antigen on membrane due to the weak immunogenicity and heterogenicity

Illustration of Immunologically targeted radiotherapy via anti-nucleus McAb this chimeric McAb can specifically bind to the histone inside the necrotising tumor cells to perform high dose local irradiation

Fig. 15. Sketch of Comparison between Immunologically Targeted Radiotherapy via anti-membrane and anti-nucleus McAb loaded ^{131}I in glioma

In collaboration with Epstein at the Department of Pathology, University of Southern California, the authors completed a phase II clinical trial in 56 MG patients in China. Of the 56 patients, 37.5% showed marked improvement and 42.8% showed mild improvement. The 1-year survival rate was 92.8%.

The recommended intrathecal administration resulted in accumulation of radioactive isotopes in the subarachnoid space and cerebral cistern rather than in the tumor tissue (Fig. 16). Additionally, intrathecal administration induced adverse effects on thyroid and bone marrow.

By contrast, when drugs were administered to the tumor via the Li Anmin I reservoir, the adverse effects on the thyroid and bone marrow were reduced (Fig. 17).

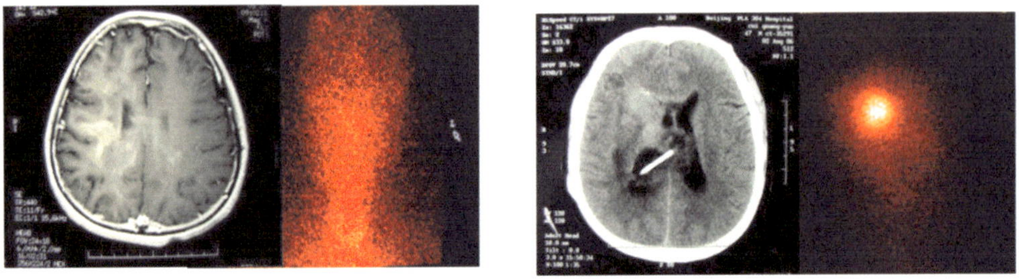

48 hours after intrathecal administration, ECT showed that radioactive isotopes mainly in the thyroid and cerebral cistern, not in the tumor

48 hours after local administration, ECT showed that radioactive isotopes mainly in the tumor, not in the thyroid and cerebral cistern

Fig. 16. ECT images of 2 methods of treatment

In May 2004, the China Cooperation Team Conference of Immune Targeted Radiotherapy was held in Shanghai. The authors proposed the local administration with LiAnmin I reservoir, which got extensive affirmation and widely accepted as the general method of immune targeted radiotherapy for MG in China.

Typical case:

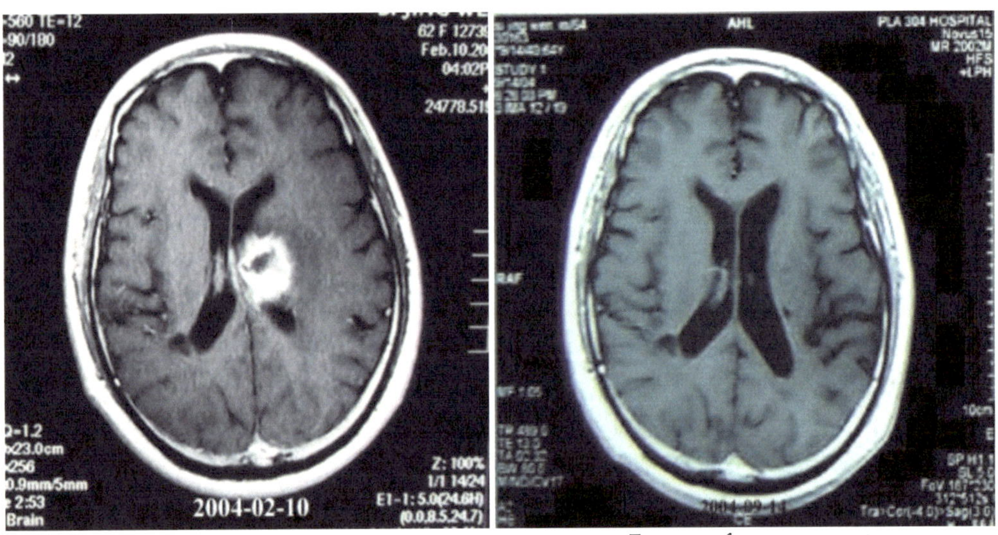

Before treatment

7 years after treatment

Fig. 17. Male, 62 years old, GBM

Treatment:

1. Immunologically targeted radiotherapy via McAb loaded 131I
2. Selective interventional chemotherapy via cerebral artery

Following positive reception at the China Cooperation Team Conference of Immune Targeted Radiotherapy (Shanghai, May 2004), local administration of anti-nucleus McAb loaded with ^{131}I via the Li Anmin I reservoir gained wide acceptance, and has become the golden standard of immune targeted radiotherapy for MG in China.

9. Peritumoral brachytherapy for MG in the brain stem/spinal cord

MG accounts for 59% of tumors in the brain stem and approximately 15% of the tumors in the spinal cord. Their survival rate is not correlated to the extent of surgical resection, but to the aggressiveness and postoperative proliferation of the residual tumor. Because of the infiltrative growth of the tumor, surgical resection has the risk of damaging the brain stem and spinal cord and threatening the quality of life. Conventional radiotherapy only inhibits tumor growth for ~3 months and does not affect the recurrent tumor.

Between Sept 2005 and Dec 2008, 15 patients were treated with peritumoral brachytherapy. In a follow-up of 1-3 yr, tumor control was seen in all cases. In 4 cases, the tumor disappeared. Shrinkage of the tumor was seen in 7 cases and maintained in 6 cases for 6-12 months. In the remaining 4 cases, tumor size remained stable for 1 year.

9.1 Methods

The treatment consisted of surgery and postoperative brachytherapy. For brain stem MG, the occipital squama and posterior arch of the atlas were removed. In spinal cord MG, laminectomy was performed for decompression in the two adjacent normal vertebral plates. Biopsies were conducted as needed. The intra-tumoral sack of the reservoir (Li Anmin I reservoir) was implanted near the tumor (Fig. 18). After 7 d, liquid 30 mCi ^{125}I/^{131}I was injected via the reservoir valve into the intra-tumoral sack. Radioactive isotope was administered every four months (2 half lives of ^{125}I) or 16-21 days (2-3 half lives of ^{131}I) for four doses in one cycle. Most of the 15 patients received three treatment cycles. Two patients with brain stem MG received two 30 mCi ^{131}I treatments. MRI examination was performed at 4 months after therapy.

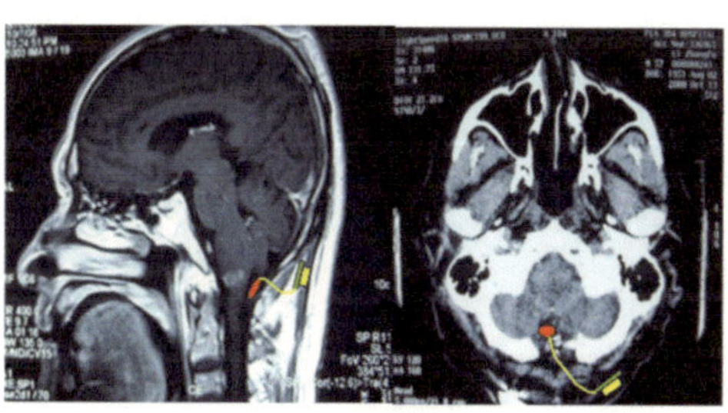

Illustration of peritumoral brachytherapy for brain stem glioma

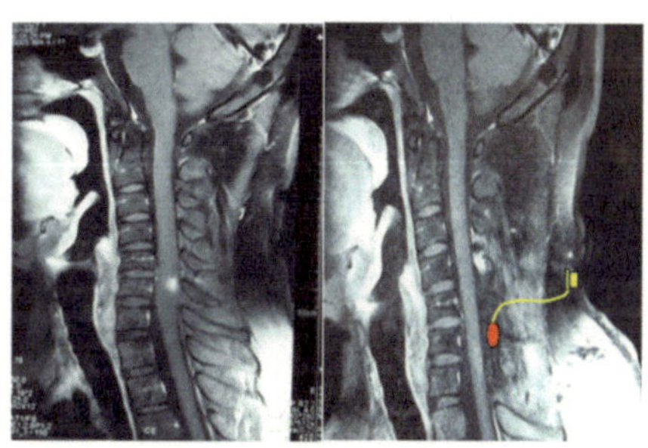

Illustration of peritumoral brachytherapy for spinal cord glioma

Fig. 18. The sketch of peritumoral brachytherapy for brain stem/spinal cord glioma

9.2 Efficacy

Brachytherapy has the advantages of localized high-absorption, long treatment cycles, and low radioactive injury to normal neural tissue, and therefore is suitable for patients with MG the brain stem or spinal cord [12,13]. The 15 patients receiving this therapy exhibited improved short-term and long-term survival. Two patients survived for >3 years. Post-treatment MRI revealed that all primary tumors were under control or in partial remission (Figs. 19 and 20).

Typical case:

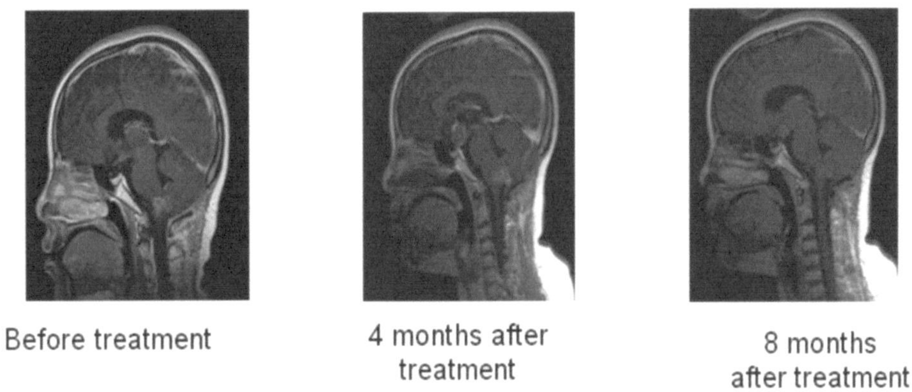

Fig. 19. Female, 11 years old, medulloblastoma

Treatment: peritumoral Brachytherapy for brain stem glioma

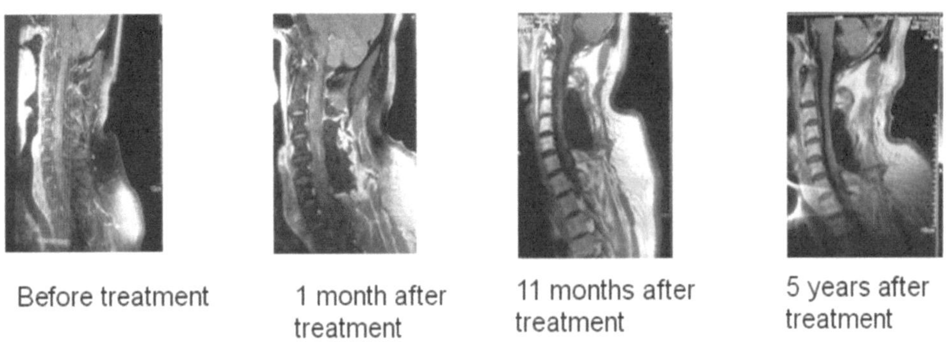

Fig. 20. Male, 46 years old, anaplastic astrocytoma in the cervical cord

Treatment: peritumoral brachytherapy for spinal cord glioma

9.3 Clinical application of new regional tumor therapy

Traditional treatments ignore the fact that MG is a localized tumor and target the entire body or the entire brain. Such treatments impair the immune and hemotopoeitic systems, and drastically reduce the quality of life. Based on pathogenesis, proliferation, pathological types, recurrence mode, and age at onset, MG is classified into six categories: primary glioma, recurrent glioma, cystic glioma, glioma in functional zones, low-grade glioma, and brain stem/spinal cord glioma.

With the goal of improving the quality of life for MG patients, the authors developed seven new regional therapeutic methods. Long-term therapeutic plan was individualized for each patient.
Intra-tumoral brachytherapy and selective/super-selective interventional chemotherapy were commonly used in combination in our practice. A second common treatment combination included brachytherapy, intra-tumor interstitial chemotherapy, and selective/super-selective interventional chemotherapy via cerebral artery. (Table 2).

	primary glioma	recurrent glioma	cystic glioma	glioma in functional zones	low-grade glioma	Brainstem /-spinal cord glioma
Intra-tumoral interstitial chemotherapy	⊙	⊙	⊙		⊙	
Selective/super-selective interventional chemotherapy via cerebral artery	⊙	⊙	⊙	⊙	⊙	
Autologous peripheral blood bone marrow stem cell supported high-dose chemotherapy	⊙	⊙				
Intratumoral brachytherapy	⊙	⊙	⊙		⊙	
Immunologically targeted radiotherapy via ^{131}I loaded McAb		⊙				
Intratumoral interstitial brachytherapy				⊙		
Peritumoral brachytherapy for brain stem/spinal cord glioma						⊙

Table 2. Clinical treatments of the six MG categories.

The overall 1-year, 2-year, and 3-year survival rate in our patients was 65.0%, 47%, and 16.6%, respectively. The tumor completely disappeared in 6.3% of the patients. This outcome is significantly better than previously reported (Table 3).

	country	Time	cases	Therapeutic regimen	1-year survival rate (%)	2-year survival rate (%)	3-year survival rate (%)
Bloom	UK	1966	141	Surgery + Radiotherapy	27	15	8
Fine	USA	1993	3000	Surgery + Radio/chemotherapy	53.2	25.0	-
Scott	USA	1995	747	Surgery + Radio/chemotherapy	30	8	2.5
Davis	USA	1999	146	Surgery + Radiotherapy	46	9.0	3.0
Laws	USA	2004	565	Surgery + Radio/chemotherapy	-	34.5	-
Li Anmin	CHN	2008	379	Local Therapy	65	47	16.6

Note: Above data were from following articles:

Table 3. Clinical outcome of glioma treatments.

[1] Fine HA, Dear KB, Loeffler JS, Black PM, Canellos GP. Meta-analysis of radiation therapy with and without adjuvant chemotherapy for malignant gliomas in adults. Cancer. 1993, 71(8):2585-97.

[2] Scott CB, Nelson JS, Farnan NC, Curran WJ Jr, Murray KJ, Fischbach AJ, Gaspar LE,Nelson DF.Central pathology review in clinical trials for patients with malignant glioma. A Report of Radiation Therapy Oncology Group 83-02. Cancer. 1995, 76(2):307-13.

[3] Chen P, Aldape K, Wiencke JK, Kelsey KT, Miike R, Davis RL, Liu J, Kesler-Diaz A,Takahashi M, Wrensch M. Ethnicity delineates different genetic pathways in malignant glioma. Cancer Res. 2001, 61(10):3949-54.

[4] Chang SM, Parney IF, Huang W, Anderson FA Jr, Asher AL, Bernstein M, Lillehei KO, Brem H, Berger MS, Laws ER; Glioma Outcomes Project Investigators. Patterns of care for adults with newly diagnosed malignant glioma. JAMA. 2005, 293(5):557-64.

10. Magnetic targeting chemotherapy against brain gliomas

One of the major problems in chemotherapy for MG is the lack of permeation of chemotherapeutic drugs through the BBB and tumor cell membrane. These difficulties may be overcome by novel delivery methods. For example, we developed a magnetic targeting drug delivery system between 1995 and 2008 (Fig.21). We conducted a series of experiments to examine the distribution, efficacy, and potential toxicity of this system. Results are summarized below.

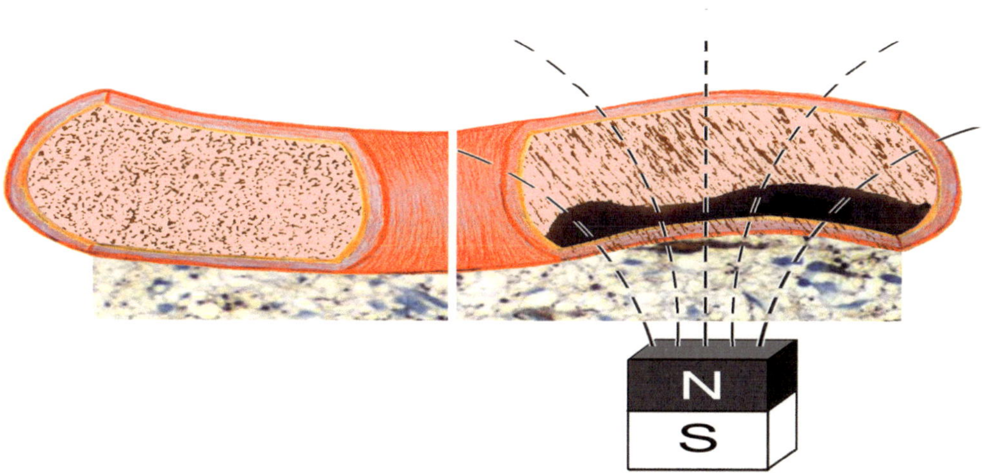

Fig. 21. The sketch of magnetic targeting delivery system

11. Toxicity of magnetic drugs on liver, kidney, and bone marrow

11.1 Methods

Sixty Kunming mice were randomly divided into three groups, and received different drugs in the presence or absence of an external magnetic field (Table 4). RBC, WBC, PLT, alamine aminotransferase (ALT), and blood urea nitrogen (BUN) were measured prior to and at 1, 7, 14, 30, and 90 d after the treatment.

Groups	Drug	External Magnetic Field
Magnetic targeting	magnetic MTX drug	0.5T, across head
MTX	MTX	Without
Control	saline	Without

Table 4. Toxicity profile.

11.2 Results

RBC, WBC, and PLT counts in the MTX group decreased significantly after the treatment, reached the lowest levels at 14 d post-injection and recovered after 90 d. In the magnetic targeting group, the RBC count was lowest at 7 d post-injection and gradually recovered after 90 d.

Remarkable difference was found among three groups, as shown in Fig. 22, demonstrating that magnetic targeting can reduce the toxicity of chemical drugs on bone marrow. Changes in ALT and BUN levels reflected the hepatic and renal injury. The magnetic targeting group had markedly lower ALT and BUN levels compared to the MTX group, indicating that magnetic targeting can reduce the side effects of chemotherapeutic drugs and protect the liver, kidneys, and bone marrow from systemic chemotherapy [14].

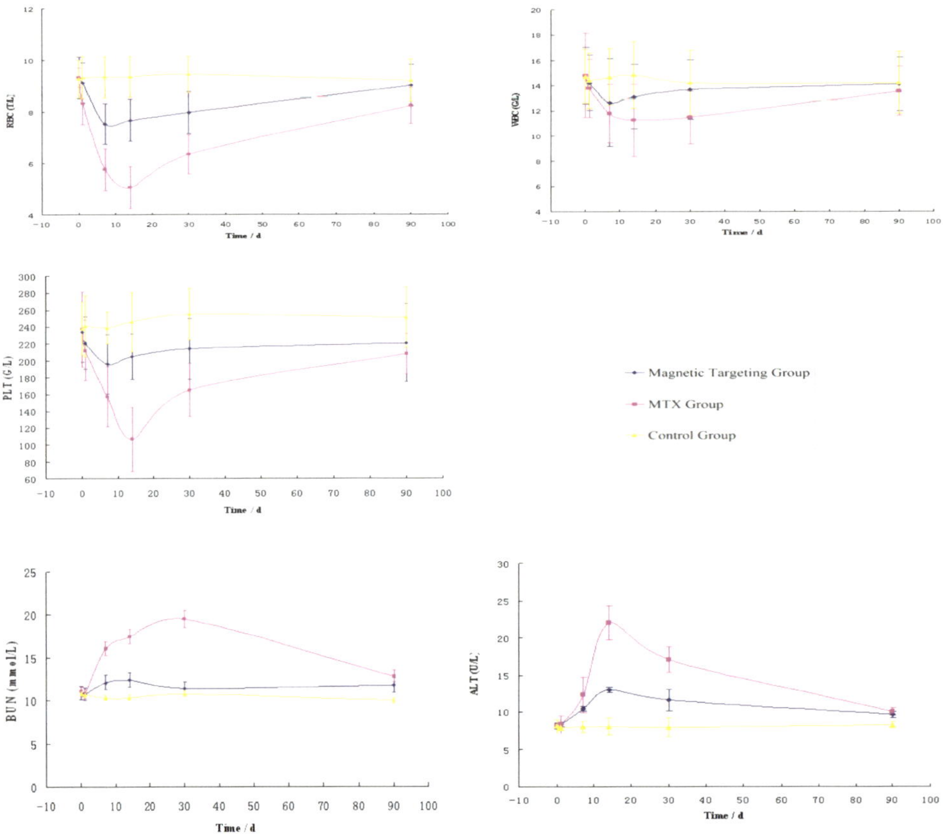

Fig. 22. Peripheral levels of RBC, WBC, PLT, ALT and BUN at pre-injection, and 1, 7, 14, 30 and 90 d after drug injection.

12. Distribution of the magnetic drugs in the brain

We investigated the distribution of magnetic drugs in the brain under magnetic drug targeting and explored magnetic targeting chemotherapy for malignant brain tumors.

12.1 Methods

Ninety SD rats were divided into three groups, and received different drugs in the presence or absence of an external magnetic field (Table 5). Ten rats from each group were randomly selected for sacrifice at 15 min intervals after drug injections. MTX levels in both sides of brain of each rat were measured.

Groups	Drug	External Magnetic Field
Magnetic targeting	magnetic MTX drug	0.5T, across head
Non-magnetic targeting	magnetic MTX drug	without
Control	MTX	0.5T , across head

Table 5. Distribution of magnetic drugs in the brain.

12.2 Results

MTX concentration in the brain was significantly higher in the magnetic targeting group. The difference between the three groups increased with time after injection.

Group	Drug content in hemispheres post-injection		
	15 min	30 min	45 min
Magnetic targeting	0.28±0.03 [a]	0.38±0.04 [a]	0.56±0.02 [a]
Non-magnetic targeting	0.10±0.02	0.14±0.01	0.06±0.02
MTX	0.13±0.12	0.11±0.02	0.07±0.05

Note: a: $P<0.01$ vs. other groups

Table 6. MTX concentration in the brain hemispheres.

12.3 Conclusions

Under magnetic targeting, magnetic drugs accumulated in the targeted area in the brain and local drug concentrations increased by 2- 9 folds.

13. Drug delivery by Superparamagnetic Paclitaxel Nanoparticles (SPPNPs)

13.1 Preparation and characteristics of SPPNPs

13.1.1 Methods

SPPNPs were synthesized with octadecyl-quaternized carboxymethyl chitosans and Fe_3O_4 ferrofluid, cholesterol, and paclitaxel at a weight ratio of 4:3:3:2 by reverse-phase evaporation. The diameters, magnetism, and drug release rates of the SPPNPs were examined with transmission electron microscope (TEM), a vibrating sample magnetometer (VSM), and high performance liquid chromatography (HPLC).

13.1.2 Results

TEM revealed an average diameter of ~20 nm with a narrow size distribution. The VSM analysis indicated that the paclitaxel nanoparticles were superparamagnetic (Fig. 23). The drug release test showed sustained drug release for >15 days (Fig. 24).

13.2 Cellular study

13.2.1 Methods

We examined intracellular distribution of FITC-labeled SPPNPs in MG cell line C6 under a fluorescent microscope. Cytotoxicity and apoptosis-inducing capacity of SPPNPs were also examined using CCK-8 kit and flow cytometry, respectively.

13.2.2 Results

The nanoparticles were taken up by the glioma cells. Confocal microscopy showed that these nanoparticles are present in the cytoplasm. C6 Cells were incubated with magnetic paclitaxel nanoparticles containing 1-80 nM paclitaxel or free paclitaxel of the same concentrations for 6-24 h. Both free placlitaxel and magnetic paclitaxel nanoparticles inhibited the proliferation of C6 cells in a dose and time-dependent manner. Cytotoxicity was comparable between free paclitaxel and paclitaxel released from the magnetic nanoparticles (Fig. 25).

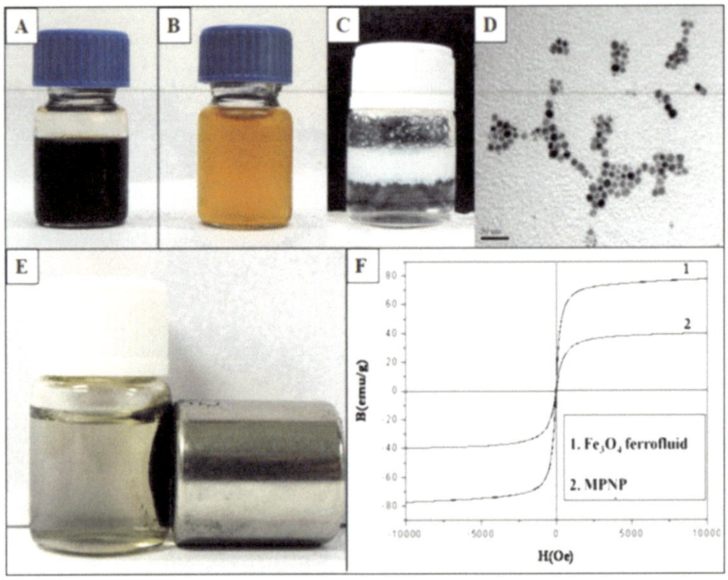

(Magnetic paclitaxel nanoparticles inhibit glioma growth and improve the survival of rats bearing glioma xenografts. Anticancer Research, 2010; 30(6): 2217-2223.)

Fig. 23. The aqueous solution of the magnetic paclitaxel nanoparticles at a concentration of 1 mg/ml (A) and 0.02 mg/ml (B) (calculated by the paclitaxel content). The same concentration of free paclitaxel (1 mg/ml) was insoluble in water (C). Under transmission electronic microscope, the magnetic paclitaxel nanoparticles showed a uniform size of 20 nm in diameter (D). After an external magnet was placed, the nanoparticles were attracted to the container wall (E). Vibrating sample magnetometry showed that these nanoparticles were superparamagnetic (F).

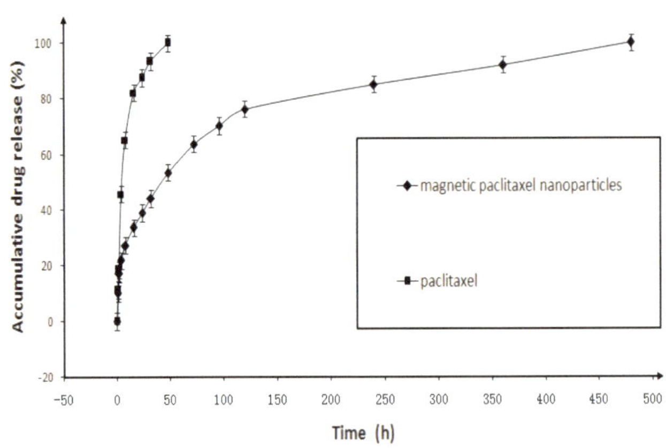

Fig. 24. In vitro paclitaxel release of free paclitaxel and the magnetic paclitaxel nanoparticles (pH 7.4 at 37°C). The results are shown as mean ± S.D.. The experiments were conducted three times independently. (*Magnetic paclitaxel nanoparticles inhibit glioma growth and improve the survival of rats bearing glioma xenografts. Anticancer Research, 2010; 30(6): 2217-2223.*)

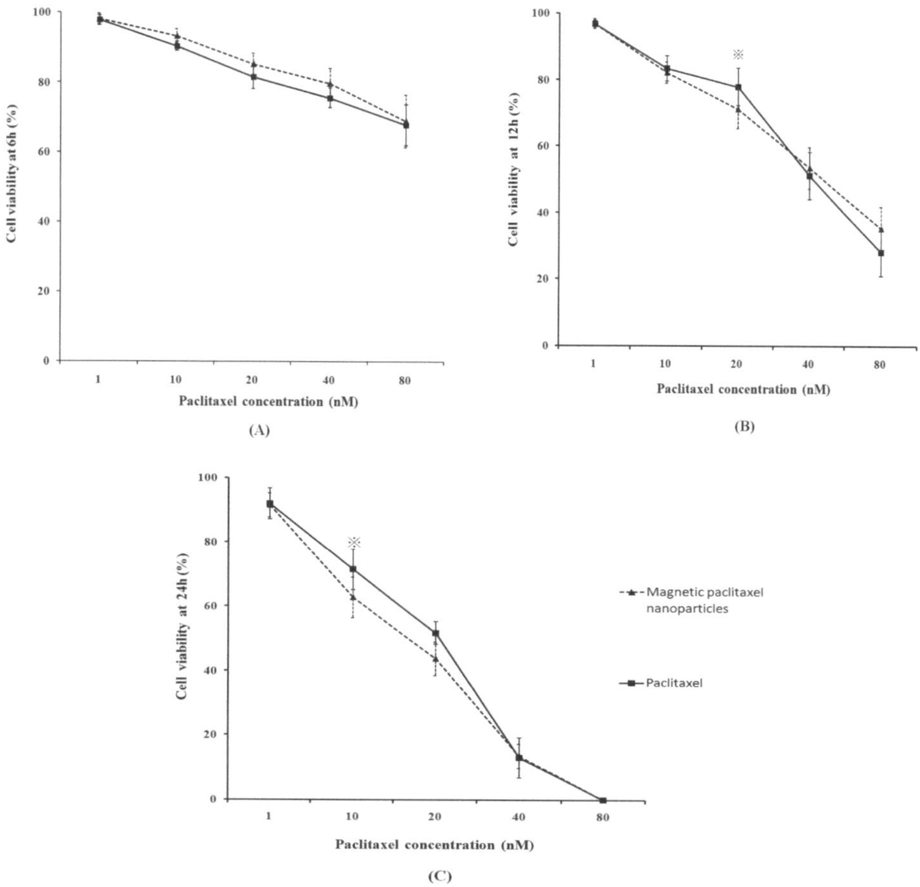

Fig. 25. The in vitro cytotoxicity of the magnetic paclitaxel nanoparticles and free paclitaxel against C6 cells at 6h (A), 12h (B) and 24h (C) post drug treatment. The cytotoxicity was determined by CCK-8 assays. The results are shown as mean ± S.D.. The experiments were conducted three times independently. * indicates $P < 0.05$. (*Magnetic paclitaxel nanoparticles inhibit glioma growth and improve the survival of rats bearing glioma xenografts. Anticancer Research, 2010; 30(6): 2217-2223.*)

13.3 Animal experiments

13.3.1 Drug concentration in rat brains after magnetic targeting

Male Wistar rats were randomly assigned into three groups, and received SPPNPs or PTX in the presence or absence of an external magnetic field (Table 7).

Groups	Drug	External Magnetic Field
Magnetic targeting	SPPNP (2.5 mL/kg)	0.5T, across head
Non-magnetic targeting	SPPNP (2.5 mL/kg)	without
Control	PTX (1.0 mg/mL)	without

Table 7. Treatment conditions in rat experiments.

The brain tissues were harvested at 1, 4, 8, and 16 h post-injection. PTX concentration was measured by HPLC.

13.3.1.1 Results

After intravenous injection of SPPNP, the PTX concentration in the non-magnetic targeting group was significantly lower compared to the magnetic targeting group, but markedly higher than that in control group (Fig. 26).

13.3.2 Inhibition of glioma cells in tumor-bearing rats after SPPNP injection and magnetic targeting

13.3.2.1 Methods

C6 cells were implanted into the rat brain stereotactically. After emergence of brain tumor symptoms, rats were divided into three groups. They were treated as shown in the following **Table 7**.

13.3.2.2 Results

The effect of free paclitaxel or the SPPNPs on the survival of rats bearing C6 glioma was depicted in Fig. 5. We found that the rats that received free paclitaxel at 10 mg/kg had a median survival of 12 d and a mean survival of 13.6 d (Tab. 2). The rats that received the magnetic paclitaxel nanoparticles and magnetic targeting had a median survival of 27 d and a mean survival of 27.4 d with the longest survival at 34 d, whose survival time increased for 1.5 times compared to those who received free paclitaxel (Fig. 27).

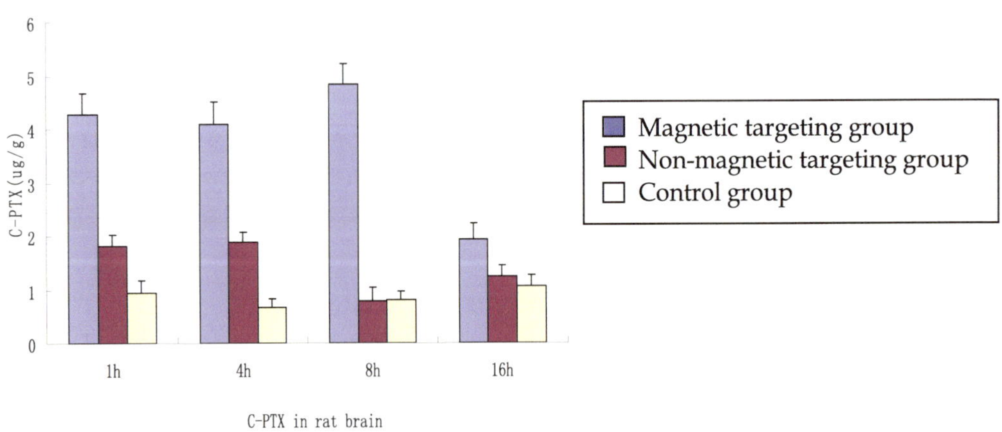

Fig. 26. Drug Concentration in Rat Brain in 3 Groups.

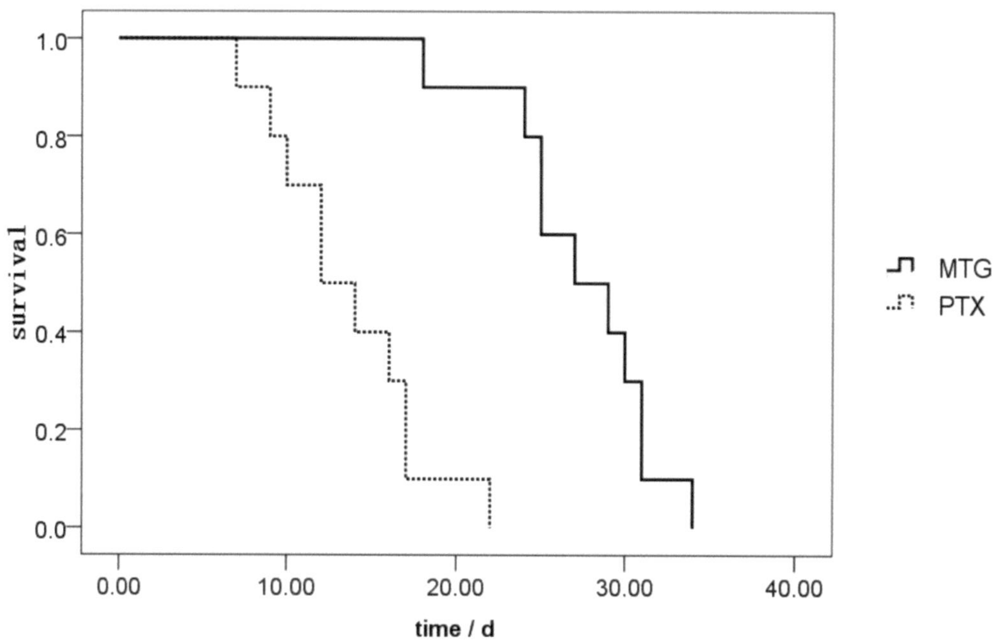

Fig. 27. Kaplan-Meier survival plots for C6 glioma-bearing rats given magnetic paclitaxel nanoparticles or free paclitaxel with or without magnetic targeting. MTG: magnetic targeting group, injection of magnetic paclitaxel nanoparticles combined with 0.5T magnetic field across the head; PTX: commercial paclitaxel was administered. Significantly prolonged survival was found in the MTG. (*Magnetic paclitaxel nanoparticles inhibit glioma growth and improve the survival of rats bearing glioma xenografts. Anticancer Research, 2010; 30(6): 2217-2223.*)

14. Conclusion

SPPNPs are safe and stable vectors to release chemotherapeutic drugs [15]. The small size allows SPPNPs to enter tumor cells. In the presence of an external magnetic field, SPPNPs can accumulate in magnetic targeted area [16,17]. This treatment inhibited tumor growth and prolonged the survival of glioma-bearing rats.

14.1 Possible mechanisms of magnetic targeting therapy against MG

1. **Increase localized drug concentration**

In the presence of an external magnetic field, magnetic chemotherapeutic drugs move within capillaries in the targeted areas of the brain and tumor. This increases the local drug concentration dramatically both around the tumor region and in the blood vessels of magnetic field [18]. Our results showed that magnetic targeting could increase the local drug concentration by 2-15 folds.

2. **Slow release of loaded drugs**

In the magnetic targeted area, the biodegradable capsule of magnetic drugs constantly degrades, slowly releasing the drugs into the vasculature or interstitial space of tumors or inside the tumor cells. This slow-release produces a sustained inhibition of the tumor cells.

3. **Thrombosis by magnetic particles**

Neoplastic deformation of tumor vasculature and ferrofluid in the magnetic field may facilitate the formation of micro-thrombi in the tumor capillary vessel and microvessel, and decrease the blood supply to the tumor [19].

4. **Improve the penetration across biological membrane**

The penetration of drugs across BBB depends on the local concentration gradient across the brain endotheliocytes. Magnetic targeting increases the drug content in the interstitial fluid of tumor. In addition to this concentration gradient, the strong magnetic field promotes the movement of the magnetic drug into the tumor from the capillary vessels and microvessels. Permeability and endocytosis permit the magnetic particles and chemotherapeutic drugs to enter the tumor cells [20].

5. **Magnetic-chemotherapeutic effects of magnetic particles**

The magnetic particles and external magnetic field may have synergistic action. In traditional Chinese medicine, magnetite has been used to generate magnetic field in tumor patients. In magnetic targeting therapy, the encapsulated ferrofluid can generate the magnetic-chemotherapeutic antineoplastic effects [21].

15. References

[1] Wen PY and Kesari S: Malignant gliomas in adults. N Engl J Med 2008, 359: 492-507. 2008, 31;359(5):492-507.

[2] Gurney JG, Kadan-Lottick N: Brain and other central nervous system tumors: rates, trends, and epidemiology. Curr Opin Oncol 13:160-166, 2001, 13(3):160-6.

[3] Mamelak AN. Locoregional therapies for glioma. Oncology (Williston Park). 2005, 19(14):1803-10.

[4] Boiardi A, Silvani A, Eoli M, Lamperti E, Salmaggi A, Gaviani P, Fiumani A,Botturi A, Falcone C, Solari A, Filippini G, Di Meco F, Broggi G. Treatment of recurrent glioblastoma: can local delivery of mitoxantrone improve survival? J Neurooncol. 2008, 88(1):105-13.

[5] Rhines LD, Sampath P, DiMeco F, Lawson HC, Tyler BM, Hanes J, Olivi A, Brem H. Local immunotherapy with interleukin-2 delivered from biodegradable polymer microspheres combined with interstitial chemotherapy: a novel treatment for experimental malignant glioma. Neurosurgery. 2003, 52(4):872-9.

[6] Engelhard HH. The role of interstitial BCNU chemotherapy in the treatment of malignant glioma. Surg Neurol. 2000, 53(5):458-64.

[7] Boiardi A, Salmaggi A, Pozzi A, Broggi G, Silvani A. Interstitial chemotherapy with mitoxantrone in recurrent malignant glioma: preliminary data. J Neurooncol. 1996, 27(2):157-62.

[8] Sato M, Iwatsuki K, Akiyama C, Masana Y, Yoshimine T, Hayakawa T. Use of Ommaya CSF reservoir for refractory chronic subdural hematoma. No Shinkei Geka. 1999, 27(4):323-8.

[9] Jimbo Y, Uzuka T, Fujii Y. A case of cerebrospinal fluid hypovolemia caused by Ommaya reservoir successfully treated by epidural blood patch. No Shinkei Geka. 2008, 36(7):639-43.

[10] Drabko K, Wiśniewska-Slusarz H, Wójcik B, Choma M, Zaucha-Prazmo A, Kowalczyk JR. Megachemotherapy followed by autologous haematopoietic stem cell rescue in children with high risk CNS tumours. Med Wieku Rozwoj. 2005, 9(3 Pt 2):439-47.

[11] Kato Y, Vaidyanathan G, Kaneko MK, Mishima K, Srivastava N, Chandramohan V, Pegram C, Keir ST, Kuan CT, Bigner DD, Zalutsky MR. Evaluation of anti-podoplanin rat monoclonal antibody NZ-1 for targeting malignant gliomas. Nucl Med Biol. 2010, 37(7):785-94.

[12] Julow J, Viola A, Major T, Valálik I, Sági S, Mangel L, Kovács BR, Repa I, Bajzik, G, Zoltán TN, Németh G.. Iodine-125 brachytherapy of brain stem tumors Strahlenther Onkol. 2004, 180(7):449-54.

[13] Chuba PJ, Zamarano L, Hamre M, Bhambhani K, Canady A, Guys MB, Matter A, Portillo G, Chung-bin S, Fontanesi J. Permanent I-125 brain stem implants in children. Childs Nerv Syst. 1998, 14(10):570-7.

[14] Alexiou C, Jurgons R, Schmid RJ, Bergemann C, Henke J, Erhardt W, Huenges E, Parak F. Magnetic drug targeting--biodistribution of the magnetic carrier and the chemotherapeutic agent mitoxantrone after locoregional cancer treatment. J Drug Target. 2003, 11(3):139-49.

[15] McBain SC, Yiu HH, Dobson J. Magnetic nanoparticles for gene and drug delivery. Int J Nanomedicine. 2008;3(2):169-80.

[16] Sakamoto J, Annapragada A, Decuzzi P, Ferrari M. Antibiological barrier nanovector technology for cancer applications. Expert Opin Drug Deliv. 2007, 4(4):359-69.

[17] Laquintana V, Trapani A, Denora N, Wang F, Gallo JM, Trapani G: New strategies to deliver anticancer drugs to brain tumors. Expert Opin Drug Deliv. 2009, 6(10):1017-32.

[18] Pulfer SK, Ciccotto SL, Gallo JM: Distribution of small magnetic particles in brain tumor-bearing rats. J Neurooncol. 1999, 41(2):99-105.

[19] Alexiou C, Jurgons R, Seliger C, Brunke O, Iro H, Odenbach S. Delivery of superparamagnetic nanoparticles for local chemotherapy after intraarterial infusion and magnetic drug targeting. Anticancer Res. 2007, 27(4A):2019-2022.

[20] Hillaireau H, Couvreur P. Nanocarriers' entry into the cell: relevance to drug delivery. Cell Mol Life Sci. 2009, 66(17):2873-2896.

[21] Chertok B, David AE, Huang Y, Yang VC. Glioma selectivity of magnetically targeted nanoparticles: a role of abnormal tumor hydrodynamics. J Control Release. 2007, 122(3):315-323.

11

Novel Pharmacological and Magnetic Resonance Strategies to Enhance Boron Neutron Capture Therapy (BNCT) Efficacy in the Clinical Treatment of Malignant Glioma

Paola Porcari[1], Silvia Capuani[2] and Francesco Saverio Pastore[3]
[1]*Sapienza University of Rome, Rome,*
[2]*Sapienza University of Rome, CNR-IPCF UOS Rome, Physics Department, Rome*
[3]*University of Rome Tor Vergata, Neuroscience Department,*
Institute of Neurosurgery, Rome,
Italy

1. Introduction

High-grade glioma, such as anaplastic astrocitomas (AA, WHO grade 3) and glioblastomas multiforme (GBM, WHO grade 4) are extremely aggressive and highly infiltrative brain tumours (Kleihues & Cavenee, 2000; Louis et al., 2007). In most cases they recur locally after applying the standard multimodality treatment based on surgical resection, followed by radiotherapy and/or chemotherapy. Despite advances in medicine, malignant gliomas continue to carry a dismal prognosis, even though a modest increase (by 4.5 months) in median survival and quality of life has been achieved. The main limitation to the effectiveness of surgery and radiotherapy in patients suffering from high-grade glioma is that these techniques, based on the geometric definition of tumour volume, are not suitable to eradicate tumour infiltrating cells within normal brain tissue. Moreover adjuvant chemotherapy has little effect on prolonging survival in patients with GBM (Stupp et al., 2005). As a consequence, novel therapeutic approaches, based on a better understanding of cancer biology, are needed. To this end, experimental therapies such as gene therapy (Mischel et al., 2003), antiangiogenic therapy (Van Meir et al., 2010), monoclonal antibodies (Zhu et al. 2010), cancer immunotherapy (Keunen et al., 2011), vaccines (Hickey et al., 2010), boron neutron capture therapy (BNCT) (Barth et al., 1992, 2005) and radioimmunotherapy (Joensuu, 2000) are under investigation. Among these, BNCT represents a promising adjuvant therapy for malignant glioma, and for other forms of cancer such as head/neck cancer. It is a binary form of radiation therapy based on the selective accumulation of boronated compounds within tumour cells which are then irradiated by low-energy thermal neutrons. The nuclear reaction that occurs between the stable isotope, ^{10}B, and thermal neutrons, yields high-energy alpha particles and recoiling lithium nuclei which release most of their ionizing energy within a few microns (about one cell diameter), therefore limiting radiation damage only to ^{10}B-containing cells. Thus, BNCT can be considered as a biologically targeted form of radiation therapy because of its ability to target tumour cells through boron compounds which selectively accumulate within them. Given this selectivity of BNCT, infiltrating tumour cells, as well as subclinical lesions, can be targeted by ^{10}B compounds and underwent the therapeutic effect.

For effective BNCT a large amount of ^{10}B nuclei (about 10^9 atoms of ^{10}B per cell) (Barth & Soloway, 1997) should be selectively accumulated within tumour cells, whilst ^{10}B concentration levels in blood and in normal brain tissues should be the lowest. At the same time, a tumour-to-brain (T:Br) ^{10}B concentration ratio of at least 3:1 must be achieved to ensure the optimal therapeutic dose to the tumour. Furthermore a sufficient number of thermal neutrons (thermal neutron fluences should be greater than 10^{12} $n \cdot cm^{-2}$) must be captured by ^{10}B atoms into the target volume during irradiation (Barth & Soloway, 1997).

BNCT therapy has been evaluated for safety and efficacy in several centres around the world. So far, no severe effects of BNCT-related toxicity have been observed (Phase I), whilst little evidence of therapeutic effectiveness has been evaluated (Phase II) in patients with GBM (Diaz, 2003). Presently the therapy is under experimentation in Phase II clinical trials, while a randomized Phase III study has not yet been justified because of previous disappointing results.

Currently, the boron carrier most widely used for clinical purpose is the boronated derivative of the essential amino acid L-phenylalanine, *p*-boronophenylalanine (BPA). Due to its poor solubility at physiological pH, it is administrated as a complex with fructose (BPA-fr complex). It is widely accepted that BPA is actively transported across the blood brain barrier (BBB) into the normal glia, while its uptake within the tumour is due to an increased rate of L-amino acid transport across the tumour cell membrane (Wittig et al., 2000). In addition, BPA accumulation within tumour cells increases during the cell cycle (S-phase) so that its use in treating aggressive GBM might be an advantage. Furthermore it has been demonstrated that pre-treatment with L-tyrosine (Papaspyrou et al. 1994), or other molecules targeted by L or A amino acid transport systems, can enhance intracellular BPA accumulation (Wittig et al., 2000). Previous *in vitro* (Wittig et al., 2000) and *in vivo* (Capuani et al., 2008, 2009) studies have demonstrated that preloading with L-DOPA (a well-known molecule with chemical structure similar to those of L-tyrosine and BPA) improves the accumulation of BPA. As a consequence, more interest is being devoted to the potential clinical application of L-DOPA preloading. Indeed, due to the wide clinical experience with the administration of L-DOPA for the treatment of Parkinson's disease, its use as a potential enhancer of BPA accumulation in BNCT clinical trials could be immediately applied.

The main limitations for BNCT effectiveness are due to: a) insufficient ^{10}B intake within tumour cells, even if the most efficient methods of ^{10}B administration are utilised; b) the lack of reliable imaging methods for monitoring the bio-distribution of ^{10}B-carriers in order to estimate both the effectiveness of the carrier and the optimal timing for neutron irradiation (that is when T:Br ^{10}B concentration ratio achieves the maximum value whilst at the same time the ^{10}B concentration in blood is the lowest).

Our research work has focused on developing solutions to overcome these BNCT limitations, in order to make it a clinically useful treatment modality in the near future. Specifically, we have evaluated *in vivo* (using C6 glioma model) the pharmacokinetics of BPA, and the effect of L-DOPA preloading on BPA accumulation both in the tumour and normal tissues. Pharmacokinetic data were helpful in determining the optimal irradiation time, as well as to develop computational strategies in order to define as accurately as possible the radiation dose released within tumour and surrounding healthy tissues.

In order to determine the best fitting curve of BPA pharmacokinetics (used to extrapolate the BPA concentration over time after infusion), *in vivo* monitoring of ^{10}B-carrier was performed using nuclear magnetic resonance (NMR), either by imaging (MRI) or by spectroscopy (MRS). In both cases, the fluorinated analogue of BPA, F-labelled BPA, was investigated using ^{19}F-MRI and ^{19}F-MRS (Porcari et al., 2006, 2008, 2009). All previously mentioned methodologies and strategies designed to overcome some fundamental limitations of BNCT therapy have been developed to ensure a straightforward transfer from pre-clinical to clinical applications.

2. Principles of boron neutron capture therapy

BNCT is an experimental, radio-therapeutic modality able to biologically target malignant cells. It theoretically allows a *selective* delivery of the radiation damage within an infiltrating cancer cell while preserving the surrounding healthy tissues.

BNCT has been preferentially employed in clinical trials designed for the treatment of GBM (Henriksson et al., 2008; Yamamoto et al., 2008, 2011; van Rij et al., 2005). This high grade tumour of the central nervous system is highly malignant and extremely infiltrative, characterized by rapid tumour growth with a wide microscopic invasion of malignant cells within the normal parenchyma. It is extremely resistant to all current therapies, including surgery, chemotherapy, radiotherapy, immunotherapy and gene therapy. Despite advances in medicine, its prognosis is still very poor with a median survival time of less than one year (Ohgaki & Kleihues, 2005). Thus, GBM remains one of the challenges to be faced by physicians and scientists worldwide. BNCT holds therapeutic promise for these incurable tumours. Clinical interest in BNCT has also been focused on high-grade gliomas (Chanana et al., 1999), as well as the treatment of malignant meningiomas (Tamura et al., 2006) and cutaneous melanomas (Mishima & Kondoh, 2000). More recently, interest has been extended to other forms of neoplasms such as head-neck cancers (Kankaanranta et al., 2007), liver (Wittig et al., 2008a) and lung tumours (Suzuki et al., 2007), as well as undifferentiated thyroid cancers (Dagrosa et al., 2007).

The treatment is binary and is carried out following two distinct phases. Firstly, an intravenous infusion of ^{10}B-enriched compounds is given to the patient, allowing the selective uptake of ^{10}B-carriers within neoplastic cells. Subsequently, when the T:Br ^{10}B concentration ratio has achieved its highest value (at least 3:1) and, at the same time, the ^{10}B concentration in blood is the lowest, the patient is irradiated with low energy ($E < 0.4eV$, thermal) or higher energy ($0.4eV \leq E \leq 10$ keV, epithermal) neutrons.

BNCT is based on the nuclear reaction $^{10}B(n,\alpha)^{7}Li$ (1) (Sauerwein, 1993) that occurs when the stable isotope, ^{10}B (characterized by a high thermal neutron capture cross section) captures a thermal neutron (n_{th}) to yield $^{11}B^{*}$ in an unstable form, which decays in highly cytotoxic alpha ($^{4}_{2}H$) and lithium ($^{7}_{3}Li$) particles (Fig. 1.a). Due to their high Linear Energy Transfer (LET) (ICRU, 1998), these heavy charged particles release along their paths (comparable with the cell diameter, 5-9 μm) a great density of ionization responsible for elevated Relative Biological Effectiveness (RBE) (ICRU, 1998). Thus, the dose delivered and the radiation damage is mostly confined within the ^{10}B-loaded tumour cell (Fig. 1.b).

$$ {}^{10}_{5}\mathrm{B} + \mathrm{n}_{th}(0.025\mathrm{eV}) \rightarrow \left[{}^{11}_{5}\mathrm{B}^{*}\right] \rightarrow \begin{cases} {}^{4}_{2}\mathrm{H} + {}^{7}_{3}\mathrm{Li} + 2.79\mathrm{MeV} \quad (6\%) \\ {}^{4}_{2}\mathrm{H} + {}^{7}_{3}\mathrm{Li}^{*} + 2.31\mathrm{MeV}\ (94\%) \\ \quad\downarrow \\ {}^{7}_{3}\mathrm{Li}^{*} + \gamma(0.48\mathrm{MeV}) \end{cases} \qquad (1) $$

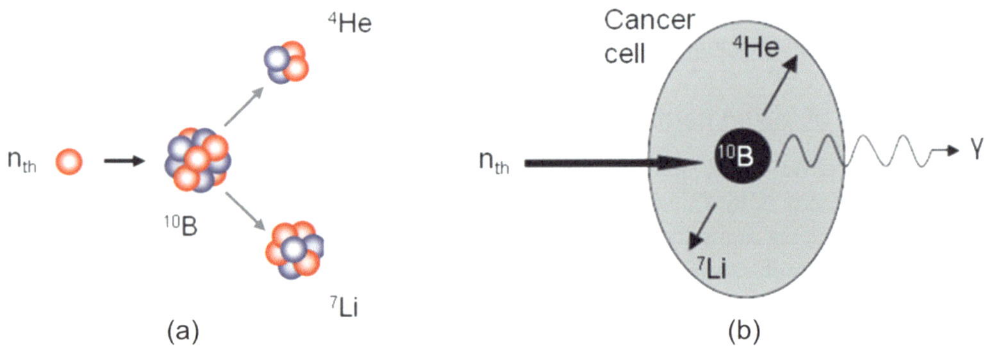

Fig. 1. $^{10}B(n,\alpha)^{7}Li$ reaction (a); cellular damage of BNCT (b).

The effectiveness of the therapy is dependent on two conditions:

- a high number of ^{10}B atoms must be selectively localized within neoplastic cells (at least 20-35 μg/g ~10^9 atoms of ^{10}B per targeted cell) (Barth et al., 1996; Barth & Soloway, 1997);
- a sufficient number of thermal neutrons has to reach and be captured by the ^{10}B atoms into the target volume during irradiation (thermal neutron fluences should be greater than 10^{12} n·cm^{-2}) (Barth et al., 1996; Barth & Soloway, 1997).

Although theoretically only a few alpha particles, releasing their energy within a cancer cell, assure the cell death, both of the above conditions should be satisfied because of the low probability of interaction between a single ^{10}B atom with a thermal neutron.

The therapeutic gain of BNCT is strictly dependent on the achievable T:Br ^{10}B concentration ratio between tumour and normal tissue. It has been established that the higher the T:Br ^{10}B concentration ratio is, the better the therapeutic gain of BNCT. Moreover, the tolerance dose of normal tissues should not be exceeded. It is mainly dependent on the neutron capture reactions, $^{1}H(n,\gamma)^{2}H$ and $^{14}N(n,p)^{14}C$ (2) (Soloway et al., 1997), that occur when hydrogen, ^{1}H, and nitrogen, ^{14}N, isotopes (with relative abundances of 3% and 10%, respectively, in normal tissue) capture thermal neutrons yielding low LET γ rays and high LET protons (2), respectively.

$$ \begin{aligned} {}^{1}\mathrm{H}(\mathrm{n},\alpha)^{2}\mathrm{H} &\rightarrow {}^{1}\mathrm{H} + \mathrm{n}_{th} \rightarrow \left[{}^{2}\mathrm{H}\right] \rightarrow {}^{2}\mathrm{H} + \gamma(2.23\mathrm{MeV}) \\ {}^{14}\mathrm{N}(\mathrm{n},\mathrm{p})^{14}\mathrm{C} &\rightarrow {}^{14}\mathrm{N} + \mathrm{n}_{th} \rightarrow \left[{}^{15}\mathrm{N}\right] \rightarrow {}^{14}\mathrm{C} + \mathrm{p}(0.63\mathrm{MeV}) \end{aligned} \qquad (2) $$

Due to the small neutron capture cross-sections of ^{1}H and ^{14}N (σ_H = 0.332 and σ_N = 1.82 barns; 1 barn = 10^{-24} cm^2) compared with that of ^{10}B (σ_B = 3838 barns), the dose released within surrounding healthy tissues is, in most of cases, much smaller than that delivered within the tumour, even though its value is dependent on neutron fluences. Thus, the upper limit of the neutron fluences is determined by the normal tissue tolerance dose for protons and γ rays. As a consequence, for the best therapeutic result the T:Br ^{10}B concentration ratio should be as high as possible.

In order to satisfy the previous conditions, intensive investigations have been performed since the introduction of BNCT in most of the research centres worldwide. Considerable efforts have been directed towards the design and synthesis of new efficient boron agents, as well as in developing strategies to maximize the tumour boron uptake whilst minimizing, at the same time, ^{10}B levels in blood and in normal brain. The disappointing outcomes of early BNCT clinical trials in the United States (Slatkin, 1991) were mainly due to the inability of thermal neutrons to deliver therapeutic neutron fluences to deep-sited brain tumours. To overcome this, the use of higher energy epithermal neutron beams was pursued because of their greater tissue penetrating properties. Indeed, when epithermal neutrons penetrate tissues, they are slowed down into the thermal neutron range (Seppälä et al., 2002, Coderre et al., 1997) by means of collisions with atoms (Fig. 2). Epithermal neutrons, therefore, allow delivery of therapeutic fluences of thermal neutrons at greater depths in the brain without reflecting the scalp or doing a craniotomy as required by using thermal fluences.

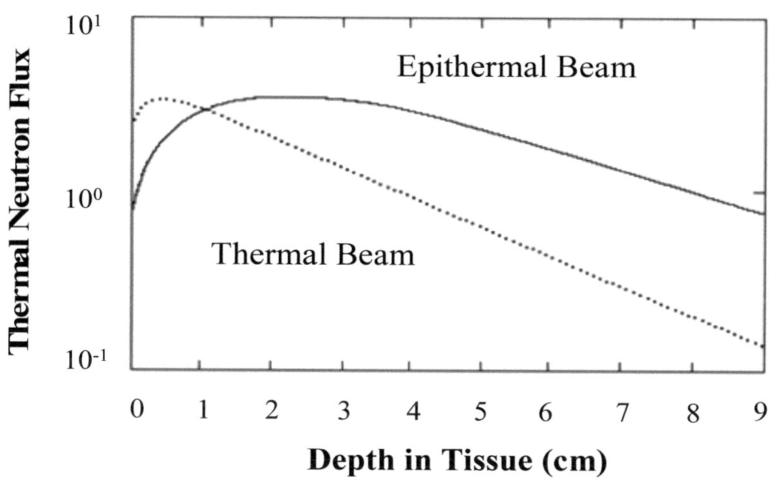

Fig. 2. Variation of the thermal neutron fluence with tissue depth using a thermal or epithermal neutron beam (Coderre & Morris, 1999).

Currently, nuclear reactors are the only sources of neutrons for clinical BNCT. The neutrons are produced by the fission process in the core of the reactor and are classified according their energy as thermal (E_{th} < 0.025eV), epithermal (0.4eV < E_{epi} < 10 keV) or fast (E_{fast} > 10k eV). Since it is highly unlikely that the reactors can be sited in the main medical centres, alternative sources of thermal and epithermal neutrons for BNCT are being sought (Blue & Yanch, 2003). Among these, low-energy proton accelerators with low z targets are the most attractive.

At present several reactors creating optimal epithermal neutron beams for BNCT are being used clinically worldwide. They include the Massachusetts Institute of Technology Reactor (MITR) (Busse et al., 2003) in the USA, the Kyoto University Research Reactor (KURR) and JRR4 at the Japan Atomic Energy Research Institute (Nakagawa, 2003) in Japan, and the RA-6 CNEA reactor in Bariloche (Riley et al., 2008), Argentina. In Europe there are several clinical BNCT nuclear reactors: the FiR1 clinical reactor in Helsinki (Finland) (Joensuu et al.,

2003), the LVR-15 reactor at the Nuclear Research Institute in Rez (Czech Republic) (Burian et al., 2004) and the clinical reactor at Studsvik Medical AB (Sweden) (Capala et al., 2003).

2.1 Boron agents

Since its inception, the development of boron delivery agents for BNCT therapy has been one of the most important topics to fulfil. For BNCT to be successful ^{10}B carriers should satisfy the following requirements:

- selectivity for malignant cells (with preferential ^{10}B intracellular localization) compared with blood and contiguous normal tissue;
- achievement of tumour boron concentrations of at least 20-35 $\mu g^{10}B/g$ (approximately 10^9 boron atoms per cell);
- permanence (at a constant concentration) within tumour during the BNCT radiation procedure and rapid clearance from both blood and normal tissues. This is necessary to estimate the radiation dose delivered to tumour, brain and vascular endothelium;
- minimal systemic toxicity in order to achieve adequate tumour concentrations *in vivo* assuring, at the same time, favourable T:Br and tumour-to-blood (T:Bl) concentration ratios (at least 3:1);

So far, two ^{10}B carriers have been used clinically: the polyhedral borane, sodium borocaptate ($Na_2B_{12}H_{11}SH$ or BSH) (Fig. 3), and the dihydroxyboryl derivate of phenylalanine, boronophenylalanine ($C_9H_{12}BNO_4$ or BPA) (Fig. 3).
Both compounds are characterized by low toxicities, selective tumour cell uptake, long tumour persistence and safety after their intravenous (i.v.) administration.

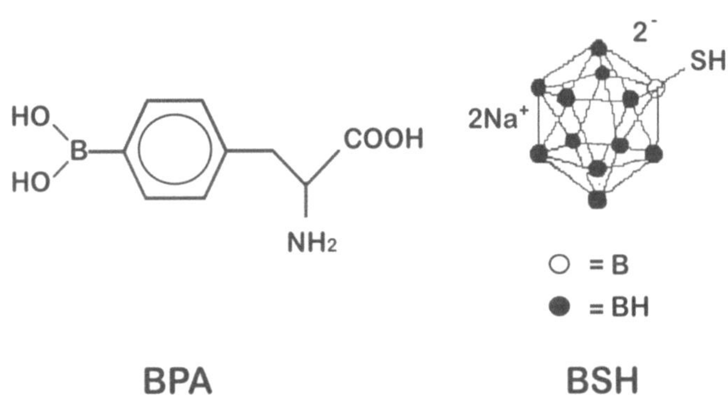

Fig. 3. Chemical structures of BPA and BSH.

Moreover, it has been demonstrated that either BPA or BSH may be able to target both proliferating and non-proliferating cells. This is of major importance for GBM treatment because of the relatively small percentage of GBM cells in the proliferative status at any time.
Previously, BPA and BSH have been employed as boron agents in clinical trials designed for brain tumour treatments in the United States of America (Chanana et al.,1999; Coderre et al.,1999), in Europe (Phase I) (Capala et al., 2003; Joensuu et al., 2003, Burian et al., 1994) and in Japan (Phase II) (Nakagawa et al., 2003). The results of these trials confirmed the therapeutic efficacy of BNCT and provided the basis of the subsequent experimental clinical trials. However, the design of BNCT clinical protocols carried out using both mentioned ^{10}B-carriers was also influenced by the findings on animal model studies (Nakagawa et al., 2007; Smith et al., 1996).

In recent years, the clinical use of BPA for the GBM treatment has aroused great interest (Coderre et al., 1997; Capala et al., 2003; Joensuu et al., 2003) because of its encouraging results in experimental brain tumour therapy. Due to its low solubility in aqueous solutions at physiological conditions (pH ~ 7.4) it is administered as a complex with fructose (BPA–fr complex) (Yoshino et al., 1989). It was observed that BPA can be selectively accumulated either in the main tumour mass or in the microscopic cluster of tumour cell invading the normal parenchyma, even though the measured ^{10}B concentration in the isolated cluster was only about 50% of that obtained in the main tumour mass (Smith et al., 1996). This result is of great importance for the efficacy of BNCT because the isolated clusters represent potential sites of tumour re-growth. Furthermore the ability of BPA to target the microscopic cluster within the normal brain suggests that it is actively transported through the BBB.
Although the details of BPA accumulation into tumour cells are not completely understood, it is accepted that it is due to an elevated rate of amino acid transport across the tumour cell membrane (Wittig et al., 2000). Furthermore, there is evidence that BPA accumulation is enhanced by a pre-treatment with molecules vehiculated through L or A amino acid transport systems (Wittig et al., 2000). The increase of BPA intracellular accumulation was also demonstrated in mouse melanoma cells (Papaspyrou et al., 1994) using L-tyrosine pre-administration.
In addition, it has also been demonstrated that BPA accumulation within tumour cells increases during the cell cycle (S phase) (Nichols et al., 2002) so that its use in the treatment of aggressive brain gliomas might be an advantage.

3. Main limitations for BNCT effectiveness

BNCT is one of the most complex therapeutic modalities used to treat malignant brain tumours. Its success or failure is highly dependent on a combination of several chemical, physical and biological factors. Up to now, BNCT has been trialled to investigate its safety and efficacy in several centres worldwide. However, to date, the results of Phase I and II clinical trials have not shown therapeutic responses to justify Phase III trials.
These disappointing results are mainly due to the following limitations.
The first limitation was mostly due to insufficient uptake of ^{10}B-labelled compound within tumour cells even though the most advanced methods of ^{10}B administration were used (Chanana et al., 1999; Elowitz et al., 1998).
Normally, the ^{10}B uptake within brain tumours may be influenced by several factors such as the BBB permeability to the ^{10}B-carrier, the plasma concentration profile of the ^{10}B-agent (which is dependent on either the drug dose or the way of administration), the blood flow within tumour as well as the drug lipophilicity.
So far, some strategies have been proposed to improve BNCT effectiveness by increasing BPA and BSH tumour intake. Some of these, including the use of pharmacological agents such as mannitol (Barth et al., 2000) or Cereport (RMP-7) (Yang et al., 1997) to disrupt the BBB, have been experimented on animal models (Barth et al., 2000; Yang et al., 1997). Although the results showed an increase in T:Br and T:Bl indices, the potential toxicities were not completely investigated. Moreover these methodologies have been classified as invasive, so numerous investigations are needed before considering them as potential applications in future clinical trials.
The second main limitation for BNCT effectiveness was due to the lack of efficient imaging methods to monitor the spatial bio-distribution of ^{10}B-labelled compounds and their

pharmacokinetics, in order to estimate the efficacy of the carrier and the optimal timing of neutron irradiation. This ideal time is when the ^{10}B concentration in tumour is higher than the concentration in blood and surrounding healthy tissues to prevent damage to these regions. Previous studies carried out in order to estimate brain-to-blood (Br:Bl), T:Br and T:Bl ^{10}B concentration ratios using kinetic models (Ryynanen et al., 2000; 2002) and Inductively Coupled Plasma-Atomic Emission Spectrometry (ICP-AES) (Laakso et al., 2001) techniques, gave different results.
Up to now several techniques (Wittig et al., 2008b) have been used to determine the spatial distribution and pharmacokinetics of ^{10}B agents (Elowitz et al., 1998; Ryynanen *et al* 2000, 2002, Laakso et al., 2001, Kabalka et al., 2003, Wang et al., 2004). Among these, MRI and MRS provide useful methods for non-invasive and non-destructive real-time monitoring of ^{10}B compounds during BNCT treatment *in vivo*. Given the low sensitivity of the ^{10}B NMR method (Bendel et al., 2001; Bendel 2005) and the intense proton background signal that makes ^{1}H-MRS (Zuo et al., 1999) and Magnetic Resonance Spectroscopy Imaging (MRSI) (Bendel et al., 2005) techniques problematic *in vivo*, new strategies to detect BPA by NMR are in progress.

4. Strategies to improve the efficacy of the therapy

In order to make BNCT a clinical useful treatment modality in the near future, our work aims at investigating solutions to overcome the main limitations to the efficacy of the current methodology.
Firstly, with the aim of improving the effectiveness of the therapy by increasing BPA tumour intake, the strategy used was to assess the effect of L-DOPA pre-loading on BPA accumulation within the tumour.
L-DOPA is a well-known molecule with a chemical structure similar to those of L-tyrosine and BPA. Its use as a potential enhancer of BPA accumulation was suggested by previous encouraging results obtained on both mouse melanoma (Papaspyrou et al., 1994) and 9L rat gliosarcoma cells by pre-administration of L-tyrosine (Wittig et al., 2000). The enhancement of BPA accumulation in 9L rat gliosarcoma cells has been also replicated by using pre-treatment with both molecules targeted by L and A aminoacid transport system. These findings suggest that the substrate-coupled antiport (exchange) mechanism of these transporters is enhanced by the preloading of specific aminoacids. Previous *in vitro* (Wittig et al., 2000) and *in vivo* (Capuani et al., 2008; 2009) studies have demonstrated that L-DOPA preloading improves the accumulation of BPA in the tumour. Specifically it was demonstrated *in vivo* (Capuani et al., 2008; 2009) that L-DOPA pre-administration on C6 glioma model gave rise to an increase of BPA tumour accumulation of 2.7 times with respect to those of controls. Conversely, no significant difference was evaluated by using the High Performance Liquid Chromatography (HPLC) method in both blood and normal brain between L-DOPA preloaded rats and controls. These findings are of fundamental importance for their impact on potential clinical applications. Indeed, the introduction of L-DOPA as a potential enhancer of BPA accumulation in BNCT clinical trials could be of immediate application because of its established clinical use as a treatment for Parkinson's disease.
Then, with the aim of investigating the pharmacokinetic behaviour of ^{10}B carriers and their boron bio-distribution, both of them essential to evaluate the efficiency of the carrier and the optimal irradiation time, a novel approach to detect BPA was proposed. The strategy used was to map the fluorinated analogue of BPA (^{19}F–BPA–fr complex) (Fig. 4) using ^{19}F NMR in a way

similar to Positron Emission Tomography (PET) studies (Kabalka et al., 2003; Wang et al., 2004). The feasibility of the method was previously demonstrated *in vitro* (Porcari et al., 2006).

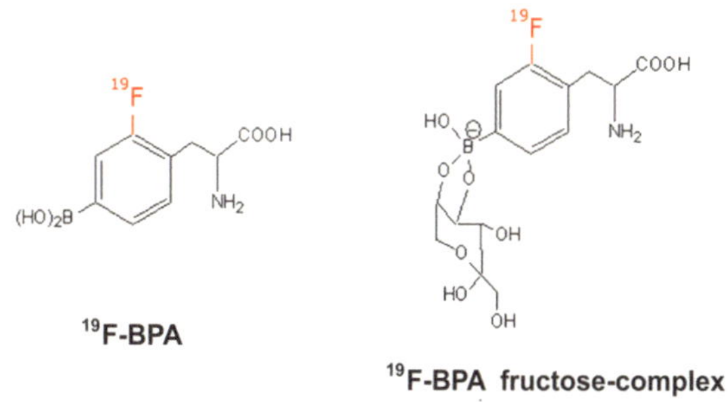

Fig. 4. Chemical structures of ^{19}F-BPA and ^{19}F-BPA-fr complex.

Specifically, selective bio-distribution (Fig. 5.) (Porcari et al., 2008; 2009) of ^{19}F-BPA-fr complex in C6 tumour-bearing rats as compared with normal brain has been demonstrated using ^{19}F MRI. In addition, a better understanding of ^{19}F-BPA pharmacokinetic was achieved because of the correlation between the results obtained by using both ^{19}F MRI and ^{19}F MRS methodologies. Indeed the correlation between ^{19}F MR monitoring on rat brain over 4h after ^{19}F-BPA-fr complex infusion and the quantification of ^{19}F spectra collected from blood samples showed a maximum uptake of ^{19}F-BPA in C6 glioma at 2.5h after infusion. Thus, 2.5h after infusion is the optimal time of neutron irradiation according to previous results (Hsieh et al., 2005) obtained by using PET measurements of ^{19}F - BPA.

These findings suggest the potential future application of ^{19}F MRI and ^{19}F MRS using ^{19}F-BPA in clinical trials. Indeed, the correlation of both techniques allows the mapping with the high spatial resolution characteristics of MRI of the distribution of ^{10}B compounds and at the same time to follow the pharmacokinetic of ^{10}B agents. Moreover, since ^{19}F NMR can be performed using an ^{1}H MR scanner by suitably tuning RF coils, only minor improvements in the MRI clinical scanner are required for future clinical applications.

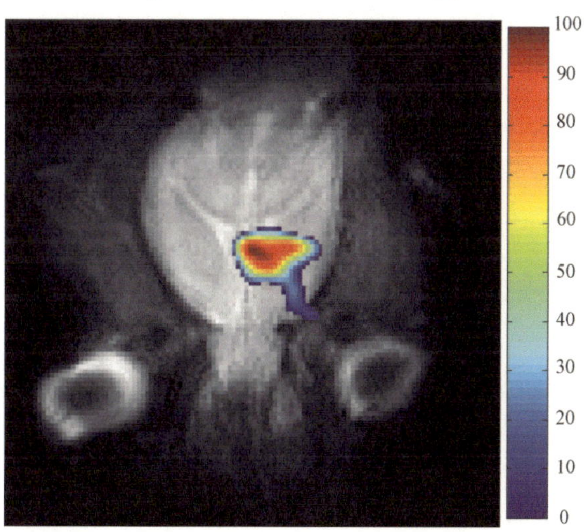

Fig. 5. ^{19}F-BPA-fr complex bio-distribution map in C6 glioma model at 2.5h after infusion (Porcari et al., 2008)

5. Conclusion

It is apparent from previous sections that BNCT is one of the most complex therapeutic modalities for brain tumour treatment. Due to the lack of progress in developing more effective treatments for high grade gliomas, the main challenge for BNCT in the near future, is to become a clinically useful treatment modality. Our work in optimizing the therapy has just this aim. Our research has been focused in overcoming some of the major limitations of BNCT effectiveness.

Firstly, in order to improve ^{10}B accumulation within the tumour, we demonstrated, both *in vitro* and *in vivo*, the potential of L-DOPA to enhance tumour uptake of BPA (Capuani et al., 2008, 2009). The most interesting findings of this work were the increased BPA tumour uptake *in vitro*, with C6 glioma cells, as well as *in vivo*, with C6 glioma model. Indeed, the L-DOPA preloading increased the BPA intracellular accumulation in C6 glioma cells 5 times with 4-hours of L-DOPA incubation (Capuani et al., 2008). The BPA tumour uptake in C6 glioma model (Capuani et al., 2008) increased 2.7 times. Interestingly, there was no increasing of BPA uptake in a normal brain. These stimulating results encourage the potential use of L-DOPA in BNCT of brain tumours because of L-DOPA ability to induce a significant enhancement of BNCT effectiveness without remarkable associated side effects. Moreover, the use of L-DOPA in BNCT clinical trials could be also facilitated because of its long-standing clinical use as a treatment for Parkinson's disease.

In order to determine the optimal irradiation time improving the BNCT efficiency, ^{19}F MR imaging and spectroscopy methodologies were proposed for investigating the pharmacokinetics and bio-distribution of BPA (Porcari et al., 2008; 2009). The correlation between both imaging and spectroscopic results obtained on glioma model highlights a better understanding of ^{19}F–BPA uptake either in the tumour or in systemic circulation confirming evidence of maximum BPA uptake within the tumour at 2.5 hours after infusion (Porcari et al., 2008). These results demonstrate that both ^{19}F MRI and ^{19}F MRS are feasible and practical methodologies with potential future clinical application. Indeed, ^{19}F NMR can be performed with an ^{1}H MR clinical scanner with only minor hardware and software improvements. Both of the solutions proposed to improve BNCT effectiveness will help the therapy to overcome its main hindrances to become a clinically useful modality in the near future.

6. Some standard abbreviations and symbols

^{10}B	Boron-10 isotope
BBB	Blood Brain Barrier
BNCT	Boron Neutron Capture Therapy
BPA	*p*-boronophenylalanine
BPA-fr complex	*p*-boronophenylalanine-fructose complex
Br:Bl	brain-to-blood
BSH	sodium borocaptate
^{14}C	Carbon-14 isotope
γ rays	gamma rays
ICP-AES	Inductively Coupled Plasma-Atomic

	Emission Spectrometry
^{19}F-BPA	fluorinated analogue of BPA
^{19}F-BPA-fr complex	^{19}F-BPA-fructose complex
^{19}F-MRI	Fluorine Magnetic Resonance Imaging
^{19}F-MRS	Fluorine Magnetic Resonance Spectroscopy
^{19}F-NMR	Fluorine Nuclear Magnetic Resonance
GBM	Glioblastomas Multiforme
^{1}H, ^{2}H	Hydrogen isotopes
$^{4}_{2}H$	Alpha particle
HPCL	High Performance Liquid Chromatography
^{7}Li	Lithium-7 isotope
L-DOPA	L-3,4-dihydroxyphenylalanine
LET	Linear Energy Transfer
MRI	Magnetic Resonance Imaging
MRS	Magnetic Resonance Spectroscopy
MRSI	Magnetic Resonance Spectroscopy Imaging
n_{th}	thermal neutron
^{14}N, ^{15}N	Nitrogen isotopes
NMR	Nuclear Magnetic Resonance
p	proton
PET	Positron Emission Tomography
σ	cross-sections
RBE	Relative Biological Effectiveness
T:Bl	tumour-to-blood
T:Br	tumour-to-brain
WHO	World Health Organization

7. Acknowledgment

We acknowledge support from Italian Institute of Technology under the Seed project BACT-MOBIL.

8. References

Barth, R.F., Coderre, J.A., Vicente, M.G. & Blue, T.E. (2005). Boron neutron capture therapy of cancer: current status and future prospects. *Clinical Cancer Research*, Vol. 11, No. 11, (June 2005), pp. 3987-4002, ISSN 1557-3265

Barth, R.F., & Soloway, A.H. (1997). Boron neutron capture therapy of brain tumors-current status and future prospects. *Journal of Neuro-Oncology*, Vol. 33, No. 1-2, (May 1997), pp. 3-7, ISSN 0167-594X

Barth, R.F., Soloway, A.H. & Brugger, R.M. (1996). Boron neutron capture therapy of brain tumors: past history, current status, and future potential *Cancer Investigation*, Vol. 14, No 6, pp. 534-50, ISSN 0735-7907

Barth, R.F., Soloway, A.H., Fairchild, R.G. & Brugger, R.M. (1992). Boron neutron capture therapy for cancer: Realities and prospects. *Cancer*, Vol. 70, No. 12, (December 1992), pp. 2995-3007, ISSN 0008-543X

Barth, R.F., Yang, W., Rotaru, J.H., Moeschberger, M.L., Boesel, C.P., Soloway, A.H., Joel, D.D., Nawrocky, M.M., Ono, K. & Goodman, J.H. (2000). Boron neutron capture therapy of brain tumurs: Enhanced survival and cure following blood-brain barrier disruption and intracarotid injection of sodium borocaptate and boronophenylalanine. *International Journal of radiation, oncology, biology, physics*, Vol. 47, No. 1, (April 2000), pp. 209-18, ISSN 0031-9155

Bendel, P. (2005). Biomedical application of ^{10}B and ^{11}B NMR. *NMR in Biomedicine,* Vol. 18, No. 2, (April 2005), pp. 74-82, ISSN 0952-3480

Bendel, P., Koudinova, N. & Salomon, Y. (2001). *In vivo* imaging of the neutron capture therapy agent BSH in mice using ^{10}B-MRI. *Magnetic Resonance in Medicine,* Vol. 46, No. 1, (July 2001), pp. 13-7, ISSN 1522-2594

Bendel, P., Margalit, R. & Salomon, Y. (2005). Optimized 1H MRS and MRSI methods for the *in vivo* detection of boronophenylalnine. *Magnetic Resonance in Medicine,* Vol. 53, No. 5, (May 2005), pp. 1166-71, ISSN 1522-2594

Blue, T.E. & Yanch, J.C. (2003). Accelerator-based epithermal neutron sources for boron neutron capture therapy of brain tumors. *Journal of Neuro-Oncology*, Vol. 62, No. 1-2, (March-April 2003), pp. 19-31, ISSN 0167-594X

Burian, J., Marek, M., Rataj, J., Flibor, S., Rejchrt, J., Viererbl, L., Sus, F., Honova, H., Petruzelka, L., Prokes, K., Tovarys, F., Dbaly, V., Benes, V., Kozler, P., Honzatko, J., Tomandl, I., Mares, V., Marek, J. & Syrucek, M. (2004). Report on the first patient group of the phase I BNCT trial at the LVR-15 reactor. (2004) *Proceeding of the 11th World Congress on Neutron Capture Therapy,* pp. 27-32, Boston, USA, October 11-15, 2004

Busse, P.M., Harling, O.K., Palmer, M.R., Kiger, W.S., Kaplan, J., Kaplan, I., Chuang, C.F., Goorley, J.T., Riley, K.J., Newton, T.H., Santa, Cruz, G.A., Lu, X.Q. & Zamenhof, R.G. (2003). A critical examination of the results from the Harvard-MIT NCT program phase I clinical trial of neutron capture therapy for intracranial disease. *Journal of Neuro-Oncology*, Vol. 62, No. 1-2, (March-April 2003), pp. 111-21, ISSN 0167-594X

Capala, J., Stenstam, B.H., Sköld, K., Munck af Rosenschöld, P., Giusti, V., Persson, C., Wallin, E., Brun, A., Franzen, L., Carlsson, J., Salford, L., Ceberg, C., Persson, B., Pellettieri, L. & Henriksson, R. (2003). Boron neutron capture therapy for glioblastoma multiforme: clinical studies in Sweden. *Journal of Neuro-Oncology*, Vol. 62, No. 1-2, (March-April 2003), pp. 135-44, ISSN 0167-594X

Capuani, S., Gili, T., Bozzali, M., Russo, S., Porcari, P., Cametti, C., D'Amore, E., Colasanti, M., Venturini, G., Maraviglia, B., Lazzarino, G. & Pastore, F.S. (2008). L-DOPA preloading increases the uptake of borophenylalanine in C6 glioma rat model: a new strategy to improve BNCT efficacy. *International Journal of Radiation, Oncology, Biology, Physics*, Vol. 72, No. 2, (October 2008), pp. 562-7, ISSN 0031-9155

Capuani, S., Gili, T., Bozzali, M., Russo, S., Porcari, P., Cametti, C., Muolo, M., D'Amore, E., Maraviglia, B., Lazzarino, G. & Pastore, F.S. (2009). Boronophenylalanine uptake in C6 glioma model is dramatically increased by L-DOPA preloading. *Applied Radiation and Isotopes,* Vol. 67, Suppl. 7-8, (March 2009), S.34-6, ISSN 0969-8043

Chanana, A.D., Capala, J., Chadha, M., Coderre, J.A., Diaz, A.Z., Elowitz, E.H., Iwai, J., Joel, D.D., Liu, H.B., Ma, R., Pendzick, N., Peress, N.S., Shady, M.S., Slatkin, D.N., Tyson, G.W. & Wielopolski, L. (1999). Boron neutron capture therapy for glioblastoma multiforme: interim results from the phase I/II dose-escalation studies. *Neurosurgery,* Vol. 44, No. 6, (June 1999), pp. 1182-93, ISSN 0148-396X

Coderre, J.A., Elowitz, E.H., Chandha, M.D., Bergland, R., Capala, J., Joel, D.D., Liu, H.B., Statkin, D.N. & Chanana, A.D. (1997). Boron neutron capture therapy for glioblastoma multiforme using p-boronophenyalanine and the epithermal neutrons: trial design and early clinical results. *Journal of Neuro-Oncology,* Vol. 33, No. 1-2, (May 1997), pp. 141-52, ISSN 0167-594X

Coderre, J.A. & Morris, G.M. (1999). The radiation biology of boron neutron capture therapy. *Radiation Research,* Vol. 151, No. 1, (January 1999), pp. 1-18, ISSN 0033-7587

Dagrosa, M.A., Thomasz, L., Longhino, J., Perona, M., Calzetta, O., Blaumann, H., Rebagliati, R.J., Cabrini, R., Kahl, S., Juvenal, G.J. & Pisarev, M.A. (2007). Optimization of boron neutron capture therapy for the treatment of undifferentiated thyroid cancer. *International Journal of Radiation, Oncology, Biology, Physics,* Vol. 69, No. 24, (November 2007), pp. 1059-66, ISSN 0031-9155

Diaz, A.Z. (2003). Assessment of the results from the phase I/II boron neutron capture therapy trials at the Brookhaven National Laboratory from a clinician's point of view. *Journal of Neuro-Oncology,* Vol. 62, No. 1-2, (March-April 2003), pp. 101-9, ISSN 0167-594X

Elowitz, E.H., Bergland, R.M., Coderre, J.A., Joel, D.D., Chadha, M. & Chanana, A.D. (1998). Biodistribution of p-boronophenylalanine in patients with glioblastoma multiforme for use in boron neutron capture therapy. *Neurosurgery,* Vol. 42, No. 3, (March 1998), pp. 463-93, ISSN 0148-396X

Henriksson, R., Capala, J., Michanek, A., Lindahl, S.A., Salford, L.G., Franzén, L., Blomquist, E., Westlin, J.E., Bergenheim, A.T. & Swedish Brain Tumour Study Group (2008). Boron neutron capture therapy (BNCT) for glioblastoma multiforme: a phase II study evaluating a prolonged high-dose of boronophenylalanine (BPA). *Radiotherapy and Oncology,* Vol. 88, No. 2, (March 2008), pp. 183-91, ISSN 0167-8140

Hickey, M.J., Malone, C.C., Erickson, K.L., Jadus, M.R., Prins, R.M., Liau, L.M. & Kruse, C.A. (2010). Cellular and vaccine therapeutic approaches for gliomas. *Journal of translational medicine,* Vol 14, No 8, pp.100, ISSN 1479-5876

Hsieh, C.H., Chen, Y.F., Chen, F.D., Hwang, J.J., Chen, J.C., Liu, R.S., Kai, J.J., Chang, C.W., & Wang, H.E. (2005). Evaluation of pharmacokinetics of 4-borono-2-(18)F-fluoro-L-phenylalanine for boron neutron capture therapy in a glioma-bearing rat model with hyperosmolar blood-brain barrier disruption. *Journal of Nuclear Medicine,* Vol. 46, No. 11, (November 2005), pp. 183-91, ISSN 1858-65

International Commission on Radiation Units and Measurements. (1998). *ICRU Report No. 60 - Fundamental Quantities and Units for Ionizing Radiation,* In ICRU Publications, (Ed.), ISBN 09-13394599, Bethesda, Maryland, U.S.A

Joensuu, H. (2000). Novel cancer therapies: more efficacy, less toxicity and improved organ preservation. *Annals of Medicine,* Vol. 32, No. 1, (February 2000), pp. 31-3, ISSN 0785-3890

Joensuu, H., Kankaanranta, L., Seppälä, T., Auterinen, I., Kallio, M., Kulvik, M., Laakso, J., Vähätalo, J., Kortesniemi, M., Kotiluoto, P., Serén, T., Karila, J., Brander, A., Järviluoma, E., Ryynänen, P., Paetau, A., Ruokonen, I., Minn, H., Tenhunen, M., Jääskeläinen, J., Färkkilä, M. & Savolainen, S. (2003). Boron neutron capture therapy of brain tumors: clinical trials at the finnish facility using boronophenylalanine. *Journal of Neuro-Oncology,* Vol. 62, No. 1-2, (March-April 2003), pp. 123-34, ISSN 0167-594X

Kabalka, W. G., Nichols, T. L., Smith, G. T., Miller, L. F., Khan, M. K. & Busse, P. M. (2003). The use of positron emission tomography to develop boron neutron capture therapy treatment plans for metastatic malignant melanoma. *Journal of Neuro-Oncology,* Vol. 62, No. 1-2, (March-April 2003), pp. 187-95, ISSN 0167-594X

Kankaanranta, L., Seppälä, T., Koivunoro, H., Saarilahti, K., Atula, T., Collan, J., Salli, E., Kortesniemi, M., Uusi-Simola, J., Mäkitie, A., Seppänen, M., Minn, H., Kotiluoto, P., Auterinen, I., Savolainen, S., Kouri, M., & Joensuu, H. (2007). Boron neutron capture therapy in the treatment of locally recurred head and neck cancer. . *International Journal of Radiation, Oncology, Biology, Physics,* Vol. 69, No. 2, (October 2007), pp. 475-82, ISSN 0031-9155

Keunen, O., Johansson. M., Oudin. A., Sanzey. M., Rahim, S.A., Fack, F., Thorsen, F., Taxt, T., Bartos, M., Jirik, R., Miletic, H., Wang, J., Stieber, D., Stuhr, L., Moen, I., Rygh, C.B., Bjerkvig, R. & Niclou, S.P. (2011). Anti-VEGF treatment reduces blood supply and increases tumor cell invasion in glioblastoma. *Proceedings of the National Academy of science of the United States of America,* Vol 108, No. 9, (March 2011), pp 3749-54, ISSN:0027-8424

Kleihues, P. & Cavenee, W.K. (2000). *Pathology and genetics of tumours of the nervous system, World Health Organization classification of tumours.* In Kleihues, P., Cavenee, W.K., (Ed.), IARC Press, ISBN 9283224094, Lyon, France

Laakso, J., Kulvik, M., Ruokonen, I., Vahatalo, J., Zilliacus, R., Farkkila, M. & Kallio, M. (2001) Atomic emission method for total boron in blood during neutron capture therapy. *Clinical Chemistry,* Vol. 47, No. 10. (October 2001), pp. 1796 - 803 ISSN 0009-9147

Louis, D.N., Ohgaki, H., Wiestler, O.D., Cavenee, W.K., Burger, P.C., Jouvet, A., Scheithauer, B.W. & Kleihues, P. (2007). The 2007 WHO classification of tumours of the central nervous system. *Acta Neuropathologica,* Vol. 114, No. 2, (July 2007), pp. 97-109, ISSN 1432-0533

Mischel, P.S., Shai, R., Shi, T., Horvath, S., Lu, K.V., Choe, G., Seligson, D., Kremen, T.J., Palotie, A., Liau, L.M., Cloughesy, T.F. & Nelson, S.F. (2003). Identification of molecular subtypes of glioblastoma by gene expression profiling. *Oncogene*, Vol. 22, No. 15, (April 2003), pp. 2361-73, ISSN 1476-5594

Mishima, Y. & Kondoh, H. (2000). Dual control of melanogenesis and melanoma growth: overview molecular to clinical level and the reverse. *Pigment Cell Research*, Vol. 13, Suppl. 8, pp. 10-22, ISSN 0893-5785

Nakagawa, N., Akai, F., Fukawa, N. Fujita, Y., Suzuki, M., Ono, K. & Taneda, M. (2007). Early effects of boron neutron capture therapy on rat glioma models. *Brain Tumor Pathology*, Vol. 24, No. 1, (May 2007), pp. 7-13, ISSN 1433-7398

Nakagawa, Y., Pooh, K., Kobayashi, T., Kageji, T., Uyama, S., Matsumura, A. & Kumada, H. (2003). Clinical review of the Japanese experience with boron neutron capture therapy and a proposed strategy using epithermal neutron beams. *Journal of Neuro-Oncology*, Vol. 62, No. 1-2, (March-April 2003), pp. 87-99, ISSN 0167-594X

Nichols, T.L, Kabalka, G.W., Miller, L.F., Khan, M.K. & Smith, G.T. (2002). Improved treatment planning for boron neutron capture therapy for glioblastoma multiforme using fluorine-18 labeled boronophenylalanine and positron emission tomography. *Physics in Medicine and Biology*, Vol. 29, No. 10, (October 2002), pp. 2351-8, ISSN 1361-6560

Ohgaki, H. & Kleihues, P. (2005). Population-based studies on incidence, survival rates, and genetic alterations in astrocytic and oligodendroglial gliomas. *Journal of Neuropathology and Experimental Neurology*, Vol. 64, No. 6, (June 2005), pp. 479-89, ISSN 0022-3069

Papaspyrou, M., Feinendegen, L.E. & Müller-Gärtner, H.W. (1994). Preloading with L-tyrosine increases the uptake of boronophenylalanine in mouse melanoma cells. *Cancer Research*, Vol. 54, No. 24, (December 1994), pp. 6311-4, ISSN 1538-7445

Porcari, P., Capuani, S., Campanella, R., La Bella, A., Migneco, L.M. & Maraviglia, B. (2006). Multi-nuclear MRS and ^{19}F-MRI of ^{19}F-labelled and ^{10}B-enriched p-boronophenylalanine-fructose complex to optimize boron neutron capture therapy: phantom studies at high magnetic fields. *Physics in Medicine and Biology*, Vol. 51, No. 12, (June 2006), pp. 3141-54, ISSN 1361-6560

Porcari, P., Capuani, S., D'Amore, E., Lecce, M., La Bella, A., Fasano, F., Campanella, R., Migneco, L.M., Pastore, F.S. & Maraviglia, B. (2008). *In vivo* ^{19}F-MRI and ^{19}F-MRS of ^{19}F-labelled boronophenylalanine-fructose complex on a C6 rat glioma model to optimize boron neutron capture therapy. *Physics in Medicine and Biology*, Vol. 53, No. 23, (December 2008), pp. 6979-89, ISSN 1361-6560

Porcari, P., Capuani, S., D'Amore, E., Lecce, M., La Bella, A., Fasano, F., Migneco, L.M., Campanella, R., Maraviglia, B. & Pastore, F.S. (2009). In vivo ^{19}F MR imaging and spectroscopy for the BNCT optimization. *Applied Radiation and Isotopes*, Vol. 67, Suppl. 7-8, (March 2009), S.365-8, ISSN 0969-8043

Riley, K.J., Binns, P.J., Harling, O.K., Kiger, W.S., González, S.J., Casal, M.R., Longhino, J., Larrieu, O.A. & Blaumann, H.R. (2008). Unifying dose specification between clinical BNCT centers in the Americas. *Medical Physics*, Vol.35, No. 4, (April 2008), pp. 1295-8, ISSN 0094-2405

Ryynanen, P., Kangasmaki, A., Hiismaki, P., Coderre, J. A., Diaz, A. Z., Kallio, M., Laakso, J., Kulvik, M., & Savolainen, S. (2002). Non linear models for the kinetics of 10B in blood after BPA-fructose complex infusion *Physics in Medicine and Biology*, Vol. 47, No. 7, (March 2002), pp. 737-45, ISSN 1361-6560

Ryynanen, P., Kortesnieni, M., Coderre, J. A., Diaz, A. Z., Hiismaki, P. & Savolainen, S. (2000). Models for estimation of the ^{10}B concentration after BPA-fructose complex infusion in patient during epithermal neutron irradiation in BNCT *International Journal of Radiation, Oncology, Biology, Physics*, Vol. 48, No. 1 , (November 2000), pp. 1145-54, ISSN 0031-9155

Sauerwein, W. (1993). Principles and history of neutron capture therapy. *Strahlentherapie und Onkologie*, Vol. 169, No. 1, (January 1993), pp.1-6, ISSN 0179-7158

Seppälä, T., Auterinen, I., Aschan, C., Serén, T., Benczik, J., Snellman, M., Huiskamp, R., Ramadan, U.A., Kankaanranta, L., Joensuu, H. & Savolainen, S. (2002). Dose planning with comparison to in vivo dosimetry for epithermal neutron irradiation of the dog brain. *Medical Physics*, Vol.29, No. 11, (November 2002), pp. 2629-40, ISSN 0094-2405

Slatkin, D.N. (1991). A history of neutron capture therapy of brain tumours. Postulation of a brain radiation dose tolerance limit. *Brain*, Vol. 114, No. Pt4, (August, 1991), pp. 1609-29, ISSN 0006-8950

Smith, D.R., Chandra, S., Coderre, J.A. & Morrison, G,H. (1996). Ion microscopy imaging of 10B from p-boronophenylalanine in a brain tumor model for boron neutron capture therapy. *Cancer Research*, Vol. 56, No. 19, (October 1996), pp. 4302-6, ISSN 1538-7445

Soloway, A.H., Barth, R.F., Gahbauer, R.A., Blue, T.E. & Goodman, J.H. (1997) The rationale and requirements for the development of boron neutron capture therapy of brain tumors. *Journal of Neuro-Oncology*, Vol. 33, No. 1-2, (May 1997), pp. 9-18, ISSN 0167-594X

Stupp, R., Mason, W.P., van den Bent, M.J., Weller, M., Fisher, B., Taphoorn, M.J., Belanger, K., Brandes, A.A., Marosi, C., Bogdahn, U., Curschmann, J., Janzer, R.C., Ludwin, S.K., Gorlia, T., Allgeier, A., Lacombe, D., Cairncross, J.G., Eisenhauer, E., Mirimanoff, R.O., European Organisation for Research and Treatment of Cancer Brain Tumor & Radiotherapy Groups; National Cancer Institute of Canada Clinical Trials Group & et al. (2005). Radiotherapy plus concomitant and adjuvant temozolomide for glioblastoma. *The New England Journal of Medicine*, Vol. 352, No. 4, (March 2005), pp. 987-996, ISSN 1533-4406

Suzuki, M., Sakurai, Y., Hagiwara, S., Masunaga, S., Kinashi, Y., Nagata, K., Maruhashi, A., Kudo, M. & Ono, K. (2007). First attempt of boron neutron capture therapy (BNCT) for hepatocellular carcinoma. *Japanese Journal of Clinical Oncology*, Vol. 37, No. 5, (May 2007), pp. Vol. 352, No. 4, (March 2005), pp. 987-996, ISSN 0368-2811

Tamura, Y., Miyatake, S., Nonoguchi, N., Miyata, S., Yokoyama, K., Doi, A., Kuroiwa, T., Asada, M., Tanabe, H. & Ono, K. (2006). Boron neutron capture therapy for recurrent malignant meningioma. Case report. *Journal of Neurosurgery*, Vol. 105, No. 6, (December 2006), pp. 898-903, ISSN 00223085

Van Meir, E.G., Norden, A.D., Hadjipanayis, C.G., Shu, H.K., Wen, P.Y. & Olson, J.J. (2010). Exciting New Advances in Neuro-Oncology: The Avenue to a Cure for Malignant Glioma. *CA: A Cancer Journal for Clinicians*, Vol. 60, No.3, (May-June 2010), pp. 166-93, ISSN 1542-4863

van Rij, C.M., Wilhelm, A.J., Sauerwein, W.A. & van Loenen, A.C. (2005). Boron neutron capture therapy for glioblastoma multiforme. *Pharmacy world & Science*, Vol 27, No. 2, pp 92-5, ISSN 2210-7703

Wang, H.E., Liao, A.H., Deng, W.P., Chang, P.F., Chen, J.C., Chen, F.D., Liu, R.S., Lee, J. S. & Hwang, J.J. (2004). Evaluation of 4-Borono-2-18F-Fluoro-L-Phenylalanine-Fructose as a probe for boron neutron capture therapy in a glioma-bearing rat model. *Journal of Nuclear Medicine*, Vol. 45, pp. 302-8, ISSN 0161-5505

Wittig, A., Malago, M., Collette, L., Huiskamp, R., Bührmann, S., Nievaart, V., Kaiser, G.M., Jöckel, K.H., Schmid, K.W., Ortmann, U. & Sauerwein, W.A. (2008a) Uptake of two ^{10}B-compounds in liver metastases of colorectal adenocarcinoma for extracorporeal irradiation with boron neutron capture therapy (EORTC Trial 11001). *International Journal of Cancer*, Vol. 122, No. 5, (March 2008), pp. 1164-71, ISSN 1097-0215

Wittig, A., Michel. J., Moss. R.L., Stecher-Rasmussen. F., Arlinghaus, H.F., Bendel, P., Mauri, P. L., Altieri, S., Hilger, R., Salvadori, P.A., Menichetti, L., Zamenhof, R. & Sauerwein, W.A.G. (2008b). Boron analysis and boron imaging in biological materials for Boron Neutron Capture Therapy. *Critical Reviews in Oncology/. Hematology*, Vol. 68, No. 1, (October 2008), pp. 66-90, ISSN 1040-8428

Wittig, A., Sauerwein, W.A. & Coderre, J.A. (2000). Mechanisms of transport of p-borono-phenylalanine through the cell membrane in vitro. *Radiation Research*, Vol. 153, No. 2, (February 2000), pp. 173-80, ISSN 1938-5404

Yamamoto, T., Nakai, K. & Matsumura, A. (2008). Boron neutron capture therapy for glioblastoma. *Cancer Letters*, Vol. 262, No. 2, (January 2008), pp. 143-52, ISSN 0340-3835

Yamamoto, T., Nakai, K., Nariai, T., Kumada, H., Okumura, T., Mizumoto, M., Tsuboi, K., Zaboronok, A., Ishikawa, E., Aiyama, H., Endo, K., Takada, T., Yoshida, F., Shibata, Y. & Matsumura, A. (2011). The status of Tsukuba BNCT trial: BPA-based boron neutron capture therapy combined with X-ray irradiation. *Applied Radiation and Isotopes*, Vol. 15, (February 2011), [Epub ahead of print], ISSN 0969-8043

Yang, W., Barth, R.F., Rotaru, J.H., Moeschberger, M.L., Joel, D.D., Nawrocky, M.M., Goodman, J.H. & Soloway, A.H. (1997). Boron neutron capture therapy of brain tumors: enhanced survival following intracarotid injection of sodium borocaptate with or without blood-brain barrier disruption. *International Journal of Radiation, Oncology, Biology, Physics*, Vol. 37, No. 3, (February 1997), pp. 663-72, ISSN 0031-9155

Yoshino, K., Suzuki, A., Mori, Y., Kakihana, H., Honda, C., Mishima, Y., Kobayashi, T. & Kanda, K. (1989). Improvement of solubility of p-boronophenylalanine by complex formation with monosaccharides. *Strahlentherapie und Onkologie*, Vol. 165, No. 2-3, (Febrary-March 1989), pp.127-9, ISSN 1439-099X

Zhu, X., Fujita, M., Snyder, L.A. & Okada, H. (2010). Systemic delivery of neutralizing antibody targeting CCL2 for glioma therapy. *Journal of Neuro-Oncology*, [Epub ahead of print], (Nov 2010), ISSN 0167-594X

Zuo, C.S., Prasad, P.V., Busse, P., Tang, L. & Zamenhof, R.G. (1999). Proton nuclear magnetic resonance measurement of *p*-boronophenylalnine (BPA): a therapeutic agent for boron neutron capture therapy. *Medical Physics*, Vol.26, No. 7, (July 1999), pp. 1230-

Part 8

Chemotherapy in CNS Tumors

12

Research the Mechanism of Various Antineoplastic Agents with Use of Flow Cytometry *in Vitro* Glioma Cells

Hideyuki Oshige, Yoshihiro Numa, Takuya Kawaguchi, Kunikazu Yoshimura, Akio Asai, and Keiji Kawamoto
Kansai Medical University
Japan

1. Introduction

Nowadays, steady progress like in endovascular, microsurgical, neuroendoscopic fields, affect deeply neurosurgergical field, too. But in spite of arising so many innovations, average survival time in glioma is a year and five year survival rate is 8%. These results have not slightly changed for 30 years.(*1)
For us to continue research glioma in future, our purpose discloses what we should be going to do for improve prognosis and needs to analyze data about tumor cells in the various views. In our laboratory, we research brain tumor with flow cytometory. In this chapter, we describe how to analyze the mechanism of various antineoplastic agents for tumor cells centered glioma and research results with flow cytometry.

2. Chemotherapy for central nerves system

There is Blood Brain Barrier, as you know, in central nervous system like a brain and a spinal cord. We can easy to understand the Blood Brain Barrier referred to fig 1(*2). Arteries and veins from subarachnoid space feed the brain after perforating vertically brain pia matter and extending into brain substance. In extending into brain substance, micro perivascular space is formed around vessels in brain substance. It is for us to observe a section of vessels in brain substance (Fig1-2). Vascular endothelium cells adhered to basement membrane form the structure like a tube with tight junction constituted by astrocyte and pericyte adhered outside of basement membrane. This structure formed the group of cells around basement membrane and tight junction between each endothelium around vessels is, so to speak, the Blood Brain Barrier.
The Blood Brain Barrier is hard to absorb aqueous solution. So This is the difference central nervous system from body except it. This property has been the limitation for developing chemotherapeutic drugs. According to same above reasons, chemotherapeutic drugs for glioma also were limited. But, recently, it has produced starting from ACNU, BCNU, CCNU, MCNU, bleomycin , IFN etc, via PCZ, VCR, to TMZ approved. Especially TMZ has been a standard drugs for glioma in the world. Though it gradually has progressed,

variation for combination therapy for glioma has increased too. In this time, we analyzed these chemotherapeutic drugs with FCM, LSC as below.

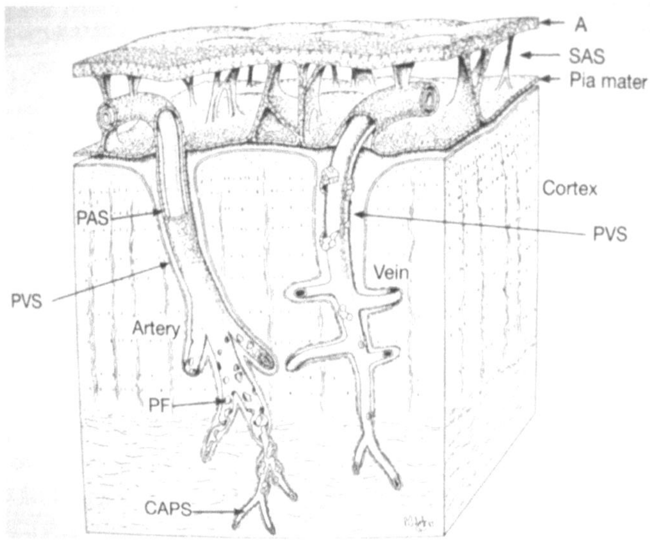

Abbreviation: A: Arachnoid membrane, SAS: Subarachnoid space, PAS: Periarterial space, PVS: Perivenous space, PF: Perforater foramen, CAPS: Capillary artery perispace

Fig. 1-1. Shows blood brain barrier.

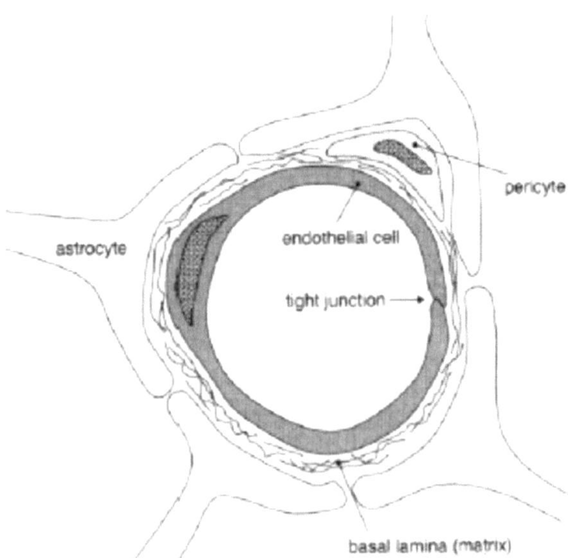

Fig. 1-2. Reveal tomography around of micro vessels in the brain.

2.1 Prostaglandin J2α(PGJ2α)

PGJ2α is one of eicosanoid producing in the body. In the beginning of 1980, it cleared up that PGD2 was produced after dehydration need to no enzyme. From the late of 1980 to the beginning of 1990, it was reported the very effective inhibition of tumor cells and viruses. So we expect to have thought of one of new antineoplasitc agent and antiviral drug. But it doesn't attains to apply clinically the glioma therapy, because it is unstable in the body. (*3)

2.2 Interferon (IFN)

IFN belongs to glycoprotein family. IFN has been reported it has direct effect for inhibition tumor growth, indirect effect with immune system and the synergy effect with other antineoplastic agents(*4). Though IFN has subtypes $\alpha \sim \gamma$, as shown our experimental result, IFNβ is the most effective for glioma(*5). But direct tumor suppression effect about IFN is only 18%. In the reports until now, IFN usually has effects combined with other antineoplastic agents. The famous report as for IFN combined with other drugs is about IAR(IFNβ+ACNU+Radiation) therapy. Median survival time about only radiation therapy, radiation+ACNU and IAR therapy were each 15.2 months, 19.7 months and 25.3 months. Initial response rate about radiation +ACNU, IAR therapy were each 35.7%, 60.5%. As this result, IAR therapy showed clearly better result than the other (level 4 evidence) (*28). Response rate in recent report about IAR therapy is 33%(*29).

2.3 ACNU

ACNU is the drug belonging to nitrosourea. This drug easily can pass through BBB. So this was standard drug against glioma until TMZ appeared. Though BCNU, CCNU, MCNU is developed in the West, ACNU is developed and used in Japan. As for metaanalysis, ACNU extended survival time to about one or two year and survival rate increased 6-10% and Median survival time extended to about two months. But this results were unsatisfied with us (*6,7).

2.4 CDDP, CBDCA

Cisplatin isn't general therapeutic drug against glioma.
Rosenberg et al reported it in 1965(*8). CDDP is one of the antineoplastic agent had very wide spectrum for various solid tumors. On the other hand, CDDP has high percentage of side effect like a toxicity of kidney, the digestive system and auditory system. Carboplatin (CBDCA) induced from CDDP was developed in order to reduce the toxicity CBDCA is platinum antineoplastic agent in second generation and was developed in England by Harrap. Though CBDCA has less antineoplastic effect than CDDP, CBDCA reduces clearly side effect like the toxicity for kidney, the digestive system and auditory system(*9).

2.5 As_2O_3 (Arsenic trioxide)

As_2O_3, which is originally used to treat acute promyelocytic leukemia (APL) since the early 1970s at Harbin Medical University in China, has drawn attention to treat solid tumors including gliomas. As_2O_3 enhanced radiation response and increase cure rate of glioma patients.Mechanisms that might explain the anti-tumor cytotoxicity of As_2O_3 include its ability to induce cellular differentiation, tumor apoptosis, the degradation of specific APL transcripts, and inhibition of tumor cell growth by modulating redox balance and/or mitochondrial membrane potential.(*24)

2.6 Temozolomide (TMZ)

Temozolomide belongs to the second generation of alkylating agents, and it can be orally. This drug has become a standard antineoplastic agent against malignant glioma. The effectiveness of this drug has been verified with much evidence. From 1995 to 1997, Yung et al. studied the first endpoint of 6 months without tumor progression in cases of recurrent anaplastic astrocytoma after addition of 200mg/m2 TMZ during the first 5 days. They analyzed about 111 of 162 anaplastic astrocytoma or anaplastic oligodendrocytoma cases diagnosed in their pathology center. As a result of these analyses, over all response rate (RR) is 66%; for anaplastic astrocytoma, RR is 62%. The complete response rate is 6% and the partial response rate is 28%. At present, relatively good outcomes are ensured and have been accumulated in phase studies such as those by the RTOG Group. One of the representative phase Ⅲ study is the research that ,so to speak, Stupp regimentation was added against cohort of 573 cases caught initially GBM by EORTC (European Organization for Research and Treatment of Cancer) and NCIC(national cancer institute of Canada). In summary, induction therapy is GBM after tumor resection is irradiated 60Gy and given TMZ (75mg/m2/day) for 6 week. Maintenance therapy is they gave 6 courses, when one course is TMZ (150～200mg/m2/day) for 5 days on and 23 days off. In the result from this comparison only irradiation with this regimentation, MST (median survival time) is 14.6 months in 247 cases administrated TMZ and irradiated, 12.1 months in 286 cases only irradiated. 2 year's survival rate is 26.5% in TMZ group, 10.4% in irradiated group. Hazard ratio for death is 38% statistically dominant decrease. In spite of excellent result like these, incidence of blood toxicity was only 7%.TMZ prized a level Ⅰ evidence.

As above, we used flow cytometer and laser cytometer for tools of analysis the drugs for pharmacological mechanism already known on the basis of cell kinetics.

3. History of flow cytometry (Fig2) and laser cytometry

Flow cytometer was developed for cancer research in Los Alamos institute in 1959, simultaneously, for immune system research in Stanford University. Then, various flow cytometer are developed as fig2. Recently, a serious of FACS made in BD corporation and Epix made in Coulter company and so on are familiarized. These developments caused we can measure amount of various kinds of ingredients like intracellular DNA and of protein, can easy to analyze cell cycle too. In addition, it could see, measure amount of antigens on cell surface, major progress with immunology field.

On the other hand, it had developed image cytometry of analyses about cell figures and so on. In 1976, Kawamoto in our institution started the measure intracellular DNA of brain tumors, in his being in Monte Fiore Hospital in New York. In 1976, he used with the prototype of Fluorograph (Fig3-1), which could measure amount of DNA and its histogram, not analyze cell cycles. In 2011, we use, in our institution, FACS Calivur (Fig3-2), which can analyze simultaneously and automatically histogram, cell cycle, DNA index (DI) calculate. In 1991, Kamentsky et al invented Laser Scannning Cytometer(LSC) which was the machine having dual character of FCM and image cytometory. LSC can analyze automatically amount of DNA and grasp cell figures, after put above the slide prepared for a microscope.

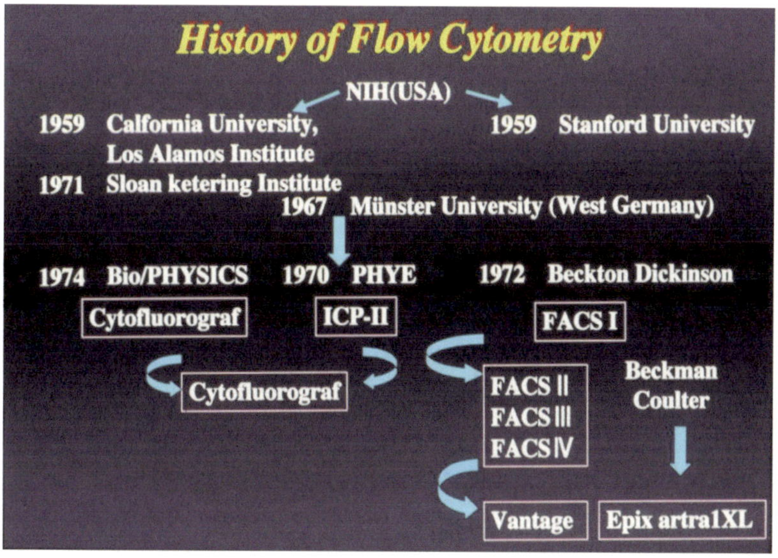

Fig. 2. History of Flow Cytometry

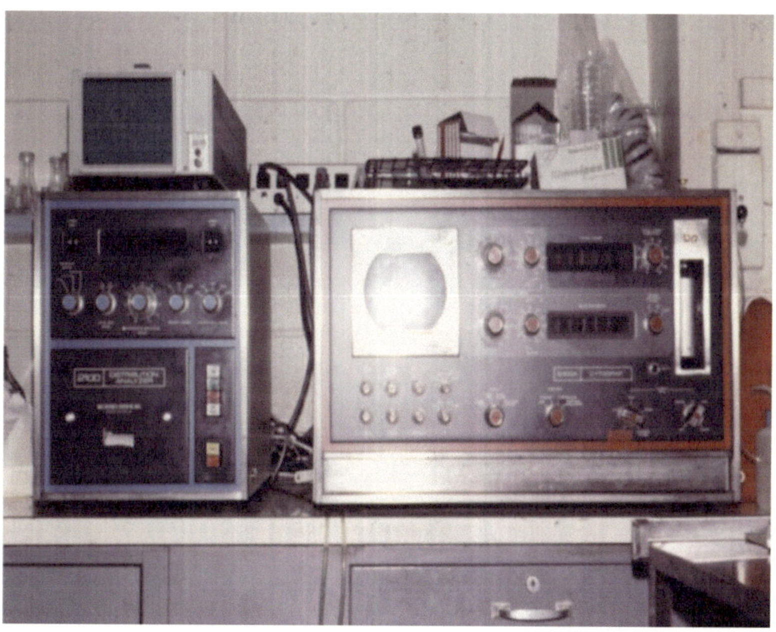

Fig. 3-1. Prototype of Fluorograph could measure amount of DNA and its histogram, not analyze cell cycles (in1976, Monte Fiore Hospital, New York).

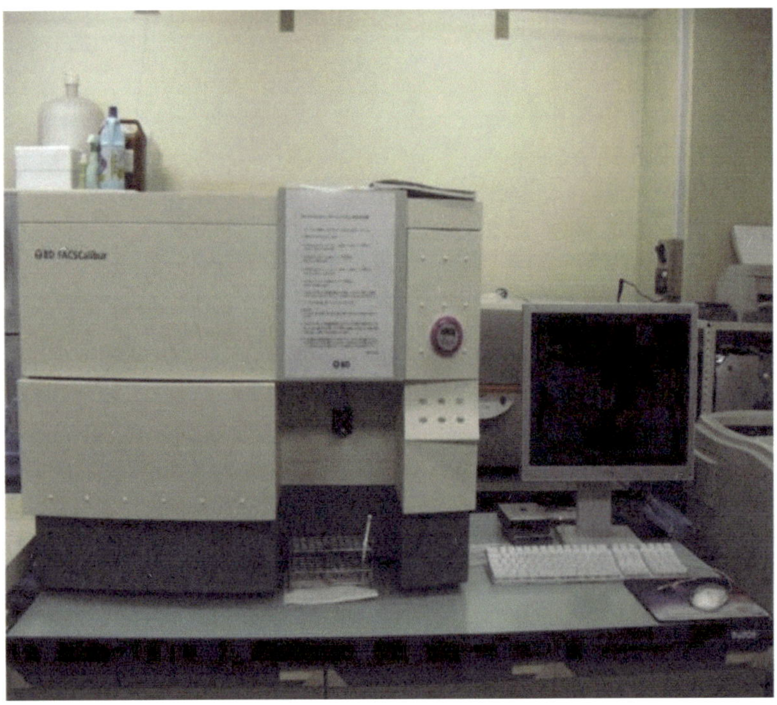

Fig. 3-2. FACS Calivur in our institution can analyze simultaneously and automatically histogram, cell cycle, DNA index (DI) calculated .

4. The principle of flowcytometry (Fig4)

Isolated cell stained with fluorescent pigment dropped from the nozzle. After laser hit each cells, it can identify fluorescence dividing into two directions. These fluorescences are frontal scatter fluorescence meaning cell size (figure) and lateral scatter fluorescence meaning biological property (=relative amount of DNA). Sensors on each direction translate these intensities into electric signals depending on amount of DNA, and conduct electric circuit (*10). We can analysis passing these signals from 1000 to 5000 cells per second with computer. More advanced machine can sort cells through making dropped cells plus or minus charge, so to speak, cell sorting (*11,12). Because these machines are delicate, we have to adjust repeatedly for reliable datum. Mainly, these adjustments include flow system, the axis of laser. It is important to line up stable laser and water pressure for continue to flow isolated cells with regular speeds and orderly from the nozzle. As it repeats the adjustments on two or three times with, for example, micro beads, calculates coefficient of variation: CV of histogram. In this time, CV with micro beads hopes to be less than 2%. About how to adjust in detail, you had better refer to texts and papers (*13,14)

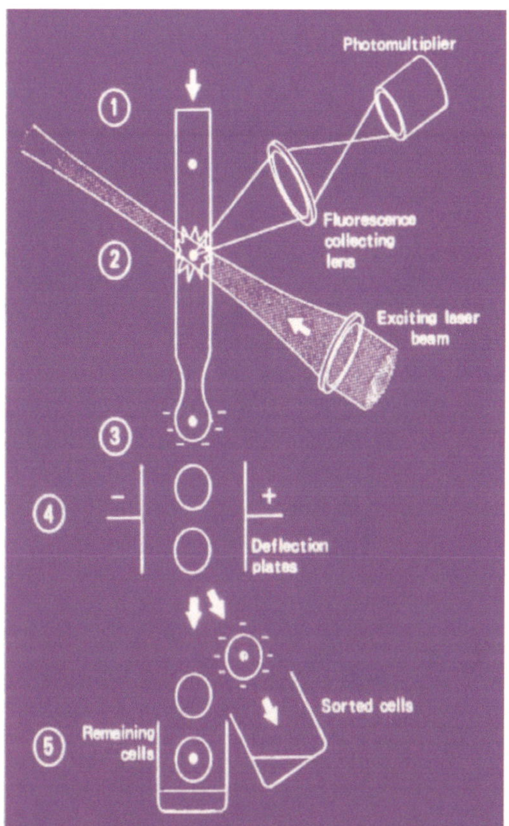

Fig. 4. Figure reveals principle of flow cytometory. Isolated cell droped from the nozzle. Laser hit each cells. We can analysis passing this laser from 1000 to 5000 cells. More advanced machine can sort cells through making dropped cells plus or minus charge. This technique can choose cells we can point out free.

5. About scattergram (dotgram)

The data analyzed with flowcytometer good adjusted reveals a scattergram (dotgram) like fig 5. Scattergram (dotgram) is consist of x axis set frontal scatter concentration of fluorescence and y axis set lateral scatter concentration of fluorescence, is the aggregation result from plotting on the basis of each value. Because this aggregation includes debris of cells and unnecessary cells, we need to narrow moreover aiming cells. What we do to narrow aiming cells is called gating procedure. Gate is the procedure sort a aiming group of cells on the basis of wavelength of beam, from whole group of cells. Fig 5 reveals dotgram consisted of X axis set 7-AAD used in measuring amount of DNA and Y axis set BrdU used in measuring amount of cells in S phase. Revealing concretely with Fig 5, the procedure of gating is surrounding square each group of cells. If it sets up gating on same condition, you can measure the percentage of any cell groups in whole of objective group (In fig.5, you can measure how percentage of each cell in each cell cycle). In addition, if you stain cells with monoclonal antigen with FITC (BrdU with FITC in fig5), can response differentially antigen on cell surface, you can measure quickly and objectively not only whether antigen stained with fluorescence or not, but also measure that densities.

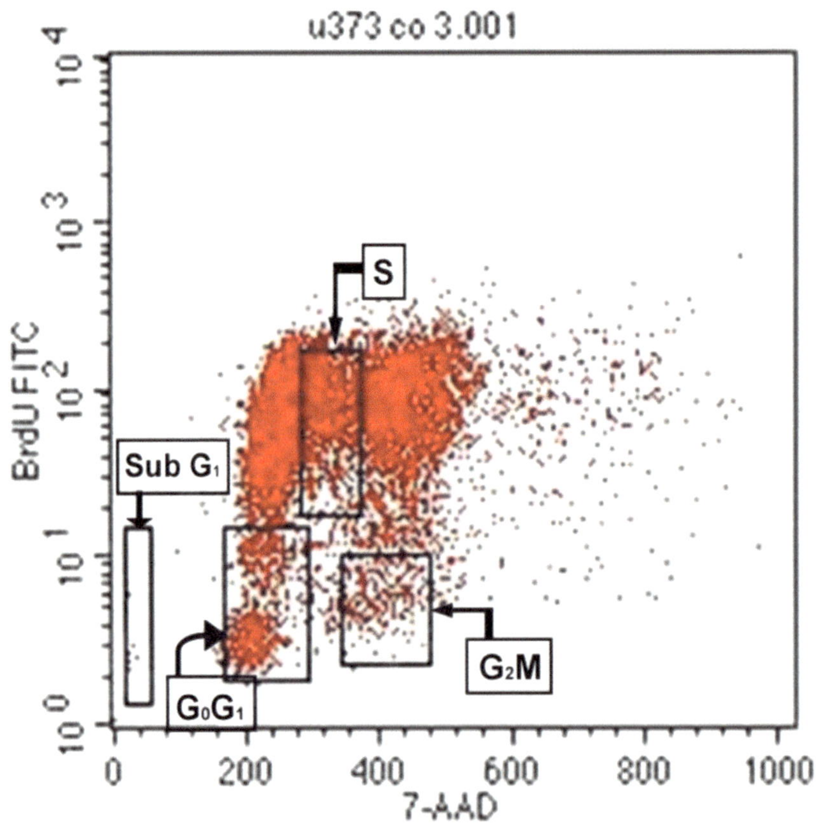

Fig. 5. This is the dotgram consisted of X axis set 7-AAD and Y axis set BrdU with FITC.

6. About histogram

Various kinds of fluorescence stain are used in measuring amount of nuclear DNA. It is hoped that these amount of fluorescence pigment in linear proportion to amount of DNA. In our institution, we use PI (Propidum iodide), 7-AAD (Actinomycin D). As s result of measure amount of DNA depending on amount of fluorescence pigment, it reveals DNA histogram. Generally, there are G_0G_1 phase cells having DNA amount of 2C, G_2M phase cells having DNA amount of 4C and S (=synthesis) phase cells between G_0G_1 and G_2M phase. Because in S phase the reason of overlap a group of cells in early S phase with a group of cells in G_0G_1 phase and the reason of overlap a group of cells in late S phase with a group of G_2M phase, we have difficulty in identifying a group cells in S phase. Various mathematical models for calculate each division of S, G_0G_1, S, G_2M on cell cycles, were reported. For example, Baisch.H et al(*15), Bariogie B et al(*19), Fried et al(*17,18) were reported. In this time, we adopted three-division method (Kawamoto et al) (*16) (Fig6).

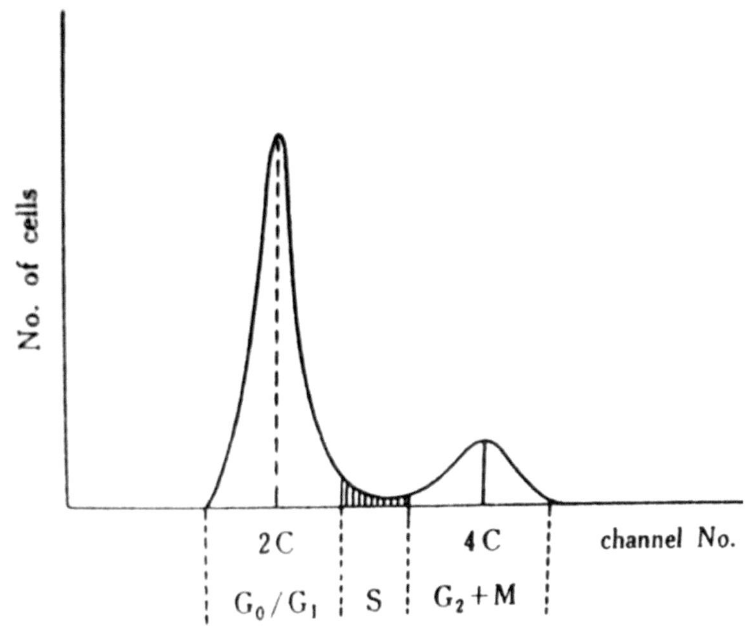

First peak, G_0G_1 phase; second peak G_2M phase; between two peaks, S phase

Fig. 6. The three-division histogram method (Kawamoto et al.).

7. Clinical material and method

We used the target cells as follow: human glioma cell lines like U373, U251, U87MG, KMU100, rat glioma cell lines like 9-LMG, C6 and KB cell line (nasopharyngeal carcinoma. Depending on each experiment, we added each cell line to medium concentration dose near ED50 (effective dose 50%) and high concentration dose more than ED 50. ED50 was decided on the basis of result from basic experiment like phase I study. Cell killing effect depending on concentration of dose was assessed with cell count depending on process of times and days. Simultaneously, we analyzed the histograms with FCM (or LSC) depending on process of days. When we make the specimen for FCM, we can easy to understand in sight through sometimes using double staining (BrdU, PI, 7AAD etc.) method depending on process of days. Drugs our analyses histogram in this chapter are ACNU, IFN, PGJ2 α, DCCP, A2O3, TMZ.

7.1 Culture method

The established cell lines were subjected to monolayer culture in minimum essential medium (MEM) and dMEM(Dulbecco's modified Eagle's medium)(Gibco:high glucouse with L-glutamine with pyridoxine hydrochloride without sodium pyruvate or sodium bicarbonate) supplemented with 10% fetal bovine serum(FBS) in a 5% CO2 incubator.

7.2 How to make specimen for FCM

A single suspended cell according to method our draw above was fixed by 70% ethanol. After it was made reaction of 0.5% RNAse treatment under 37℃ for 30 minutes, 7AAD or PI staining treated cells went into FCM owing to measure amount of DNA. Flow cytometers we used were FACStar and FACS Calivur supported by Becton Dickinson (BD) Corporation. For example, FACStar's laser has wavelength of 488nm, wave strength of 200-500mW and long pass filter of 520nm.

7.3 Double staining method

For example, in the case that you want to ensure specifically S phase cell, you make reaction monoclonal antibody to BrdU with IgG labeled FITC. Everyone has understood DNA uptake BrdU (Bromodeoxyuridine) as thymidine (*20). After monoclonal antibody ensured BrdU which was developed by Gratzner et al (*21) in 1982, we can analyze cell growth with BrdU. Though BrdU is taken into intranuclear DNA in synthesis (S) phase, we can identify cells taken anti BrdU antibody by stain after short time treatment. If Z axis are set the density of dots in dotgram in addition to X axis set PI or 7AAD and Y axis set BrdU, we can get 3D expression of histogram. 3D histogram makes us easy to sight cell distribution in S phase (fig7).

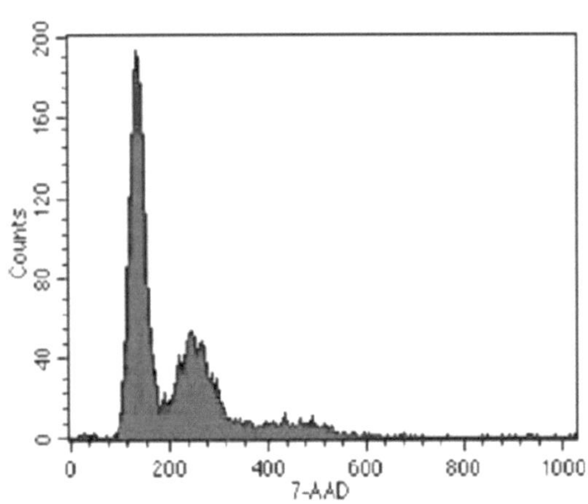

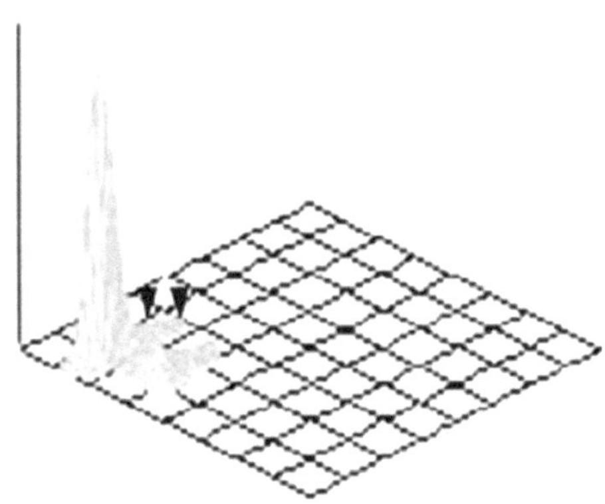

Fig. 7. Example of exchange 2D (left graph) for 3D expression (right graph) It is hard to identify S-phase cell accumulation with 3D expression (arrowheads)

On the other hand, when you want to check the cell viability, you had better stain with Fluorescein diacetate (FDA). Like these examples, when it identifies specifically the relationship between cell cycles and cell distributions, this technique is inducted.
Studies and results about each antineoplastic agents.
Summary of our results are below.

1. PGJ2 blocks cell cycle at G_0G_1.
2. IFN 、ACNU 、CDDP、As_2O_3 、TMZ block cell cycle at S phase.
3. ACNU、CDDP、As_2O_3、TMZ blocks at G_2M phase.

7.3.1 Prostaglandin J2α(PGJ2α)

We tried to analyze the mechanism of PGJ2α with FCM after addition for PGJ2α to tumor cells(Fig8). The cells distribution in S phase are disappeared after addition for PGJ2α to tumor cells. In other words, cells accumulate in G_0G_1phase and G_2M phase. So PG is effective to G_0G_1 phase.

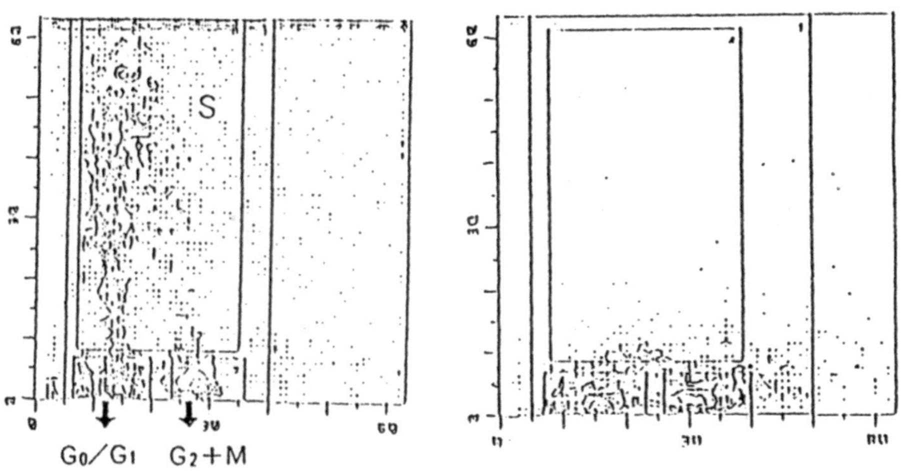

Left graph is control. Right graph is in case of add PG. Cells in S phase are disappear and cells accumulate in G_0G_1, G_2M phase. Results from the above, we thought, PGJ2α effect for GoG1 phase.

Fig. 8. Reveals dotgram meaning the mechanism of PGJ2α's antineoplastic effect.

7.3.2 Interferon (IFN)

In the case of IFN, after we added each α, β, γ IFN(low~high dose like 10^2~10^5IU/ml) to U373MG(10^5/dish), counted cells on 1st ,3rd,5th day. Results of that, we studied the suppression effect of propagate. When studied the graph about cell count after addition of IFN α, β, γ as figure 9, we can observe the suppression of cell count depending on the IFN concentration .

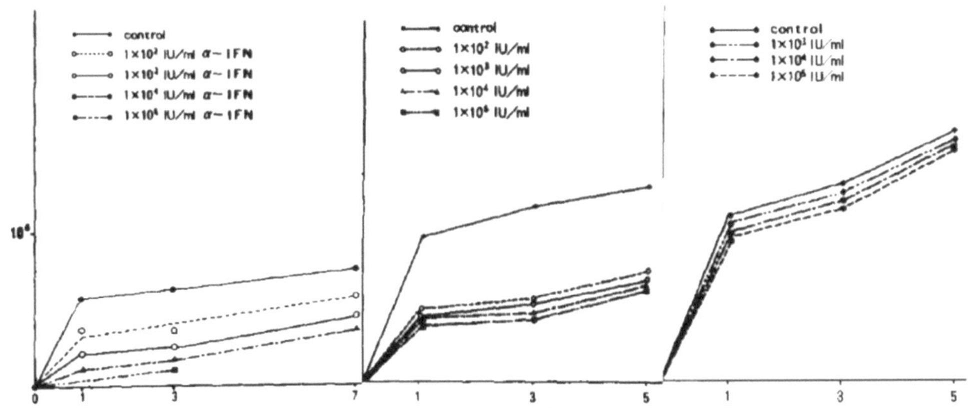

Fig. 9. Graphs from left to right reveal graph of α,β,γ. Concentrations are heighen increasing from upper to lower. The drug having the biggest subtraction from control was IFN βwhich had the highest suppression of propagation. IFN α had second suppression of propagation. In this experiment, IFN γ has not almost suppression of propagation.

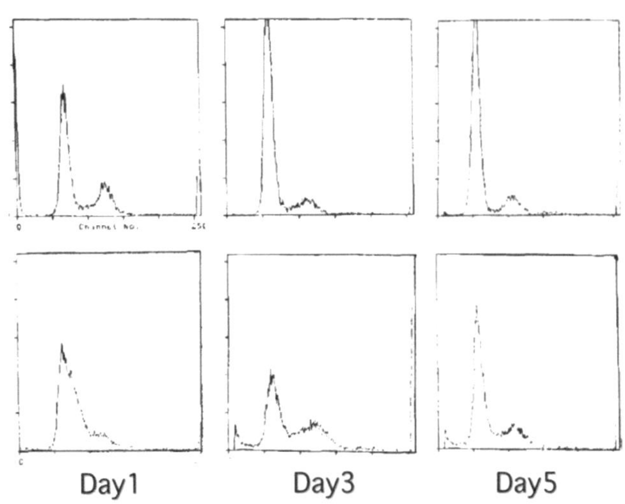

Fig. 10. Upper row is control. Lower row is histograms of IFNβ. IFNβ has early S phase block earlier than control group. Then, S phase block was clarified on 3rd day. On 5th day, it was observed recruitment.

The drug having the biggest subtraction from control was IFN βwhich had the highest suppression of propagation. IFN α had second suppression of propagation. In this experiment, IFN γ has not almost suppression of propagation. As a result of this, we studied cell kinetics with IFNβ. After 104IU/ml IFNβ was added to U373MG(105/dish), we counted cells on 1st ,3rd,5th day and analyzed histogram with FCM. These results are like Fig10. IFNβ has early S phase block earlier than control group. Then, S phase block was clarified on 3rd day. On 5th day, it was observed recruitment.

7.3.3 ACNU

It reveals a DNA histogram resulted from the addition 5μg/ml 、10μg/ml ACNU to U251MG cell lines(fig 11). Standard histogram is revealed in the group of control without the addition ACNU. The histogram a day after addition 10μg/ml ACNU reveals DNA accumulation in S phase meaning S phase block. Moreover, histogram two days after addition 5μg/ml ACNU reveals DNA accumulation in G_2M phase and these cells were dead. So ACNU has effect both S and G_2M phase.

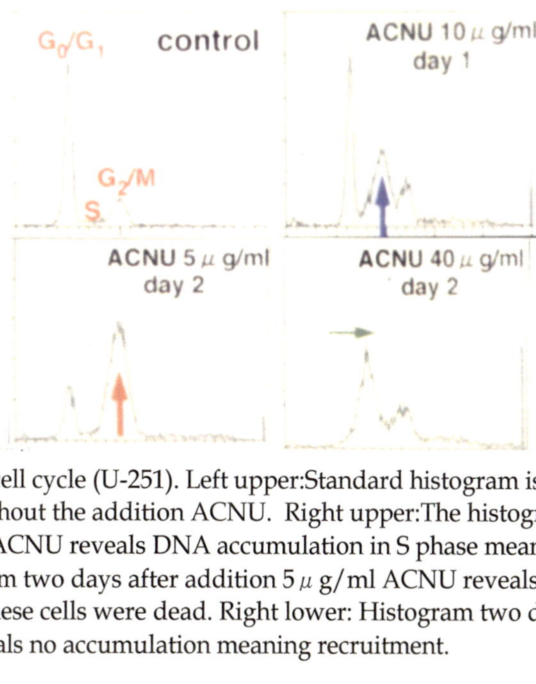

Fig. 11. Analysis of cell cycle (U-251). Left upper:Standard histogram is revealed in the group of control without the addition ACNU. Right upper:The histogram a day after addition 10μg/ml ACNU reveals DNA accumulation in S phase meaning S phase block. Left lower: Histogram two days after addition 5μg/ml ACNU reveals DNA accumulation in G_2M phase and these cells were dead. Right lower: Histogram two days after addition 40 μg/ml ACNU reveals no accumulation meaning recruitment.

7.3.4 CDDP, CBDCA

After it contacted KB cells with 2μg/ml thought ED50 for KB cells CBDCA for 24 hours or with 0.5μg/ml CDDP for 24 hours, KB cells were rinsed with PBS two times. It continued cell culture and analyzed with FCM, in case of CBDCA on 1st, 2nd, 3rd, in case of CDDP on 1st, 3rd, 5th, 7th day. In addition, it was performed double staining with BrdU and 3D analysis. In case of CBDCA, the peak in S phase of cell accumulation on 1st day transferred into the peak in G_2M phase of cell accumulation on 2nd and 3rd day (fig12). In case of CDDP, the peak in S phase on 1st, 3rd day transferred tended to migrate gradually into G_2M phase according to the progression like 5th, 7th day (fig13).

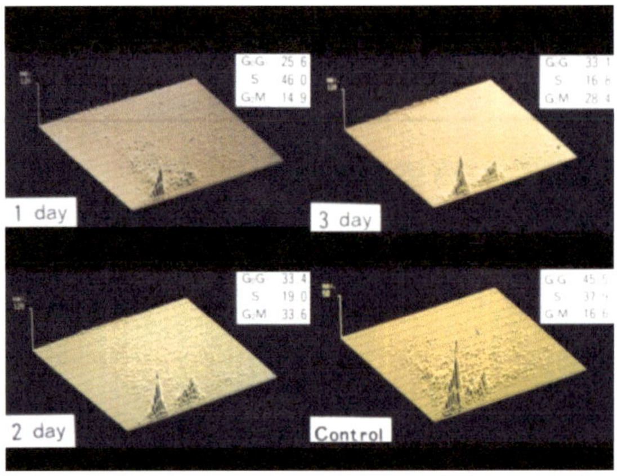

Fig. 12. 3D expression of Carboplatin reveals the peak in S phase of cell accumulation on 1st day transferred into the peak in G_2M phase of cell accumulation on 2nd -3rd day.

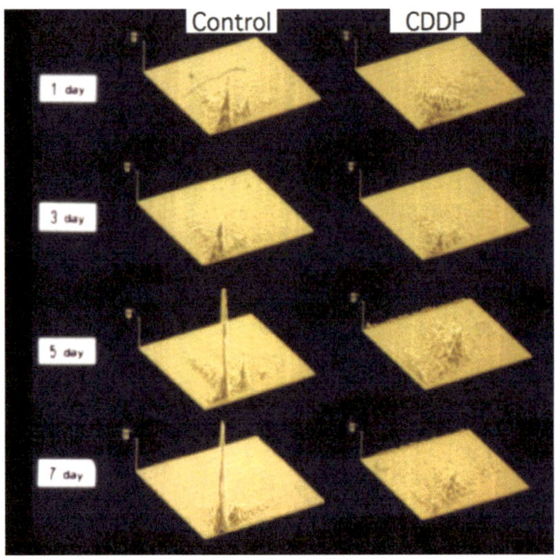

Fig. 13. 3D expression of cisplatin reveals the peak in S phase on 1st, 3rd day transferred tended to migrate gradually into G_2M phase according to the progression like 5th, 7th day .

Result from above, CBDCA has effect in S phase and G_2M phase. In case of CDDP, it has the same tendency. So CDDP has also effect in S phase and G_2M phase (*22)

7.3.5 As_2O_3

It analyzed the change depending on passing time after the addition As_2O_3 to U87MG and T98G cell lines with LSC (fig14).

In case of U87MG, it observed a DNA accumulation tendency in S phase until 24 hours from the addition, this peak immigrated into G_2M phase from 24 hours to 72 hours and it observed slight accumulation in sub G1 phase from 24 hours to 48 hours. Though the same tendency was in case of T98G, this tendency of cell accumulation was slight different from U87MG like fig 14. Result from the above, As_2O_3 has effective in S and G_2M phase (*23).

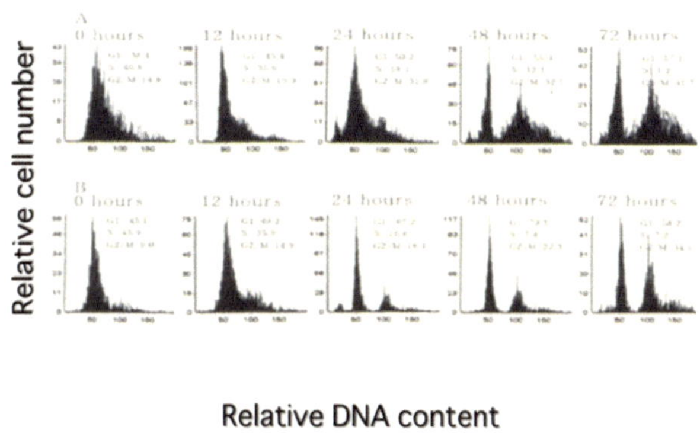

Fig. 14. Cellular DNA content frequency histograms demonstrating As_2O_3-induced changes in cell cycle distribution and apoptosis of U87MG(A) and T98G(B) cells.

7.3.6 Temozolomide(TMZ)

Each U373MG (human glioma cell line), U87MG (human) and 9L (rat) cell line was divided into three groups: a control group, a low-dose temozolomide group [addition,100～200 μg/ml temozolomide; near ED 50], and an high-dose temozolomide group [addition, 300～500 μg/ml]. On day 1, temozolomide was added to each cell line. Then, we counted the number of cells on days 2,3,4 and 5. In the U87MG line, we counted the number of cells on days 8 and 9. Simultaneously, we performed flow cytometric analysis with the double staining (7-AAD and BrdU)(fig 15).

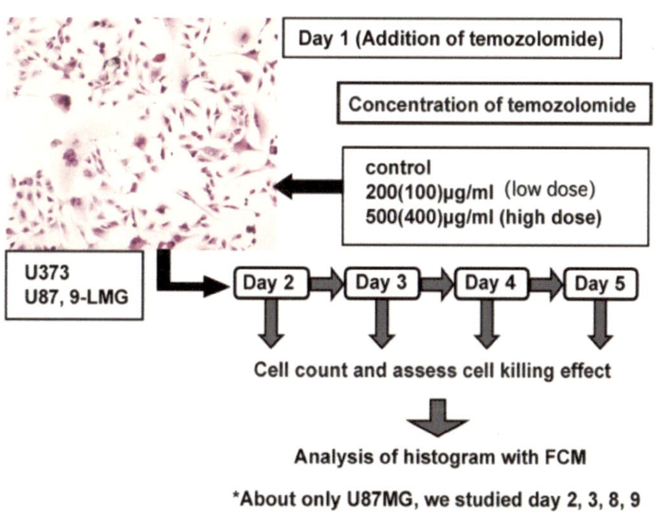

Fig. 15. This is experimental method about TMZ. Each cell line was divided into three groups, control group, low-dose TMZ group, high-dose TMZ group. On Day 1, TMZ was added to each cell line. Then, we counted the number of cells on Day 2, 3, 4, and 5. In U87MG, we counted the number of cells on Day 8 and 9. Simultaneously, we performed flow cytometric analysis with single and double staining methods.

7.4 Result 1

Suppression of cell proliferation with TMZ

Growth curves of all cell lines showed suppression of cell growth depended on TMZ concentration. A 50% cell-killing effect was obtained with 200-500 μg/ml TMZ in U373 and 100-400 μg/ml TMZ in U87MG and 9LMG. This concentration is considered the ED50 (fig16) In the U373MG cell line, a significant decrease(χ square test) in the growth curve was observed with 200 μg/ml and 500 μg/ml TMZ on day5. In the 9-LMG cell line, a significant decrease was observed in 100 μg/ml and 400 μg/ml TMZ after day 3.Tumor cells (in all cell lines) to which TMZ was added showed morphologically shrinkage of cell processes, ligetening of the nucleus and cell atrophy (fig 17).

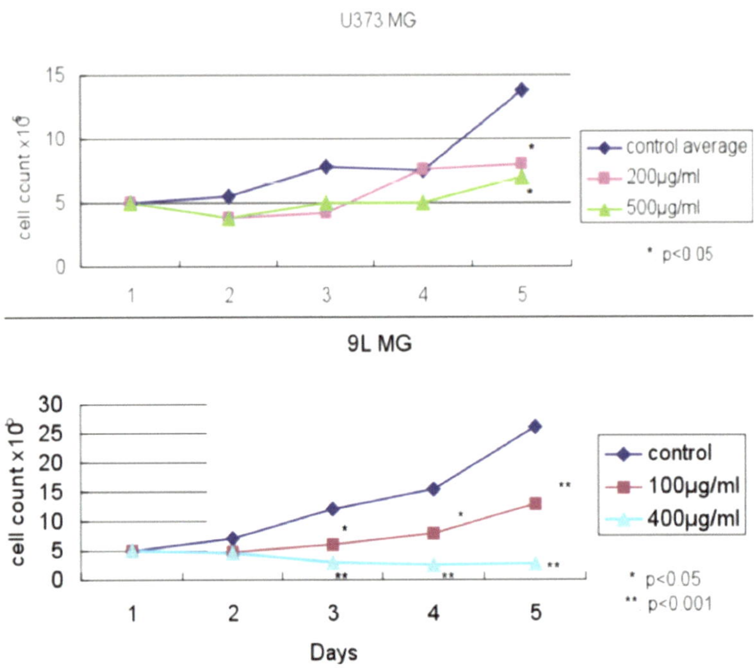

Fig. 16. Results of cell counts for U373MG and 9LMG. Both cell lines show that the cell killing effect depends on dose concentration.

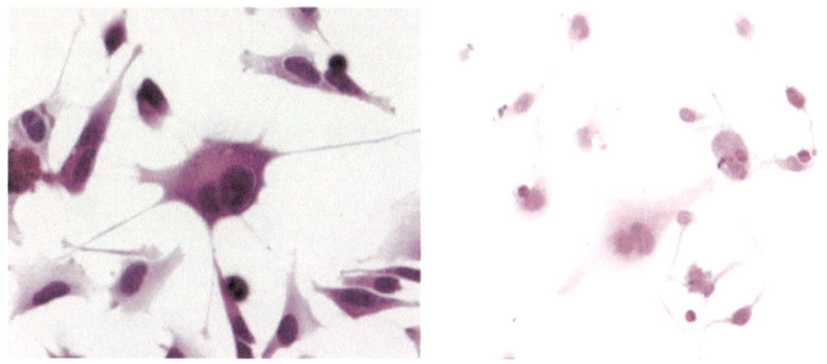

Left: normal glioma cells (before TMZ addition)
Right:Glioma cells after addtion of TMZ show shrinkage of cell processes pale nuclei, and call atrophy

Fig. 17. Morphological change of U373 cells with hemaatoxylin and eosin (H&E) stain before and after addition of TMZ

7.5 Result 2

Analyses of effect of TMZ on cell cycle with FCM: The U373MG cell line had a tendency to accumulate in the G_0G_1 and S phases on day2 though 4. On day 4 in the group with 200μg/ml TMZ added, or days 1 through 4 in the group with 500μg/ml TMZ added, we observed significant accumulation (fig 18-19). On days 4 though 5, there was a tendency for cells to accumulate in the G_2M phase. Especially on day 5, for 200μg/ml TMZ and on days 4 through 5, for 500μg/ml TMZ we observed significant accumulation (see fig19-1,2 and fig 18-3). The 9-L cell line also accumulated in the S phase from days 2 through 3 and then accumulated in the G_2M phase (see fig 19-3). The U87 MG cell line also accumulated in S phase on days 2 through 3, and then accumulation in G_2M phase, and finally in sub-G1 phase on days 8 through 9(see figs 18-5,6)
Result 3: The dominant morphological changes observed in U87MG were confined to the nuclei (fig 20), with positive terminal deoxynucleotidyl transferase-mediated dUTP-biotin nick-end labeling (TINEL) staining. These changes suggested apoptosis (*25).

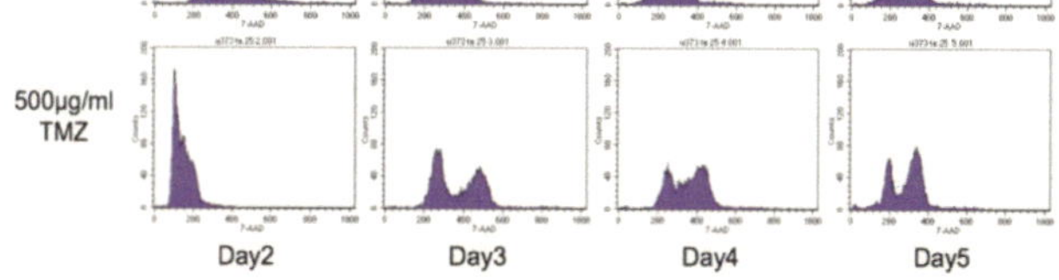

Fig. 18-1. Histogram for U373MG shows changing amount of DNA after addition of TMZ. By this histogram, we can see the G_2M-phase block after S-phase block. In addition, it shows clearly that the G_2M-phase block depends on TMZ concentration.

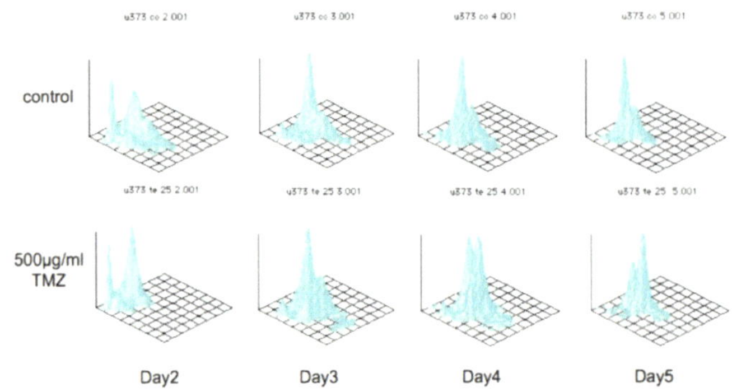

Fig. 18-2. For U373MG: 3D expression of changing amount of DNA by using TMZ. The G_2M-phase block after S-phase block is easily seen

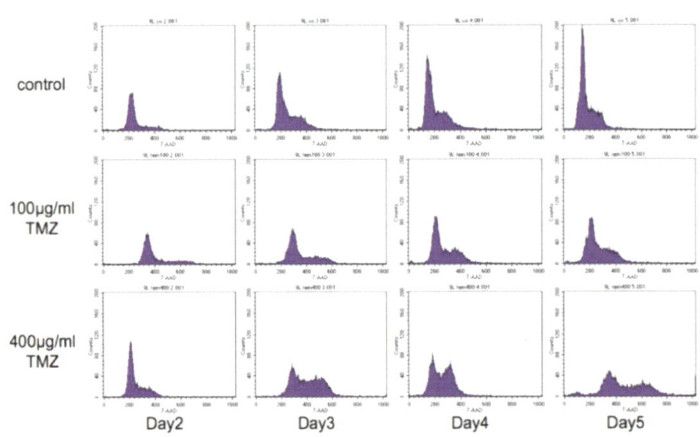

Fig. 18-3. Histogram for 9L MG shows changing amount of DNA after addition of TMZ. By this histogram, we can see the G2- phase block after S-phase block. In addition, it shows clearly that the G_2M-phase block after S-phase block depends on TMZ concentration.

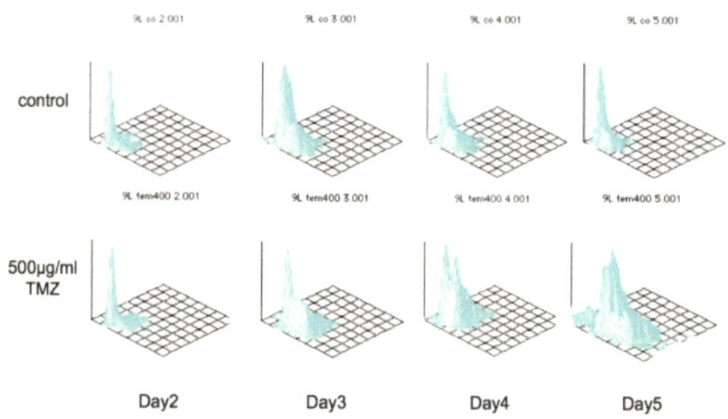

Fig. 18-4. 9LMG: 3D expression of changing amount of DNA by using TMZ. The G_2M - phase block after S-phase block is easily seen.

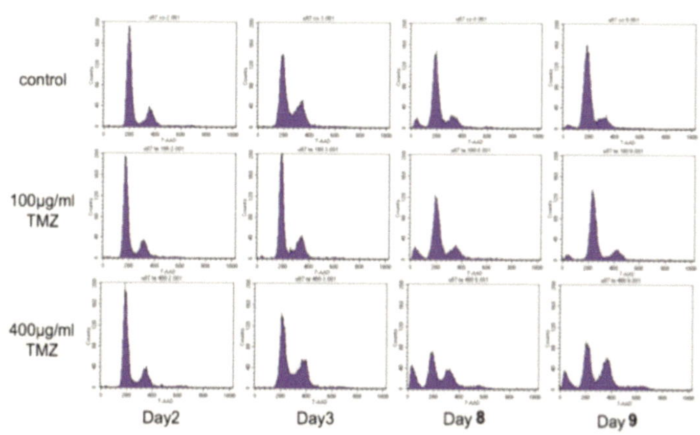

Fig. 18-5. Histogram for U87MG shows changing amount of DNA after addition of TMZ. The sub-G1 phase peak after S-phase block is easily seen.

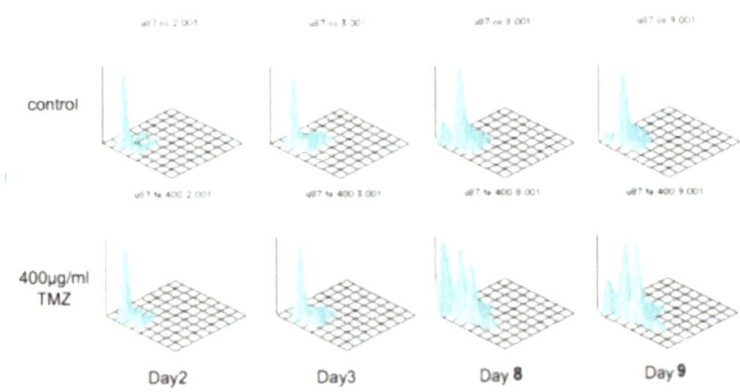

Fig. 18-6. U87MG: 3D expression of changing amount of DNA by using TMZ. The sub-G1 phase peak after S phase block is easily seen.

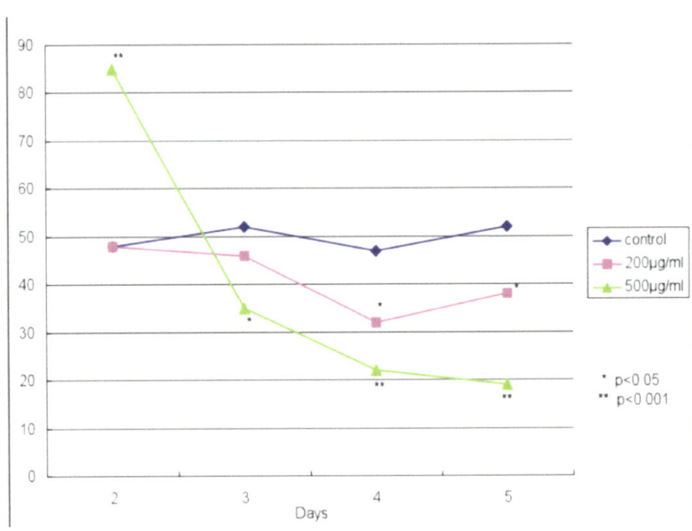

Fig. 19-1. Amount of DNA in G_0G_1 phase with U373MG. On day 2 of addition of 500µg/ml TMZ, we observed a statistically significant increase of DNA. On days 4 and 5 of addition of 200 and 500µg/ml TMZ, we observed a statistically significant decrease of DNA. We called this pattern left peak.

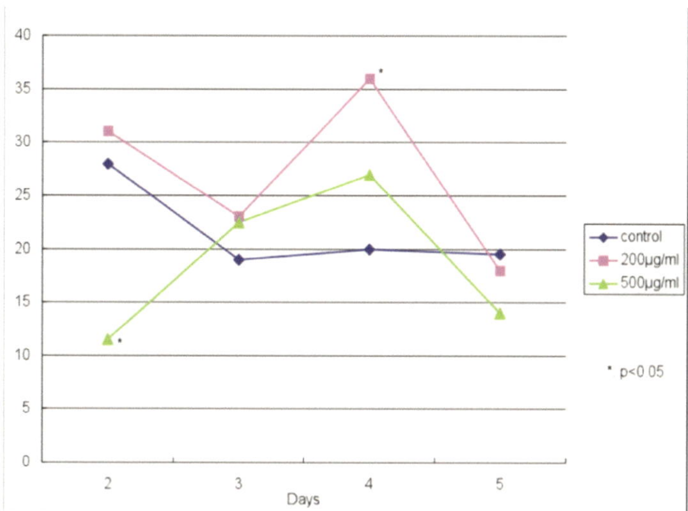

We called this pattern center peak.

Fig. 19-2. Amount of DNA in S phase with U373MG. On day 2 of addition of 500 µg/ml TMZ., We observed a statistically significant decrease of DNA. On day 4 of addition of 200mg/ml TMZ., we observed a statistically significant increase of DNA.

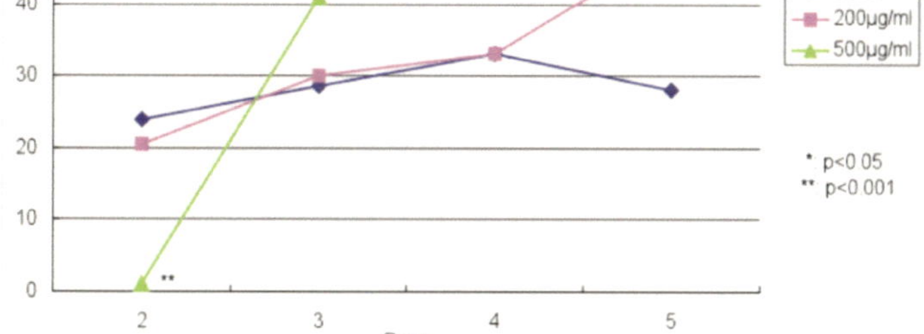

Fig. 19-3. Amount of DNA in G_2M phase with U373MG. On day 2 of addition of 500µg/ml TMZ, we observed a statistically significant decrease of DNA. On days 4 and 5 of addition of 500µg/ml TMZ and 200µg/ml TMZ, we observed statistically significant increase of DNA. We called this pattern right peak.

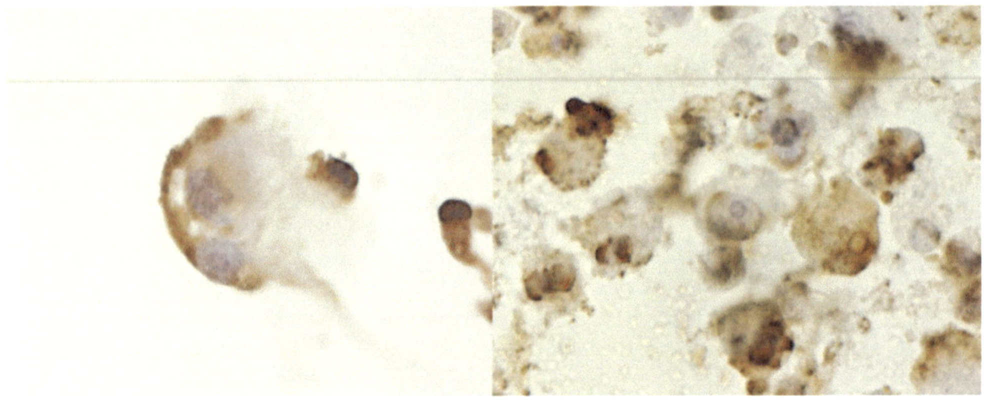

Fig. 20. Apoptotic cells shown by TUNEL stain (left ×600; right×400)

8. Discussion

Each antineoplasitic agent has each pharmacological mechanism. The all reasons of tumor cell killing weren't explained from view in cell kinetics. However, because we can imagine the strategy of treatment on the basis of cell kinetics about each antineoplastic agent, it is truth that information about cell kinetics has important profile.

For example, as the radiation that was used with various types of antineoplastic agents, it has reported the result of analyses from the view of cell kinetics. Though Yokoyama et al reported the slight accumulation in G_2M phase at 24 hours after low dose radiation like 5Gy, 7Gy, it is no subtraction at 48 hours after radiation. We considered this reversible change. But, in case of radiation more than 10Gy, this accumulation in G_2M phase decreased additionally. We considered this tendency irreversible change (*26). Especially, in case of a study about the radiation more than 15 Gy, it reported almost complete G_2M block our considered. In addition, Kubota et al, with HeLa cells, reported the observation of considerable cell accumulation in S phase at 5 hours after 10Gy radiation, then, that accumulation in S phase migrated quickly G_2M phase meaning considerable G_2M block (*27).

As a result of above, low dose radiation made reversible effect and weak cell cycle block, and high radiation made irreversible effect, you know, cell cycle block in S phase migrate in G_2M phase. These results from radiation are similar to the result from drugs like some antineoplastic agents having constant clinical effect. In other word, drugs having weak clinical effect have reversible tendency and showed partially cell cycle block.

What is important in analyze experimentally these cell kinetics, set the cell line and the concentrations of drugs. If it is same antineoplastic agent, these drugs tend to have different results depends on the difference from kind of cell line, drug concentration, addition methods. From the view of clinical application, we might have better choice proper how to add and proper drugs.

For example, as my mentioned before, though S phase block was observed in the result from the addition only IFN to glioma, such block effect tended to reversible. However, the clinical studied effect for glioma cell with using IFN with TMZ is ensured (COG:Japan Clinical Oncolgy Group 0911). In the view of cell kinetics, those mechanisms were considered S and G_2M blocks in radiation, in addition to the synergy effect between temporary S phase block in IFN and S and G_2M blocks in TMZ. From now on everyone expects these effects that IFN made the sensitivity of TMZ up via p 53 via the suppression of MGMT gene, in the view of pharmacology.

It might be hard to ensure, even if experimentally, clinically and also in view of cost, these synergy effects between radiation and antineoplastic agents. However, when we consider the combination of therapeutic alternations and additional methods, we concluded that the study of cell kinetics with FCM and LSC, one of data considered like these, is very effective.

9. Abbreviation

ACNU (nimusutine hydrochloride) ,
BCNU (1,3-Bis (2-Chloroethyl)-1-Nitrosourea),
CCNU(1-(2-chloroethyl)-3-cyclohexyl-l-nitrosourea),
MCNU,(1-(2-chloroethyl)-3-(trans-4-methylcycloethyl)-1-nitrosourea),
IFN (Interferon),
PCZ(Procarbazine),
VCR(Vincristine),
TMZ (Temozolomide),
CDDP(Cisplatin),
CBDCA(Carboplatin),
BBB: Blood Brain Barrier,
APL : acute promyelocytic leukemia

10. References

[1] Hensley ML, Schuchter LM, Lindley C, et al: American Society of Clinical Oncology clinical practice guidelines for the use of chemotherapy and radiotherapy protectants. J Clin Oncol 17:3333-3335,1999.
[2] Saeki et al: neurological surgery Vol 34 No9 Sep 2006 p885-598
[3] Yoshikazu Miwa, Yoji Taba,Megumi Miyagi、Toshiyuki Sasaguri Physiology and pharmacology of the prostaglandin J2 family. Folia Pharmacol. Jpn.（Nippon Yakurigaku Zasshi）123,34～40(2004)
[4] Borden EC, Sen GC, Uze G, et al: Interferons at age 50:past, current and future impact on biomedicine. Nat Rev Drug Discov 6: 975-990, 2007
[5] Yoshihiro Numa, Keiji Kawamoto, Nobuyuki Sakai,Heroshi Matsumura:Flow cytometric analysis of antineoplastic effects of interferon-α,β and γ labeled with fluoroscein isothiocyanate on cultured brain tumors. Journal of Neuro-Oncology 11:225-234,1991
[6] Yoshida J, Kajita Y, Wakabayashi T, et al: Long-term follow-up results of 175 patients with malignant glioma:importance of radical tumour resection and postoperative adjuvant therapy with interferon, ACNU and radiation.:Acta neurochirurgica 127:55-59,1994
[7] Walker MD、et al：Randomized comparisons of radiotherapy and nitrosourea for the treatment of malignant glioma after surgery.:N Eng J Med 303：1323-1329,1980
[8] Rosenberg, B. et al：Nature,205：698−699,1965・
[9] Harrap,K,R, et al: Current status and new development(ed, by Prestayko, A,W, et al.). Academic Press, New York, 1980, pp. 193-212.
[10] Melamed,M.R.,Mullaney,P.F. & Mendelsohn,M.L.,:(eds):Flow cytometry and sorting, John Wiley and Sons.Inc,New York,1979.

[11] Merrill,J.Y.:Investigations in high-precision sorting J.Histochem.Cytochem.27:280-283,1979.

[12] Dean,P.N.:High resolution dual laser cytometry. J.Histochem. Cytochem.26:622-627,1978

[13] Pinkel,D.& Steen,H.B.:Simple methods to determine and compare the sensitivity of flow cytometry. Cytometry 3:220-223,1982

[14] Thornthwaite,J.T.,Sugarbaker,E.V.:Preparation of tissues for DNA flow cytometric analysis. Cytometry 1:229-237,1980.

[15] Baisch,H.,Gohde,W.& Linden,W.:Analysis of PCP-date to determine the fraction of cells in the vari Phases of cell Cycle.Radiat.Environ. Biophys. 12:31 1975.

[16] Kawamoto,K.,Herz.F.,Wolley,R.C.,Girano,A,Kajikawa,H,Koss,K.G.:Flow cytometric analysis of the DNA distribution in human brain tumors. Acta Beuropath.46:39-45,1979.

[17] Fried,J:Analysis of deoxyribonucleic acid histogram from flow cytometry estimation of the distribution of cells within S phase. The J.of Histochem. And Cytohem. 25:972-951,1977.

[18] Fried,J.,Perez,A.G.& Clarkson,B.D.:Flow Cytometric Analysis of cell Cycle Distribution Using Propidium Iodide.Properties of the Method and Mathematical Analysis of the date.The J.of cell Biology.71 : 172-181, 1976.

[19] Baisch,H.et al.:A comparison of mathematical methods for the analysis of DNA histograms obtained by flow cytometry. Cell Tissue Kinet. 15: 235-249, 1982.

[20] Goz, B.:The effects of incorporation of 5-halogenated deoxyuridines into the DNA of eukaryotic cells. Pharmacol. Rev. 29:249-272,1978

[21] Gratzner,H.G.:Monoclonal antibody to 5-bromo-and 5-iododeoxyuridine: a new reagent for detection DNA replication. Science 218: 474-476,1982.

[22] Fujiwara T, Nakasone S,Matsumoto K, Ohnishi R, Tabuchi K, Nishimoto A:Effect of ACNU, a water-soluble nitrosourea, on cell cycle of cultured glioma cells-flow cytometric analysis.:Gan To Kagaku Ryoho,1983 Sep;10(9):2055-61

[23] Zhao S,Tsuchida T, Kawakami K et al(2002) Effect of As203 on cell cycle progression and cyclins D1 and B1 expression in Two glioma cell lines differing in p53 status. Int J Oncol 21(1):49-55

[24] Zhao S, Zhang J, Zhang X et al(2007) Arsenic trioxide induces different gene expression profiles of gene related to growth and apoptosis in glioma cells dependent on the p53 status. Mol Biol Rep

[25] Oshige H, Yamahara T, Oishi T et al(2010) Flow cytometric analysis for the mechanism of the new antineoplastic agent temozolomide in glioma cells. Brain Tumor Pathol (2010) 27:7-15

[26] Yokoyama H et al, A study of irradiation-caused changes in cancerous cell kinetics. Advances in obstetrics and gynecol- -ogy 17-25,1986.

[27] Kubotal: Effect of hyperthermia Radiation on the cell cycle progression of HeLa Cells. Nihon Housyasen gakkai zassi 42:188-199,1981.

[28] Yoshida J, Kajita Y, Wakabayashi T, et al: Long-term follow-up results of 175 patients with malignant glioma: importance of radical tumor resection and postoperative adjuvant therapy with interferon, ACNU and radiation. Acta neurochirurgica 127:55-59,1994

[29] Watanabe T, Katayama Y, Yoshino A, et al: Human interferon beta, nimusutine hydrochloride, and radiation therapy in the treatment of newly diagnosed malignant astrocytomas. J Neurooncol 72: 57-62, 2005

13

Anti-Angiogenic Therapy for Malignant Glioma: Insights and Future Directions

Paula Province, Xiaosi Han, L. Burt Nabors and
Hassan M. Fathallah-Shaykh
The University of Alabama at Birmingham
United States of America

1. Introduction

Malignant gliomas comprise a significant number of new cases of brain cancer diagnosed in the United States each year. Despite recent therapeutic advances, they remain associated with high morbidity and mortality rates. The current standard of care for newly diagnosed malignant gliomas includes surgical resection followed by radiotherapy with concomitant and adjuvant Temozolomide. Bevacizumab, a humanized anti-VEGF (vascular endothelial growth factor) monoclonal antibody, has recently gained FDA approval for use in the treatment of recurrent glioblastoma multiforme (GBM), based on clinical trials that revealed both efficacy and favorable side-effects. Anti-angiogenic therapy has raised new hopes, new basic and clinical questions, and has uncovered new insights into the biological and clinical behavior of these tumors. Here, we review the medical, social, and economic significance of gliomas, discuss briefly the evolution of therapeutic modalities leading to anti-angiogenesis, depict the basic mechanisms of angiogenesis, detail data from Bevacizumab clinical trials, and address new clinical issues leading to the revision of the Macdonald criteria. We close with unresolved questions and potential future directions.

2. Significance of malignant gliomas

2.1 Demographics

The annual incidence of malignant gliomas is approximately 4 to 5 per 100 thousand; they account for approximately 70% of the total number of new cases of malignant primary brain tumors diagnosed in adults in the United States each year (Wen and Kesari 2008; Wen, Macdonald et al. 2010). The overall incidence of gliomas is higher among males as compared to females (7.2 per 100,000 person-years in males versus 5.0 per 100,000 person-years in females); it is highest among Caucasians and it also increases with age (Peak and Levin 2010). Glioblastoma multiforme (GBM) is the most aggressive glioma. Stupp and colleagues reported overall survival at 2 years to be 26.5 percent among patients who received combination treatment with radiotherapy and Temozolomide and 9.8 percent at 5 years (Stupp, Mason et al. 2005; Stupp, Hegi et al. 2009). For patients diagnosed with anaplastic astrocytoma, a malignant glioma subtype, the median survival is higher at approximately 2 to 5 years (Wen and Kesari 2008). It is worth mentioning that the aforementioned survival statistics do not take into account the therapeutic effects from the current use of anti-angiogenic agents.

2.2 Economic impact

The economic impact of cancer is significant. At the present time, cancer is the second leading cause of death in the United States and, as a result of high mortality and morbidity, cancer is also a major cause of loss of productivity among American adults. In the year 2000, the U.S. annual productivity cost from cancer mortality was estimated to be 115.8 billion dollars and the projected cost for the year 2020 is 147.6 billion dollars. Death from brain cancer was estimated to be the third most costly cancer per death in the year 2010, preceded by testicular and Non-Hodgkin Lymphoma, respectively. Furthermore, death from brain cancer in men younger than 35 years of age caused the most negative impact on productivity. Another important factor to consider is the impact of cancer on caregivers and on households in general. In particular, the costs increased significantly to 232.4 billion dollars in 2000 when the value of care-giving and household activities were included; the numbers are projected to be even higher in 2020 at 308 billion dollars (Bradley, Yabroff et al. 2008). Because of its neurological morbidity, patients with brain cancer require significant care-giving and are the focus of many household activities, thus contributing to the overall cost. In particular, because almost 10 percent of GBM patients survive 5 or more years (Stupp, Hegi et al. 2009), the survivors require significant care. For example, Steinbach and colleagues have reported that patients with GBM experience neurologic impairment, psychiatric symptoms, neuro-cognitive deficits, and severe fatigue that result in significant impairment of function, including inability to work and participate in day-to-day and social activities (Steinbach, Blaicher et al. 2006). Furthermore, Hottinger and colleagues found that 85 percent of long-term survivors of GBM had at least one significant neurological deficit leading to a decline of the median Karnofsy Performance Scale (KPS) value from that at the time of initial diagnosis (from 90 to 70). This decline ultimately results in impaired day-to-day function (Hottinger, Yoon et al. 2009).

2.3 Evolution of the therapeutic strategies

In the 1970s, the Brain Tumor Study Group (BTSG), a group of neurosurgeons, neuropathologists, and radiotherapists, in conjunction with the National Cancer Institute, performed a clinical trial that evaluated the use of BCNU, 1,3-bis(2-chloroethyl)-1-nitrosurea, versus radiotherapy (both alone and in combination) versus supportive care alone. The results of this trial, published in 1978, showed only a slight but statistically-insignificant increase in the median survival times of patients treated with BCNU alone (18.5 weeks) as compared to those who received best supportive care (14 weeks). However, those who received radiotherapy alone experienced a statistically significant improvement in the median survival times (36 weeks). Moreover, as compared to the radiotherapy alone arm, the combination of radiotherapy and BCNU did not yield a statistically-significant effect on survival times. Nonetheless, the data showed a trend for better survival at 2 years (Walker, Alexander et al. 1978). After this trial, BCNU became the drug most commonly used as adjuvant therapy with radiation. Since then, many trials were conducted to investigate the effects of the addition of various chemotherapeutic agents to radiotherapy (Levin, Wara et al. 1985; Prados, Scott et al. 1999). The standard of care for newly diagnosed GBM changed in 2005, after the results of a large phase III clinical trial of post-operative radiotherapy with concomitant and adjuvant Temozolomide (Stupp, Mason et al. 2005).

Temozolomide is a second generation alkylating agent developed in the 1980s which is rapidly and completely absorbed via oral administration; it also has excellent penetration into many tissues, including the brain. Another key advantage of Temozolomide is that it does not require enzymatic demethylation in the liver in order to be converted into its active species. Instead, it is spontaneously activated at physiological pH in aqueous solution (Stupp, Gander et al. 2001).

Three key phase II clinical trials collectively supported the conclusion that Temozolomide is effective against malignant gliomas (Stupp, Gander et al. 2001). The first was conducted by Yung and colleagues in patients with malignant astrocytomas at first relapse. The results revealed 6- and 12-month progression-free survival (PFS) rates of 46 and 24 percent, respectively; the median PFS time was 5.4 months. This study not only supported the use of Temozolomide as a single agent in the treatment of malignant astrocytoma, but it also revealed that it is well-tolerated. The most commonly reported adverse events were nausea and vomiting, which were easily controlled with standard anti-emetic therapy (Yung, Prados et al. 1999). Brada and colleagues studied Temozolomide in patients with GBM at first relapse. The results showed a 6-month PFS rate of 18 percent and a median PFS time of 2.1 months. This study also revealed that Temozolomide has a favorable side-effect profile (Brada, Hoang-Xuan et al. 2001). In 2000, Yung and colleagues compared Procarbazine versus Temozolomide in GBM patients at first relapse. This trial revealed a statistically-significant improvement in 6-month PFS rates, 21 percent for Temozolomide verses 8 percent for Procarbazine (Yung, Albright et al. 2000).

In 2005, Stupp and colleagues published the results of a randomized, multi-center, phase III clinical trial that compared concomitant and adjuvant Temozolomide with radiotherapy to radiotherapy alone in patients with newly diagnosed GBM. This study demonstrated an increase in mean survival time of 2.5 months, which was both clinically and statistically significant. It also demonstrated that at 2 years, the radiotherapy plus Temozolomide group had a survival rate of 26.5 percent, as opposed to a 10.4 percent survival rate in the radiotherapy group alone (Stupp, Mason et al. 2005). Again, the 5 year survival rate for the combination therapy group was 9.8 percent versus 1.9 percent for the radiotherapy alone group (Stupp, Hegi et al. 2009). Alkylating chemotherapeutic agents, including Temozolomide, induce DNA lesions that are repaired by the O^6-methylguanine-DNA methyltransferase (*MGMT*) protein. Thus, high levels of *MGMT* activity diminish their therapeutic effects. Interestingly, Temozolomide-treated patients whose *MGMT* promoter elements were epigenetically silenced by methylation, had a statistically-significant improvement in overall survival times (Hegi, Diserens et al. 2005). Promoter methylation lowers *MGMT* levels/activity, thus impairing the ability of the cancer cells to repair and survive the DNA damage.

3. Angiogenesis

3.1 History

The idea of anti-angiogenesis as a concept for therapy of tumors was first proposed by Dr. Folkman in the 1970s (Folkman 1972). This subject has continued to be studied in terms of the development of targeted therapies and by elucidating the mechanism of action.

3.2 Summary of angiogenesis

Angiogenesis is the process by which the vascular system is formed through growth of new capillaries from pre-existing vessels. Angiogenesis plays a critical role in key physiologic

processes such as embryogenesis, regeneration, and wound healing. And although angiogenesis is usually regarded as a formative process, it is also involved in various pathologic processes, including age-related macular degeneration, rheumatoid arthritis, and tumor growth and development, which is the focus of this chapter (Wang, Fei et al. 2004).
Of note, there are 2 types of angiogenesis: sprouting and splitting, and in this discussion, the term "angiogenesis" will refer to the sprouting type. The process of angiogenesis can be briefly summarized as follows. First, there is vasodilation, in response to nitric oxide, and increased permeability of the existing vessels. This step is then followed by degradation of the existing vessel's basement membrane and subsequent migration of endothelial cells to this area. After the endothelial cells arrive, they begin to proliferate and mature into capillaries via a balance of both growth and inhibition. The final steps involve the recruitment of pericytes and vascular smooth muscle cells that form a new network of mature vessels (Shinkaruk, Bayle et al. 2003).

3.3 Molecular signals of angiogenesis, VEGF

Although there is a great diversity in the factors and signals that contribute to angiogenesis, the chemical signal that seems to play the most critical role in the process is Vascular Endothelial Growth Factor, or VEGF. VEGF is a pro-angiogenic growth factor that is secreted by many cells, including mesenchymal, stromal, and especially tumor cells. VEGF induces the migration of the endothelial precursor cells to sites of angiogenesis and is also responsible for the proliferation and differentiation of these cells. The VEGF gene is located on chromosome 6p12 and the gene family is composed of 5 members, namely VEGF-A, VEGF-B, VEGF-C, VEGF-D, and placental-derived growth factor (PIGF). Of these, VEGF-A, B, and PIGF are involved in proliferation of the vascular system and VEGF-C and D are involved in the development of the lymphatic system (Ahluwalia and Gladson 2010). VEGF primarily signals through its receptor VEGFR2, which is a tyrosine kinase receptor, expressed by many cells, including endothelial cells, endothelial cell precursors, and tumor cells. The interaction between VEGF and VEGFR2 is heavily involved in both the physiologic and pathologic effects of VEGF (Jain, di Tomaso et al. 2007)

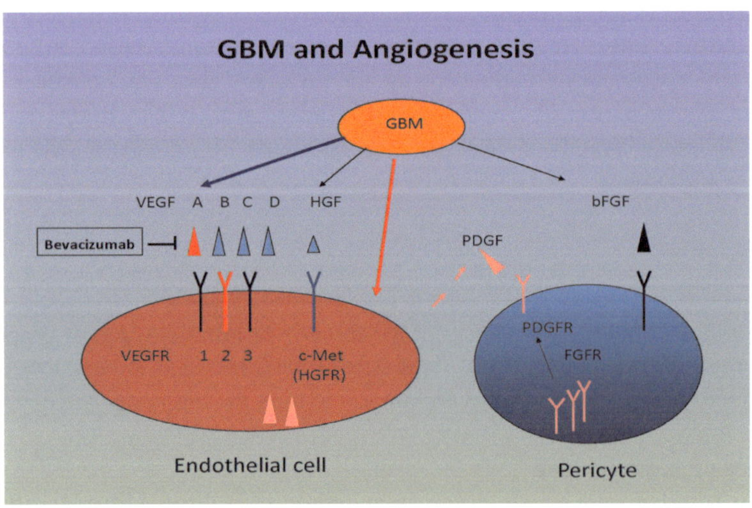

Fig. 1. GBM tumors influence multiple pathways of angiogenesis.

GBM cells secrete angiogenic molecules including VEGF, Hepatocyte Growth Factor (HGF), and basic Fibroblast Growth Factor (bFGF), which interact with their respective receptors on either endothelial cells or pericytes. Specifically, VEGFA interacts with VEGFR2, HGF with c-Met, and bFGF with FGFR. Bevacizumab is believed to block the interaction of VEGF with its receptors. Endothelial cells secrete PDGF, which promotes recruitment of pericytes. bFGF/FGFR interaction promotes PDGFR expression leading to enhanced recruitment of pericytes. The red arrow illustrates the fact that tumor-derived endothelial cells arise from the GBM tumor.

Other chemical signals that play an important role in angiogenesis are fibroblast growth factor, HGF, tumor necrosis factor-alpha (TNF-α), transforming growth factor-beta (TGF-β), angiopoietins, and platelet derived growth factor (PDGF). The function of these signals ranges from involvement in extracellular matrix degradation to endothelial proliferation and migration and then ultimately to neo-vessel stabilization and maturation (Martin and Jiang 2010; Ucuzian, Gassman et al. 2010).

3.4 Details of angiogenesis

In the first steps of angiogenesis, the vessels become leaky and dilate. Then, there is proteolytic degradation of the endothelial cell's basement membrane. This degradation is mainly carried out by matrix metalloproteinases (MMPs), which are zinc-dependent extracellular matrix (ECM) endopeptidases that work to expose the endothelial cells to other signaling factors important for regulation of angiogenesis and migration of endothelial cells (Ahluwalia and Gladson 2010; Gialeli, Theocharis et al. 2011). These factors bind to specific receptors on the endothelial cells, such as the integrin cell adhesion receptors, which promote endothelial cell survival, proliferation, and migration. This process proceeds through specific cooperation with other angiogenic pathways that originate from VEGFR2 and FGFR. Next, pericytes are recruited to help form a new endothelial cell basement membrane and provide stabilization of the growing neo-vessel (Ahluwalia and Gladson 2010). Please see Figure.

The controlled and precise development of endothelial cells into patterned vessels is thought to be controlled by the fundamental Notch pathway that regulates cell differentiation in many mammalian cell-types. Delta-Notch signaling is a form of cell-to-cell communication that plays a role in determining differentiation of cells within similar groups. The Notch pathway in mammals is comprised of 4 Notch trans-membrane receptors (Notch 1-4) and 5 membrane-bound Notch ligands. Of these, Notch 1, 3, and 4 receptors and ligands Delta-like 1 (DLL1), Delta-like 4 (DLL4), and Jagged1 play a role in angiogenesis (Thurston and Kitajewski 2008). Of note, Notch signaling regulates angiogenesis by simultaneously activating and repressing vessel sprouting. In particular, DLL4 is a selective inhibitor of VEGF; signals downstream from DLL4 and Notch 1 repress vessel sprouting by restricting the response of tip cells to VEGF. Tip cells are specialized endothelial cells located at the leading edge of blood-vessel sprouting (Jain, di Tomaso et al. 2007).

Circulating endothelial precursors (CEPs), which are bone marrow-derived, were previously recognized as the main source of vascular endothelial cells. Recently, Soda and colleagues examined endothelial cells in tumor samples collected from human GBM xenografts implanted in immunodeficient mice as well as in GBM tumors induced in $p53^{+/-}$ heterozygous mice by lentiviral delivery of oncogenes. Unexpectedly, their findings showed the presence of tumor derived endothelial cells (TDECs) suggesting that the endothelial cells transdifferentiated from the neuroectoderm, not from the CEPs. This data also suggests that this process may be independent of signaling from VEGF and FGF and may help to explain resistance mechanisms to anti-VEGF therapy (Soda, Marumoto et al. 2011).

3.5 Targeting angiogenesis

Dr. Folkman observed that brain tumors appear to be highly dependent on endothelial cell proliferation and hypothesized that anti-angiogenic therapy may be particularly useful in the treatment of brain cancer (Folkman 1972). Angiogenesis is crucial for supplying tumors with nutrients, oxygen, and growth factors time (Khasraw and Lassman 2010). Malignant tumors in general, and gliomas in particular, are very vascular and they secrete VEGF (Peak and Levin 2010). Thus, VEGF is a prime target for anti-angiogenic therapy, leading to the development of Bevacizumab (Ahluwalia and Gladson 2010).

4. Anti-angiogenesis

4.1 Introduction to bevacizumab

Bevacizumab (Avastin) is a recombinant humanized monoclonal antibody that targets VEGF; it was the first anti-angiogenesis agent to be approved by the United States Food and Drug Administration (FDA) in 2004. Bevacizumab was initially approved for use in metastatic colorectal cancer. Nevertheless, its clinical use has been extended to other cancers, including lung, breast, renal cell, and glioblastoma (Van Meter and Kim 2010).

Study and Publication Year	Agents Studied	No of Patients	Radiographic Response Rate, %	6-mo PFS, %	Median PFS Time (months)	Median OS Time (months)
Vredenburgh, Desjardins et al. 2007	Bevacizumab + Irinotecan	35	57	46	6	10.5
Friedman, Prados et al. 2009	Bevacizumab + Irinotecan	82	37.8	50.3	5.6	8.7
Reardon, Desjardins et al. 2009	Bevacizumab + Etoposide	27	23	44.4	4.5	11.6
Gutin, Iwamoto et al. 2009	Bevacizumab + Radiation	20	50	65	7.3	12.5
Sathornsumetee, Desjardins et al. 2010	Bevacizumab + Erlotinib	25	48	29.2	4.5	11.2
Verhoeff, Lavini et al. 2010	Bevacizumab + dose-intense Temozolomide	23	20	6.7	2.6	3.9
Hasselbalch, Lassen et al. 2010	Bevacizumab + Cetuximab + Irinotecan	43	26	33	4	7.5

Table 1. Prospective Phase II Clinical Trials of Bevacizumab + Other Therapies for Recurrent GBM. PFS = Progression Free Survival, OS = Overall Survival.

4.2 Mechanism of action of bevacizumab

Bevacizumab has 6 VEGF binding residues that neutralize the ability of VEGF to bind to its target receptors on endothelial cells. This neutralization has been shown to have efficacy not only in *in vitro* studies, but also in *in vivo*. In 2004, Willet and colleagues treated 6 patients with primary and non-metastatic colorectal cancer with adjuvant Bevacizumab in a phase I clinical trial. The results revealed significant reduction in tumor blood volume and perfusion and micro-vascular density (MVD) (Willett, Boucher et al. 2004); thus yielding positive evidence of the anti-angiogenic effects of Bevacizumab in human cancer.

The therapeutic effects of Bevacizumab against cancer have been illustrated by several clinical trials. In 2004, Hurwitz conducted a randomized double-blinded phase III clinical trial of Bevacizumab plus irinotecan, fluorouracil, and leucovorin (IFL) versus IFL plus placebo in colorectal cancer. Subjects treated with Bevacizumab experienced significant prolongation in 1-year survival rates (74.3 percent vs. 63.4 percent), in the median duration of PFS time (10.6 months vs. 6.2 months), in response rates (44.8 percent vs. 34.8 percent), and in the median duration of response time (10.4 months vs. 7.1 months) (Hurwitz, Fehrenbacher et al. 2004). In 2007, Giantonio reported that the addition of Bevacizumab led to a significant prolongation of the median duration of survival time of patients with recurrent metastatic colorectal cancer (12.9 months versus 10.8 months) (Giantonio, Catalano et al. 2007).

Study and Publication Year	Agents Studied	No of Patients	Overall Radiographic Response Rate, %	6-mo PFS, %	Median PFS Time (months)	Median OS Time (months)
Kreisl, Kim et al. 2009	Bevacizumab single agent	48	35	29	4	7.8
Friedman, Prados et al. 2009	Bevacizumab single agent	85	28.2	42.6	4.2	9.2
Raizer, Grimm et al. 2010	Bevacizumab single agent	50	NA	25	NA	6.5

Table 2. Prospective Phase II Clinical Trials of Single-agent Bevacizumab for Recurrent GBM. PFS = Progression Free Survival, OS = Overall Survival.

4.3 Clinical activity of bevacizumab against recurrent GBM

Stark-Vance treated 21 patients, 11 with GBM and 10 with other high-grade gliomas, with the combination of Bevacizumab and Irinotecan, a topoisomerase 1 inhibitor. Interestingly, 1 patient had a complete response (CR), 8 patients had partial responses (PR), and 11 patients had stable disease (SD) (Stark-Vance 2005). This observation suggested that Bevacizumab may be active against high-grade gliomas and led to prospective clinical trials (Chamberlain 2010).

Since the initial work by Stark-Vance, several phase II clinical trials have studied the therapeutic efficacy of Bevacizumab as a single-agent or in combination with chemotherapy or radiation for recurrent GBM (see Tables 1 and 2). The results support the conclusion that Bevacizumab is effective as a single-agent for recurrent GBM. In particular, the prospective studies, detailed in Table 2, reveal 6-month PFS rates ranging from 25 to 42.6 percent and median OS times from 6.5 to 9.2 months; these outcomes are statistically significant as compared to historical controls of salvage chemotherapy (Friedman, Prados et al. 2009; Kreisl, Kim et al. 2009; Raizer, Grimm et al. 2010). Retrospective studies have also supported the same conclusion. Agha and colleagues reviewed 18 patients diagnosed with recurrent malignant gliomas with Bevacizumab alone versus salvage chemotherapy. Half of the patients in the Bevacizumab arm remained progression-free at 12 months, while all patients treated with salvage chemotherapy died within 6 months. It is also important to note that 7 of 8 patients in the group treated with Bevacizumab alone showed a radiological response as compared to 4 of 10 patients in the group treated with salvage chemotherapy (Agha, Ibrahim et al. 2010). In another retrospective analysis of 50 adult patients with GBM treated with single-agent Bevacizumab, the results revealed efficacy with 6- and 12- month PFS rates of 42 and 22 percent, respectively (Chamberlain and Johnston 2010).

On the other hand, data from prospective studies also support the idea that the addition of chemotherapy or radiation therapy to Bevacizumab does not yield a clear therapeutic benefit for recurrent GBM (see Table 1). In particular, the 6-month PFS rates ranged from 6.7 to 65 percent, the median PFS time ranged from 2.6 to 7.3 months, and the median OS time ranged from 3.9 to 12.5 months (Vredenburgh, Desjardins et al. 2007; Friedman, Prados et al. 2009; Gutin, Iwamoto et al. 2009; Reardon, Desjardins et al. 2009; Hasselbalch, Lassen et al. 2010; Sathornsumetee, Desjardins et al. 2010; Verhoeff, Lavini et al. 2010). Notably, the BRAIN study evaluated the efficacy of Bevacizumab alone and in combination with Irinotecan in patients with recurrent GBM in a phase II, non-comparative trial. The 6-month PFS rates were 42.6 percent (97.5 percent CI, 29.6 percent to 55.5 percent) and 50.3 percent (97.5 percent CI, 36.8 percent to 63.9 percent) in the Bevacizumab arm and the Bevacizumab plus Irinotecan arm, respectively. Both groups exceeded the historical 15 percent 6-month PFS rate for salvage chemotherapy and Irinotecan alone ($p<0.0001$) (Friedman, Petros et al. 1999; Cloughesy, Filka et al. 2003; Raymond, Fabbro et al. 2003; Prados, Lamborn et al. 2006; Friedman, Prados et al. 2009). The objective response (OR) rates were 28.2 percent (97.5 percent CI, 18.5 percent to 40.3 percent) and 37.8 percent (97.5 percent CI, 26.5 percent to 50.8 percent) for the Bevacizumab and the combination groups, respectively (Friedman, Prados et al. 2009). Therefore, it is unclear whether the therapeutic benefits of adding Irinotecan exceed those of single-agent Bevacizumab. The possibility of a small therapeutic benefit may be resolved by future studies that include a larger number of patients.

4.4 Bevacizumab for treatment of primary GBM

Because of the positive results in recurrent GBM, recent research has focused on the therapeutic benefits of Bevacizumab in conjunction with Temozolomide for newly-diagnosed GBM. Lai and colleagues conducted a prospective phase II study evaluating Bevacizumab in combination with radiation therapy and Temozolomide in 70 newly diagnosed GBM patients. They compared the results to a retrospectively reviewed cohort of patients treated with standard of care of radiation therapy and Temozolomide. The findings reveal a statistically-significant improvement in PFS time, 13.6 months (95 percent CI, 11.1 to 16.5 months) versus 7.6 months (95 percent CI, 5.9 to 10.8 months) in the control group, but lack of benefit in OS times (Lai, Tran et al. 2011). These results have paved the way for 2 large, prospective, randomized phase III clinical trials in newly diagnosed GBM, sponsored by the Radiation Therapy Oncology Group (RTOG, trial RTOG-0825) and Roche (AVAglio) (Chamberlain 2010; Chinot, de La Motte Rouge et al. 2011).

4.5 Bevacizumab associated toxicities

Bevacizumab is generally well-tolerated. Nevertheless, its potential side effects include hypertension, thrombo-embolic events, bleeding complications (including intracranial hemorrhage), fatigue, proteinuria, impaired wound healing, and bowel perforation (Dietrich, Norden et al. 2008). Hypertension appears to be related to the physiologic role of VEGF in regulating vasomotor tone and blood pressure, possibly through regulation of nitric oxide synthase expression (Facemire, Nixon et al. 2009).

In the BRAIN study discussed above, fatigue, headache, and hypertension were the most common adverse events in the Bevacizumab group, while fatigue, diarrhea, and nausea were the most common adverse events in the Bevacizumab plus Irinotecan group. The rate of grade 3 adverse events was 46.4 percent in the Bevacizumab-alone arm and 65.8 percent in the combination arm (Friedman, Prados et al. 2009). There is some evidence to suggest that the rate of grade 3 adverse events is lower when Bevacizumab is used as a single-agent, rather than in combination based regimens (Friedman, Prados et al. 2009; Chamberlain 2010). Rare complications affecting the central nervous system have been observed in GBM patients treated with Bevacizumab, namely Posterior Reversible Leuko-encephalopathy Syndrome (PRES) and optic neuropathy (Hinchey, Chaves et al. 1996; Glusker, Recht et al. 2006; Sherman, Aregawi et al. 2009).

4.6 Bevacizumab and assessment of tumor response

The Macdonald criteria, developed for 2-dimensional CT (computed tomography) scans, have been considered the standard to assess response or progression of malignant gliomas since 1990. These criteria have since been applied to MRIs (magnetic resonance images), which have replaced CT scans as the standard imaging modality. The Macdonald criteria are useful because they provide an objective radiologic assessment of tumor response and allow response rates to be compared between clinical trials, both ongoing and historical, in a standardized manner. However, their limitations have been recently noted, in particular, inter-observer variability, the difficulty of measuring irregularly shaped tumors, failure to assess the non-enhancing portion of the tumor, and the difficulty of measuring enhancing lesions in the walls of cystic or surgical cavities without also including the cyst or cavity in the tumor measurement. For example, the Macdonald criteria define tumor progression as at least a 25 percent increase in the contrast-enhancing lesion. However, enhancement is influenced by many factors, including corticosteroid dosages, anti-angiogenic agents, seizure activity, surgery, radiation-induced changes, and treatment-related inflammation, to name a few, and therefore it is problematic to equate changes in contrast-enhancing areas with tumor progression (Wen, Macdonald et al. 2010).

Other important considerations include pseudoprogession and the changes in tumor vasculature permeability caused by anti-angiogenic agents. Pseudoprogression describes a treatment-related increase in contrast enhancement that usually occurs within 12 weeks of the completion of radiation therapy; it is believed to be mediated by a transient increase in tumor vasculature permeability (Chamberlain, Glantz et al. 2007; Taal, Brandsma et al. 2008; Roldan, Scott et al. 2009; Wen, Macdonald et al. 2010). On the other hand, Bevacizumab and other anti-angiogenic drugs may cause a pseudoresponse, as early as 1 to 2 days, because of a marked decrease in contrast enhancement due to the normalization of abnormally permeable tumor vasculature. Furthermore, by the same mechanism, Bevacizumab-treated tumors may progress by increased T2/FLAIR (fluid attenuation inversion recovery) signal without an associated increase in contrast uptake/blood brain barrier disruption (Wen, Macdonald et al. 2010). In order to address the above-mentioned limitations, the Response Assessment in Neuro-Oncology (RANO) Working Group has proposed modifications to the original Macdonald Criteria. In the modified criteria, measurements of T2/FLAIR lesions are included in the determination of response or progressive disease (see Tables 3-4). Notably, progression is defined not only by increases in enhancing lesions, but also by increases in non-measurable disease and by significant increases in non-enhancing T2/FLAIR lesions, though the term "significant" is not quantifiable (Wen, Macdonald et al. 2010). Agha and colleagues have suggested a rule for progressive disease, that is if the MRI shows greater than 25 percent increase in FLAIR then the consecutive MRI, done at one month or later, must show an increase in FLAIR or enhancing volume on a stable or higher dose of corticosteroids (Agha, Ibrahim et al. 2010)

	Macdonald Criteria	RANO Criteria
CR	Requires all of the following: 1.1 Complete disappearance of all enhancing measurable and non-measurable disease sustained for at least 4 weeks, 1.2 No new lesions, 1.3 No corticosteroids, 1.4 Stable or improved clinically	Requires all of the following: 1.1 Same as MacDonald 1.1, 1.2 Same as MacDonald 1.2, 1.3 Patient must be off corticosteroids or on physiologic replacement doses only, 1.4 Same as McDonald 1.4, 1.5 Stable or improved non-enhancing (T2/FLAIR) lesions.
PR	Requires all of the following: 2.1 $\geq 50\%$ decrease compared with baseline in the sum of products of perpendicular diameters of all measurable enhancing lesions sustained for at least 4 weeks, 2.2 No new lesions, 2.3 Stable or reduced corticosteroid dose, 2.4 Stable or improved clinically.	Requires all of the following: 2.1 Same as MacDonald 2.1, 2.2 Same as MacDonald 2.2, 2.3 Stable or improved non-enhancing (T2/FLAIR) lesions on same or lower dose of corticosteroids, compared with baseline scan and corticosteroid dose must not be greater than the dose at time of baseline scan, 2.4 Same as McDonald 2.4, 2.5 No progression of non-measurable disease.
SD	Requires all of the following: 3.1 Does not qualify for complete response, partial response, or progression, 3.2 Stable clinically.	Requires all of the following: 3.1 Same as MacDonald 3.1, 3.2 Same as MacDonald 3.2, 3.3 Stable non-enhancing (T2/FLAIR) lesions on same or lower dose of corticosteroids compared with baseline scan.

CR: complete Response, PR: Partial response, SD: Stable Disease.

Table 3. Comparison of Response Criteria, CR, PR, and SD.

In the absence of a confirming scan 4 weeks later, a CR or PR response is considered stable disease. In the RANO SD criteria, in the event that the corticosteroid dose was increased for new symptoms and signs without confirmation of disease progression on neuroimaging, and subsequent follow-up imaging shows that this increase in corticosteroids was required because of disease progression, the last scan considered to show stable disease will be the scan obtained when the corticosteroid dose was equivalent to the baseline dose.

	Macdonald Criteria	RANO Criteria
PD	Any of the following: 4.1 ≥ 25% increase in sum of the products of perpendicular diameters of enhancing lesions 4.2 New lesion, 4.3 Clinical deterioration.	Any of the following: 4.1 Same as MacDonald 4.1 but compared with smallest tumor measurement at baseline or best response on stable or increasing doses of corticosteroids, 4.2 Same as McDonald 4.2 4.3 Same as McDonald 4.3 not attributable to other causes apart from the tumor or to changes in corticosteroid dose 4.4 Clear progression of non-measurable disease 4.5 Significant increase in T2/FLAIR non-enhancing lesions on stable or increasing doses of corticosteroids compared with baseline scan or best response after initiation of therapy, not due to co-morbid events. 4.6 Failure to return for evaluation as a result of death or deteriorating condition.

Table 4. Comparison of Response Criteria, PD. PD: Progressive Disease.

4.7 Bevacizumab and patterns of GBM recurrence

Interestingly, the use of Bevacizumab has raised many questions about patterns of recurrence. Unfortunately, the data from several retrospective reviews have produced conflicting conclusions that appear to be secondary to such issues as poor design (retrospective analyses) and small numbers. On one side of the argument, Wick and colleagues (n = 44), Norden and colleagues (n = 26), and Chamberlain (n = 80) argue that the majority of patients who receive Bevacizumab exhibit no change in patterns of recurrence (Norden, Young et al. 2008; Chamberlain 2011; Wick, Dorner et al. 2011). However, Norden and colleagues argue that the likelihood of diffuse or distant recurrence was higher in Bevacizumab-treated patients (Norden, Young et al. 2008). Furthermore, the results of Chamberlain reveal that the number of patients with diffuse disease increases from 5/80 (6.25 percent) at the time of first recurrence, to 9/80 (11.25 percent) at the time of second recurrence while on single-agent Bevacizumab (Chamberlain 2011). On the other end of the spectrum, Pope and colleagues reported that the incidence of diffuse disease increased from 14/67 (21 percent) to 26/67 (39 percent) and from 12/57 (21 percent) to 36/57 (63 percent) in patients treated by single-agent Bevacizumab and Bevacizumab plus Irinotecan, respectively (Pope, Xia et al. 2011). Zuniga and colleagues have also reported a diffuse pattern of recurrence of 7/38 (18.42 percent) in patients treated with Bevacizumab and Irinotecan (Zuniga, Torcuator et al. 2009). These conflicting conclusions appear to arise from the fact that the aforementioned studies are not powered to detect differences in patterns of diffuse recurrence, which are not very large. The aforementioned ongoing phase III prospective studies that include much larger numbers of patients may address this question for newly diagnosed GBM.

The biological explanation of a change in patterns of recurrence may be justified by the "Go or Grow" mechanism as a possible explanation for the switch between a proliferative tumor phenotype and an invasive one that occurs when the tumor is exposed to a hypoxic environment (Hatzikirou, Basanta et al. 2010). The basic idea is that some GBM tumors have a molecular system that allows them to infiltrate outward in search of nutrients and, in turn, may help explain the diffuse radiographic patterns of relapse seen in patients treated with Bevacizumab.

4.8 Other anti-angiogenic agents

Other anti-angiogenic agents that have been evaluated in GBM include Vandetanib, Cediranib, Tamoxifen, Enzastaurin, and Cilengitide, to name a few. These and others have been investigated in early trials. For example, Cediranib has been shown to reduce edema and the amount of tumor enhancement on contrasted studies. Cilengitide, an inhibitor of integrin receptors, has shown activity in clinical trials, both as a single agent and in combination with other, standard chemotherapeutic regimens (Reardon, Fink et al. 2008; Ahluwalia and Gladson 2010; Khasraw and Lassman 2010; Reardon, Neyns et al. 2011).

5. Future directions

Anti-angiogenic therapies, especially Bevacizumab, offer new options and hope for better outcomes to patients, caregivers, and clinicians. However, many new important questions have been raised and remain unanswered. For example, there is evidence that abrupt discontinuation of Bevacizumab may result in rebound tumor growth and rapid clinical decline (median OS of 47.5 days after discontinuation) (Zuniga, Torcuator et al. 2009). These preliminary results should be investigated in the future as they leave the clinician with the dilemma of how to discontinue Bevacizumab. In addition, more research is needed to address treatment options when patients fail Bevacizumab. For example, with other anti-angiogenic therapies in the pipeline, it is unknown if Bevacizumab-treated patients will respond to these agents. Furthermore, recent evidence suggest that gliomas, heavily treated with chemotherapy, mutate at a fast rate; this hypermutation phenotype is daunting as it may enhance resistance and aggressiveness (Chen, Delaloye et al. 2007).

The fact that Bevacizumab normalizes the blood-brain barrier leads to clinical conundrums, namely, the inability to judge tumor response, the possibility of decreased delivery of crucial chemotherapeutic agents, and changes in recurrence patterns (Thompson, Frenkel et al. 2011). Results by Chen and colleagues suggest that positron emission tomography (PET) using [18F] fluorothymidine (FLT) may help differentiate the anti-tumor effects of Bevacizumab from its effects on the BBB as well as serve as a predictor for survival (Chen, Cloughesy et al. 2005; Chen, Delaloye et al. 2007).

As noted above, patients with malignant gliomas experience significant morbidity related to neurologic impairment, psychiatric symptoms, neuro-cognitive deficits, and fatigue. Assessment of quality of life and, in particular, of neuro-cognitive functioning, is an important end-point in clinical trials of patients with malignant gliomas and was analyzed in the BRAIN study. The findings reveal that the majority of patients treated with Bevacizumab experienced stable or improved neuro-cognitive function during the first 6 weeks of treatment, suggesting that Bevacizumab either preserves or improves neuro-cognitive function, and thus positively affects quality of life among patients with GBM (Friedman, Prados et al. 2009; Henriksson, Asklund et al. 2011). Future studies are needed to investigate the effects of Bevacizumab on neuro-cognitive functioning and on other aspects affecting quality of life. Notably, there is recent recognition of the need to adopt new clinical endpoints including, PFS at defined intervals, development of alternative imaging approaches, and validated metrics of patient function and well-being (Reardon, Galanis et al. 2011).

6. Conclusion

In this chapter, we discuss the financial and social impacts caused by the significant morbidity and poor prognosis that remain to be associated with malignant gliomas, despite recent advances in basic sciences and the introduction of novel therapeutic strategies, including anti-angiogenesis. Bevacizumab has therapeutic efficacy against recurrent malignant gliomas; its role in the treatment of newly-diagnosed GBM is being investigated. Importantly, the use of Bevacizumab has raised new and novel questions about the basic biology of malignant gliomas and has led to a revision of the Macdonald criteria. We expect future research to answer important clinical questions about the "Go or Grow" phenotype, the patterns of recurrence of newly diagnosed and recurrent GBM treated by anti-angiogenic drugs, the importance of rebound growth when Bevacizumab is discontinued, chemotherapeutic drug delivery when used in combination with anti-angiogenic drugs, and the hypermutation phenotype. Additional clinical questions that remain open include therapeutic options when patients fail anti-angiogenic therapy and cross-sensitivity to various anti-angiogenic agents.

7. References

Agha, C. A., S. Ibrahim, et al. (2010). "Bevacizumab is active as a single agent against recurrent malignant gliomas." Anticancer Res 30(2): 609-611.

Ahluwalia, M. S. and C. L. Gladson (2010). "Progress on anti-angiogenic therapy for patients with malignant glioma." J Oncol 2010: 689018.

Brada, M., K. Hoang-Xuan, et al. (2001). "Multicenter phase II trial of temozolomide in patients with glioblastoma multiforme at first relapse." Ann Oncol 12(2): 259-266.

Bradley, C. J., K. R. Yabroff, et al. (2008). "Productivity costs of cancer mortality in the United States: 2000-2020." J Natl Cancer Inst 100(24): 1763-1770.

Chamberlain, M. C. (2010). "Emerging clinical principles on the use of bevacizumab for the treatment of malignant gliomas." Cancer 116(17): 3988-3999.

Chamberlain, M. C. (2011). "Radiographic patterns of relapse in glioblastoma." J Neurooncol 101(2): 319-323.

Chamberlain, M. C., M. J. Glantz, et al. (2007). "Early necrosis following concurrent Temodar and radiotherapy in patients with glioblastoma." J Neurooncol 82(1): 81-83.

Chamberlain, M. C. and S. K. Johnston (2010). "Salvage therapy with single agent bevacizumab for recurrent glioblastoma." J Neurooncol 96(2): 259-269.

Chen, W., T. Cloughesy, et al. (2005). "Imaging proliferation in brain tumors with 18F-FLT PET: comparison with 18F-FDG." J Nucl Med 46(6): 945-952.

Chen, W., S. Delaloye, et al. (2007). "Predicting treatment response of malignant gliomas to bevacizumab and irinotecan by imaging proliferation with [18F] fluorothymidine positron emission tomography: a pilot study." J Clin Oncol 25(30): 4714-4721.

Chinot, O. L., T. de La Motte Rouge, et al. (2011). "AVAglio: Phase 3 trial of bevacizumab plus temozolomide and radiotherapy in newly diagnosed glioblastoma multiforme." Adv Ther.

Cloughesy, T. F., E. Filka, et al. (2003). "Two studies evaluating irinotecan treatment for recurrent malignant glioma using an every-3-week regimen." Cancer 97(9 Suppl): 2381-2386.

Dietrich, J., A. D. Norden, et al. (2008). "Emerging anti-angiogenic treatments for gliomas - efficacy and safety issues." Curr Opin Neurol 21(6): 736-744.

Facemire, C. S., A. B. Nixon, et al. (2009). "Vascular endothelial growth factor receptor 2 controls blood pressure by regulating nitric oxide synthase expression." Hypertension 54(3): 652-658.

Folkman, J. (1972). "Anti-angiogenesis: new concept for therapy of solid tumors." Ann Surg 175(3): 409-416.

Friedman, H. S., W. P. Petros, et al. (1999). "Irinotecan therapy in adults with recurrent or progressive malignant glioma." J Clin Oncol 17(5): 1516-1525.

Friedman, H. S., M. D. Prados, et al. (2009). "Bevacizumab alone and in combination with irinotecan in recurrent glioblastoma." J Clin Oncol 27(28): 4733-4740.

Gialeli, C., A. D. Theocharis, et al. (2011). "Roles of matrix metalloproteinases in cancer progression and their pharmacological targeting." FEBS J 278(1): 16-27.

Giantonio, B. J., P. J. Catalano, et al. (2007). "Bevacizumab in combination with oxaliplatin, fluorouracil, and leucovorin (FOLFOX4) for previously treated metastatic colorectal cancer: results from the Eastern Cooperative Oncology Group Study E3200." J Clin Oncol 25(12): 1539-1544.

Glusker, P., L. Recht, et al. (2006). "Reversible posterior leukoencephalopathy syndrome and bevacizumab." N Engl J Med 354(9): 980-982; discussion 980-982.

Gutin, P. H., F. M. Iwamoto, et al. (2009). "Safety and efficacy of bevacizumab with hypofractionated stereotactic irradiation for recurrent malignant gliomas." Int J Radiat Oncol Biol Phys 75(1): 156-163.

Hasselbalch, B., U. Lassen, et al. (2010). "Cetuximab, bevacizumab, and irinotecan for patients with primary glioblastoma and progression after radiation therapy and temozolomide: a phase II trial." Neuro Oncol 12(5): 508-516.

Hegi, M. E., A. C. Diserens, et al. (2005). "MGMT gene silencing and benefit from temozolomide in glioblastoma." N Engl J Med 352(10): 997-1003.

Hinchey, J., C. Chaves, et al. (1996). "A reversible posterior leukoencephalopathy syndrome." N Engl J Med 334(8): 494-500.

Hottinger, A. F., H. Yoon, et al. (2009). "Neurological outcome of long-term glioblastoma survivors." J Neurooncol 95(3): 301-305.

Hurwitz, H., L. Fehrenbacher, et al. (2004). "Bevacizumab plus irinotecan, fluorouracil, and leucovorin for metastatic colorectal cancer." N Engl J Med 350(23): 2335-2342.

Jain, R. K., E. di Tomaso, et al. (2007). "Angiogenesis in brain tumours." Nat Rev Neurosci 8(8): 610-622.

Khasraw, M. and A. B. Lassman (2010). "Advances in the treatment of malignant gliomas." Curr Oncol Rep 12(1): 26-33.

Kreisl, T. N., L. Kim, et al. (2009). "Phase II trial of single-agent bevacizumab followed by bevacizumab plus irinotecan at tumor progression in recurrent glioblastoma." J Clin Oncol 27(5): 740-745.

Lai, A., A. Tran, et al. (2011). "Phase II study of bevacizumab plus temozolomide during and after radiation therapy for patients with newly diagnosed glioblastoma multiforme." J Clin Oncol 29(2): 142-148.

Levin, V. A., W. M. Wara, et al. (1985). "Phase III comparison of BCNU and the combination of procarbazine, CCNU, and vincristine administered after radiotherapy with hydroxyurea for malignant gliomas." J Neurosurg 63(2): 218-223.

Martin, T. A. and W. G. Jiang (2010). "Hepatocyte growth factor and its receptor signalling complex as targets in cancer therapy." Anticancer Agents Med Chem 10(1): 2-6.

Norden, A. D., G. S. Young, et al. (2008). "Bevacizumab for recurrent malignant gliomas: efficacy, toxicity, and patterns of recurrence." Neurology 70(10): 779-787.

Peak, S. J. and V. A. Levin (2010). "Role of bevacizumab therapy in the management of glioblastoma." Cancer Manag Res 2: 97-104.

Pope, W. B., Q. Xia, et al. (2011). "Patterns of progression in patients with recurrent glioblastoma treated with bevacizumab." Neurology 76(5): 432-437.

Prados, M. D., K. Lamborn, et al. (2006). "A phase 2 trial of irinotecan (CPT-11) in patients with recurrent malignant glioma: a North American Brain Tumor Consortium study." Neuro Oncol 8(2): 189-193.

Prados, M. D., C. Scott, et al. (1999). "Procarbazine, lomustine, and vincristine (PCV) chemotherapy for anaplastic astrocytoma: A retrospective review of radiation therapy oncology group protocols comparing survival with carmustine or PCV adjuvant chemotherapy." J Clin Oncol 17(11): 3389-3395.

Raizer, J. J., S. Grimm, et al. (2010). "A phase 2 trial of single-agent bevacizumab given in an every-3-week schedule for patients with recurrent high-grade gliomas." Cancer 116(22): 5297-5305.

Raymond, E., M. Fabbro, et al. (2003). "Multicentre phase II study and pharmacokinetic analysis of irinotecan in chemotherapy-naive patients with glioblastoma." Ann Oncol 14(4): 603-614.

Reardon, D. A., A. Desjardins, et al. (2009). "Metronomic chemotherapy with daily, oral etoposide plus bevacizumab for recurrent malignant glioma: a phase II study." Br J Cancer 101(12): 1986-1994.

Reardon, D. A., K. L. Fink, et al. (2008). "Randomized phase II study of cilengitide, an integrin-targeting arginine-glycine-aspartic acid peptide, in recurrent glioblastoma multiforme." J Clin Oncol 26(34): 5610-5617.

Reardon, D. A., B. Neyns, et al. (2011). "Cilengitide: an RGD pentapeptide alphanubeta3 and alphanubeta5 integrin inhibitor in development for glioblastoma and other malignancies." Future Oncol 7(3): 339-354.

Roldan, G. B., J. N. Scott, et al. (2009). "Population-based study of pseudoprogression after chemoradiotherapy in GBM." Can J Neurol Sci 36(5): 617-622.

Sathornsumetee, S., A. Desjardins, et al. (2010). "Phase II trial of bevacizumab and erlotinib in patients with recurrent malignant glioma." Neuro Oncol 12(12): 1300-1310.

Sherman, J. H., D. G. Aregawi, et al. (2009). "Optic neuropathy in patients with glioblastoma receiving bevacizumab." Neurology 73(22): 1924-1926.

Shinkaruk, S., M. Bayle, et al. (2003). "Vascular endothelial cell growth factor (VEGF), an emerging target for cancer chemotherapy." Curr Med Chem Anticancer Agents 3(2): 95-117.

Soda, Y., T. Marumoto, et al. (2011). "From the Cover: Feature Article: Transdifferentiation of glioblastoma cells into vascular endothelial cells." Proc Natl Acad Sci U S A 108(11): 4274-4280.

Stark-Vance, V. (2005). "Bevacizumab (Avastin) and CPT-11 (Camptosar) in the treatment of relapsed malignant glioma." Neuro-oncol 7(369): Abstract 342.

Steinbach, J. P., H. P. Blaicher, et al. (2006). "Surviving glioblastoma for more than 5 years: the patient's perspective." Neurology 66(2): 239-242.

Stupp, R., M. Gander, et al. (2001). "Current and future developments in the use of temozolomide for the treatment of brain tumours." Lancet Oncol 2(9): 552-560.

Stupp, R., M. E. Hegi, et al. (2009). "Effects of radiotherapy with concomitant and adjuvant temozolomide versus radiotherapy alone on survival in glioblastoma in a randomised phase III study: 5-year analysis of the EORTC-NCIC trial." Lancet Oncol 10(5): 459-466.

Stupp, R., W. P. Mason, et al. (2005). "Radiotherapy plus concomitant and adjuvant temozolomide for glioblastoma." N Engl J Med 352(10): 987-996.

Taal, W., D. Brandsma, et al. (2008). "Incidence of early pseudo-progression in a cohort of malignant glioma patients treated with chemoirradiation with temozolomide." Cancer 113(2): 405-410.

Thurston, G. and J. Kitajewski (2008). "VEGF and Delta-Notch: interacting signalling pathways in tumour angiogenesis." Br J Cancer 99(8): 1204-1209.

Ucuzian, A. A., A. A. Gassman, et al. (2010). "Molecular mediators of angiogenesis." J Burn Care Res 31(1): 158-175.

Van Meter, M. E. and E. S. Kim (2010). "Bevacizumab: current updates in treatment." Curr Opin Oncol 22(6): 586-591.

Verhoeff, J. J., C. Lavini, et al. (2010). "Bevacizumab and dose-intense temozolomide in recurrent high-grade glioma." Ann Oncol 21(8): 1723-1727.

Vredenburgh, J. J., A. Desjardins, et al. (2007). "Bevacizumab plus irinotecan in recurrent glioblastoma multiforme." J Clin Oncol 25(30): 4722-4729.

Walker, M. D., E. Alexander, Jr., et al. (1978). "Evaluation of BCNU and/or radiotherapy in the treatment of anaplastic gliomas. A cooperative clinical trial." J Neurosurg 49(3): 333-343.

Wang, Y., D. Fei, et al. (2004). "Biological activity of bevacizumab, a humanized anti-VEGF antibody in vitro." Angiogenesis 7(4): 335-345.

Wen, P. Y. and S. Kesari (2008). "Malignant gliomas in adults." N Engl J Med 359(5): 492-507.

Wen, P. Y., D. R. Macdonald, et al. (2010). "Updated response assessment criteria for high-grade gliomas: response assessment in neuro-oncology working group." J Clin Oncol 28(11): 1963-1972.

Wick, A., N. Dorner, et al. (2011). "Bevacizumab does not increase the risk of remote relapse in malignant glioma." Ann Neurol 69(3): 586-592.

Willett, C. G., Y. Boucher, et al. (2004). "Direct evidence that the VEGF-specific antibody bevacizumab has antivascular effects in human rectal cancer." Nat Med 10(2): 145-147.

Yung, W. K., R. E. Albright, et al. (2000). "A phase II study of temozolomide vs. procarbazine in patients with glioblastoma multiforme at first relapse." Br J Cancer 83(5): 588-593.

Yung, W. K., M. D. Prados, et al. (1999). "Multicenter phase II trial of temozolomide in patients with anaplastic astrocytoma or anaplastic oligoastrocytoma at first relapse. Temodal Brain Tumor Group." J Clin Oncol 17(9): 2762-2771.

Part 9

CNS Tumor Associated Disorders

14

Syndromes Associated with Intracranial Tumours: A Paediatric Neurosurgeon's Perspective

Adrianna Ranger
Children's Hospital, London Health Sciences Center
University of Western Ontario,
Canada

1. Introduction

Cancer is the leading disease-related cause of death among children and adolescents(Centers for Disease Control and Prevention (CDC), 2007); and cancer involving the central nervous system (CNS) is among the most common cancers seen in infancy through adolescence, ranking either first or second only to leukaemia in Canada(Ellison *et al.*, 2009), the USA(Linet *et al.*, 1999;Bunin *et al.*, 1996;Centers for Disease Control and Prevention (CDC), 2007) and Mexico(Rendón-Macías *et al.*, 2008). In the year 2004, for example, there were 555 confirmed cases of CNS cancer-related death among children in the United States, versus 566 for leukemia, representing 25.0% and 25.5% of the total number of cancer deaths in individuals less than 20 years old(Centers for Disease Control and Prevention (CDC), 2007). Nevertheless, survival from cancer has improved dramatically over the past forty years, presumably due to a combination of improved treatments and earlier detection(Chatenoud *et al.*, 2010).

Most CNS cancers occur sporadically, outside the context of a familial disorder or multi-systemic syndrome. However, a certain percentage occurs in children who have a recognizable risk of CNS malignancy. Such cases are important for several reasons. From a research perspective, understanding risk factors for cancer brings us all closer to understanding its underlying cause or causes. In those cases where there is familial clustering, chromosomal alterations that are common to cases but not unaffected relatives lead to an improved understanding of the genetics behind neoplastic disease (Bondy *et al.*, 1994). Perhaps first and foremost from a clinical perspective is that children and youths with a known risk of CNS malignancy may be more likely to be diagnosed earlier in the course of their disease, potentially leading to earlier treatment and, thereby, enhanced outcomes. Even outside of the potential for earlier diagnosis and treatment, in certain syndromes, the cancer itself behaves differently, sometimes tending toward better, and at other times, worse outcomes. Moreover, whereas most CNS malignancies are intracranial, with cancers primarily involving the spine much less common(Koeller *et al.*, 2000), extra-cranial tumours are much more common in certain syndromes.

Another reason such malignancies are important is that syndrome-affiliated malignancies often may be multiple, sometimes involving several different tumours of the same tissue type or within the same body system; and sometimes involving malignancies ranging across different histological types and tissues. And, finally, patients who have CNS malignancies that occur within the context of some greater syndrome often have health problems beyond that of the malignancy, some of which may be as problematic.

This chapter reviews CNS cancers that occur within a broad range of clinical syndromes, starting with what some consider the prototype CNS tumour syndromes - neurofibromatosis, types I and II. In the next section, other skin conditions that, along with neurofibromatosis, are collectively known as the *phakomatoses*, will be examined. These additional syndromes include disorders like tuberous sclerosis, Von Hippel-Lindau Disease and basal cell nevus syndrome. Then, other familial disorders like Li-Fraumeni syndrome, a congenital condition linked to germ-line mutations of the p53 tumour suppressor gene, and familial polyposis disorders, like Turcot syndrome, will be examined. To conclude, the author's own findings regarding the associations between CNS tumours and dyschondroplasia syndromes, in particular Ollier's disease and Maffucci's syndrome, will be discussed.

- Phakomatosis syndromes
    - Neurofibromatosis (types 1 and 2, and segmental forms)
    - Tuberous sclerosis
    - Von Hippel-Lindau disease
    - Basal cell nevus syndrome
- Other familial syndromes
    - Li Fraumeni syndrome
    - Familial polyposis syndromes (e.g., Turcot syndrome)
    - Rubenstein-Taybi syndrome
- Dyschondroplasia syndromes
    - Ollier's disease
    - Maffucci's syndrome

Table 1. Syndromes Associated with CNS Malignancies

This discussion will focus primarily on recognizing and diagnosing both the syndrome and the tumour; and, where appropriate, on differences in the management and prognosis of such patients, relative to those who present with the same tumour alone.

2. Phakomatosis syndromes

The phakomatoses are characterized by the presence of pathological lesions involving the skin, eyes and central and peripheral nervous system (CNS)(Korf, 2005), all tissues of ectodermal origin. The phakamotoses otherwise share the features of being autosomal dominant, with variable expression, but high penetrance; and all involving mutations of a tumour suppressor gene. Initially conceptualized by the ophthalmologist van der Hoeve in the early nineteenth century(Van der Hoeve, 1920), they were assumed to primarily consist of three disorders: neurofibromatosis, tuberous sclerosis, and what we now know as von Hippel-Lindau syndrome. Over time, each of these three disease labels has been recognized as a collective term for multiple disorders; for example, as will be described in the next section, neurofibromatosis is not one disease, but a collection of quite distinct diseases. On occasion, two distinct phakomatosis syndromes (for example, neurofibromatosis and tuberous sclerosis) have been described in the same patient(Alaraj *et al.*, 2007); but this is rare and may be the result of chance rather than some increased risk for both conditions. In terms of the current chapter, these three disorders, as well as more-recently described phakomatoses, share the property of being associated with an increased risk of malignancies involving the central and, sometimes, peripheral nervous system.

2.1 Neurofibromatosis

Neurofibromatosis (NF) is the most common of all the phakomatosis syndromes, having been initially described by Frederick von Recklinghausen in the year 1882(Crump, 1981). Also initially called von Recklinghausen's disease, the disorder received public attention in the highly-acclaimed 1981 movie, *The Elephant Man*, which portrayed the life of Joseph Merrick (who was erroneously called John in the film); though some controversy exists as to whether Merrick truly suffered from neurofibromatosis, another condition called Proteus syndrome, or some combination of the two(Legendre *et al.*, 2011). For the purposes of this chapter, what is most significant is that, whereas CNS tumours are the rule in both types of neurofibromatosis, Proteus Syndrome generally is not associated with CNS tumours(Satter, 2007). Proteus syndrome is also much less common than neurofibromatosis, with a prevalence of less than one in one million(Legendre *et al.*, 2011).

In fact, neurofibromatosis is now recognized not to be one, but at least two distinct disorders: neurofibromatosis type 1 (NF-1) and neurofibromatosis type 2 (NF-2)(Ferner, 2007). Each of these two syndromes has its own diagnostic criteria that are very different; and whereas the characteristic lesion in NF-1 is the neurofibroma, the characteristic lesion in NF-2 is a peripheral nerve Schwannoma or neurolemoma(Pearce, 2003;Ferner, 2007;Lu-Emerson and Plotkin, 2009a;Lu-Emerson and Plotkin, 2009b). Neurofibromatosis has been further subcategorized beyond just neurofibromatosis types 1 and 2, into milder and more severe forms of NF-2 (Gardner syndrome and Wishart or Lee-Abbott Syndrome, respectively); segmental NF-1 and NF-2; and other variants of NF, including mixed NF. All forms of the disease appear to be autosomal dominant, though they are phenotypically highly variable, in terms of the presenting features and syndrome severity, even within a given family and when comparing monozygotic twins, suggesting the involvement of other disease-modifying genes and/or additional non-hereditary influences like second hit somatic events, environmental agents, epigenetic modification, and post-zygotic mutations(Rieley *et al.*, 2011). This makes it difficult to advise parents regarding the risk to their future offspring, because a parent with very mild disease may have a child with severe involvement, or vice versa.

2.1.1 Neurofibromatosis type 1

Neurofibromatosis type 1 (NF-1) is the most common form of disease, affecting one in roughly 2500 to 5000 live births(Evans *et al.*, 2010;Ferner *et al.*, 2007;Legendre *et al.*, 2011). This renders it more than ten times more common than NF-2(Evans *et al.*, 2010;Ferner *et al.*, 2007). Though autosomal dominant, up to 50% of cases arise spontaneously from a gene mutation that occurs on chromosome 17q11.2, which encodes for a large protein called *neurofibromin* (Evans *et al.*, 2010;Legendre *et al.*, 2011). This NF-1 gene is a classical tumour suppressor gene, with tumour growth requiring the loss of BOTH alleles. Neurofibromatosis type 1 has a classical combination of clinical signs(Ferner, 2010), for which the mnemonic CHANSOR has been used. These signs include **C**afé au lait macules; **H**amartomas of the iris (called Lisch nodules); **A**xillary and Inguinal Freckling;

Neurofibromas; **S**keletal lesions – like sphenoid wing dysplasia and thinning of long bone cortices; **O**ptic gliomas; and in increased **R**isk of other CNS and systemic tumours. The disorder is diagnosed using National Institutes of Health (NIH) Consensus Criteria for the Diagnosis of NF-1(Ferner *et al.*, 2007).

A diagnosis of NF-1 requires that at least TWO of the following be documented within a given patient:

- SIX or more café au lait spots with a maximum diameter
    - > 5 mm in pre-pubertal patients
    - > 15 mm in post-pubertal patients
- TWO or more neurofibromas of any type, or one plexiform neurofibroma
- Freckling in the axillary or inguinal areas
- An optic glioma
- TWO or more Lisch nodules
- A characteristic skeletal lesion, like
    - Sphenoid wing dysplasia
    - Thinning of long bone cortex, with or without pseudoarthrosis
- A first-degree relative (i.e., parent, sibling, or child) with confirmed NF-1

Table 2. National Institutes of Health (NIH) Consensus Criteria for the Diagnosis of NF-1

The requirement for no fewer than two of these findings means that NF-1 often only is confirmed after some passage of time, since certain features, like Lisch nodules, may not be present in infancy. Consequently, only about half (54%) of children meet the diagnostic criteria for NF-1 by the age of one year. This number rises to 90% by 7 years; and virtually 100% of cases are diagnosed by 20 years old(DeBella et al., 2000). The Committee on Genetics of the American Academy of Pediatrics has published guidelines for the baseline/screening and follow-up evaluations of confirmed or presumed NF-1(Hersh and American Academy of Pediatrics Committee on Genetics, 2008).

- An annual physical examination, including thorough skin and neurological exams
- Annual eye exams
- Magnetic resonance imaging (MRI) of the head for
    - Children diagnosed BEFORE age 5
    - Children with NEW neurological deficits, vision loss or endocrinopathy
- MRI of the spine and plain X-rays for
    - Children with scoliosis
    - Children with back pain, radiculopathy, or long tract signs referable to the spine
- Neuropsychological and developmental testing for
    - Children with learning, speech or social difficulties OR impaired motor skills
- Genetic counselling for the family
    - At diagnosis and as needed, on an ongoing basis.

Table 3. Published Committee on Genetics of the American Academy of Pediatrics guidelines for the baseline/screening and follow-up of confirmed or presumed NF-1

Roughly 5% of NF-1 cases are segmental, in that they involve only segments of the body(Sezer *et al.*, 2006). Such cases usually are the result of mosaicism, with mutations in the

NF-1 gene occurring AFTER fertilization, within the developing embryo(Morais *et al.*, 2010). Such mutations are not necessarily transmissible. For example, if gonadal progenitors are spared, the transmission risk is virtually zero. If, on the other hand, gonadal progenitors are affected, the risk of transmission to the next generation ranges from near zero to 50%, depending upon the percentage of gonadal cells involved. Phenotypically, one not atypical presentation of segmental NF-1 is café au lait spots affecting one limb or one side of the body and Lisch nodules in the ipsilateral eye(Morais *et al.*, 2010;Mansur *et al.*, 2011); others have been described with multiple localized cutaneous neurofibromas in the absence of all other sequelae(Arfan-ul-Bari, 2003). Serious sequelae, like malignancy, have been reported, but appear to be rare(Dang and Cohen, 2010).

2.1.2 Neurofibromatosis type 2

Neurofibromatosis type 2 (NF-2) is much less common than NF-1, with a prevalence that has been estimated as roughly one in 25,000 to 50,000(Ferner, 2010;Evans *et al.*, 2010;Ferner *et al.*, 2007). Although it shares the same name, it is entirely different than NF-1, in terms of the underlying cause, its presentation, its characteristic lesion, and its course(Baser *et al.*, 2003;Bance and Ramsden, 1999).

Typically, NF-2 is caused by a mutation affecting chromosome 22q12 and the gene product *merlin* (a moesin-, erzin-, and radixin-like protein), which sometimes is called *schwannomin.* Merlin encodes for a polypeptide that may affect cell growth and motility; more interesting, in terms of its presence in NF-2, is that it is a tumour inhibitor that often is absent in brain tumours(Evans, 1999;Fontaine *et al.*, 1991b;Fontaine *et al.*, 1991a). In addition, the same chromosomal abnormality is found in spontaneous spinal schwannomas, which suggests that a single location causes Schwann cell tumour growth(Jacoby *et al.*, 1999).

Clinically, NF-2 is a combination of features that always entails at least one eighth cranial nerve (CN-VIII) neurilemoma, in addition to a variety of other tumours (e.g., neurofibromas, meningiomas, gliomas, neurilemomas), juvenile posterior sub-capsular cataracts, and occasional other lesions, like café au lait spots. Like NF-1, it is diagnosed using NIH Consensus Criteria, initially proposed in 1988(Neurofibromatosis Conference Statement, 1988), but modified in 1997(Gutmann *et al.*, 1997). To meet these most recent criteria, for either definite or presumptive NF-2, a person must have:

- Definite diagnosis of NF2
  - The patient has bilateral CN VIII Schwannomas on MRI or CT scan (no biopsy necessary)
  - The patient has a first-degree relative with NF2 AND personally has either unilateral early-onset (age <30 years) CN VIII Schwannoma or any 2 of the following:
    - Meningioma
    - Glioma
    - Schwannoma
    - Juvenile posterior subcapsular lenticular opacity (juvenile cortical cataract)
- Presumptive diagnosis of NF2
  - The patient has early-onset (age <30 years) unilateral CN VIII Schwannomas detected on MRI or CT scan; AND one of the following:
    - Meningioma

    - Glioma
    - Schwannoma
    - Juvenile posterior subcapsular lenticular opacity
- The patient has >2 meningiomas and a unilateral CN VIII Schwannoma, OR one of the following:
    - Glioma
    - Schwannoma
    - Juvenile posterior subcapsular lenticular opacity

Table 4. Modified NIH Consensus Criteria for Neurofibromatosis type 2

As for NF-1, the diagnosis of NF-2 may be suspected for some time before being confirmed, given that cranial nerve VIII (acoustic) Schwannomas may present unilaterally, with the other side only becoming affected considerably later. It has been estimated, for example, that roughly 10% of individuals presenting with a unilateral acoustic Schwannoma ultimately will be diagnosed as having NF-2, a percentage high enough to warrant concern, but too low to allow for any sort of prediction(Evans *et al.*, 2007). Similarly, juvenile cortical cataracts may antedate the confirmation of any other lesion(s). In fact, the somewhat elusive nature of both NF-1 and NF-2 (given that lesions may be small and subclinical, and/or family histories unobtainable) make it somewhat difficult to estimate the true prevalence of these disorders. What is clear is that the presentation especially of a young patient with any of the lesions described in the preceding paragraphs warrants somewhat heightened vigilance. Consequently, also as for NF-1, the Committee on Genetics of the American Academy of Pediatrics has published guidelines for the baseline screening and follow-up evaluations of confirmed or presumed NF-2, which include:

- Neurological exam
- Eye exam
- Audiogram
- MRI of head and spine
- Genetic counselling for the family, at diagnosis and as needed, on an ongoing basis.

Table 5. Committee on Genetics of the American Academy of Pediatrics guidelines for the baseline/screening and follow-up of confirmed or presumed NF-2

Finally, as for NF-1, NF-2 might present in a segmental form, though it is less well defined, and whether or not it truly exists remains somewhat controversial. Segmental NF-2 has been defined as multiple discrete neurilemomas in peripheral nerves within an extremity without any central features of NF-2. In general, segmental forms of NF-1 and, especially, NF-2 are less problematic than systemic disease, including fewer of the associated features(Hager *et al.*, 1997). This said, some cases of segmental NF-1 can be extremely disfiguring, and malignancies have been reported(Dang and Cohen, 2010).

2.1.3 Neurological manifestations of NF-1 AND NF-2

All forms of neurofibromatosis, and especially neurofibromatosis type 1, are associated with numerous non-neurological, as well as neurological signs and symptoms. But it is beyond the scope of this chapter to discuss these, as they have been well described elsewhere(Hersh and American Academy of Pediatrics Committee on Genetics, 2008;Committee on Genetics, 1995;Lu-Emerson and Plotkin, 2009a;Lu-Emerson and Plotkin, 2009b).

2.1.3.1 Neurological manifestations of neurofibromatosis type 1

2.1.3.1.1 Cognitive impairment

Various degrees and forms of intellectual and social impairment are common in those with NF, affecting up to fifty percent of patients(Ferner, 2007;Ferner, 2010;Ferner *et al.*, 2007;Hersh and American Academy of Pediatrics Committee on Genetics, 2008;Lopes Ferraz Filho *et al.*, 2008;Committee on Genetics, 1995;NF1 Cognitive Disorders Task Force., 1997;Lu-Emerson and Plotkin, 2009a;Huson *et al.*, 1988;Rieley *et al.*, 2011). Specific abnormalities that have been noted include mental retardation , learning disabilities, and speech disorders(Arun and Gutmann, 2004;Lu-Emerson and Plotkin, 2009a;Rieley *et al.*, 2011;North *et al.*, 1997).

Of these, learning disabilities are the most common, present in roughly one third to one half of patients(North *et al.*, 1995;Denckla *et al.*, 1996). Mental retardation, once thought to be almost ubiquitous in neurofibromatosis(Crowe *et al.*, 1956), in fact only affects less than five percent(North *et al.*, 1997). The etiology of these impairments may be multi-factorial, including seizures; but there is some, albeit conflicting(Hyman *et al.*, 2003), evidence that cognitive impairment and/or the learning disabilities correlate with focal hyper-intensities that are present on magnetic resonance images(NF1 Cognitive Disorders Task Force., 1997;North *et al.*, 1994;Joy *et al.*, 1995). These areas of focal hyper-intensity are known as unidentified bright objects.

2.1.3.1.2 Unidentified Bright Objects (UBOs)

Of the myriad of neurological lesions that can be seen in patients with NF-1, unidentified bright objects (UBOs) are, by far, the most common lesion seen on MRI(Lopes Ferraz Filho *et al.*, 2008). They are characterized as foci of increased signal on T2-weighted images in the absence of any mass effect, accompanied by changes on T1-weighted images and contrast enhancement. Their appearance on MR spectroscopy is different than normal brain and neoplasms. What they actually represent remains unknown, however, as well as whether or not they have any clinical relevance. There is some evidence that they correlate with learning disabilities(NF1 Cognitive Disorders Task Force., 1997), but published evidence is conflicting. In general, UBOs are considered benign. Atypical lesions generally are deemed to require further work-up, to rule out some other potentially-relevant lesion; but UBOs typically are merely noted and left alone. Left alone, many UBOs regress spontaneously over time. Lesions that correlate with neurological symptoms and new lesions in older patients require more extensive work-up.

2.1.3.1.3 Optic-hypothalamic glioma

Optic-hypothalamic gliomas comprise the second most common imaging abnormality seen in NF-1, being detectable in roughly 15% of NF-1 patients. In 1958, Dodge et al published a classification scheme for these lesions, with lesions allocated to one of three main categories dependent upon the extent of the tumour(Dodge *et al.*, 1958). In essence, lesions were categorized into those involving just the optic nerve(s), lesions also involving the optic chiasm, and lesions extending all the way into the hypothalamus. These descriptions are expanded somewhat in Table 6.

Vision loss is characteristic of all categories of lesion(Massimi *et al.*, 2007), but it often only is diagnosed late in younger children, who will not complain of decreased vision until losses are severe. Loss of vision usually progresses slowly, with sudden visual loss reported, but quite uncommon(Valdueza *et al.*, 1995;Giuffré *et al.*, 1982). Not uncommon signs with optic nerve gliomas are exophthalmos, optic nerve atrophy, painless ocular proptosis, papilledema, nystagmus, strabismus and conjunctival redness(Massimi *et al.*, 2007). Optic nerve atrophy and/or papilledema, nystagmus and visual field defects are more classic for chiasmic lesions, the visual field defects often incongruous due to the irregular infiltration of the chiasm with tumour.

- Mild thickening of one or both optic nerves
  - Sometimes is a low-grade glioma
  - Sometimes is hyperplasia of the optic nerve sheath
- Globular thickening of the optic nerves and chiasm
- A large mass lesion involving the optic chiasm and hypothalamus

Table 6. Variants of optic-hypothalamic gliomas

Lesions that also involve the hypothalamus generally present with a more complicated clinical picture, that may include hydrocephalus (due to foramina of Monroe obstruction); various endocrinopathies (especially growth hormone deficiency and precocious puberty); diencephalic syndrome, characterized by nystagmus and profound emaciation, despite normal caloric intake, and only subtle deterioration of muscles, level of alertness, and hyperkinesis (Poussaint *et al.*, 1997); and other neurological deficits like hemiparesis or ataxia.

Management is somewhat controversial, though there is evidence that, though an aggressive lesion in children (often infants) without NF-1, the course is much more indolent in neurofibromatosis(Massimi *et al.*, 2007;Oh *et al.*, 2011). Newer imaging techniques now allow for the detection of asymptomatic lesions and, among those with NF-1, many lesions progress slowly, if at all. The major difficulty is that, once vision is lost, blindness is irreparable. This is particularly catastrophic in those with bilateral or chiasmic lesions, because the blindness will involve both eyes.

Monitoring of optic-hypothalamic gliomas in children who are less than 5 years old is particularly problematic, because they often experience considerable vision loss before anything is detected. However, no firm or universally-accepted guidelines exist for monitoring. Some doctors advise annual MRIs. Meanwhile, others recommend annual neurological and ophthalmological exams, with MRIs limited to those patients who have new symptoms or findings.

Treatment is likewise controversial and lacking firm guidelines(Massimi *et al.*, 2007). Surgery generally is restricted to those patients in whom only a single optic nerve is involved and severe vision loss already exists. It is avoided in patients with bilateral lesions or lesions involving the optic chiasm, because this generally results in total blindness. Radiation usually is effective, but it is not advised in younger children because radiation often causes significant loss of cognitive and endocrine function(Ellenberg *et al.*, 2009;Boman *et al.*, 2009). It also increases the risk of intracranial malignancies and vasculopathies, like moyamoya disease. Chemotherapy also is often effective, and typically selected for younger children, due to the risk of radiation-induced cognitive deficits mentioned earlier(Massimi *et al.*, 2007). In general, combination therapy is used, involving two or more drugs. Unfortunately, chemotherapy itself is associated with an increased risk of secondary malignancies, like leukemia.

As stated earlier, those who have optic-hypothalamic gliomas in the context of NF-1 generally have a much more indolent course than those in whom NF-1 does not exist(Massimi *et al.*, 2007;Oh *et al.*, 2011). This said, the prognosis is quite variable, depending upon the lesion, and may be better than for those with pure optic gliomas (again, in the absence of NF-1).

2.1.3.1.4 Gliomas of the cerebral and cerebellar hemispheres

In NF-1, hemispheric and cerebellar gliomas are less common than lesions involving the optic tract(Hottinger and Khakoo, 2009a). Most are benign or only exhibit low-grade malignant potential; but all grades of malignancy have been reported(Hottinger and Khakoo, 2009a). They differ in appearance from the UBOs mentioned earlier, in that there generally is a mass effect, and the signal on T1-weighted images is decreased, not increased. Most are resectable. Consequently, management usually starts with surgical excision. If total excision is achieved and the lesion is low-grade, monitoring may be all that is required. Partial excisions usually require adjuvant radiation therapy and/or chemotherapy(Hottinger and Khakoo, 2009a); though, as stated earlier in this chapter, radiation generally is avoided or delayed for as long as possible in younger children, especially those who are less than 3 years old, because of the risk of radiation-induced cognitive deficits. Recurrence is managed as for similar lesions in patients without neurofibromatosis.

2.1.3.1.5 Brainstem gliomas

Brainstem gliomas comprise a heterogeneous group of lesions, with at least three main subtypes: (1) a diffuse area of brainstem enlargement; (2) focal enhancing nodules with or without cystic areas; and (3) peri-aqueductal gliomas. All subtypes generally have a very indolent course. Most do not require treatment, though MRI monitoring is indicated until their indolent course is confirmed. Some lesions regress on their own(Hottinger and Khakoo, 2009a).

When there is a diffuse area of brainstem enlargement, it is somewhat similar in appearance to UBOs, except that a mass effect usually is evident. Such lesions also typically are quite a bit larger than most UBOs. Like UBOs, they exhibit abnormal signals on T1-weighted images. What the diffuse enlargement represents is controversial. Presumed to be gliomas, they have a more indolent course than brainstem gliomas seen outside of NF-1, such that adjuvant treatment only is required in the minority of patients whose lesions progress. However, ongoing monitoring is required to detect the few who do progress, before neurological deficits ensue, which often are irreversible. Rarely, these gliomas progress to more malignant forms of astrocytoma, including glioblastoma(Leonard *et al.*, 2006;Hottinger and Khakoo, 2009a).

The focal enhancing nodules, with or without cystic areas, generally are thought to represent pilocytic astrocytomas, given their imaging characteristics. Like pilocytic astrocytomas elsewhere, they generally are indolent; but their course is unpredictable and the brainstem so susceptible to major deficits, relative to the cerebral hemispheres, that ongoing monitoring is required. Small, focal intrinsic lesions may enlarge and then regress spontaneously. Exophytic tumours often are more aggressive and require treatment.

Periaqueductal gliomas occur adjacent to the aqueduct of Sylvius between the 3rd and 4th ventricles in the midbrain. They typically manifest with late-onset aqueductal stenosis, leading to hydrocephalus. Presumably, they represent low-grade gliomas or glial hamartomas, and typically are indolent. However, because of their location, shunting often is necessary. Resection is usually not necessary for any of the brainstem gliomas seen in NF-1(Hottinger and Khakoo, 2009a;Leonard *et al.*, 2006).

2.1.3.1.6 Neurofibromas

Neurofibromas are one of the hallmark lesions of NF-1, occurring both in paraspinal areas and in peripheral nerves(Ferner, 2010;Hersh and American Academy of Pediatrics Committee on Genetics, 2008;Lu-Emerson and Plotkin, 2009a). They are histologically distinct from the neurilemomas that are the hallmark of NF-2, being composed of Schwann cells, fibroblasts, mast cells, axons and abundant extracellular matrix, with both myelinated and unmyelinated zones(Lu-Emerson and Plotkin, 2009a). Neurofibromas within the central nervous system are best visualized by MRI, which can document each lesion's size, pattern of growth, and proximity to adjacent structures, like nerves and other tissues. These tumours may be few in number or seemingly everywhere. They can be small or grow to enormous sizes that may be extremely and tragically disfiguring. Conventional wisdom states that the more cutaneous (external) lesions there are, the fewer lesions there will be in deeper (internal) tissues; but this is not necessarily the case.

Neurofibromas can be subdivided in several ways. One way is to subdivide them, according to their pattern of growth, into fusiform and plexiform lesions. Fusiform lesions are discrete lesions that involve a well-circumscribed area of a single nerve. As such, they generally are easy to resect, when necessary or indicated. In contrast, plexiform lesions often are found in nerve trunks and extend over long distances, diffusely invading the nerve tissue(Korf, 1999). They also are highly vascular and induce diffuse hypertrophy of adjacent connective tissues. Because they are so extensive and invasive, they are virtually impossible to resect without causing major neurological deficits (Hottinger and Khakoo, 2009a;Korf, 1999). Moreover, though incidence estimates vary, at least two percent of neurofibromatosis patients experience malignant transformation of a neurofibroma into a neurofibrosarcoma (Woodruff, 1999), and plexiform neurofibromas generally are perceived to be more likely to do this, with a risk as high as ten percent per lesion(Hottinger and Khakoo, 2009a).

Another way to categorize neurofibromas is by their location, into subcutaneous, peripheral nerve, plexus, paraspinal, craniofacial, and visceral lesions.

Subcutaneous neurofibromas (NFs) can be fusiform or plexiform(Hottinger and Khakoo, 2009a). Both types tend to recur after resection. Consequently, resection usually is limited to lesions that are cosmetically intolerable, unacceptably painful, growing rapidly, prone to irritation due to their location (e.g., at the patient's beltline), or undergoing malignant change.

Peripheral nerve NFs may be asymptomatic. They can, however, produce symptoms if they irritate the involved nerve, resulting in pain, paresthesias, and/or other neurological dysfunction. As stated above, they tend to be fusiform, rather than plexiform. Hence, resection generally is feasible without producing major neurological deficits if not all the nerve fascicles are involved, by starting at the proximal and distal poles of the tumour and identifying all the fascicles from which the tumour arises. If all the fascicles are involved, *en bloc* resection often does result in major deficits, so a subtotal resection must be performed. Follow-up of any residual tumour is necessary because approximately 15% undergo malignant transformation.

Plexus NFs are plexiform and, consequently, virtually always non-resectable without causing major neurological deficits. Resection generally is limited to tumours with evidence of malignant transformation or those causing intractable severe symptoms from pain or compression of adjacent structures. Many actually run an indolent course and need only be followed. Various chemotherapy protocols are being tested for those with progressive neurological impairment.

Paraspinal NFs usually are fusiform or nodular lesions that involve nerve roots as they enter the spinal canal. They occasionally involve multiple nerve roots; there even are reported cases where ALL the nerve roots were found to be involved. Generally, these lesions are slowly progressive, if at all. Monitoring often is all that is required, and there is considerable debate as to whether routine imaging even is needed, versus clinical examination alone(Khong *et al.*, 2003). However, some do cause progressive spinal encroachment such that surgical resection is indicated(Sarica *et al.*, 2008). When resection is necessary, various surgical approaches are used, depending on the spinal level and the tumour's relationship to surrounding paraspinal anatomy, to access and resect these tumours(Cherqui *et al.*, 2007).

Craniofacial NFs typically are plexiform lesions that involve peripheral nerves of the face(Greig *et al.*, 2009;Baujat *et al.*, 2006;Visrutaratna *et al.*, 2004;Jacquemin *et al.*, 2003;Park *et al.*, 2002;Jackson, 2001). Either the tumour itself or surgery to resect it can compromise the facial nerve, leading to facial paralysis and resultant cosmetic deformity. The lesions also can become massive, resulting in horrific cosmetic deformity(Greig *et al.*, 2009;Park *et al.*, 2002). Many involve the orbit, where they can be extremely invasive and destructive; and sometimes extend intra-cranially (Jacquemin *et al.*, 2003). Resection of orbital lesions often requires enucleation; consequently, if they are stable, orbital lesions are usually just monitored closely.

Finally, visceral NFs tend to be plexiform and, hence, cannot be completely resected. They may occur in almost any tissue (e.g., bladder, the gastrointestinal tract), where symptoms relate to their location and size(Cheng *et al.*, 1999;Kaefer *et al.*, 1997;Hahn *et al.*, 1992). Malignant transformation is a recognized, long-term risk.

2.1.3.2 Neurological manifestations of neurofibromatosis type 2

2.1.3.2.1 Vestibular neurolemomas

Vestibular neurolemomas are tumours of the eighth cranial nerve (CN-VIII) that occur in roughly 95% of patients with NF-2, often bilaterally(Ferner, 2010;Lu-Emerson and Plotkin, 2009b). They are diagnostic of NF-2 when bilateral. Typically, these lesions present in late adolescence or adulthood, but they can be seen in children. They should be suspected in any patient with a posterior cataract and multiple spinal cord or peripheral nerve tumours, when in the absence of café au lait spots or Lisch nodules. In such a patient, an MRI of the head clearly is indicated to rule out NF-2. In fact, the cataract could be a red herring; if the MRI shows an optic glioma, NF-1 should be considered.

Magnetic resonance imaging is the optimum screening tool for these lesions(Lu-Emerson and Plotkin, 2009b), because it is relatively sensitive at detecting them, even when they are asymptomatic. Symptomatic tumours in childhood suggest a more aggressive course. If a vestibular neurolemoma is, or bilateral neurolemomas are present, regular hearing tests are indicated, because of the risk of progressive bilateral hearing loss.

The primary goals of treatment are, first of all, to preserve hearing, recognizing that unilateral disease may become bilateral later on; and second, to prevent brainstem dysfunction or frank damage secondary to compression by tumour. However, the best way to achieve these two objectives remains both unproven and controversial. Significant brainstem compression is an indication for immediate surgical resection, despite the risk of lost hearing. However, if the tumour is small and not compressing the brainstem, opinions vary. Some recommend early surgery to remove tumours while small, lowering the risk of post-operative hearing loss; but the course of these tumours is variable. Hence, others recommend a wait-and-see approach, delaying surgery for as long as possible. The risk of this latter approach is that *en bloc* surgery ultimately may be necessary, ensuring deafness in that ear, and placing the adjacent facial nerve (CN-VII) at risk.

Stereotactic surgery MAY reduce the risk of deafness; and, if deafness occurs, it tends to be delayed one to two years, allowing for the patient to learn sign language and/or lip reading. However, the benefits of this approach over others remain unproven. Another approach is partial (sub-capsular) resection, leaving some residual tumour adherent to the auditory and facial nerves to reduce the risk of injury to both; however, residual tumour may grow and become problematic at some later date.

Especially in those with bilateral lesions, learning sign language or how to lip read ultimately may prove beneficial. And the placement of a cochlear or auditory brainstem implant may preserve some hearing, even in those who have undergone bilateral resections.

2.1.3.2.2 Intracranial meningiomas

Intracranial meningiomas are found in approximately 50% of patients with NF-2(Lu-Emerson and Plotkin, 2009b). They can occur singly, but commonly there are multiple lesions in a given patient with NF-2. They also often occur along with one or more non-auditory cranial nerve neurolemomas. They tend to be more aggressive in children versus adults with NF-2. As with non-auditory cranial nerve neurolemomas, because they often are multiple, it is not unusual for surgery to be deferred.

2.1.3.2.3 Meningioangiomatosis

Meningioangiomatosis is a rare, benign, focal lesion of the leptomeninges and underlying cerebral cortex, which is characterized by leptomeningeal and meningovascular proliferation(Omeis *et al.*, 2006;Deb *et al.*, 2006). Histologically, it appears as hamartomatous proliferation of capillary-sized vessels, meningothelial cells, and fibroblasts within cerebral cortex. It may occur in either the presence or absence of an adjacent meningioma. Though sporadic cases have been reported, meningioangiomatosis most often occurs in patients with NF-2. As with most neurofibromatosis lesions, they can be multifocal, especially in NF-2. Though histologically benign, they can produce seizures(Jallo *et al.*, 2005), though this is more common in sporadic than in NF-2 cases(Omeis *et al.*, 2006).

In cases of intractable seizures, resection is indicated(Jallo *et al.*, 2005). At least one case of sudden death, presumably secondary to a fatal seizure, has been reported involving a previously-asymptomatic 13-year old boy(Wixom *et al.*, 2005).

2.1.3.2.4 Non-vestibular cranial nerve neurolemomas

Non-vestibular cranial nerve neurolemomas are found in more than 30% of NF-2 patients. Like auditory neurilemomas, they usually are benign, but their course is more unpredictable. Some grow very slowly, if at all, and cause no problems. Others grow rapidly and are quite problematic, both due to damage of the involved nerve and because of their mass effect. And, on occasion, malignant transformation of a non-vestibular neurolemoma has been reported(Hanada *et al.*, 1982). Because they often are multifocal, surgery usually is deferred unless they are unacceptably symptomatic, endangering function, or growing rapidly.

2.1.3.2.5 Intraparenchymal gliomas

As a rule, spinal lesions are more common in NF-2 than in NF1, while brain lesions are less common in NF-2 than NF-1. And ependymomas are the most common malignancy in NF-2, versus astrocytomas in NF-1(Lu-Emerson and Plotkin, 2009a;Hottinger and Khakoo, 2009a;Lu-Emerson and Plotkin, 2009b). As opposed to astrocytomas, which rapidly invade surrounding neural tissue, sending multiple tumour fronds in all directions, ependymomas usually are well-circumscribed, and therefore often quite resectable. Their surgical and post-operative management (like the use of adjuvant therapy) is the same as for intramedullary spinal tumours in patients without neurofibromatosis.

2.1.3.2.6 Extracranial neurilemomas and meningiomas

Benign intraspinal tumours of the nerve sheath or meningeal cells are more common in NF-2 than in the general population, though still rare. In NF-2, however, they often are multiple, occurring at many different spine levels. As they are when they are intra-cranial, both neurilemomas and meningiomas are well-circumscribed tumours that displace, rather than invade adjacent tissues; and most grow slowly(Lu-Emerson and Plotkin, 2009b;Zhang *et al.*, 2007). They also can occlude up to 90% of the spinal canal before neurological deficits occur. Hence, most remain asymptomatic for years. However, once deficits start to appear, minimal growth can cause significant reductions in function. Surgical outcomes generally are better if such tumours are removed before neurological dysfunction is detected. Management, therefore, consists of close monitoring with repeat neurological exams and MRI; and surgical resection before neurological function starts to deteriorate. Sometimes, they must be removed because of intractable, unacceptable pain. Because they generally involve a single nerve fascicle, they often can be resected without significant neurological deterioration, if any at all(Lu-Emerson and Plotkin, 2009b;Zhang *et al.*, 2007).

2.1.3.2.7 Neurofibromas

In NF-2, neurofibromas are much as they are in NF-1, except that they are much less common(Lu-Emerson and Plotkin, 2009b). Because many neurofibromas, especially plexiform lesions, are not as well-encapsulated as neurilemomas, they are more problematic, and more difficult to resect. Consequently, surgical outcomes generally are worse than for neurilemomas.

2.1.4 Summary: Neurofibromatosis

Neurofibromatosis is a collection of disorders, which can be systemic or segmental. Systemic neurofibromatosis types 1 and 2 are the most common and best recognized syndromes, though segmental and overlap syndromes exist. Both NF-1 and NF-2 are autosomal dominant, but spontaneous mutations are not uncommon, and there is tremendous phenotypic variability even within a given family or between twins. Type 1 is at least ten times as common as type 2 disease, with all other types less common still. The two classic forms of neurofibromatosis, NF-1 and NF-2, are very different. Whereas the characteristic lesion of NF-1 is a neurofibroma, the characteristic lesion of NF-2 is a neurilemoma, which involves either one or both auditory nerves (CN-VIII) in 95% of cases. Both NF-1 and NF-2 are associated with numerous other CNS and peripheral nervous system tumours. These are summarized in Table 11.

Neurofibromatosis type 1

- Non-neurological lesions:
  - Skin and retinal hamartomas (café au lait spots, axillary freckling and Lisch nodules)
  - Various bone abnormalities, including cortical thinning, sphenoid dysplasia, and bowing of long bones
  - Segmental hypertrophy of skin, bone and subcutaneous tissues
  - Hypothalamic tumours
  - Neoplasms involving other body systems, including pheochromacytomas, rhabdomyosarcomas, adenocarcinomas, melanomas, non-Hodgkin's lymphomas, and lymphoblastic leukemias
- Neurological lesions
  - Neurofibromas
  - Neurofibrosarcoma (malignant transformation of a neurofibroma)
  - Unidentified bright objects (UBOs) on MRI
  - Optic-hypothalamic gliomas
  - Cerebral, cerebellar and brainstem gliomas

Neurofibromatosis type 2

- Non-neurological lesions:
  - Posterior subcapsular cataracts
- Neurological lesions
  - Vestibular neurolemomas
  - Intracranial meningiomas
  - Meningioangiomatosis
  - Non-vertebral cranial nerve neurolemomas
  - Extracranial neurolemomas and meningiomas
  - Intraparenchymal gliomas, especially of the spine

Table 7. Lesions classically associated with neurofibromatosis types 1 and 2

Both NF-1 and NF-2 are diagnosed using published diagnostic criteria that, like the syndromes themselves, are highly different from one another. The diagnostic process requires patient and family histories, detailed physical examinations (especially dermatological and neurological), and imaging studies (especially MRI). The course of many tumours and of the disease itself is often hard to predict. Most tumours are slow-growing and relatively indolent, but many have the potential to undergo malignant change and others may cause neurological impairment, either by compression or invasion. Especially in NF-1, neurofibromas can be tragically disfiguring. Management of the neurofibromatosis syndromes includes regular close monitoring; genetic counselling of families; and surgery, which typically is deferred until absolutely necessary. Surgical outcomes generally are better with NF-2 than with NF-1.

2.2 Tuberous sclerosis (Bourneville's disease)

Tuberous sclerosis, which also is called tuberous sclerosis complex (TSC) and Bourneville's disease, is the second most common phakomatosis syndrome, after neurofibromatosis type 1. It affects anywhere from one in 6000 to one in 30,000 people(Osborne *et al.*, 1991;Hong *et al.*, 2009;Morrison, 2009), with marked variations in penetrance rendering all estimates somewhat unreliable.

Like neurofibromatosis, it initially was described by von Recklinghausen, in 1862; however, it is named after a French physician, Désiré-Magloire Bourneville, who coined the term 'sclerose tubereuse' in 1880, likening the cerebral lesions he detected at autopsy to small potatoes. The physical manifestations of tuberous sclerosis largely are due to the formation of hamartia (malformed tissue, like cortical tubers), hamartomas (like facial angiofibroma and subependymal nodules) and, very rarely, cancerous hamartoblastomas. The effect of these various lesions on the brain includes various neurological symptoms, such as seizures, developmental delay, and behavioural problems. The initially-described triad of features was epilepsy, low intelligence, and skin lesions, though the condition is now recognized to involve numerous other organ systems, as well, including the kidneys, lungs, heart and eyes. And many cases of 'low intelligence' have since been recognized as learning disabilities, autism, and pervasive development disorders, rather than low intelligence, per se(Ridler *et al.*, 2006;Harrison and Bolton, 1997).

Tuberous sclerosis (TS) is autosomal dominant, but up to 60% of cases arise from spontaneous mutations(Orlova and Crino, 2010;Osborne *et al.*, 1991;Morrison, 2009). Two tumour-suppressor genes, TSC-1 (tuberous sclerosis complex-1) and TSC-2, are responsible for TS. Roughly 80-90% of mutations involve TSC-2, while just 10-20% of mutations involve TSC-1(Orlova and Crino, 2010). The genetic locus for TSC-1 is chromosome 9q34, and the TSC-1 gene product is called *hamartin.* The genetic locus for TSC-2 is chromosome 16p13.3, and the TSC-2 gene product is called *tuberin.* Both hamartin and tuberin appear to have roles in cell differentiation, proliferation and migration. The disorder effects cellular differentiation, proliferation and migration during early development, leading to various diffuse hamartomas and neoplastic lesions affecting virtually every body organ(Grajkowska *et al.*, 2010;Orlova and Crino, 2010). It can present at any age, but most commonly appears during childhood, especially late childhood.

2.2.1 Non-neurological involvement in tuberous sclerosis

A broad spectrum of skin lesions are associated with tuberous sclerosis, with skin lesions the most common and recognizable feature of this syndrome. They include ash-leaf spots; facial angiofibromas; lumbosacral angiofibromas (Shagreen patches); café au lait spots; periungual fibromas (Koenen tumours); forehead plaques; skin tags (molluscum fibrosum pendulum); confetti macules; and poliosis, with ash-leaf spots the most characteristic lesion, seen in 5% of the general population, but 97% of TS patients. The ash-leaf spot is a hypomelanotic macule, of variable size but up to several inches in length, which is found on the trunk and/or the buttocks. It is recognized by the axis of the leaf, which tends to line up perpendicular to the axis of the spine. This usually is the only sign of TS that is visible at birth. Because they are characterized by decreased pigmentation, a Wood's lamp may be required to see ash-leaf spots in fair-skinned individuals.

Facial angiofibromas, also called *adenoma sebaceum,* are reddish macules or papules, though they may appear dark brown in darker-skinned individuals. Classically, they are clustered around the nose and cheeks in a butterfly distribution, and may be mistaken for acne, especially in teenagers, except that they do not contain purulent material and, hence, cannot be drained. Histologically, they consist of blood vessels and fibrous tissue. Because they can be cosmetically displeasing, they can be removed either by dermabrasion or laser treatments(Verma *et al.*, 2001).

Lumbosacral angiofibromas also are called shagreen patches. These are areas of thick leathery skin that are dimpled like an orange peel, usually found on the lower back or nape of the neck. They, like ash-leaf spots, are of variable size, but can be quite sizeable. Café au lait spots are as previously described for neurofibromatosis. Periungual fibromas (Koenen tumours) are very rare in childhood, but common by middle age. They are small, fleshy tumours that grow around and under the toenails and/or fingernails. They sometimes need to be surgically removed if they enlarge or cause bleeding. Forehead plaques are as they sound: raised, discoloured areas on the forehead. Skin tags (molluscum fibrosum pendulum) are very non-specific, commonly seen in healthy individuals. Confetti macules are clusters of small, punctate, hypopigmented macules that look like confetti (hence, the name). They are fairly specific for TS, commonly found symmetrically on the limbs. Poliosis is a tuft or patch of white hair on the patient's scalp or eyelids, and patients may have several.

Intraventricular rhabdomyomas are the most common cardiac manifestation of tuberous sclerosis. These are benign tumours of striated muscle that, in TS, may be multiple. In fact, multiple tumours affecting multiple chambers are common, though most are found within the ventricles. They are detectable by echocardiography in roughly 50% of TS patients. However, their incidence ranges from up to 90% in newborns to as low as 20% in adults. They generally grow during the second half of pregnancy and regress after birth. Many disappear entirely. Alternatively, tumour size may remain constant as the heart grows, with much the same effect. Most remain asymptomatic, detected on peri-natal ultrasound after 20 weeks of gestation, and never become clinically manifest. Some produce a murmur. Potential problems include obstruction of blood flow if the tumour impedes proper valve opening; and arrhythmia. However, most cardiac complications occur before the child reaches one year old. Why they are clinically important is that this rare tumour is a strong indicator of TS in a child, especially if there is a positive family history of TS.

Kidney involvement is the second most common cause of morbidity and mortality in TS, after neurological disease. It is the most common cause of death in patients who are greater than 30 years old. A host of renal lesions exist, which include angiomyolipomas, renal cysts, renal cell carcinomas, and oncocytomas. Renal cell carcinomas are rare, relative to anygiomyolipomas and cysts, but still affect up to 3% of patients, making them considerably more common in TS patients than in the general population. Oncocytomas are a benign adenomatous hamartoma that are even more uncommon. Conversely, angiomyolipomas are indentified in 60 to 80% of TS patients. They usually are benign; but they also usually are multiple and bilateral and frequently cause haematuria. Histologically, they are composed of vascular tissue, smooth muscle, and fat. And, although benign, a lesion larger than 4 cm in diameter is at risk for a potentially catastrophic haemorrhage, either spontaneously or with minimal trauma. These lesions are not exclusive to TS, being found in about 1 in 300 people without TS. However, lesions in non-TS patients usually are solitary. Renal cysts can be identified in between 20 and 30% of TS patients, but they usually cause few if any problems. Having said this, 2% of TS have autosomal dominant polycystic kidney disease which commonly leads to renal failure.

Lung involvement in tuberous sclerosis usually affects women in their third and fourth decades of life, implicating some hormonal influence. The classic lesion is lymphangioleiomyomatosis (LAM), which is progressive replacement of the lung parenchyma with multiple cysts, generally measuring 2-20 mm in diameter, with equal involvement of all lobes. These cysts are formed by hyperplastic smooth muscle. Recent genetic analysis suggests that this proliferative bronchiolar smooth muscle represents monoclonal metastases from a coexisting renal angiomyolipoma. There have been cases of TSC-related LAM recurring following lung transplantation, confirming the concept of an 'external' source. The prevalence of LAM in patients with TS is roughly 1-5%, making it vastly more common than the one per million prevalence observed in the general population. Nonetheless, it often is misdiagnosed as asthma, emphysema, or some other pulmonary disease. Plain radiographs reveal the superimposition of cysts, producing the reticulonodular pattern typical of interstitial lung disease. High-resolution CT is more specific for the diagnosis, and better at assessing the degree of pulmonary involvement. Prognostically, LAM is slowly progressive. It also, interestingly, tends to be associated with less severe TS, accompanied by less intellectual impairment and fewer seizures. Roughly 90% of patients with LAM remain alive 15 to 20 years after diagnosis.

Retinal phakomas, gray or yellow retinal plaques that may be single or multiple, are the classic ocular lesion seen in TS, being present in up to 87% of patients. They rarely affect vision and, hence, usually do not warrant any treatment.

2.2.2 Neurologic involvement in tuberous sclerosis

Neurological involvement is the most common cause of morbidity and mortality from TS, and the most common cause of death in patients under 30 years old. Problems stem from a broad variety of intra-cerebral tumours, which include cortical tubers, subependymal nodules, and subependymal giant cell astrocytomas (SEGA).

Cortical tubers can be identified in more than 80% of patients. Recall that they are what Bourneville first described, and the reason behind the disease's name. They are formed from aberrant neuronal migration during the development of the cerebral cortices, and primarily affect the frontal and parietal lobes. Although non-malignant, they are problematic, because they may result in life-long, intractable seizures. Unfortunately, resection of these tumours often does NOT lead to any major reduction in seizures, though large tumours may need to be resected due to their mass effect.

Subependymal nodules are the hallmark lesion for TS on computed tomography (CT) scans. They may be either calcified or non-calcified, and may number from one to as many as 20 lesions. Some have described their appearance on CT as looking like the drippings of a candle. They are composed of abnormal, swollen glial cells and bizarre multinucleated cells that are indeterminate, in terms of glial versus neuronal origin. There is no interposed neural tissue. These nodules have a tendency to calcify as the patient ages. More ominously, any nodule that markedly enhances and enlarges over time should be considered suspicious for transformation into a subependymal giant cell astrocytoma (SEGA).

Subependymal giant cell astrocytomas (SEGA) develop in between 5 and 15% of TS patients(Goh *et al.*, 2004), typically developing in the region of the foramen of Monro, where they frequently cause obstructive hydrocephalus. Though they are slow-growing and rarely undergo malignant transformation, these tumours are problematic because of their location and relative inaccessibility for resection.

Problems related to the various neurological lesions of TS include intractable seizures, which ultimately present in 97% of patients with cortical tubers and in 75% of patients with cortical tubers before one year old. Various forms of intellectual, social and behavioural impairment are other sequelae of these tumours, including autism in roughly 20 to 60%, learning disabilities in about 50%, and mental retardation and self-mutilation, both in roughly 10%. These effects often are progressive; in fact, many neonates are neurologically normal. Table 8 lists the various complications related to cortical tubers and other CNS lesions in tuberous sclerosis.

- Seizures, often intractable
- Progressive intellectual impairment
- Learning disabilities
- Impaired social and communication skills
- Behavioural impairment
- Purposeful self-injury / self-mutilation
- Autism
- Hyperactivity
- Obsessive behaviours
- Obstructive hydrocephalus
- Mass effects from tumour growth
- Death, primarily from intractable seizures or SEGA-induced obstructive hydrocephalus

Table 8. Complications related to cortical tubers and other CNS lesions in tuberous sclerosis

These CNS lesions are diagnosed by various imaging techniques, including CT, CT with contrast, and MRI. Gadolinium-enhanced MRI is the most sensitive radiographic study. Electroencephalograms (EEG) are useful to document and identify the foci of seizures. The diagnosis of tuberous sclerosis as a syndrome, however, is made using published criteria that include a wide range of both major and minor criteria(Roaches *et al.*, 1998).

Management essentially consists of monitoring and supportive measures. Magnetic resonance imaging of the head every 1-2 years is indicated to assess for tumour growth, mass effects, and impending outflow obstruction. Anti-epileptic drugs are used to control seizures, since the resection of tumours is difficult, dangerous and of uncertain benefit; surgery to control seizures rarely results in complete seizure resolution.

Surgery may be performed to relieve increased intracranial pressure and focal deficits from tumours, and hydrocephalus from obstruction, primarily at the foramen of Munro. Complete resection of intra-ventricular tumours often is difficult, if not impossible, because of their origins in the caudate nucleus and septum pellucidum. Also, though relatively avascular, the tumours invade surrounding tissue and can be quite large. Finally, incomplete resection risks tumour re-growth. Recently, rapamycin has demonstrated some promise for SEGA in patients with tuberous sclerosis(Franz *et al.*, 2006). Overall, however, the long-term prognosis is poor. The rate of mortality is increased relative to age-matched population, with the #1 cause of death being renal disease, and the #1 cause of morbidity CNS disease, primarily related to seizures, cognitive impairment, and SEGA-induced obstructive hydrocephalus.

2.3 Von Hippel-Lindau disease

With angiomas in the eye first described by the German ophthalmologist Eugen Von Hippel in 1904, and the association between these retinal with CNS tumours first noted by the Swedish pathologist Arvid Lindau in 1927, the disease that Lindau first called 'angiomatosis of the central nervous system', and which for years was known just as Lindau syndrome, is now named for both men. Also known as retinocerebellar angiomatosis, its incidence has been estimated as roughly 1 in 31-36,000 live births(Hottinger and Khakoo, 2009b), though it is not usually manifested in infancy. The average age at first presentation is 26 years, and the average age at diagnosis 31 years(Hottinger and Khakoo, 2009b). Nonetheless, paediatric cases are not uncommon, and certainly seen by the paediatric neurosurgeon as a challenging disorder to treat.

Von Hippel-Lindau disease is autosomal dominant, with 97-99% of cases familial and only 1-3% occurring as a result of spontaneous mutations. It is associated with inactivation of the tumour-suppressor gene VHL (Von Hippel Lindau), which is found on chromosome 3p25(Hottinger and Khakoo, 2009b;Seizinger *et al.*, 1988). Decreased levels of the VHL protein, which is important in a critical pathway helping cells to adapt to hypoxic stress, lead to over-expression of a hypoxia-inducible transcription factor (HIF-1) which, in turn, results in increased cell proliferation, and the over-expression of several growth factors, ultimately manifesting as multiple, multi-systemic benign and malignant tumours, which sometimes are bilateral (e.g., both eyes)(Glasker, 2005). These tumours include haemangioblastomas of the cerebellum, spine, brainstem and retina (the most common tumour identified); renal clear cell carcinomas; pheochromocytomas; pancreatic and renal cysts; endolymphatic sac tumours (ELSTs, of the petrous bone at the cerebellopontine angle)(Hassard *et al.*, 1984); papillary cystadenomas of the epididymus or broad ligament; and haemanigiomas of the adrenal glands, liver and lungs. The diagnosis is made on clinical grounds using established, published criteria:

- Two or more haemangioblastomas; OR
- One haemangioblastoma PLUS some visceral lesion, like pheochromocytoma, pancreatic or renal cyst, or renal cell carcinoma; OR
- One retinal or CNS haemangioblastomas or some other visceral lesion PLUS a positive family history of CNS or visceral manifestations of the disease.

Table 9. Classification criteria for Von Hippel-Lindau disease

The disease is subdivided into various clinical subtypes, based upon genotype-phenotype correlations within families, with type 1 families having pheochromocytomas, and three sub-classes of type 2 disease, all lacking pheochromocytomas but a familial risk of other tumour typess: type 2a, with a low familial risk of renal cell carcinoma and pancreatic tumours; type 2b, with a high familial risk of renal cell carcinoma and pancreatic tumours; and type 2c, with a high familial risk of isolated pheochromocytomas(Ong *et al.*, 2007)

Central nervous system manifestations are highly prevalent(Butman *et al.*, 2008;Richard *et al.*, 1998), with CNS haemangioblastomas occurring in 60 to 80% of patients. Moreover, they are more likely to be multiple and present at an earlier age than when they occur sporadically, being a presenting feature in roughly 60% of VHL patients(Wanebo *et al.*, 2003). These lesions may occur anywhere along the cranioaxial axis, but only 1% of these tumours are supratentorial(Wanebo *et al.*, 2003). The site of lesion determines the symptoms with which the patient presents. The cerebellum and brainstem are the most common sites of haemangioblastomas in VHL syndrome(Wanebo *et al.*, 2003), where patients present with headaches, vomiting, lethargy, dysmetria, ataxia, papilloedema, polycythemia from tumour production of erythropoietin, and/or enlarging cysts that may cause brainstem compression (solid tumours generally do not cause such compression in VHL syndrome).

Conversely, spinal haemangioblastomas present with neck, chest and back pain, sensory losses, and various signs and symptoms of cord compression depending upon tumour location. Patients with cervical haemangioblastomas typically present with neck pain, signs and symptoms of cord compression and, sometimes, severe infratentorial and supratentorial subarachnoid haemorrhage. Finally, retinal haemangioblastomas present with vision loss secondary to haemorrhage, exudation, and retinal detachment.

Haemangioblastomas typically are cystic, and, thus, enhance with contrast. Contrast-enhanced T1-weighted MRI is largely considered the diagnostic test of choice to detect and monitor CNS lesions. The optimum treatment of CNS haemangioblastomas is complete surgical excision, whenever possible, since residual tumour may cause severe bleeding(Schimke *et al.*, 2009). Pre-surgical endovascular embolization may reduce operative complications and morbidity; while small asymptomatic lesions may be monitored with repeat MRIs.

Alternative treatments have been developed that include gamma knife radiosurgery(Wang *et al.*, 2005;Tago *et al.*, 2005), which seems to be effective for small to medium-sized nodular, but not cystic lesions, which bleed. Linear-accelerator (LINAC)-based cranial stereotactic radiation therapy also has proven effective with some tumours. And multiple agents that target gene products downstream from pVHL and HIF-1, like platelet-derived growth factor (PDGF), have recently become available and are being tested(Hottinger and Khakoo, 2009b).

Despite all these surgical advances, and the fact that haemangioblastomas are considered 'benign', the average patient succumbs in their fifth decade of life(Niemela *et al.*, 1999), with the main causes of mortality being metastatic renal cell carcinoma and cerebellar haemangioblastomas(Hes *et al.*, 2001;Niemela *et al.*, 1999).

2.4 Basal cell nevus syndrome (Gorlin-Goltz syndrome)

As with almost all the disorders described so far in this chapter, basal cell nevus syndrome (BCNS) is autosomal dominant, the offending gene, called PTCH1, localized to chromosome 9q31 in about 85% of cases. The PTCH1 gene product is a trans-membrane receptor that binds to and regulates a protein called Sonic the hedgehog homolog (SHH), one of three proteins in the mammalian signalling pathway family called 'hedgehog', and one which plays a key role in the regulation of organ development in vertebrates, including the growth of fingers and toes and the organization of the central nervous system. It also controls cell division in adult stem cells and has been implicated in oncogenesis. Mutations in the PTCH1 gene result in uncontrolled SHH activation(Thayer *et al.*, 2003).

This rare condition, which affects roughly one in 50 to 60 thousand live births(Hottinger and Khakoo, 2009b), is characterized by multiple basal cell cancers, often presenting in adolescence. Despite the relatively innocuous-sounding name, there is a wide range of non-neurological manifestations, as listed in Table 10, including numerous other benign and malignant tumours, both non-CNS and CNS, including melanomas, leukaemia, lymphoma, lung and breast cancers, medulloblastoma and meningiomas(Shanley *et al.*, 1994).

Odontogenic keratocysts (jaw cysts) are often the first sign of the syndrome, commonly becoming manifest early in childhood. These are cysts lined with keratinized epithelium that originate in dental lamina and locally erode all the way to the teeth, to cause dental displacement and loss, if they are not completely excised. Medulloblastomas are the most common CNS tumour, and they too present early, in roughly 3 to 5% of children with BCNS(Evans *et al.*, 1991). The medulloblastomas seen in BCNS tend to occur earlier than in sporadic cases and often are histologically distinct from classic medulloblastomas, being defined by the presence of several prominent nodules, or 'pale islands', of tumour. These areas are of lower cellularity, which are reticulin-free, exhibit nuclear uniformity and are in a background of collagen-rich, highly-proliferative tumour. Desmoplastic medulloblastomas also tend to be more discrete than the classic variety and often are located in the cerebellar hemispheres. Given their location in the posterior fossa and the fact that they can become quite large, hydrocephalus is a common complication of medulloblastomas in BCNS, and may be a presenting sign.

- Multiple Nevoid Basal Cell Cancers
- Odontogenic keratocysts (jaw cysts)
- Other bone cysts
- Calcified falx cerebri / dural calcifications
- Pitting of plantar or palmar surfaces
- Congenital skeletal abnormalities including:
  - Hypertelorism
  - High scapulae (Sprengel's Deformity)
  - Frontal bossing (that also may involve parietal area)
  - Synostosis of various cranial sutures
  - Bifid ribs
  - Cleft lip and/or palate
  - Eye disorders
    - Colobomas
    - Cataracts
    - Glaucoma
  - Non-CNS benign and malignant tumours
    - Melanoma
    - Chronic lymphocytic leukaemia
    - Non-Hodgkin's lymphoma
    - Lung cancer
    - Breast cancer
    - Myocardial fibromas
    - Lyomesenteric cysts
    - Ovarian fibromas and dermoids
    - Rhabdomyoma
  - CNS tumours
    - Medulloblastoma
    - Meningioma

Table 10. Clinical characteristics of basal cell nevus syndrome

Like virtually all the familial cancer syndromes, basal cell nevus syndrome is diagnosed using diagnostic criteria. More advanced imaging, like MRI or CT, is necessary for CNS tumours. Again, jaw and other bone cysts plus medulloblastomas may present before nevi on the skin, so the absence of nevi does not rule out the condition. Interestingly, a recently-diagnosed 10-year old child was found to have café au lait spots(Balasundrum *et al.*, 2010), emphasizing the considerable phenotypic variability evident in virtually all of the phakomatosis syndromes(Hottinger and Khakoo, 2009b). The diagnostic criteria are summarized in Table 11(Amlashi *et al.*, 2003).

The diagnosis is established in the presence of TWO or more major criteria or ONE major criterion plus TWO or more minor criteria:

- Major criteria
    - Calcification of the falx cerebri
    - Bifid or fused ribs
    - Jaw cysts
    - Palmar and plantar pits
    - First-degree relatives with the same syndrome
- Minor criteria
    - Medulloblastoma
    - Ovarian fibroma
    - Macrocephaly
        - Congenital facial or skeletal abnormalities like cleft lip or palate; hypertelorism; frontal bossing; syndactyly; and radiological bone abnormalities like bridging of the sella turcica.

Table 11. 2003 Diagnostic Criteria for Basal Cell Nevus Syndrome

Treatment of BCNS is largely supportive and as for others with similar tumours, of the CNS and elsewhere. However, it is complicated by current failures to accurately predict the course of medulloblastomas, in general and in BCNS, since no histological grading system has yet been identified that accurately predicts prognosis. This is confounded further by concerns as to the potentially increased risk of radiation-induced secondary malignancies, especially in children who have the potential for very long-term survival (e.g., the child who develops secondary osteosarcoma in the radiation field for a previously-treated medulloblastoma). The general impression that medulloblastomas have a more indolent course in BCNS than otherwise has led to some to suggest that the dose of radiation can be reduced(Stavrou *et al.*, 2001). As with many of the familial cancer syndromes described in this chapter, better understanding of the underlying genetics of cancers like medulloblastoma has led to more directed chemotherapies that hold some promise(Taipale *et al.*, 2000).

3. Other familial syndromes associated with pediatric CNS malignancies

3.1 Li-Fraumeni syndrome

Li-Fraumeni Syndrome (LFS) is another very rare autosomal dominant disease that is caused by a germ line mutation of chromosome p53 in roughly 70% of families in which the syndrome is diagnosed(Kleihues *et al.*, 1997). Patients exhibit an increased risk of variety of carcinomas and sarcomas, including premenopausal breast cancers, osteosarcomas, soft tissue sarcomas, acute leukaemia, cancer involving the adrenal cortex, and primitive neuroectodermal tumours (PNET) like medulloblastoma. This increased risk of a wide variety of malignancies likely stems from deactivation of p53, which normally controls apoptosis and the repair of damaged DNA.

Patients present not only with a variety of cancers, but with cancers at a very early age. The mean age at presentation in LFS patients with brain tumours is about 25 years. The diagnosis of so-called 'classic LFS' is made in any patient under 45 years who presents with a bone or soft-tissue sarcoma, plus one first-degree relative who presents with any cancer before age 45, plus one further first or second-degree relative of the same lineage who has had any cancer before age 45 or a sarcoma at any age(Li *et al.*, 1988). More recently, a related syndrome, called Li-Fraumeni-like syndrome, has been described, defined as a proband with any childhood tumour or any sarcoma, brain or adrenocortical tumour before 45 years of age, who has a first- or second-degree relative with any cancer before the age of 60(Birch, 1994;Evans *et al.*, 2008). Interestingly, whereas p53 germ-line mutations are found in 70% to 80% of families with classic Li-Fraumeni syndrome, they only are identified in between 20% and 40% of families with Li-Fraumeni-like syndrome(Hottinger and Khakoo, 2009b). The CHK2 checkpoint homolog gene, CHEK2, which is located on the long (q) arm of chromosome 22, also has been implicated in some families with classic Li-Fraumeni syndrome. Recently, mutation of another gene, which encodes for the breast cancer 2 (BRCA2) susceptibility protein, has been found with increased frequency in the non-classic syndrome(Evans *et al.*, 2008). It should be noted that p53 mutations are rare in sporadically occurring medulloblastomas.

Overall, about 10% of LFS patients will develop a glioma before the age of 45, and another 5% a supratentorial primitive neuroectodermal tumour (PNET), like a medulloblastoma, or choroid plexus carcinoma(Taylor et al., 2000). Since LFS is so rare, no clinical trials document the optimum treatment; but it generally is agreed that incident tumours should be treated as for sporadic cases, albeit with increased vigilance for additional tumours, both within the proband patient due to the increased risk of second cancers(Birch et al., 2001), and the family.

3.2 Familial polyposis / Turcot syndrome

A Canadian surgeon named Jacques Turcot is accredited with having characterized Turcot syndrome, one of the several familial polyposis syndromes associated with familial, in this case autosomal recessive, inheritance and the presence of multiple colonic adenomas and adenocarcinomas(Foulkes, 1995). An additional feature of Turcot syndrome is its association with several different neuroepithelial tumours of the central nervous system, including astrocytomas, medulloblastomas, pineoblastomas, gangliogliomas, and ependymomas(Hottinger and Khakoo, 2009b).

Turcot syndrome has been categorized into types 1 and 2, with type 1 characterized by glioblastoma, no familial adenomatous polyposis, but often hereditary non-polyposis-related colorectal carcinoma. Germ-line mutations in a few DNA mismatch repair genes - PMS2, MLH1 and MSH2 - are associated with type-1 Turcot syndrome. Interestingly, type-1 Turcot syndrome also is associated with café au lait spots(Hottinger and Khakoo, 2009b). Conversely, type-2 Turcot syndrome families have medulloblastomas as their most common CNS malignancy, and multiple adenomatous polyps that often undergo malignant transformation(Hamilton *et al.*, 1995). Unfortunately, medulloblastomas, glioblastomas and anaplastic astrocytomas are the most common CNS tumours observed in Turcot's syndrome, the three combined accounting for 95% of all CNS tumours in these families(Paraf *et al.*, 1997); and the latter two are inevitably fatal. In addition, they tend to occur early, with medulloblastomas typically diagnosed in children less than 10 years old, and gliomas in those under age 30(Hottinger and Khakoo, 2009b;McLaughlin *et al.*, 1998;Jamjoom *et al.*, 1989;Schroder *et al.*, 1983).

As such, and because some die of metastatic colon cancer that sometimes presents quite early in childhood or the second decade of life, many die as adolescents or young adults. In one tragic case, for example, doctors in Pittsburgh reported the case of a girl who developed a medulloblastoma at the age of 5 years. Ten years later, she developed adenocarcinoma of the colon. Then, seven months after resection of a Dukes' C2 adenocarcinoma, she presented with a second primary CNS tumour, this time a glioblastoma multiforme(McLaughlin *et al.*, 1998). Presumably, she died shortly thereafter from her glioblastoma.

3.3 Rubenstein-Taybi syndrome

Rubenstein-Taybi syndrome is an autosomal dominant disorder that is associated with numerous anatomical/functional abnormalities that include abnormal facies, microcephaly, broad thumbs, big toes and moderate to severe intellectual impairment. There also is an increased incidence of neuroepithelial tumours; in particular medulloblastomas, meningiomas, and oligodendrogliomas(Taylor *et al.*, 2001), though other CNS tumours have been described(Burton *et al.*, 1997). A germ-line mutation in one allele of CRE binding protein (CBP, a transcriptional co-activator for several c-AMP regulated genes) has been implicated in many cases. CBP binds to the activated form of GLI, a transcription factor that is important in the regulation of the Sonic hedgehog homolog (SHH) that, as stated earlier, controls cell division in adult stem cells and has been implicated in oncogenesis. The GLI gene is downstream of the PTCH1 gene that is mutated in basal cell nevus syndrome.

4. Ollier's disease and Maffucci syndrome

Enchondromatosis, also called dyschondroplasia, is a hamartomatous proliferation of chondrocytes within the metaphysis of bone (2008). Enchondromatosis often is asymptomatic and only diagnosed as an incidental X-ray finding. On the other hand, it can lead to significant deformities, reduced bone length(Baumgart *et al.*, 2005;Shapiro, 1982), and occasional pathologic fractures(Shapiro, 1982). Moreover, enchondromas appear to have an association with malignancy. This includes both chondrosarcomas that result from sarcomatous transformation of the enchondromas themselves, and other histologically-distinct malignancies, including angiosarcomas, osteosacrcomas, a variety of central nervous system tumours, ovarian tumours, and various leukaemias(Ranger *et al.*, 2009b). This association with malignancy appears to be particularly true in instances of multiple enchondromatoses, as in Ollier's disease and Maffucci's syndrome(Schwartz *et al.*, 1987).
In 1881, an Italian pathologists named Angelo Maffucci first described a patient with enchondromatosis and venous angiomas on the skin(Maffucci, 1881), though others followed suit within a decade(Kast and von Recklinghausen, 1889). For years, the apparent 'dual discovery' of this combination of clinical findings led to the alternative use of the labels Maffucci's syndrome and Maffucci-Kast syndrome, though the latter label ultimately largely was discarded. The term Ollier's disease entered into use after 1889, when a French surgeon, Louis Léopold Ollier, described a patient with enchondromatosis in the absence of any evident vascular abnormalities(Ollier, 1899). Since then, a line largely has been drawn between those with accompanying vascular abnormalities, primarily haemangiomas, and those without. Debate continues as to whether these two 'syndromes' are distinct clinical entities, versus variations in the expression of the same disease(Mellon *et al.*, 1988). This debate has been fuelled by the late discovery of vascular abnormalities in some patients previously considered to have Ollier's disease(Ahmed *et al.*, 1999;Bertucci and Krafchik, 1995). Both conditions are considered very rare, with Ollier's disease having a reported prevalence of roughly one in 100,000(Silve and Jüppner, 2006); and fewer than 200 total cases of Maffucci's syndrome reported in the literature since it first was reported in 1881(Balcer *et al.*, 1999).

The first report of a CNS malignancy in a patient with multiple enchondromatosis was published in 1904, by Boinet, who diagnosed a chondrosarcomatous lesion of the skull base in a 37-year old gentleman with Maffucci's syndrome who was living in France(Boinet, 1904). Since that time, 45 additional patients with either Ollier's disease (OD) or Maffucci's syndrome (MS) and some form of intracranial malignancy have been reported in the medical literature, ranging from 6 to 58 years old(Ranger *et al.*, 2009a).

The combination of enchondromatosis and an intracranial malignancy is rare, but this is because both conditions are relatively rare in themselves(Balcer *et al.*, 1999;Silve and Jüppner, 2006). This combination is not likely to be a coincidence(Ranger *et al.*, 2009a). Moreover, though traditionally it has been thought that Maffucci's syndrome is the more likely syndrome of the two to be associated with a malignancy, in fact, the combination of Ollier's disease and an intracranial malignancy is at least as common, albeit allowing for our lack of knowledge regarding the baseline prevalence rates of OD and MS. Ollier's disease patients also appear to contract their neoplasm at an earlier age, including very young childhood(Ranger *et al.*, 2009b). This is true for both chondrosarcomas and non-sarcomatous neoplasms (NSN). In another study using the same subject pool, for example, patients with OD and malignancy were more than 10 years younger than their MS counterparts (24.7 vs. 34.9 years; $p = 0.002$), as were patients with OD and chondrosarcoma versus those with MS and chondrosarcoma (24.7 vs. 36.2; $p = 0.035$)(Ranger *et al.*, 2009a). Among those with NSN, the difference in mean age approached statistical significance (24.7 vs. 32.6; $p = 0.092$). Also, seven of 24 with OD were 18 years old or younger, versus just 2 of 22 with MS.

However, other than youths tending towards being more likely to have the combination of OD and malignancy than MS and malignancy, no other significant differences seem to exist between youths and adults, with respect to the demographic characteristics of patients or the clinical characteristics of their intracranial tumours(Ranger and Szymczak, 2009). What this implies is that the underlying enchondromatosis is associated with at least a reasonably lifelong increased risk of malignancy, which persists into the sixth decade, if not beyond, rather than there being distinct characteristics of childhood/adolescence and adulthood that predispose such patients to risk.

What causes that persistent increase in malignancy potential is not yet known. We do know that single enchondromas, outside some greater syndrome, are associated with an elevated risk of malignant change. Altay *et al*(Altay *et al.*, 2007), for example, conducted an 18-year retrospective analysis of 627 cartilage-forming benign bone tumours, and found that 32 patients had experienced malignant transformation, with 14 of these 32 patients initially having had a solitary osteochondroma, ten multiple osteochondromas, six a solitary enchondroma, one Ollier's disease, and one Maffucci's syndrome. The one patient with Ollier's disease had two chondrosarcomas; and the single patient with multiple osteochondroma had three chondrosarcomas. The overall rate of malignant transformation for cartilage-originating tumours was 5.1%, being 4.2% for solitary osteochondromas, 9.2% for multiple osteochondromas, and 4.2% for solitary enchondromas.

A variety of chromosomal abnormalities also have been reported in isolated cases of OD or MS and chondrosarcoma. These abnormalities include, for example, the interstitial deletion, del(1)(p11p31.2), as the only chromosomal abnormality identified in a low-grade chondrosarcoma in a patient with Ollier's disease(Ozisik *et al.*, 1998). Also, Bovée *et al*(Bovee *et al.*, 2000) identified (1) the loss of heterozygosity (LOH) in a tibial chondrosarcoma and its metastases, exclusively on chromosome bands 13q14 and 9p21, with the LOH not identified in a femoral enchondroma that was analyzed; and (2) p53 over-expression in a tibial chondrosarcoma and its metastases, not present in a femoral enchondroma. Meanwhile, Chang *et al*(Chang and Prados, 1994) identified identical male twins with OD who both developed astrocytomas within their cerebral cortex during their early twenties; and Robinson *et al*(Robinson *et al.*, 1994) found evidence of mitogenic neurotransmitters within both enchondromas and soft tissue hemangiomas in a patient with Maffucci's syndrome, implying that the bone and vascular lesions, and possibly malignant tumours, might be related to an underlying neural abnormality. Having said all this, to date, no consistent chromosomal abnormalities have been identified in these patients, and all theories regarding the cause of malignancies in these syndromes remain unproven.

Just like the phakomatoses and familial syndromes like Li-Fraumeni and Turcot syndrome, enchondromatosis appears to confer a substantial increased risk of a variety of CNS and other malignancies, at least through the sixth decade of life and as early as the first decade; and children, adolescents and adults appear not to differ substantially in this risk. These two points have implications for both primary physicians and specialists, including surgeons; because it means that the risk of intracranial malignancy should not be ignored in any patient with enchondromatosis, whether they have accompanying vascular lesions or not. In fact, those without vascular lesions may have higher risk over the first few decades of life than those with. Ideally, further research one day will clarify the cause or causes of this increased risk. Moreover, as we gain a better understanding of the genetics behind the various familial disorders associated with malignancy, improved and more precisely targeted therapies will be developed, to more successfully treat malignancies once they arise, and perhaps even to prevent them in those who are at significantly increased risk.

5. References

(2008) Enchondromatosis: In The Free Dictionary by Farlex at http://medical-dictionary.thefreedictionary.com/enchondromatosis. In.

Ahmed,S.K., Lee,W.C., Irving,R.M., Walsh,A.R. (1999) Is Ollier's disease an understaging of Maffucci's syndrome? *J Laryngol Otol* 113(9): 861-864.

Alaraj,A.M., Valyi-Nagy,T., Roitberg,B. (2007) Double phakomatosis; neurofibromatosis type-1 and tuberous sclerosis. *Acta Neurochir (Wien).* 149(5): 505-509.

Altay,M., Bayrakci,K., Yildiz,Y., Erekul,S., Saglik,Y. (2007) Secondary chondrosarcoma in cartilage bone tumors: report of 32 patients. *J Orthop Sci* 12(5): 415-423.

Amlashi,S.F., Riffaud,L., Brassier,G., Morandi,X. (2003) Nevoid basal cell carcinoma syndrome: relation with desmoplastic medulloblastoma in infancy. A population-based study and review of the literature. *Cancer* 98(3): 618-624.

Arfan-ul-Bari,S.-R. (2003) Segmental neurofibromatosis [NF type - v]. *J Coll Physicians Surg Pak.* 13(12): 717-718.

Arun,D., Gutmann,D.H. (2004) Recent advances in neurofibromatosis type 1. *Curr Opin Neurol.* 17(2): 101-105.

Balasundrum,S., Kovilpillai,F.J., Hopper,C. (2010) Nevoid basal cell carcinoma syndrome presenting with neck pits and café au lait patches. *J Clin Pediatr Dent.* 35(1): 95-100.

Balcer,L.J., Galetta,S.L., Cornblath,W.T., Liu,G.T. (1999) Neuro-ophthalmologic manifestations of Maffucci's syndrome and Ollier's disease. *J Neuroophthalmol* 19(1): 62-66.

Bance,M., Ramsden,R.T. (1999) Management of neurofibromatosis type 2. *Ear Nose Throat J.* 78(2): 91-94, 96.

Baser,M.E., R Evans,D.G., Gutmann,D.H. (2003) Neurofibromatosis 2. *Curr Opin Neurol.* 16(1): 27-33.

Baujat,B., Krastinova-Lolov,D., Blumen,M., Baglin,A.C., Coquille,F., Chabolle,F. (2006) Radiofrequency in the treatment of craniofacial plexiform neurofibromatosis: a pilot study. *Plast Reconstr Surg.* 117(4): 1261-1268.

Baumgart,R., Bürklein D, Hinterwimmer,S., Thaller,P., Mutschler,W. (2005) The management of leg-length discrepancy in Ollier's disease with a fully implantable lengthening nail. *J Bone Joint Surg Br* 87(7): 1000-1004.

Bertucci,V., Krafchik,B.R. (1995) What syndrome is this? Ollier disease + vascular lesions: Maffucci syndrome. *Pediatr Dermatol* 12(1): 55-8.

Birch,J.M. (1994) Li-Fraumeni syndrome. *Eur J Cancer* 30A(13): 1935-1941.

Birch,J.M., Alston,R.D., McNally,R.J., et al. (2001) Relative frequency and morphology of cancers in carriers of germline TP53 mutations. *Oncogene* 20(34): 4621-4628.

Boinet,E. (1904) Enchondrose rachitiforme. *Arch Gen de Med* 194: 2689-2717.

Boman,K.K., Hoven,E., Anclair,M., Lannering,B., Gustafsson,G. (2009) Health and persistent functional late effects in adult survivors of childhood CNS tumours: a population-based cohort study. *Eur J Cancer* 45(14): 2552-2561.

Bondy,M., Wiencke,J., Wrensch,M., Kyritis,A.P. (1994) Genetics of primary brain tumors: a review. *J Neurooncol.* 18(1): 69-81.

Bovee,J.V.M.G., Graadt van Roggen,J.F., Cleton-Jansen,A.M., Taminiau,A.H.M., Woude,H.J., van der Hogendoorn,P.C.W. (2000) Malignant progression in multiple enchondromatosis (Ollier"s disease): An autopsy-based molecular genetic study. *Human Pathol* 31(10): 1299-1303.

Bunin,G.R., Feuer,E.J., Witman,P.A., Meadows,A.T. (1996) Increasing incidence of childhood cancer: report of 20 years experience from the greater Delaware Valley Pediatric Tumor Registry. *Paediatr Perinat Epidemiol* 10(3): 319-338.

Burton,B.J., Kumar,V.G., Bradford,R. (1997) Granular cell tumour of the spinal cord in a patient with Rubenstein-Taybi syndrome. *Br J Neurosurg.* 11(3): 257-259.

Butman,J.A., Linehan,W.M., Lonser,R.R. (2008) Neurologic manifestations of von Hippel-Lindau disease. *JAMA* 300(11): 1334-1342.

Centers for Disease Control and Prevention (CDC) (2007) Trends in childhood cancer mortality--United States, 1990-2004. *MMWR Morb Mortal Wkly Rep.* 56(48): 1257-1261.

Chang,S., Prados,M.D. (1994) Identical twins with Ollier's disease and intracranial gliomas: case report. *Neurosurg* 34(5): 903-906.

Chatenoud,L., Bertuccio,P., Bosetti,C., Levi,F., Negri,E., La Vecchia,C. (2010) Childhood cancer mortality in America, Asia, and Oceania, 1970 through 2007. *Cancer* 116(21): 5063-5074.

Cheng,L., Scheithauer,B.W., Leibovich,B.C., Ramnani,D.M., Cheville,J.C., Bostwick,D.G. (1999) Neurofibroma of the urinary bladder. *Cancer* 86(3): 505-513.

Cherqui,A., Kim,D.H., Kim,S.H., Park,H.K., Kline,D.G. (2007) Surgical approaches to paraspinal nerve sheath tumors. *Neurosurg Focus* 22(6): E9.

Committee on Genetics (1995) Health Supervision for children with neurofibromatosis. *Pediatrics* 96: 368-372.

Crowe,F.W., Schull,W.J., Neel,J.V. (1956) Crowe FW, Schull WJ, Neel JV. A clinical, pathological and genetic study of multiple neurofibromatosis. Springfield, IL.

Crump,T. (1981) Translation of case reports in Ueber die multiplen Fibrome der Haut und ihre Beziehung zu den multiplen Neuromen by F. v. Recklinghausen. *Adv Neurol.* 29: 259-275.

Dang,J.D., Cohen,P.R. (2010) Segmental neurofibromatosis and malignancy. *Skinmed.* 8(3): 156-159.

Deb,P., Gupta,A., Sharma,M.C., Gaikwad,S., Singh,V.P., Sarkar,C. (2006) Meningioangiomatosis with meningioma: an uncommon association of a rare entity--report of a case and review of the literature. *Childs Nerv Syst.* 22(1): 78-83.

DeBella,K., Szudek,J., Friedman,J.M. (2000) Use of the National Institutes of Health criteria for diagnosis of neurofibromatosis 1 in children. *Pediatrics* 105: 608-614.

Denckla,M.D., Hofman,K., Mazzocco,M.M.M., et al. (1996) Relationship between T2-weighted hyperintensities (unidentified bright objects)and lower IQs in children with neurofibromatosis-1. *Am J Med Genet.* 67: 98-102.

Dodge,H.W., Lowe,J.G., Craig,W.M., et al. (1958) Gliomas of the optic nerves. *Arch.Neurol.Psychiatr.* 79: 607-621.

Ellenberg,L., Liu,Q., Gioia,G., Yasui,Y., Packer,R.J., Mertens,A., Donaldson,S.S., Stovall,M., Kadan-Lottick,N., Armstrong,G., Robison,L.L., Zeltzer,L.K. (2009) Neurocognitive status in long-term survivors of childhood CNS malignancies: a report from the Childhood Cancer Survivor Study. *Neuropsychology* 23(6): 705-717.

Ellison,L.F., De,P., Mery,L.S., Grundy,P.E., Canadian Cancer Society's Steering Committee for Canadian Cancer Statistics. (2009) Canadian cancer statistics at a glance: cancer in children. *CMAJ.2009 Feb 17;180(4):422-4.* 180(4): 422-424.

Evans,D.G. (1999) Neurofibromatosis type 2: genetic and clinical features. *Ear Nose Throat J.* 78(2): 97-100.

Evans,D.G., Famdon,P.A., Burnell,L.D., Gattamaneni,H.R., Birch,J.M. (1991) The incidence of Gorlin syndrome in 173 consecutive cases of medulloblastoma. *Br J Cancer* 64(5): 959-961.

Evans,D.G., Howard,E., Giblin,C., et al. (2010) Birth incidence and prevalence of tumour prone syndromes: estimates from a UK genetic family register service. *Am J Med Genet.* 152A: 327-332.

Evans,D.G., Ramsden,R.T., Gokhale,C., Bowers,N., Huson,S.M., Wallace,A. (2007) Should NF2 mutation screening be undertaken in patients with an apparently isolated vestibular schwannoma? *Clin Genet.* 71(4): 354-358.

Evans,D.G., Wu,C.L., Birch,J.M. (2008) BRCA2: a cause of Li-Fraumeni-like syndrome. *J Med Genet.* 45: 62-63.

Ferner,R.E. (2007) Neurofibromatosis 1 and neurofibromatosis 2: a twenty first century perspective. *Lancet Neurol.* 6(4): 340-351.

Ferner,R.E. (2010) The neurofibromatoses. *Pract Neurol.* 10(2): 82-93.

Ferner,R.E., Huson,S.M., Thomas,N., Moss,C., Willshaw,H., Evans,D.G., Upadhyaya,M., Towers,R., Gleeson,M., Steiger,C., Kirby,A. (2007) Guidelines for the diagnosis and management of individuals with neurofibromatosis 1. *J Med Genet.* 44(2): 81-8.

Fontaine,B., Hanson,M.P., VonSattel,J.P., et al. (1991a) Loss of chromosome 22 alleles in human sporadic spinal schwannomas. *Ann Neurol.* 29(2): 183-186.

Fontaine,B., Sanson,M., Delattre,O., et al. (1991b) Parental origin of chromosome 22 loss in sporadic and NF2 neuromas. *Genomics* 10(1): 280-283.

Foulkes,W.D. (1995) A tale of four syndromes: familial adenomatous polyposis, Gardner syndrome, attenuated APC and Turcot syndrome. *QJM* 88(12): 853-863.

Franz,D.N., Leonard,J., Tudor,C., et al. (2006) Rapamycin causes regression of astrocytomas in tuberous sclerosis complex. *Ann Neurol.* 59(3): 490-498.

Giuffré,R., Bardelli,A.M., Taverniti,L., Barberi,I. (1982) Anterior optic pathways glioma. The dilemma of treatment. *J.Neurosurg.Sci.* 26: 61-72.

Glasker,S. (2005) Central nervous system manifestations in VHL: genetics, pathology and clinical phenotypic features. *Fam Cancer* 4(1): 37-42.

Goh,S., Butler,W., Thiele,E.A. (2004) Subependymal giant cell tumors in tuberous sclerosis complex. *Neurology* 63(8): 1457-1461.

Grajkowska,W., Kotulska,K., Jurkiewicz,E., Matyja,E. (2010) Brain lesions in tuberous sclerosis complex. Review. *Folia Neuropathol.* 48(3): 139-149.

Greig,A.V., Kirkpatrick,N.A., Joshi,N., Kelly,M., Waterhouse,N. (2009) Giant hemifacial plexiform neurofibroma arising from trigeminal ganglion. *J Craniofac Surg.* 20(3): 833-836.

Gutmann,D.H., Aylsworth,A., Carey,J.C., et al. (1997) The diagnostic evaluation and multidisciplinary management of neurofibromatosis 1 and neurofibromatosis 2. *JAMA* 278(1): 51-57.

Hager,C.M., Cohen,P.R., Tschen,J.A. (1997) Segmental neurofibromatosis: case reports and review. *J Am Acad Dermatol.* 37((5 Pt 2)): 864-869.

Hahn,J.S., Chung,J.B., Han,S.H., Lee,S.W., Noh,S.H., Lee,J.T., Chun,S.I., Kim,S.H. (1992) Intestinal neurofibromatosis in von Recklinghausen's disease: presenting as chronic anemia due to recurrent intestinal hemorrhage. *Korean J Intern Med.* 7(2): 137-142.

Hamilton,S.R., Liu,B., Parsons,R.E., et al. (1995) The molecular basis of Turcot's syndrome. *N Engl J Med.* 332(13): 839-847.

Hanada,M., Tanaka,T., Kanayama,S., Takami,M., Kimura,M. (1982) Malignant transformation of intrathoracic ancient neurilemoma in a patient without von Recklinghausen's disease. *Acta Pathol Jpn.* 32(3): 527-536.

Harrison,J.E., Bolton,P.F. (1997) Annotation: Tuberous sclerosis. *J Child Psychol Psychiatry* 38(6): 603-614.

Hassard,A.D., Boudreau,S.F., Cron,C.C. (1984) Adenoma of the endolymphatic sac. *J Otolaryngol.* 13: 213-216.

Hersh,J.H., American Academy of Pediatrics Committee on Genetics (2008) Health supervision for children with neurofibromatosis. *Pediatrics* 121(3): 633-642.

Hes,F.J., van der Luitj,R.B., Lips,C.J. (2001) Clinical management of Von Hippel-Lindau (VHL) disease. *Neth J Med.* 59(5): 225-234.

Hong,C.H., Darling,T.N., Lee,C.H. (2009) Prevalence of tuberous sclerosis complex in Taiwan: a national population-based study. *Neuroepidemiology* 33(4): 335-341.

Hottinger,A.F., Khakoo,Y. (2009a) Neuro-oncology of Neurofibromatosis Type 1. *Curr Treat Options Neurol.* 11(4): 306-314.

Hottinger,A.F., Khakoo,Y. (2009b) Neurooncology of familial cancer syndromes. *J Child Neurol..* 24(12): 1526-1535.

Huson,S.M., Harper,P.S., Compston,D.A. (1988) Von Recklinghausen neurofibromatosis. A clinical and population study in south-east Wales. *Brain* 111((Pt 6)): 1355-1381.

Hyman,S.L., Gill,D.S., Shores,E.A., Steinberg,A., Joy,P., Gibikote,S.V., North,K.N. (2003) Natural history of cognitive deficits and their relationship to MRI T2-hyperintensities in NF1. *Neurology* 60(7): 1139-1145.

Jackson,I.T. (2001) Management of craniofacial neurofibromatosis. *Facial Plast Surg Clin North Am.* 9(1): 59-75.

Jacoby,L.B., MacCollin,M., Parry,D.M., et al. (1999) Allelic expression of the NF2 gene in neurofibromatosis 2 and schwannomatosis. *Neurogenetics* 2(2): 101-108.

Jacquemin,C., Bosley,T.M., Svedberg,H. (2003) Orbit deformities in craniofacial neurofibromatosis type 1. *AJNR Am J Neuroradiol.* 24(8): 1678-1682.

Jallo,G.I., Kothbauer,K., Mehta,V., Abbott,R., Epstein,F. (2005) Meningioangiomatosis without neurofibromatosis: a clinical analysis. *J Neurosurg.* 103((4 Suppl)): 319-324.

Jamjoom,Z.A., Sadiq,S., Mofti,A.B., al-Mofleh,I., Ajarim,D. (1989) Turcot syndrome: report of a case and review of the literature. *Int Surg.* 74(1): 45-50.

Joy,P., Roberts,C., North,K.N., de Silva,M. (1995) Neuropsychological function and MRI abnormalities in neurofibromatosis type 1. *Dev Med Child Neurol.* 37(10): 906-914.

Kaefer,M., Adams,M.C., Rink,R.C., Keating,M.A. (1997) Principles in management of complex pediatric genitourinary plexiform neurofibroma. *Urology* 49(6): 936-940.

Kast,A., von Recklinghausen,F.D. (1889) Ein Fall von Enchondrom mit ungewöhnlicher Multiplikation. *Virchows Archiv für pathologische Anatomie und Physiologie und für klinische Medicin, Berlin* 118: 1-118.

Khong,P.L., Goh,W.H., Wong,V.C., Fung,C.W., Ooi,G.C. (2003) MR imaging of spinal tumors in children with neurofibromatosis 1. *AJR Am J Roentgenol.* 180(2): 413-417.

Kleihues,P., Schauble,B., zur Hausen,A., Esteve,J., Ohgaki,H. (1997) Tumors associated with p53 germline mutations: a synopsis of 91 families. *Am J Pathol.* 150(1): 1-13.

Koeller,K.K., Rosenblum,R.S., Morrison,A.L. (2000) Neoplasms of the spinal cord and filum terminale: radiologic-pathologic correlation. *Radiographics* 20(6): 1721-1749.

Korf,B.R. (1999) Plexiform neurofibromas. *Am J Med Genet.* 89(1): 31-37.

Korf,B.R. (2005) The phakomatoses. *Clin Dermatol.* 23(1): 78-84.

Legendre,C.M., Charpentier-Cote,C., Drouin,R., Bouffard,C. (2011) Neurofibromatosis type 1 and the "elephant man's" disease: the confusion persists: an ethnographic study. *PLoS One* 6(2): e16409.

Leonard,J.R., Perry,A., Rubin,J.B., et al. (2006) The role of surgical biopsy in the diagnosis of glioma in individuals with neurofibromatosis-1. *Neurology* 67(8): 1509-1512.

Li,F.P., Fraumeni,J.F.J., Mulvihill,J.J., et al. (1988) A cancer family syndrome in twenty-four kindreds. *Cancer Res.* 48(18): 5358-5362.

Linet,M.S., Ries,L.A., Smith,M.A., Tarone,R.E., Devesa,S.S. (1999) Cancer surveillance series: recent trends in childhood cancer incidence and mortality in the United States. *J Natl Cancer Inst* 91(12): 1051-1058.

Lopes Ferraz Filho,J.R., Munis,M.P., Soares Souza,A., Sanches,R.A., Goloni-Bertollo,E.M., Pavarino-Bertelli,E.C. (2008) Unidentified bright objects on brain MRI in children as a diagnostic criterion for neurofibromatosis type 1. *Pediatr Radiol.* 38(3): 305-310.

Lu-Emerson,C., Plotkin,S.R. (2009a) The Neurofibromatoses. Part 1: NF1. *Rev Neurol Dis.* 6(2): E47-E53.

Lu-Emerson,C., Plotkin,S.R. (2009b) The neurofibromatoses. Part 2: NF2 and schwannomatosis. *Rev Neurol Dis.* 6(3): E81-E86.

Maffucci,A. (1881) Di un caso encondroma ed angioma multiplo. Contribuzione alla genesi embrionale dei tumori. *Movimento medico-chirurgico, Napoli, 1881, 3: 399-412 and 565-575.* 3: 399-412-565-575.

Mansur,A.T., Goktay,F., Akkaya,A.D., Gunes,P. (2011) Segmental neurofibromatosis: report of 3 cases. *Cutis* 87(1): 45-50.

Massimi,L., Tufo,T., Rocco,C. (2007) Management of optic-hypothalamic gliomas in children: still a challenging problem. *Expert Rev Anticancer Ther.* 7(11): 1591-1610.

McLaughlin,M.R., Gollin,S.M., Lese,C.M., Albright,A.L. (1998) Medulloblastoma and glioblastoma multiforme in a patient with Turcot syndrome: a case report. *Surg Neurol.* 49(3): 295-301.

Mellon,C.D., Carter,J.E., Owen,D.B. (1988) Ollier's disease and Maffucci's syndrome: distinct entities or a continuum. Case report: enchondromatosis complicated by an intracranial glioma. *J Neurol* 235(6): 376-378.

Morais,P., Ferreira,O., Bettencourt,H., Azevedo,F. (2010) Segmental neurofibromatosis: A rare variant of a common genodermatosis. *Acta Dermatovenerol Alp Panonica Adriat.* 19(3): 27-29.

Morrison,P.J. (2009) Tuberous sclerosis: epidemiology, genetics and progress towards treatment. *Neuroepidemiology* 33(4): 343.

Neurofibromatosis Conference Statement (1988) National Institutes of Health. Consensus Development Conference. *Arch Neurol.* 45(5): 575-578.

NF1 Cognitive Disorders Task Force. (1997) Cognitive function and academic performance in neurofibromatosis 1. *Neurology* 48: 1121-1127.

Niemela,M., Lemeta,S., Summanen,P., Bohling,T., Sainio,M., Kere,J., et al. (1999) Long-term prognosis of haemangioblastoma of the CNS: impact of von Hippel-Lindau disease. *Acta Neurochir (Wien).* 141(11): 1147-1156.

North,K.N., Joy,P., Yuille,D., Cocks,N., Hutchins,P. (1995) Cognitive function and academic performance in children with neurofibromatosis type 1. *Dev Med Child Neurol.* 37(5): 427-436.

North,K.N., Joy,P., Yuille,D., Cocks,N., Mobbs,E., Hutchins,P., McHugh,K., de Silva,M. (1994) Specific learning disability in children with neurofibromatosis type 1: significance of MRI abnormalities. *Neurology* 44(5): 878-883.

North,K.N., Riccardi,V., Samango-Sprouse,C., Ferner,R.E., Moore,B., Legius,E., Ratner,N., Denckla,M.B. (1997) Cognitive function and academic performance in neurofibromatosis. 1: consensus statement from the NF1 Cognitive Disorders Task Force. *Neurology* 48(4): 1121-1127.

Oh,K.S., Hung,J., Robertson,P.L., Garton,H.J., Muraszko,K.M., Sandler,H.M., Hamstra,D.A. (2011) Outcomes of Multidisciplinary Management in Pediatric Low-Grade Gliomas. *Int J Radiat Oncol Biol Phys.2011 Apr 4.[Epub ahead of print].*

Ollier,L. (1899) Dyschondroplasia [Italian]. *Bull Soc Lyon Med* 93: 23-24.

Omeis,I., Hillard,V.H., Braun,A., Benzil,D.L., Murali,R., Harter,D.H. (2006) Meningioangiomatosis associated with neurofibromatosis: report of 2 cases in a single family and review of the literature. *Surg Neurol.* 65(6): 595-603.

Ong,K.R., Woodward,E.R., Killick,P., Lim,C., Macdonald,F., Maher,E.R. (2007) Genotype-phenotype correlations in von Hippel-Lindau disease. *Hum Mutat.* 28(2): 143-149.

Orlova,K.A., Crino,P.B. (2010) The tuberous sclerosis complex. *Ann N Y Acad Sci.* 1184(Jan): 87-105.

Osborne,J.P., Fryer,A., Webb,D. (1991) Epidemiology of tuberous sclerosis. *Ann NY Acad Sci.* 615: 125-127.

Ozisik,Y., Meloni,A.M., Spanier,S.S., Bush,C.H., Kingsley,K.L., Sandberg,A.A. (1998) Deletion 1p in a low-grade chondrosarcoma in a patient with Ollier disease. *Canc Genet Cytogen* 105(2): 128-133.

Paraf,F., Jothy,S., Van Meir,E.G. (1997) Brain tumor-polyposis syndrome: two genetic diseases? *J Clin Oncol.* 15(7): 2744-2758.

Park,B.Y., Hong,J.P., Lee,W.J. (2002) Netting operation to control neurofibroma of the face. *Plast Reconstr Surg.* 109(4): 1228-1237.

Pearce,J.M.S. (2003) Historical Note: Neurofibromatosis. *J Neurol Neurosurg Psychiatry* 74(3): 384.

Poussaint,T.Y., Barnes,P.D., Nichols,K., et al. (1997) Diencephalic syndrome: clinical features and imaging findings. *Am.J.Neuroradiol.* 18: 1499-1505.

Ranger,A., Szymczak,A. (2009) The association between intracranial tumours and multiple dyschondroplasia (Ollier's disease or Maffucci's syndrome): do children and adults differ? *J Neurooncol.* 95(2): 165-173.

Ranger,A., Szymczak,A., Hammond,R., Zelcer,S. (2009a) Do intracranial neoplasms differ in Ollier's disease and Maffucci's syndrome? - An in-depth analysis of the literature. [in press]. *Neurosurgery.*

Ranger,A., Szymczak,A., Hammond,R., Zelcer,S. (2009b) Pediatric thalamic glioblastoma associated with Ollier's disease (multiple enchondromatosis): a rare case of concurrence. *J Neurosurg Pediatr.* 4(4): 363-367.

Rendón-Macías,M.E., Ramos-Becerril,C., Bernardez-Zapata,I., Iglesias-Leboreiro,J. (2008) [Cancer epidemiology in children and adolescents at private health care (1995-2004)] [Article in Spanish]. *Rev Med Inst Mex Seguro Soc* 46(4): 353-360.

Richard,S., Campello,C., Taillandier,L., Parker,F., Resche,F. (1998) Haemangioblastoma of the central nervous system in von Hippel-Lindau disease. French VHL Study Group. *J Intern Med.* 243(6): 547-553.

Ridler,K., Suckling,J., Higgins,N.J., de Vries,P.J., Stephenson,C.M.E., Bolton,P.F., Bullmore,E.T. (2006) Neuroanatomical Correlates of Memory Deficits in Tuberous Sclerosis Complex. *Cerebral Cortex* 17(2): 261-271.

Rieley,M.B., Stevenson,D.A., Viskochil,D.H., Tinkle,B.T., Martin,L.J., Schorry,E.K. (2011) Variable expression of neurofibromatosis 1 in monozygotic twins. *Am J Med Genet A.2011 Feb 18.doi: 10.1002/ajmg.a.33851.[Epub ahead of print].*

Roaches,E.S., Gomez,M.R., Northrup,H. (1998) Tuberous sclerosis complex consensus conference: revised clinical diagnostic criteria. *J Child Neurol.* 13(12): 624-628.

Robinson,D., Tieder,M., Halperin,N., Burshtein,D., Nevo,Z. (1994) Maffucci's syndrome--the result of neural abnormalities? Evidence of mitogenic neurotransmitters present in enchondromas and soft tissue hemangiomas. *Cancer* 74(3): 949-957.

Sarica,F.B., Cekinmez,M., Tufan,K., Erdogan,B., Sen,O., Altinors,M.N. (2008) A rare case of massive NF1 with invasion of entire spinal axis by neurofibromas: case report. *Turk Neurosurg.* 18(1): 99-106.

Satter,E. (2007) Proteus syndrome: 2 case reports and a review of the literature. *Cutis.* 80(4): 297-302.

Schimke,R.N., Collins,D.L., Stolle,C.A. (2009) Von Hippel-Lindau Syndrome.Schimke RN, Collins DL, Stolle CA. In: Pagon,R.A., Bird,T.D., Dolan,C.R., Stephens,K. (eds) GeneReviews [Internet], Seattle (WA): University of Washington, Seattle.

Schroder,S., Moehrs,D., von Weltzien,J., Winkler,R., Otto,H.F. (1983) The Turcot syndrome. Report of an additional case and review of the literature. *Dis Colon Rectum* 26(8): 533-538.

Schwartz,H.S., Zimmerman,N.B., Simon,M.A., Wroble,R.R., Millar,E.A., Bonfiglio,M. (1987) The malignant potential of enchondromatosis. *J Bone Joint Surg Am* 69(2): 269-274.

Seizinger,B.R., Rouleau,G.A., Ozelius,L.J., et al. (1988) Von Hippel-Lindau disease maps to the region of chromosome 3 associated with renal cell carcinoma. *Nature* 332(6161): 268-269.

Sezer,E., Senayli,A., Sezer,T., Bicakci,U. (2006) Segmental neurofibromatosis: report of two cases. *J Dermatol.* 33(9): 635-638.

Shanley,S., Ratcliffe,J., Hockey,A., et al. (1994) Nevoid basal cell carcinoma syndrome: review of 118 affected individuals. *Am J MedGenet.* 50(3): 282-290.

Shapiro,F. (1982) Ollier's Disease. An assessment of angular deformity, shortening, and pathological fracture in twenty-one patients. *J Bone Joint Surg Am.1982 Jan;64(1):95-103.* 64(1): 95-103.

Silve,C., Jüppner,H. (2006) Ollier disease. *Orphanet J Rare Dis.2006 Sep 22;1:37.* 1: 37.

Stavrou,T., Bromley,C.M., Nicholson,H.S., et al. (2001) Prognostic factors and secondary malignancies in childhood medulloblastoma. *J Pediatr Hematol Oncol.* 23(7): 431-436.

Tago,M., Terahara,A., Shin,M., Maruyama,K., Kurita,H., Nakagawa,K., Ohtomo,K. (2005) Gamma knife surgery for hemangioblastomas. *J Neurosurg.* 102(Suppl.): 171-174.

Taipale,J., Chen,J.K., Cooper,M.K., et al. (2000) Effects of oncogenic mutations in Smoothened and Patched can be reversed by cyclopamine. *Nature* 406(6799): 1005-1009.

Taylor,M.D., Mainprize,T.G., Rutka,J.T. (2000) Molecular insight into medulloblastoma and central nervous system primitive neuroectodermal tumor biology from hereditary syndromes: a review. *Neurosurgery* 47(4): 888-901.

Taylor,M.D., Mainprize,T.G., Rutka,J.T., Becker,L., Bayani,J., Drake,J.M. (2001) Medulloblastoma in a child with Rubenstein-Taybi Syndrome: case report and review of the literature. *Pediatr Neurosurg.* 35(5): 235-238.

Thayer,S.P., di Magliano,M.P., Heiser,P.W.e.al. (2003) Hedgehog is an early and late mediator of pancreatic cancer tumorigenesis. *Nature* 425(6960): 851-856.

Valdueza,J.M., Cristante,L., Dreitag,J., Hagel,C., Hermann,H.D. (1995) Malignant chiasmal glioma: a rare cause of rapid visual loss. *Neurosurg.Rev.* 18: 273-275.

Van der Hoeve,J. (1920) Eye symptoms in tuberous sclerosis of the brain. *Trans Ophthalmol Soc UK.* 40: 329-334.

Verma,K.K., Ovung,E.M., Sirka,C.S. (2001) Extensive facial angiofibromas in tuberous sclerosis treated with carbon dioxide laserbrasion. *Dermato Surg.* 67(6): 326-328.

Visrutaratna,P., Oranratanachai,K., Singhavejsakul,J. (2004) Clinics in diagnostic imaging (96). Plexiform neurofibromatosis. *Singapore Med J.* 45(4): 188-192.

Wanebo,J.E., Lonser,R.R., Glenn,G.M., Oldfield,E.H. (2003) The natural history of hemangioblastomas of the central nervous system in patients with von Hippel-Lindau disease. *J Neurosurg.* 98(1): 82-94.

Wang,E.M., Pan,L., Wang,B.J., Zhang,N., Zhou,L.F., Dong,Y.F., Dai,J.Z., Cai,P.W., Chen,H. (2005) The long-term results of gamma knife radiosurgery for hemangioblastomas of the brain. *J Neurosurg.* 102(Suppl.): 225-229.

Wixom,C., Chadwick,A.E., Krous,H.F. (2005) Sudden, unexpected death associated with meningioangiomatosis: case report. *Pediatr Dev Pathol.* 8(2): 240-244.

Woodruff,J.M. (1999) Pathology of tumors of the peripheral nerve sheath in type 1 neurofibromatosis. *Am J Med Genet.* 89(1): 23-30.

Zhang,H., Cai,C., Wang,S., Liu,H., Ye,Y., Chen,X. (2007) Extracranial head and neck schwannomas: a clinical analysis of 33 patients. *Laryngoscope* 117(2): 278-281.

15

Brain Tumors and the Lynch Syndrome

Päivi Peltomäki and Annette Gylling
*Department of Medical Genetics, University of Helsinki,
Finland*

1. Introduction

1.1 Clinical features and tumor spectrum

Lynch syndrome (LS) (MIM No. 120435-6), previously known as hereditary nonpolyposis colorectal cancer (HNPCC) (Boland, 2005), is an autosomal dominant disorder caused by germline mutation in one of the DNA mismatch repair (MMR) genes. LS is among the most prevalent cancer syndromes in man and is estimated to account for 1-6% of all colorectal cancers (Lynch & de la Chapelle, 2003).

Before the discovery of DNA MMR gene defects responsible for LS in the 1990s, clinical diagnostic criteria known as the Amsterdam I criteria (Vasen et al., 1991) were used to identify families likely to represent LS. The original criteria were based on colorectal cancer only and were subsequently modified to include extracolonic cancers as well (Amsterdam II criteria, Vasen et al., 1999 (Table 1). Amsterdam II criteria include colorectal cancer, cancer of the endometrium, small bowel, ureter, and renal pelvis as unequivocal manifestations of the syndrome. Later experience incorporating epidemiological, clinical, and molecular information has resulted in the expansion of the list of LS-associated tumors. The revised Bethesda criteria (Umar et al., 2004) include, among others, brain tumors as LS-related tumors (Table 1). Individuals that meet at least one of the Bethesda criteria are considered to have suspected LS, and investigating tumors for microsatellite instability (MSI) is warranted as a pre-screening method prior to germline mutation testing. Currently, the definition of LS is a molecular one and the term LS is restricted to families with an identified pathogenic germline mutation in one of the DNA MMR genes (Boland, 2005).

Carriers of a pathogenic DNA MMR gene mutation have a lifetime risk of 10-53% for developing colorectal carcinoma, 15-44% for developing endometrial carcinoma, and less than 15% for other cancers (Aarnio et al., 1999; Watson & Lynch, 2001; Chen et al., 2006; Senter et al., 2008; Baglietto et al., 2010). The risk of developing cancer depends on the predisposing gene, gender and environmental factors. According to Vasen et al. (2001), the cumulative risk of developing brain tumor by 70 years is 1.2% in MSH2 mutation carriers and lower in MLH1 mutation carriers. Even if the life-time risk of brain tumor, compared to many other tumors, is low in LS families, the risk of brain tumors is unequivocally elevated compared to the general population; the calculated fold increase varies between 4 and 6 (Aarnio et al., 1999; Vasen et al., 1996).

Colorectal carcinomas in LS are often diagnosed at an early age (mean, 45-50 years) and the same applies to many extracolonic tumors, at least when compared to the corresponding sporadic tumors (Vasen, 2005). In published series of LS-associated brain tumors (mainly representing MLH1 or MSH2 mutation carriers), the average age at diagnosis ranges from 33 to 53 years (Vasen et al., 1996; Aarnio et al., 1999; Vasen et al., 2001; Gylling et al., 2008). LS-associated brain tumors may be of diverse histological types, the most common ones being glioblastoma (Aarnio et al., 1999) and astrocytoma (Vasen et al., 1996).

Amsterdam criteria II
There should be at least three relatives with a Lynch syndrome-associated cancer (colorectal cancer (CRC), cancer of the endometrium, small bowel, ureter or renal pelvis): all of the following criteria should be present:
1) one should be a first degree relative of the other two;
2) at least two successive generations should be affected;
3) at least one should be diagnosed before age 50;
4) familial adenomatous polyposis should be excluded in the CRC case (s) if any;
5) tumors should be verified by pathological examination
Revised Bethesda criteria
1) Colorectal cancer diagnosed in a patient <50 y of age.
2) Presence of synchronous, metachronous colorectal, or other Lynch syndrome-related tumors*, regardless of age.
3) Colorectal cancer with MSI-H phenotype diagnosed in a patient < 60 y of age.
4) Patient with colorectal cancer and a first-degree relative with a Lynch syndrome-related tumor, with one of the cancers diagnosed under age 50 y.
5) Patient with colorectal cancer with two or more first-degree or second-degree relatives with a Lynch syndrome-related tumor, regardless of age.
*Lynch syndrome related tumors include colorectal, endometrial, stomach, ovarian, pancreas, ureter, renal pelvis, biliary tract, and brain tumors, sebaceous gland adenomas, keratoacanthomas and carcinoma of the small bowel.

Table 1. Amsterdam II and revised Bethesda criteria

The clinical features of LS variants in which the risk of brain tumor is considerably higher than in classical LS, namely Turcot syndrome (TS) and constitutional mismatch repair deficiency syndrome (CMMR-D), will be described in section "The association of brain tumors with hereditary cancer syndromes" below.

1.2 Genetic basis

Predisposition to LS is caused by heterozygous germline mutations in one of four, possibly five genes with verified or putative DNA mismatch repair function, namely MLH1 (MutL homologue 1), MSH2 (MutS homologue 2), MSH6 (MutS homologue 6), PMS2 (Postmeiotic segregation 2), and possibly MLH3 (MutL homologue 3). The great majority of the presently known 3000 unique mutations and variants in MMR genes affect MLH1 and MSH2, with fewer changes in MSH6, PMS2 and MLH3 (http://www.insight-group.org; Peltomaki & Vasen, 2004; Woods et al., 2007). Most MSH2 and MLH1 mutations are truncating (Peltomaki & Vasen, 2004; Woods et al., 2007) and result in unstable mRNA and protein. However, one-third of MMR gene

alterations are of missense type and such changes may occasionally complicate the interpretation of immunohistochemical analyses of tumor tissues by leading to stable but non-functional protein. PMS2 and MSH6 mutations in particular may carry a high risk of brain tumors, but - because of reduced penetrance - mainly when biallelic (CMMR-D) (Wimmer & Etzler, 2008).
The mechanism behind constitutional inactivation of a MMR gene is not always genetic (point mutation or large rearrangement) but may be epigenetic (primary or secondary epimutation; Hitchins & Ward, 2009; Ligtenberg et al., 2009). To our knowledge, brain tumor has not yet been reported as part of the variable spectrum of colorectal and extracolonic cancers observed in constitutional epimutation carriers to date (Suter et al., 2004; Morak et al., 2008; Hitchins & Ward, 2009; Niessen et al., 2009) but there is no reason to suggest why brain tumors would not develop in constitutional epimutation carriers.

1.3 Tumorigenic mechanisms

LS generally complies with Knudson's two-hit mechanism of tumorigenesis (Knudson, 1971) where germline mutation in one copy of a DNA MMR gene (first hit) causes cancer susceptibility but cancer initiation additionally requires the inactivation of the remaining wild-type copy (second hit) in a tumor progenitor cell of a somatic target tissue. Somatic loss of the wild-type allele, as evidenced by loss of heterozygosity (LOH), is the predominant mechanism of the second hit (Ollikainen et al., 2007). As a result of inactivation of both allelic copies, tumor tissues from LS patients typically show the absence of the respective MMR protein by immunohistochemical analysis (and occasionally, other MMR proteins as well in a defined pattern (Hendriks et al., 2006). This has been shown to apply to almost all colorectal carcinomas and extracolonic cancers of the LS spectrum, and brain tumors are no different (Gylling et al., 2008).
Inactivation of a MMR gene is believed to initiate tumorigenesis through the failure of one or several essential functions that the MMR system is known to have, including repair of replication errors and a role in DNA damage signaling (Jiricny, 2006). Impaired repair capacity leads to an elevated rate of mutations in important growth-controlling genes as well as instability at random microsatellite sequences ("mutator phenotype", Perucho, 1996). The demonstration of microsatellite instability (MSI) serves as an important biomarker for LS cancers. A panel of five markers (so called Bethesda panel consisting of BAT25, BAT26, D2S123, D5S346 and D17S250) was recommended for screening purposes (Boland et al., 1998). Size shifts at two or more microsatellite loci indicate high-degree microsatellite instability (MSI-H). The mononucleotide repeats BAT26 and BAT25 are particularly sensitive for MSI-H in both familial and sporadic colorectal cancers, but their performance in extracolonic cancers is less well known. Consequently, as will be described below in section "The role of DNA mismatch repair defects in the pathogenesis of brain tumors", an investigation of different cancers from a nationwide cohort of LS families showed that, despite origin from verified MMR gene mutation carriers, MSI-H frequency in tumors varied between 100 and 0%, where the highest frequencies were for ureter, stomach, and colon and the lowest frequency for brain (Gylling et al., 2008).

2. The association of brain tumors with hereditary cancer syndromes

2.1 Main cancer syndromes in which brain tumors are overrepresented

Several inherited cancer predisposition syndromes are known that are associated with increased risk of brain tumors, besides malignancies of other organs (Table 2). Analysis of germline and somatic alterations in brain tumors from such syndromes may provide valuable clues to the mechanisms of brain tumor development in general. In most cases, the predisposing gene encodes a tumor suppressor protein and the disease is dominant on pedigree level but recessive on cellular level.

The list includes two syndromes that are associated with germline mutation in DNA MMR genes. Co-occurrence of brain tumor with colorectal tumor in the same individual is known as Turcot syndrome (TS) (Turcot et al., 1959). TS can be dominant or recessive. Dominant TS is due to heterozygous mutations in DNA MMR genes (Chan et al., 1999; Lebrun et al., 2007) or the Adenomatous Polyposis Coli (APC) gene (Foulkes, 1995). Recessive TS is due to biallelic mutation in DNA MMR genes (De Rosa et al., 2000; Miyaki et al., 2001; Hegde et al., 2005) and can also be classified under CMMR-D (but not vice versa: only a minority of CMMR-D cases fulfill the diagnostic criteria of TS). The predominant brain tumor in APC-associated TS is medulloblastoma whereas glioblastoma predominates in TS associated with DNA MMR gene mutations (Hamilton et al., 1995).

To date, some 100 patients have been reported who are homozygotes or compound heterozygotes for DNA MMR gene mutations. The term "constitutional mismatch repair deficiency" (CMMR-D) (Wimmer & Etzler, 2008) or "Lynch III" (Felton et al., 2007) has been proposed for such cases. The clinical picture is severe: the patients are affected by hematological malignancy or brain tumor in childhood and those who survive their first tumor are at risk to develop colorectal cancer or other typical LS-associated malignancy in adolescence or early adulthood (Wimmer & Etzler, 2008). The predominant type of brain tumor that develops in CMMR-D is astrocytoma, primarily glioblastoma (Wimmer & Etzler, 2008). The prevalence of hematological tumors may be higher in patients with biallelic MLH1 or MSH2 mutations whereas patients with MSH6 or PMS2 mutations have a higher risk of brain and LS-associated tumors (Wimmer & Etzler, 2008).

Syndrome	Predisposing gene	Mode of inheritance	Characteristic type of brain tumor
Li-Fraumeni	TP53	AD	Astrocytoma, choroid plexus tumor
Neurofibromatosis, type 1	NF1	AD	Optic pathway glioma
Neurofibromatosis, type 2	NF2	AD	Vestibular schwannoma, meningioma
Von Hippel-Lindau	VHL	AD	Hemangioblastoma
Tuberous sclerosis	TSC1, TSC2	AD	Subependymomal giant cell astrocytoma
Gorlin	PTCH	AD	Medulloblastoma
Turcot	APC	AD	Medulloblastoma
	MSH2, MLH1, MSH6, PMS2	AD or AR	Glioblastoma
Constitutional MMR deficiency	MSH2, MLH1, MSH6, PMS2	AR	Astrocytoma (glioblastoma)

AD, autosomal dominant, AR, autosomal recessive.

Table 2. Inherited cancer predisposition syndromes that are associated with increased risk to brain tumors, in addition to malignacies of various organs.

2.2 Molecular characteristics of "syndromic" brain tumors

As evident from Table 2, inherited syndromes are often associated with particular types of brain tumor (Ullrich, 2008). This is likely to reflect a combination of germline and somatic effects. Locus or allelic heterogeneity may explain some of the increased brain tumor risk in certain families. As mentioned above, among MMR genes, PMS2 mutations in particular (and when biallelic) are associated with increased brain tumor risk (Wimmer & Etzler, 2008). Germline mutation in TP53 predisposes to Li-Fraumeni syndrome, and especially families with TP53 missense mutations within the core DNA binding domain suffer from brain tumors (Birch et al., 1994). Some germline mutations may have tissue-specific effects that are mediated by unique mechanisms. For example, the tetramerization domain of the protein product of the R337H mutation in TP53, which is enriched in Brazil, was found to be less stable than that of wild-type p53 and therefore sensitive to disruption at acidic pH (DiGiammarino et al., 2002). This was proposed as an explanation for the frequent occurrence of adrenocortical carcinoma in association with this mutation.

Even in families segregating an identical germline mutation, tumors at different anatomical sites and at different ages develop, as observed in LS/TS (Peltomaki et al., 2001) or Li-Fraumeni syndrome (Malkin, 2004). This has prompted investigators to search for additional germline genetic variations or modifier genes. In carriers of TP53 mutation and especially those of them who were clinically affected, copy number variation frequencies in the germline were found to be significantly elevated compared to healthy controls (Shlien et al., 2008). Moreover, in choroid plexus tumors, germline hemizygous deletions had progressed into homozygous deletions and germline duplications had enlarged in size. It was suggested that in association with constitutional dysfunction of TP53, germline copy number variations may provide a foundation for the development of more striking chromosomal changes in tumors (Shlien et al., 2008). Inherited MMR deficiency could in theory have analogous effects on other genes by causing subtle genetic instability (Fodde & Smits, 2002), although it is yet to be proven.

Compatible with tumor suppressor function and Knudson's two-hit hypothesis, the wild-type allele of the predisposing genes of the syndromes listed in Table 2 is regularly inactivated in tumors, as shown for MMR genes in TS (Chan et al., 1999; Lebrun et al., 2007), APC in TS (Hamilton et al., 1995), and TP53 in Li-Fraumeni syndrome (Rieber et al., 2009; Seidinger et al., 2010). In the case of MMR genes, inactivation of both copies in a target tissue typically, but not always, results in MSI and a generalized "mutator" phenotype (Gylling et al., 2008). As will be discussed in greater detail below under "The role of DNA mismatch repair defects in the pathogenesis of brain tumors", brain tumors may constitute an important exception to the general rule. Apart from the inactivation of the alleles of the predisposing gene, additional somatic changes in tumor tissues may make a difference. In TS patients with (heterozygous) germline mutation in MSH2, TP53 inactivation and chromosomal instability were found to be required for the genesis of glioblastoma but not for colorectal carcinoma, which in turn seemed to require TGFβRII frameshift mutation (Leung et al., 2000).

3. The role of DNA mismatch repair defects in the pathogenesis of brain tumors

3.1 Sporadic brain tumors

With some exceptional single reports (Alonso et al., 2001), MSI is generally rare in brain tumors regardless of histology (Table 3). This is true especially when using microsatellite markers recommended for the analysis of colorectal cancers (like the Bethesda panel, Boland et al., 1998, or panels based on mononucleotide repeats exclusively). Frequencies of MSI from studies using dinucleotide repeat markers alone or in combination with tri- and tetranucleotide repeat markers vary considerably (see e.g., Gomori et al., 2002 and Wooster et al., 1994 in Table 3).

Tumor type	Markers used to study MSI (type of repeat)	Frequency of MSI	Status of MMR protein expression*	Reference
Pediatric malignant astrocytoma	BAT25, BAT26, MONO-27, NR-21, NR-24 (mono) and Penta C, Penta D (penta)	MSI-low (1 unstable marker): 4/126 (3%)	MSH6+ (other proteins not studied)	Vladimirova et al., 2008
Three sets of tumors: • Pediatric grade III & IV astrocytoma • Pediatric ganglioglioma • Adult grade III & IV astrocytoma	BAT25, BAT26 (mono)	2 unstable markers: 12/45 (27%) 4/17 (24%) 0/98 (0%)	Not studied	Alonso et al., 2001
Two sets of tumors: • Pediatric high-grade glioma • Adult high-grade glioma	BAT25, BAT26, CAT25 (mono)	MSI-high ($\geq$ 2/3 markers unstable): 0/71 (0%) 1/619 (0.16%)	MSH2+, MSH6+ in all MSH2-, MSH6- in the MSI-high tumor	Eckert et al., 2007
Glioma	DCC, D9S171, D10S541, D13S121, D17S520, D19S412 (di) and AR (tri)	1 unstable marker: 4/7 (57%) 2 unstable markers: 2/7 (29%)	Not studied (no mutation in MLH1 or MSH2)	Gomori et al., 2002
Glial and other brain tumors	vWFa, vWFb, DXS981 (tetra) and AR, DM, c-myc (tri) and D2S123, D16S413, D17S796, D16S301, D16S303, D16S588 (di)	1 unstable marker: 1/54 (1.9%)	Not studied	Wooster et al., 1994

Table 3. DNA mismatch repair defects in sporadic primary brain tumors.

Tumor type	Markers used to study MSI (type of repeat)	Frequency of MSI	Status of MMR protein expression*	Reference
Medulloblastoma	NR27, NR21, NR24, BAT25, BAT26 (mono)	MSI-high (≥ 2 unstable markers): 1/36 (2.7%) MSI-low (1 unstable marker): 3/36 (8.3%)	Among MSI cases, MSH6+ in all (other proteins not studied) and MSH6 promoter methylation in 2	Viana-Pereira et al., 2009
Meningioma (NF2 intact)	BAT25, BAT26, BAT40, MSH6 (mono) and D2S123, D5S346 (di)	No unstable markers in any of 25 tumors	Not studied	Tilborg et al., 2006

*+, expressed, -, not expressed

(Table 3., continued)

There is often no demonstration that MSI results from defective MMR. While immunohistochemical studies occasionally implicate one of the MMR proteins in brain tumors with MSI (Eckert et al., 2007; Szybka et al., 2003), correlation between MSI and MMR protein expression remains poor in many cases (Szybka et al., 2003).

Hardly any information is available of the molecular mechanisms that could lead to MMR protein inactivation in brain tumors. As for potential inactivating mechanisms, there is evidence that MSH6 is prone to promoter methylation (Viana-Pereira et al., 2009) and mutation (Yip et al., 2009) in sporadic brain tumors. Taken together, deficient MMR seems to play a less important role in brain tumors compared to e.g., sporadic colorectal cancers, among which 15 - 25% are MMR-deficient in virtually all published series (Peltomaki, 2003). As will be discussed below, this does not exclude the potential importance of MMR protein functions other than mismatch repair in various stages of brain tumor development.

3.2 Lynch syndrome-associated brain tumors

Our recent analysis of tumors arising in different organs from LS mutation carriers showed that, like other tumors, brain tumors complied with Knudson's two-hit hypothesis by displaying the absence of the MMR protein corresponding to the germline mutation, which suggests inactivation of both copies of the MMR gene in question (Gylling et al., 2008, Fig. 1). Studies published to date report frequencies of 75 - 100% for the immunohistochemical loss of MMR protein(s) in brain tumors from heterozygous carriers of MMR gene mutations (Table 4).

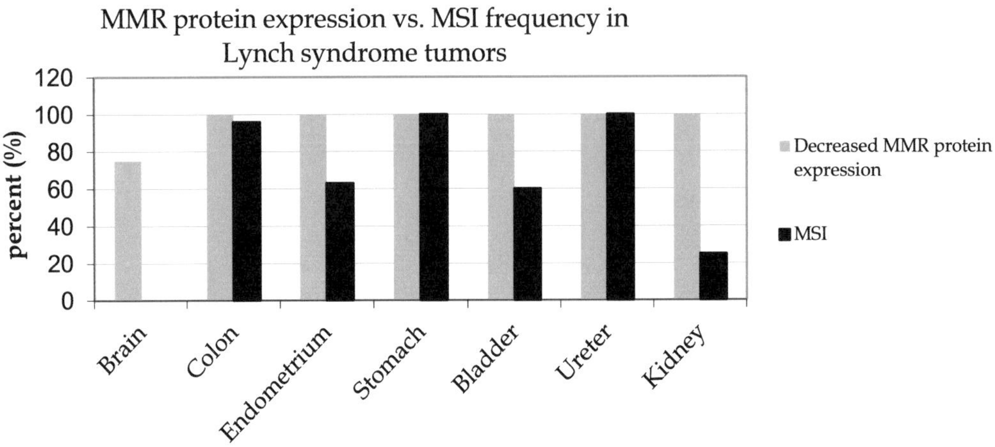

Fig. 1. Decreased MMR protein expression corresponding to germline mutation vs. microsatelite instability using Bethesda markers.

The loss of MMR protein expression may (Leung et al., 2000) or may not (Gylling et al., 2008) lead to MSI (Table 4). Since the detection of MSI by conventional techniques requires the presence of at least one major tumor clone which exhibits microsatellite repeat length deviating from the normal allele size, the apparent absence of MSI in brain tumors may have an alternative explanation based on clonal heterogeneity. Our small pool PCR experiments of brain tumors indeed supported the hypothesis since they detected MSI but it was diluted by multiple minor clones with mutant allele frequency below 30% and the high proportion of clones with normal alleles so that the pattern by conventional PCR was microsatellite-stable. The small pool PCR technique we applied is the same that has been used to detect MSI in constitutional non-neoplastic tissues from biallelic MMR gene mutation carriers in CMMR-D (see next section). Studies suggest that the presence of multiple subclones may be a general characteristic of MSI tumors from LS and sporadic settings (Fujiwara et al., 1998; Barnetson et al., 2000).

Since MSI is generally uncommon in brain tumors (see previous section), its presence may pinpoint MMR gene germline mutation carriers (Giunti et al., 2009). In a series of 34 pediatric gliomas of different grades, Giunti et al. (2009) found two with MSI and both patients subsequently revealed germline mutations in MMR genes (biallelic in one and monoallelic in the other case) compatible with TS. Interestingly, a clear qualitative difference in the MSI pattern was evident when a glioblastoma from a TS patient and a colon cancer from an affected relative were compared. Glioblastoma displayed smaller allelic shifts which may make MSI more difficult to discern and supports the idea that the type of MSI varies in tumors of different histological derivation as previously demonstrated for endometrial vs. colorectal carcinomas representing LS (Kuismanen et al., 2002) and sporadic cases (Duval et al., 2002).

Not much is known about the nature of second "hits" that may mediate MMR protein inactivation in LS-associated brain tumors. In analogy to colon cancers in LS (Ollikainen et al., 2007), LOH appears to be the predominant mechanism (Gylling et al., 2008; Chan et al., 1999) whereas promoter methylation is rare or absent (Gylling et al., 2008).

Characteristics of tumor series	Predisposing gene	Markers used to study MSI (type of repeat)	Frequency of MSI	Expression of protein corresponding to germline mutation	Reference
TS or LS (3 glioblastoma multiforme, 1 mixed glioma)	MSH2 or MLH1	BAT26, BAT40 (mono) and TP53, D18S58, D2S123 (di)	MSI-high ($\geq$ 2 unstable markers): 4/4 (100%)	MSH2- in MSH2 associated and MLH1- in MLH1 associated cases	Leung et al., 2000
LS or TS (7 brain tumors of various histology)	MLH1, MSH2, or MSH6	BAT25, BAT26 (mono) and D5S346, D2S123, D17S250 (di)	No unstable marker in any of 7 tumors*	Germline mutation-associated protein lost in 3/4 (75%)	Gylling et al., 2008
TS or LS (1 anaplastic astrocytoma grade III, 1 glioblastoma)	MSH2 or MLH1	Not studied	Not studied	MSH2- in MSH2 associated and MLH1- in MLH1 associated case	Lebrun et al., 2007
TS (2 glioblastomas)	PMS2 (biallelic) in one and MLH1 (mono-allelic) in another	BAT25, BAT26, NR21, NR22, NR24 (mono)	No. of unstable markers: 3/3 (PMS2-associated), 4/5 (MLH1-associated)	Not studied	Giunti et al., 2009

*By small-pool PCR using D5S346 and D2S123, MSI was present in 4/4 tumors tested.

Table 4. DNA mismatch repair defects in brain tumors from heterozygous carriers of MMR gene mutations, representing Lynch syndrome (LS) or Turcot syndrome (TS).

3.3 Brain tumors in constitutional mismatch repair deficiency syndrome

In individuals with homozygous or compound heterozygous germline mutations in MMR genes (CMMR-D syndrome), both alleles of a given MMR gene are inactive from birth and the corresponding MMR protein is absent not only in tumors but in normal tissue as well (Wimmer & Etzler, 2008). Since normal non-neoplastic tissues lack significant clonality which is a prerequisite for the detection of MSI, it is not surprising that conventional PCR reveals no MSI in normal tissues; however, MSI may be detectable by small-pool PCR (Parsons R et al., 1995). In regard to brain tumors from biallelic MMR gene mutation carriers, immunohistochemical studies usually show the lack of a given MMR protein, whereas MSI (by conventional techniques) is present in only a minority (Bougeard et al., 2003; Agostini et al., 2005; Poley et al., 2007; Wagner et al., 2003; Hegde et al., 2005). These observations emphasize the special nature of brain tumors when compared to other (e.g., colorectal) cancers from biallelic mutation carriers. The findings raise the question whether other functions of the MMR proteins (Jiricny, 2006), such as impaired DNA damage signaling (Agostini et al., 2005; Bougeard et al., 2003), might be more important than postreplicative mismatch repair in brain tumor development. Resistance to alkylating agents, which develops irrespective of MSI in recurrent gliomas (Yip et al., 2009) may lend further support to this possibility.

An interesting feature of CMMR-D is that almost all patients display signs of neurofibromatosis 1, mainly café-au-lait spots, in the absence of germline NF1 mutations. It was found that the NF1 gene is a mutational target in MMR-deficient cells (Wang et al., 2003), making it possible that neurofibromatosis 1 features result from early somatic mutations targeting NF1.

3.4 Therapy-induced defects in DNA mismatch repair genes

The fact that almost all glioblastomas recur and recurrent lesions are fatal within around a year has prompted comparative molecular studies between primary and recurrent brain tumors. Taking advantage of MSI as an indicator of a tumor clone (or clones), Gomori et al. (2002) found intensive clonal selection which may contribute to the recurrence of gliomas. Yip et al. (2009) observed that certain MSH6 mutations were selected in glioblastomas during temozolomide (alkylating agent) therapy and mediated temozolomide resistance, which may in part explain the poor survival associated with recurrent gliomas. Interestingly, the role of MSH6 in temozolomide response did not depend on MSI.

4. Epigenetic alterations in brain tumors

Distinct methylation profiles may accompany different histological types and subtypes of brain tumors. Studies on promoter CpG methylation of tumor suppressor and other growth-regulatory genes have revealed patterns characteristic of astrocytoma (Yu et al., 2004), various glioma subtypes (Uhlmann et al., 2003), and medulloblastoma (Lindsey et al., 2005). Epigenetic changes may correlate with grade; for example, Uhlmann et al. (2003) found that pilocytic astrocytomas, which are grade I tumors, showed no CpG island hypermethylation of growth-controlling genes as opposed to astrocytomas, oligoastrocytomas, and oligodendrogliomas (grade II – III tumors) which were associated with frequent CpG island methylation.

In analogy to sporadic brain tumors, LS-associated brain tumors that we investigated (Gylling et al., 2008, Fig. 2) may also show patterns of tumor suppressor gene promoter methylation characteristic of tumor type, which might become more distinct if larger series of brain tumors from LS patients were available for molecular studies. Furthermore, comparison of tumor suppressor promoter methylation profiles in brain tumors to those in cancers of other organs from MMR gene mutation carriers suggests the presence of organ-specific epigenetic patterns in carriers of even identical predisposing mutations (Fig. 3).

Among 24 tumor suppressor genes tested, colorectal cancers from LS patients showed the highest number of methylated genes whereas brain tumors had the lowest number (Gylling et al., 2008). Promoter methylation is expected to silence the respective tumor suppressor genes and thereby promote tumor formation. The organ-specific epigenetic patterns we observed may thus contribute to the selective tumor spectrum in LS.

Some epigenetic changes may predict treatment response in brain tumors. For example, the repair enzyme encoded by the 0^6-methylguanine-DNA methyltransferase (MGMT) gene removes alkyl groups from guanine and thereby counteracts therapy with alkylating agents. If, however, MGMT is silenced by promoter methylation, chemotherapy-induced lesions remain unrepaired in DNA and trigger apoptosis. Promoter methylation of MGMT, which occurs in approximately half of gliomas, is an independent favorable prognostic sign and confers a significant survival benefit from temozolomide treatment (Hegi et al., 2005). Moreover, recent findings indicate that methylated MGMT alleles are enriched in a subpopulation presumed to comprise glioma-initiating cells, even when the original glioblastoma may have only a minority of methylated alleles (Sciuscio et al., 2011).

Of note, besides chemotherapeutic drugs, methylated compounds may also be contained in food, and methylation tolerance due to MGMT inactivation by promoter methylation may thus have broader significance in cancer development. For example, it was proposed that MGMT field defect in colorectal mucosa may be an initiating event in colorectal carcinoma by two alternative mechanisms: first, in concert with KRAS mutation allowing a microsatellite-stable phenotype to become malignant and second, in concert with MMR deficiency facilitating the development of MSI cancers (Svrcek et al., 2010).

	TIMP3	APC	CDKN2A	MLH1	ATM	RARB	CDKN2B	HIC1	CHFR	BRCA1	CASP8	CDKN1B	PTEN	BRCA2	CD44	DAPK1	VHL	ESR1	RASSF1	TP73	FHIT	IGSF4	CDH13	GSTP1
Glioblastoma																			■					
Glioblastoma multiforme																								■
Astrocytoma											■					■			■					■
Ganglioglioma																								
Hemangiomablastoma													■						■					
Meningioma																								■
Meningioma																								■

Fig. 2. Promoter methylation in 24 tumor suppressor genes studied using methylation-specific MLPA (MS-MLPA) assay in LS brain tumors. Black boxes indicate methylation of the tumor suppressor gene, whereas no methylation is shown as a white box.

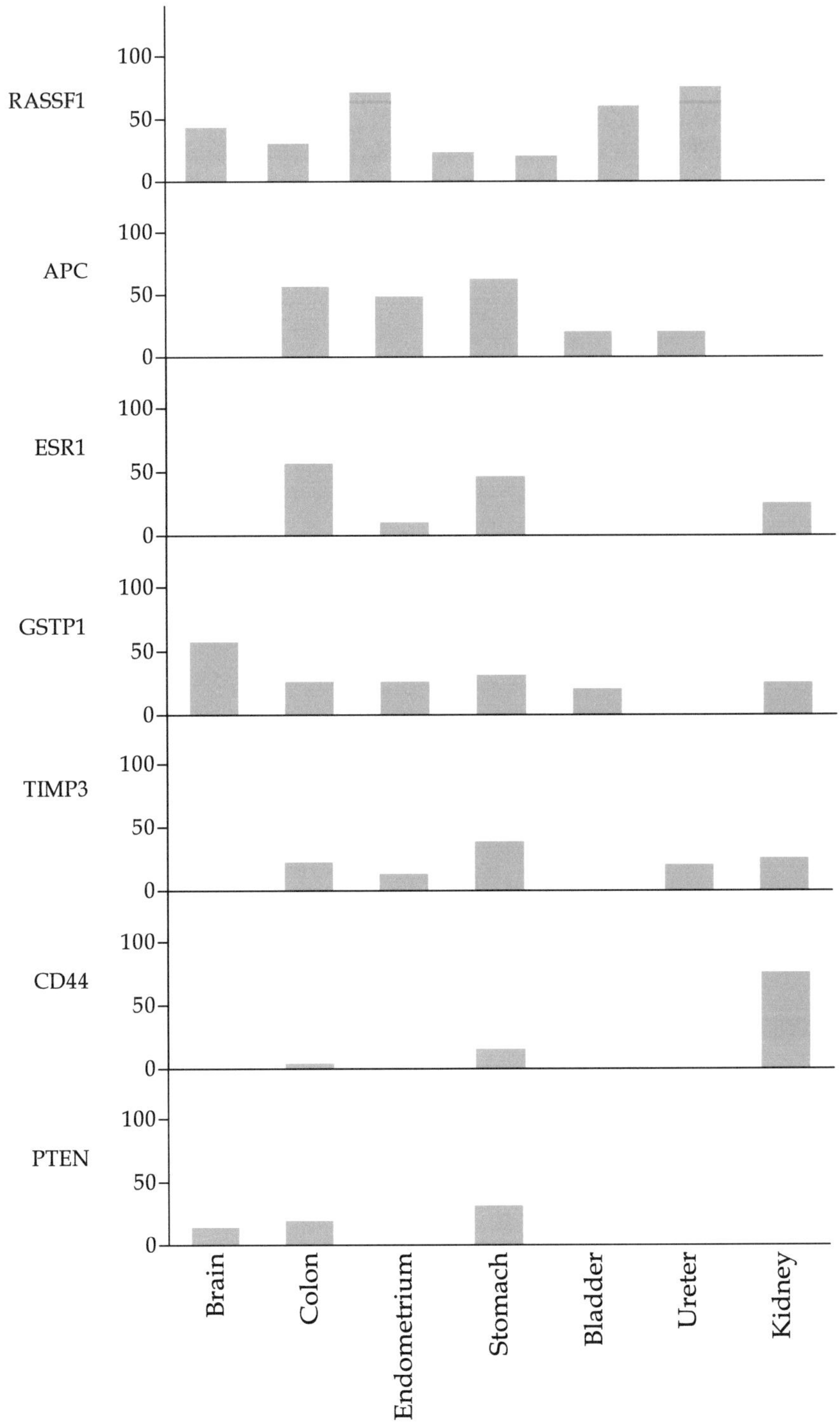

Fig. 3. Promoter methylation in Lynch syndrome patients. The height of the bar depicts percentage of tumors with methylation at a given gene promoter.

5. Concluding remarks and future directions

As multi-organ cancer syndromes, LS and its variants TS and CMMR-D provide useful models to study carcinogenesis triggered by a failure in the MMR system. Genetic and epigenetic patterns have been revealed that may help explain the organ-specific cancer susceptibility in LS and more generally, the molecular pathogenesis of cancers of different organs. Brain tumors have drawn attention to MMR gene functions beyond the mere correction of replication errors. While information of the predisposing mutation has efficiently been translated into clinical practice and a significant decrease in mortality as a result of regular surveillance has been reported for LS-associated colorectal cancer (de Jong et al., 2006; Jarvinen et al., 2009), mortality remains high for other tumors that are too rare to be screened for, such as brain tumors (de Jong et al., 2006). Biomarkers that could predict which mutation carriers are at risk for which cancers before the actual tumor develops are eagerly awaited but not yet available. Much progress has been achieved in identifying biomarkers that may predict the behavior, prognosis, and treatment response of existing tumors, including those of the brain. Inherited cancer syndromes will no doubt remain important as shortcuts to the understanding of the molecular pathogenesis of brain and other tumors also in the future. Since many such syndromes are relatively rare, collaboration between basic, epidemiological, and clinical researchers continues to be the key to sufficient numbers of cases and specimens for high-quality research.

6. Acknowledgements

This work received financial support from the Academy of Finland (grant no. 121185), Sigrid Juselius Foundation, Finnish Cancer Organizations, Biocentrum Helsinki, and European Research Council (FP7-ERC-232635).

7. References

Aarnio, M., Sankila, R., Pukkala, E., Salovaara, R., Aaltonen, L.A., de la Chapelle, A., Peltomaki, P., Mecklin, J.P. & Jarvinen, H.J. (1999). Cancer risk in mutation carriers of DNA-mismatch-repair genes. *International journal of cancer. Journal international du cancer,* 81, 2, (214-218), 0020-7136

Agostini, M., Tibiletti, M.G., Lucci-Cordisco, E., Chiaravalli, A., Morreau, H., Furlan, D., Boccuto, L., Pucciarelli, S., Capella, C., Boiocchi, M. & Viel, A. (2005). Two PMS2 mutations in a Turcot syndrome family with small bowel cancers. *The American Journal of Gastroenterology,* 100, 8, (1886-1891), 0002-9270; 0002-9270

Alonso, M., Hamelin, R., Kim, M., Porwancher, K., Sung, T., Parhar, P., Miller, D.C. & Newcomb, E.W. (2001). Microsatellite instability occurs in distinct subtypes of pediatric but not adult central nervous system tumors. *Cancer research,* 61, 5, (2124-2128), 0008-5472; 0008-5472

Baglietto, L., Lindor, N.M., Dowty, J.G., White, D.M., Wagner, A., Gomez Garcia, E.B., Vriends, A.H., Dutch Lynch Syndrome Study Group, Cartwright, N.R., Barnetson, R.A., Farrington, S.M., Tenesa, A., Hampel, H., Buchanan, D., Arnold, S., Young, J., Walsh, M.D., Jass, J., Macrae, F., Antill, Y., Winship, I.M., Giles, G.G., Goldblatt, J., Parry, S., Suthers, G., Leggett, B., Butz, M., Aronson, M., Poynter, J.N., Baron, J.A., Le Marchand, L., Haile, R., Gallinger, S., Hopper, J.L., Potter, J., de la Chapelle, A.,

Vasen, H.F., Dunlop, M.G., Thibodeau, S.N. & Jenkins, M.A. (2010). Risks of Lynch syndrome cancers for MSH6 mutation carriers. *Journal of the National Cancer Institute,* 102, 3, (193-201), 1460-2105; 0027-8874

Barnetson, R., Jass, J., Tse, R., Eckstein, R., Robinson, B. & Schnitzler, M. (2000). Mutations associated with microsatellite unstable colorectal carcinomas exhibit widespread intratumoral heterogeneity. *Genes, chromosomes & cancer,* 29, 2, (130-136), 1045-2257

Birch, J.M., Hartley, A.L., Tricker, K.J., Prosser, J., Condie, A., Kelsey, A.M., Harris, M., Jones, P.H., Binchy, A. & Crowther, D. (1994). Prevalence and diversity of constitutional mutations in the p53 gene among 21 Li-Fraumeni families. *Cancer research,* 54, 5, (1298-1304), 0008-5472; 0008-5472

Boland, C.R. (2005). Evolution of the nomenclature for the hereditary colorectal cancer syndromes. *Familial cancer,* 4, 3, (211-218), 1389-9600; 1389-9600

Boland, C.R., Thibodeau, S.N., Hamilton, S.R., Sidransky, D., Eshleman, J.R., Burt, R.W., Meltzer, S.J., Rodriguez-Bigas, M.A., Fodde, R., Ranzani, G.N. & Srivastava, S. (1998). A National Cancer Institute Workshop on Microsatellite Instability for cancer detection and familial predisposition: development of international criteria for the determination of microsatellite instability in colorectal cancer. *Cancer research,* 58, 22, (5248-5257), 0008-5472

Bougeard, G., Charbonnier, F., Moerman, A., Martin, C., Ruchoux, M.M., Drouot, N. & Frebourg, T. (2003). Early onset brain tumor and lymphoma in MSH2-deficient children. *American Journal of Human Genetics,* 72, 1, (213-216), 0002-9297; 0002-9297

Chan, T.L., Yuen, S.T., Chung, L.P., Ho, J.W., Kwan, K., Fan, Y.W., Chan, A.S. & Leung, S.Y. (1999). Germline hMSH2 and differential somatic mutations in patients with Turcot's syndrome. *Genes, chromosomes & cancer,* 25, 2, (75-81), 1045-2257

Chen, S., Wang, W., Lee, S., Nafa, K., Lee, J., Romans, K., Watson, P., Gruber, S.B., Euhus, D., Kinzler, K.W., Jass, J., Gallinger, S., Lindor, N.M., Casey, G., Ellis, N., Giardiello, F.M., Offit, K., Parmigiani, G. & Colon Cancer Family Registry. (2006). Prediction of germline mutations and cancer risk in the Lynch syndrome. *JAMA : the journal of the American Medical Association,* 296, 12, (1479-1487), 1538-3598; 0098-7484

de Jong, A.E., Hendriks, Y.M., Kleibeuker, J.H., de Boer, S.Y., Cats, A., Griffioen, G., Nagengast, F.M., Nelis, F.G., Rookus, M.A. & Vasen, H.F. (2006). Decrease in mortality in Lynch syndrome families because of surveillance. *Gastroenterology,* 130, 3, (665-671), 0016-5085; 0016-5085

De Rosa, M., Fasano, C., Panariello, L., Scarano, M.I., Belli, G., Iannelli, A., Ciciliano, F. & Izzo, P. (2000). Evidence for a recessive inheritance of Turcot's syndrome caused by compound heterozygous mutations within the PMS2 gene. *Oncogene,* 19, 13, (1719-1723), 0950-9232

DiGiammarino, E.L., Lee, A.S., Cadwell, C., Zhang, W., Bothner, B., Ribeiro, R.C., Zambetti, G. & Kriwacki, R.W. (2002). A novel mechanism of tumorigenesis involving pH-dependent destabilization of a mutant p53 tetramer. *Nature structural biology,* 9, 1, (12-16), 1072-8368; 1072-8368

Duval, A., Reperant, M., Compoint, A., Seruca, R., Ranzani, G.N., Iacopetta, B. & Hamelin, R. (2002). Target gene mutation profile differs between gastrointestinal and endometrial tumors with mismatch repair deficiency. *Cancer research,* 62, 6, (1609-1612), 0008-5472; 0008-5472

Eckert, A., Kloor, M., Giersch, A., Ahmadi, R., Herold-Mende, C., Hampl, J.A., Heppner, F.L., Zoubaa, S., Holinski-Feder, E., Pietsch, T., Wiestler, O.D., von Knebel Doeberitz, M., Roth, W. & Gebert, J. (2007). Microsatellite instability in pediatric and adult high-grade gliomas. *Brain pathology (Zurich, Switzerland),* 17, 2, (146-150), 1015-6305

Felton, K.E., Gilchrist, D.M. & Andrew, S.E. (2007). Constitutive deficiency in DNA mismatch repair: is it time for Lynch III? *Clinical genetics,* 71, 6, (499-500), 0009-9163; 0009-9163

Fodde, R. & Smits, R. (2002). Cancer biology. A matter of dosage. *Science (New York, N.Y.),* 298, 5594, (761-763), 1095-9203; 0036-8075

Foulkes, W.D. (1995). A tale of four syndromes: familial adenomatous polyposis, Gardner syndrome, attenuated APC and Turcot syndrome. *QJM : monthly journal of the Association of Physicians,* 88, 12, (853-863), 1460-2725; 1460-2393

Fujiwara, T., Stolker, J.M., Watanabe, T., Rashid, A., Longo, P., Eshleman, J.R., Booker, S., Lynch, H.T., Jass, J.R., Green, J.S., Kim, H., Jen, J., Vogelstein, B. & Hamilton, S.R. (1998). Accumulated clonal genetic alterations in familial and sporadic colorectal carcinomas with widespread instability in microsatellite sequences. *The American journal of pathology,* 153, 4, (1063-1078), 0002-9440

Giunti, L., Cetica, V., Ricci, U., Giglio, S., Sardi, I., Paglierani, M., Andreucci, E., Sanzo, M., Forni, M., Buccoliero, A.M., Genitori, L. & Genuardi, M. (2009). Type A microsatellite instability in pediatric gliomas as an indicator of Turcot syndrome. *European journal of human genetics : EJHG,* 17, 7, (919-927), 1476-5438; 1018-4813

Gomori, E., Fulop, Z., Meszaros, I., Doczi, T. & Matolcsy, A. (2002). Microsatellite analysis of primary and recurrent glial tumors suggests different modalities of clonal evolution of tumor cells. *Journal of neuropathology and experimental neurology,* 61, 5, (396-402), 0022-3069; 0022-3069

Gylling, A.H., Nieminen, T.T., Abdel-Rahman, W.M., Nuorva, K., Juhola, M., Joensuu, E.I., Jarvinen, H.J., Mecklin, J.P., Aarnio, M. & Peltomaki, P.T. (2008). Differential cancer predisposition in Lynch syndrome: insights from molecular analysis of brain and urinary tract tumors. *Carcinogenesis,* 29, 7, (1351-1359), 1460-2180; 0143-3334

Hamilton, S.R., Liu, B., Parsons, R.E., Papadopoulos, N., Jen, J., Powell, S.M., Krush, A.J., Berk, T., Cohen, Z. & Tetu, B. (1995). The molecular basis of Turcot's syndrome. *The New England journal of medicine,* 332, 13, (839-847), 0028-4793

Hegde, M.R., Chong, B., Blazo, M.E., Chin, L.H., Ward, P.A., Chintagumpala, M.M., Kim, J.Y., Plon, S.E. & Richards, C.S. (2005). A homozygous mutation in MSH6 causes Turcot syndrome. *Clinical cancer research : an official journal of the American Association for Cancer Research,* 11, 13, (4689-4693), 1078-0432; 1078-0432

Hegi, M.E., Diserens, A.C., Gorlia, T., Hamou, M.F., de Tribolet, N., Weller, M., Kros, J.M., Hainfellner, J.A., Mason, W., Mariani, L., Bromberg, J.E., Hau, P., Mirimanoff, R.O., Cairncross, J.G., Janzer, R.C. & Stupp, R. (2005). MGMT gene silencing and benefit from temozolomide in glioblastoma. *The New England journal of medicine,* 352, 10, (997-1003), 1533-4406; 0028-4793

Hendriks, Y.M., de Jong, A.E., Morreau, H., Tops, C.M., Vasen, H.F., Wijnen, J.T., Breuning, M.H. & Brocker-Vriends, A.H. (2006). Diagnostic approach and management of Lynch syndrome (hereditary nonpolyposis colorectal carcinoma): a guide for clinicians. *CA: a cancer journal for clinicians,* 56, 4, (213-225), 0007-9235; 0007-9235

Hitchins, M.P. & Ward, R.L. (2009). Constitutional (germline) MLH1 epimutation as an aetiological mechanism for hereditary non-polyposis colorectal cancer. *Journal of medical genetics,* 46, 12, (793-802), 1468-6244; 0022-2593

Jarvinen, H.J., Renkonen-Sinisalo, L., Aktan-Collan, K., Peltomaki, P., Aaltonen, L.A. & Mecklin, J.P. (2009). Ten years after mutation testing for Lynch syndrome: cancer incidence and outcome in mutation-positive and mutation-negative family members. *Journal of clinical oncology : official journal of the American Society of Clinical Oncology,* 27, 28, (4793-4797), 1527-7755; 0732-183X

Jiricny, J. (2006). The multifaceted mismatch-repair system. *Nature reviews.Molecular cell biology,* 7, 5, (335-346), 1471-0072; 1471-0072

Knudson, A.G.,Jr. (1971). Mutation and cancer: statistical study of retinoblastoma. *Proceedings of the National Academy of Sciences of the United States of America,* 68, 4, (820-823), 0027-8424

Kuismanen, S.A., Moisio, A.L., Schweizer, P., Truninger, K., Salovaara, R., Arola, J., Butzow, R., Jiricny, J., Nystrom-Lahti, M. & Peltomaki, P. (2002). Endometrial and colorectal tumors from patients with hereditary nonpolyposis colon cancer display different patterns of microsatellite instability. *American Journal of Pathology,* 160, 6, (1953-1958), 0002-9440

Lebrun, C., Olschwang, S., Jeannin, S., Vandenbos, F., Sobol, H. & Frenay, M. (2007). Turcot syndrome confirmed with molecular analysis. *European journal of neurology : the official journal of the European Federation of Neurological Societies,* 14, 4, (470-472), 1468-1331; 1351-5101

Leung, S.Y., Yuen, S.T., Chan, T.L., Chan, A.S., Ho, J.W., Kwan, K., Fan, Y.W., Hung, K.N., Chung, L.P. & Wyllie, A.H. (2000). Chromosomal instability and p53 inactivation are required for genesis of glioblastoma but not for colorectal cancer in patients with germline mismatch repair gene mutation. *Oncogene,* 19, 35, (4079-4083), 0950-9232

Ligtenberg, M.J., Kuiper, R.P., Chan, T.L., Goossens, M., Hebeda, K.M., Voorendt, M., Lee, T.Y., Bodmer, D., Hoenselaar, E., Hendriks-Cornelissen, S.J., Tsui, W.Y., Kong, C.K., Brunner, H.G., van Kessel, A.G., Yuen, S.T., van Krieken, J.H., Leung, S.Y. & Hoogerbrugge, N. (2009). Heritable somatic methylation and inactivation of MSH2 in families with Lynch syndrome due to deletion of the 3' exons of TACSTD1. *Nature genetics,* 41, 1, (112-117), 1546-1718; 1061-4036

Lindsey, J.C., Anderton, J.A., Lusher, M.E. & Clifford, S.C. (2005). Epigenetic events in medulloblastoma development. *Neurosurgical focus,* 19, 5, (E10), 1092-0684; 1092-0684

Lynch, H.T. & de la Chapelle, A. (2003). Hereditary colorectal cancer. *The New England journal of medicine,* 348, 10, (919-932), 1533-4406

Malkin, D. (2004). Predictive genetic testing for childhood cancer: taking the road less traveled by. *Journal of pediatric hematology/oncology : official journal of the American Society of Pediatric Hematology/Oncology,* 26, 9, (546-548), 1077-4114; 1077-4114

Miyaki, M., Iijima, T., Shiba, K., Aki, T., Kita, Y., Yasuno, M., Mori, T., Kuroki, T. & Iwama, T. (2001). Alterations of repeated sequences in 5' upstream and coding regions in colorectal tumors from patients with hereditary nonpolyposis colorectal cancer and Turcot syndrome. *Oncogene,* 20, 37, (5215-5218), 0950-9232; 0950-9232

Morak, M., Schackert, H.K., Rahner, N., Betz, B., Ebert, M., Walldorf, C., Royer-Pokora, B., Schulmann, K., von Knebel-Doeberitz, M., Dietmaier, W., Keller, G., Kerker, B., Leitner, G. & Holinski-Feder, E. (2008). Further evidence for heritability of an epimutation in one of 12 cases with MLH1 promoter methylation in blood cells clinically displaying HNPCC. *European journal of human genetics : EJHG,* 16, 7, (804-811), 1018-4813

Niessen, R.C., Hofstra, R.M., Westers, H., Ligtenberg, M.J., Kooi, K., Jager, P.O., de Groote, M.L., Dijkhuizen, T., Olderode-Berends, M.J., Hollema, H., Kleibeuker, J.H. & Sijmons, R.H. (2009). Germline hypermethylation of MLH1 and EPCAM deletions are a frequent cause of Lynch syndrome. *Genes, chromosomes & cancer,* 48, 8, (737-744), 1098-2264; 1045-2257

Ollikainen, M., Hannelius, U., Lindgren, C.M., Abdel-Rahman, W.M., Kere, J. & Peltomaki, P. (2007). Mechanisms of inactivation of MLH1 in hereditary nonpolyposis colorectal carcinoma: a novel approach. *Oncogene,* 26, 31, (4541-4549), 0950-9232

Parsons, R., Li, G.M., Longley, M., Modrich, P., Liu, B., Berk, T., Hamilton, S.R., Kinzler, K.W. & Vogelstein, B. (1995). Mismatch repair deficiency in phenotypically normal human cells. *Science (New York, N.Y.),* 268, 5211, (738-740), 0036-8075; 0036-8075

Peltomaki, P. & Vasen, H. (2004). Mutations associated with HNPCC predisposition -- Update of ICG-HNPCC/INSiGHT mutation database. *Disease markers,* 20, 4-5, (269-276), 0278-0240

Peltomaki, P. (2003). Role of DNA mismatch repair defects in the pathogenesis of human cancer. *Journal of clinical oncology : official journal of the American Society of Clinical Oncology,* 21, 6, (1174-1179), 0732-183X

Peltomaki, P., Gao, X. & Mecklin, J.P. (2001). Genotype and phenotype in hereditary nonpolyposis colon cancer: a study of families with different vs. shared predisposing mutations. *Familial cancer,* 1, 1, (9-15), 1389-9600

Perucho, M. (1996). Cancer of the microsatellite mutator phenotype. *Biological chemistry,* 377, 11, (675-684), 1431-6730; 1431-6730

Poley, J.W., Wagner, A., Hoogmans, M.M., Menko, F.H., Tops, C., Kros, J.M., Reddingius, R.E., Meijers-Heijboer, H., Kuipers, E.J., Dinjens, W.N. & Rotterdam Initiative on Gastrointestinal Hereditary Tumors. (2007). Biallelic germline mutations of mismatch-repair genes: a possible cause for multiple pediatric malignancies. *Cancer,* 109, 11, (2349-2356), 0008-543X; 0008-543X

Rieber, J., Remke, M., Hartmann, C., Korshunov, A., Burkhardt, B., Sturm, D., Mechtersheimer, G., Wittmann, A., Greil, J., Blattmann, C., Witt, O., Behnisch, W., Halatsch, M.E., Orakcioglu, B., von Deimling, A., Lichter, P., Kulozik, A. & Pfister, S. (2009). Novel oncogene amplifications in tumors from a family with Li-Fraumeni syndrome. *Genes, chromosomes & cancer,* 48, 7, (558-568), 1098-2264; 1045-2257

Sciuscio, D., Diserens, A.C., van Dommelen, K., Martinet, D., Jones, G., Janzer, R.C., Pollo, C., Hamou, M.F., Kaina, B., Stupp, R., Levivier, M. & Hegi, M.E. (2011). Extent and patterns of MGMT promoter methylation in glioblastoma- and respective glioblastoma-derived spheres. Clinical cancer research : an official journal of the American Association for Cancer Research, 17, 2, (255-266), 1078-0432; 1078-0432

Seidinger, A.L., Mastellaro, M.J., Fortes, F.P., Assumpcao, J.G., Cardinalli, I.A., Ganazza, M.A., Ribeiro, R.C., Brandalise, S.R., Aguiar, S.D. & Yunes, J.A. (2010). Association of the highly prevalent TP53 R337H mutation with pediatric choroid plexus carcinoma and osteosarcoma in Southeast Brazil. *Cancer,* 0008-543X; 0008-543X

Senter, L., Clendenning, M., Sotamaa, K., Hampel, H., Green, J., Potter, J.D., Lindblom, A., Lagerstedt, K., Thibodeau, S.N., Lindor, N.M., Young, J., Winship, I., Dowty, J.G., White, D.M., Hopper, J.L., Baglietto, L., Jenkins, M.A. & de la Chapelle, A. (2008). The clinical phenotype of Lynch syndrome due to germ-line PMS2 mutations. *Gastroenterology,* 135, 2, (419-428), 1528-0012; 0016-5085

Shlien, A., Tabori, U., Marshall, C.R., Pienkowska, M., Feuk, L., Novokmet, A., Nanda, S., Druker, H., Scherer, S.W. & Malkin, D. (2008). Excessive genomic DNA copy number variation in the Li-Fraumeni cancer predisposition syndrome. *Proceedings of the National Academy of Sciences of the United States of America,* 105, 32, (11264-11269), 1091-6490; 0027-8424

Suter, C.M., Martin, D.I. & Ward, R.L. (2004). Germline epimutation of MLH1 in individuals with multiple cancers. *Nature genetics,* 36, 5, (497-501), 1061-4036

Svrcek, M., Buhard, O., Colas, C., Coulet, F., Dumont, S., Massaoudi, I., Lamri, A., Hamelin, R., Cosnes, J., Oliveira, C., Seruca, R., Gaub, M.P., Legrain, M., Collura, A., Lascols, O., Tiret, E., Flejou, J.F. & Duval, A. (2010). Methylation tolerance due to an O6-methylguanine DNA methyltransferase (MGMT) field defect in the colonic mucosa: an initiating step in the development of mismatch repair-deficient colorectal cancers. Gut, 59, 11, (1516-1526), 1468-3288; 0017-5749

Szybka, M., Bartkowiak, J., Zakrzewski, K., Polis, L., Liberski, P. & Kordek, R. (2003). Microsatellite instability and expression of DNA mismatch repair genes in malignant astrocytic tumors from adult and pediatric patients. *Clinical neuropathology,* 22, 4, (180-186), 0722-5091

Turcot, J., Despres, J.P. & St Pierre, F. (1959). Malignant tumors of the central nervous system associated with familial polyposis of the colon: report of two cases. *Diseases of the colon and rectum,* 2, (465-468), 0012-3706

Uhlmann, K., Rohde, K., Zeller, C., Szymas, J., Vogel, S., Marczinek, K., Thiel, G., Nurnberg, P. & Laird, P.W. (2003). Distinct methylation profiles of glioma subtypes. *International journal of cancer.Journal international du cancer,* 106, 1, (52-59), 0020-7136; 0020-7136

Ullrich, N.J. (2008). Inherited disorders as a risk factor and predictor of neurodevelopmental outcome in pediatric cancer. *Developmental disabilities research reviews,* 14, 3, (229-237), 1940-5529; 1940-5529

Umar, A., Boland, C.R., Terdiman, J.P., Syngal, S., de la Chapelle, A., Ruschoff, J., Fishel, R., Lindor, N.M., Burgart, L.J., Hamelin, R., Hamilton, S.R., Hiatt, R.A., Jass, J., Lindblom, A., Lynch, H.T., Peltomaki, P., Ramsey, S.D., Rodriguez-Bigas, M.A., Vasen, H.F., Hawk, E.T., Barrett, J.C., Freedman, A.N. & Srivastava, S. (2004). Revised Bethesda Guidelines for hereditary nonpolyposis colorectal cancer (Lynch syndrome) and microsatellite instability. *Journal of the National Cancer Institute,* 96, 4, (261-268), 1460-2105

van Tilborg, A.A., Morolli, B., Giphart-Gassler, M., de Vries, A., van Geenen, D.A., Lurkin, I., Kros, J.M. & Zwarthoff, E.C. (2006). Lack of genetic and epigenetic changes in meningiomas without NF2 loss. *The Journal of pathology,* 208, 4, (564-573), 0022-3417; 0022-3417

Vasen, H.F. (2005). Clinical description of the Lynch syndrome [hereditary nonpolyposis colorectal cancer (HNPCC)]. *Familial cancer,* 4, 3, (219-225), 1389-9600; 1389-9600

Vasen, H.F., Stormorken, A., Menko, F.H., Nagengast, F.M., Kleibeuker, J.H., Griffioen, G., Taal, B.G., Moller, P. & Wijnen, J.T. (2001). MSH2 mutation carriers are at higher risk of cancer than MLH1 mutation carriers: a study of hereditary nonpolyposis colorectal cancer families. *Journal of clinical oncology : official journal of the American Society of Clinical Oncology,* 19, 20, (4074-4080), 0732-183X

Vasen, H.F., Watson, P., Mecklin, J.P. & Lynch, H.T. (1999). New clinical criteria for hereditary nonpolyposis colorectal cancer (HNPCC, Lynch syndrome) proposed by the International Collaborative group on HNPCC. *Gastroenterology,* 116, 6, (1453-1456), 0016-5085

Vasen, H.F., Sanders, E.A., Taal, B.G., Nagengast, F.M., Griffioen, G., Menko, F.H., Kleibeuker, J.H., Houwing-Duistermaat, J.J. & Meera Khan, P. (1996). The risk of brain tumours in hereditary non-polyposis colorectal cancer (HNPCC). *International journal of cancer.Journal international du cancer,* 65, 4, (422-425), 0020-7136

Vasen, H.F., Mecklin, J.P., Khan, P.M. & Lynch, H.T. (1991). The International Collaborative Group on Hereditary Non-Polyposis Colorectal Cancer (ICG-HNPCC). *Diseases of the colon and rectum,* 34, 5, (424-425), 0012-3706

Viana-Pereira, M., Almeida, I., Sousa, S., Mahler-Araujo, B., Seruca, R., Pimentel, J. & Reis, R.M. (2009). Analysis of microsatellite instability in medulloblastoma. *Neuro-oncology,* 11, 5, (458-467), 1522-8517; 1522-8517

Vladimirova, V., Denkhaus, D., Soerensen, N., Wagner, S., Wolff, J.E. & Pietsch, T. (2008). Low level of microsatellite instability in paediatric malignant astrocytomas. *Neuropathology and applied neurobiology,* 34, 5, (547-554), 1365-2990; 0305-1846

Wagner, A., Barrows, A., Wijnen, J., van der Klift, H., Franken, P., Verkuijlen, P.,Nakagawa, H., Geugien, M., Jaghmohan-Changur, S., Breukel, C., Meijers-Heijboer, H., Morreau, H., van Puijenbroek, M., Burn, J., Coronel, S., Kinarski, Y., Okimoto, R., Watson, P., Lynch, J., de la Chapelle, A., Henry Lynch, H., Fodde, R. (2003). Molecular analysis of Hereditary non-polyposis colorectal cancer (HNPCC) in the USA: High mutation detection rate among clinically selected families and characterization of an American founder genomic deletion of the MSH2 gene. *Familial cancer,* 2, Suppl. 1, (19), 1389-9600

Wang, Q., Montmain, G., Ruano, E., Upadhyaya, M., Dudley, S., Liskay, R.M., Thibodeau, S.N. & Puisieux, A. (2003). Neurofibromatosis type 1 gene as a mutational target in a mismatch repair-deficient cell type. *Human genetics,* 112, 2, (117-123), 0340-6717; 0340-6717

Watson, P. & Lynch, H.T. (2001). Cancer risk in mismatch repair gene mutation carriers. *Familial cancer,* 1, 1, (57-60), 1389-9600

Wimmer, K. & Etzler, J. (2008). Constitutional mismatch repair-deficiency syndrome: have we so far seen only the tip of an iceberg? *Human genetics,* 124, 2, (105-122), 1432-1203; 0340-6717

Woods, M.O., Williams, P., Careen, A., Edwards, L., Bartlett, S., McLaughlin, J.R. & Younghusband, H.B. (2007). A new variant database for mismatch repair genes associated with Lynch syndrome. *Human mutation,* 28, 7, (669-673), 1098-1004

Wooster, R., Cleton-Jansen, A.M., Collins, N., Mangion, J., Cornelis, R.S., Cooper, C.S., Gusterson, B.A., Ponder, B.A., von Deimling, A. & Wiestler, O.D. (1994). Instability of short tandem repeats (microsatellites) in human cancers. *Nature genetics,* 6, 2, (152-156), 1061-4036

Yip, S., Miao, J., Cahill, D.P., Iafrate, A.J., Aldape, K., Nutt, C.L. & Louis, D.N. (2009). MSH6 mutations arise in glioblastomas during temozolomide therapy and mediate temozolomide resistance. *Clinical cancer research : an official journal of the American Association for Cancer Research,* 15, 14, (4622-4629), 1078-0432; 1078-0432

Yu, J., Zhang, H., Gu, J., Lin, S., Li, J., Lu, W., Wang, Y. & Zhu, J. (2004). Methylation profiles of thirty four promoter-CpG islands and concordant methylation behaviours of sixteen genes that may contribute to carcinogenesis of astrocytoma. *BMC cancer,* 4, (65), 1471-2407; 1471-2407

16

Primary Central Nervous System Lymphoma

Iyavut Thaipisuttikul and Craig Nolan
Memorial Sloan-Kettering Cancer Center
United States

1. Introduction

Primary central nervous system lymphoma (PCNSL) is characterized by extranodal malignant lymphomas arising in the brain, spinal cord, CSF, and eyes in the absence of lymphoma outside the nervous system at the time of diagnosis (Deckert & Paulus, 2007). By definition, this excludes CNS involvement of systemic lymphomas and angiotropic lymphomas (Schlegel et al., 2000). The incidence of PCNSL in the United States was noted to be increasing in immunocompetent, immunosuppressed, and immunodeficient individuals over the past several decades (Schabet, 1999) with more than six-fold increase from 1973 to 1997, while the incidence of non-Hodgkin lymphoma (NHL) increased 81% during the same period (Olson et al., 2002). However, this increase in incidence seems to be leveling off in the past decade. According to the most recent Central Brain Tumor Registry Statistical Report (February 2011), PCNSL occurs at an annual incidence of 0.46 cases per 100,000 person-years in the United States during 2004-2007. PCNSL accounted for 2.4% of all primary brain tumors in the United States. There is a slight male predominance with a male-to-female ratio of 1.38. The peak incidence is between age 75 and 84. The median age in most studies is 55-65. The age at diagnosis in AIDS patients is much younger with mean age reported in the fourth decade (Deckert & Paulus, 2007; Fine et al., 1993).

2. Pathology

2.1 Histological classification

There is no generally accepted histologic classification system for PCNSL. Although the CNS in humans is devoid of B-cell and germinal center structure, more than 90% of PCNSLs are diffuse large B-cell non-Hodgkin lymphomas, while T-cell antigens are usually restricted to small reactive lymphocytes (Paulus, 1999). Primary T-cell lymphomas of the CNS, Burkitt lymphomas and other lymphoma types are rare. Although PCNSL is not specifically included in the current Revised European-American Lymphoma (REAL) classification (Harris et al., 1994), the most recent WHO Classification of Tumors of Hematopoietic and Lymphoid Tissues (2008) classified PNCSL as a separate entity under "Aggressive lymphoma/leukemia" (Jaffe, 2009).

2.2 Basic pathology features

Supratentorial locations are more common (87%) and lesions usually are located in periventricular areas involving the thalamus, basal ganglia, and corpus callosum (Bataille et al., 2000). The demarcation of the lesions from the surrounding brain is variable and this can make it resemble glioma due to diffuse borders. Necrotic areas are seen in AIDS patients (Bhagavathi & Wilson, 2008). The cells of primary diffuse large B-cell lymphoma (DLBCL) arising in the brain are morphologically similar to systemic forms. Perivascular cuffs of malignant and reactive lymphocytes are commonly seen around the larger blood vessels. They are seldom found around vessels less than 8 µm in diameter and are not present around small capillaries with a diameter less than 4 µm. This feature, however, is not specific for PCNSL but can also be seen in metastatic lymphoma to CNS (Aho et al., 1993).

2.3 Immunohistochemical profile and gene expression

Recently, three molecularly distinct forms of systemic DLBCL in immunocompetent patients were identified as germinal center B-cell-like (GCB), the activated B-cell-like (ABC) and the so-called type III (Rosenwald et al., 2002). This classification is based on immunohistochemical markers: CD10 for early germinal center, BCL-6 (which is a zinc-finger transcriptional repressor required for the formation of the GC) for early and late germinal center, MUM1 for germinal center/ early post-germinal center and CD138 for post-germinal center. Initial studies found PCNSL to be of GCB origin based on BCL-6 expression (Larocca et al., 1998) and ongoing mutational activity (Thompsett et al., 1999). BCL-6 gene mutations and BCL-6 protein expression have been reported in 50% and 100% of PCNSL, respectively. More recent studies found that most PNCL cases expressed both BCL-6 and MUM1 but lacked CD10 and CD138 which suggested late germinal center/early post-germinal center stage of differentiation (Braaten et al., 2003; Camilleri-Broet et al., 2006). Although BCL-6 expression is associated with a favorable prognosis in systemic DLBCL, its prognostic significance is less clear in PCNSL with studies showing favorable prognosis (Braaten et al., 2003; Song et al., 2011), poor prognosis (Chang et al., 2003) and no impact on outcome (Camilleri-Broet et al., 2006). The fact that PCNSL has poorer prognosis compared with systemic DLBCL and its high-grade nature may contribute to this finding. Recent studies aiming to find a "CNS signature" by comparing molecular features of PNCSL with nodal large B-cell NHL found different expression in several genes (Rubenstein et al., 2006; Tun et al., 2008). Interleukin-4 (IL-4) was found to be highly expressed by tumor vasculature as well as by tumor cells in CNS lymphomas. Moreover, expression of activated form of STAT6, a mediator of IL-4 signaling, was also found in PCNSL and was associated with short survival in patients treated with a high-dose intravenous methotrexate-containing regimen (Rubenstein et al., 2006).

3. Pathogenesis

The most important risk factor for PCNSL is immunodeficiency, whether inherited or acquired, which includes Wiskott-Aldrich syndrome, AIDS, immunosuppressive therapy following organ transplantation and other immunosuppression for cancer and autoimmune treatments. Evidence of EBV genome is present in more than 95% of AIDS-related PCNSL which suggests its major role in lymphoma pathogenesis in this group. It was hypothesized that EBV infection leads to polyclonal B-cell activation in the context of aberrant B-cell regulation and that the inherent genetic instability of the EBV-infected and immortalized B-cells eventually leads to MYC gene rearrangement and the development of malignant lymphoma (Knowles, 2003). However, the etiology of PCNSL in immunocompetent patients is still unclear. Three hypotheses have been proposed to explain how lymphomas arise and grow primarily in the CNS:

1. B-cells may be transformed outside the CNS and then develop adhesion molecules specific for CNS tropism (Deckert & Paulus, 2007). The expression of BCL-6 found in most patients suggests that PCNSL has been exposed to a germinal center microenvironment outside the CNS. Recently, some specific genes are thought to be involved in CNS tropism of PNCSL. SPP1, a member of the extracellular matrix (ECM)-related genes associated with various aspects of cancer biology, and DDR1, a member of a family of receptor tyrosine kinases involved in cell adhesion in several brain tumors, were found to be up-regulated in PCNSL (Tun et al., 2008). In one study, lymphoma cells from a PCNSL patient were implanted subcutaneously in an athymic mouse. At 16 weeks, the lymphoma cells were shown to home to CNS blood vessels through autopsy while there was no evidence of lymphoma cells at any sites including the subcutaneous implantation site (Jiang et al., 2010). This study supports the theory of highly selective tropism of PCNSL.
2. Systemic lymphoma cells may be eradicated by an intact immune system. The B-cell–activating factor of the TNF family (BAFF), produced locally by astrocytes, together with the shielding of the brain from the immune system, might provide a safe environment for PCNSL while systemic lymphoma cells outside CNS are not protected (Krumbholz et al., 2005).
3. Polyclonal inflammatory cells in the brain may transform to monoclonal PNCSL. This theory is supported by occasional reports of "sentinel lesions" which are biopsy-proven demyelinating or non-neoplastic lesions but ultimately lead to PCNSL months to years later (Alderson et al., 1996; Ng et al., 2007; Yang & Wu., 2007; Habek et al., 2008). However, infectious or inflammatory CNS diseases are rarely reported preceding PCNSL (Deckert & Paulus, 2007).

4. Clinical features

Most patients present with neurological symptoms and signs rather than systemic "B" symptoms (Batchelor et al., 2006). Neurological symptoms depend primarily on the location of the tumor and the rapidity of tumor progression with cerebral symptoms being most common followed by ocular, leptomeningeal and spinal cord. In the largest retrospective analysis of 248 immunocompetent patients with PCNSL, the most common type of clinical signs on admission was focal neurological deficit (70%). Neuropsychiatric symptoms (43%), increased intracranial pressure (33%), seizures (14%) and vitreous involvement (4%) were noted. In 7% of patients, neurological signs were preceded by systemic manifestations such as gastrointestinal symptoms or febrile respiratory illnesses (Bataille et al., 2000).

5. Neuroimaging

Recognizing the radiographic features of PCNSL is crucial as corticosteroids should not be used before biopsy and unnecessary surgical resection can be avoided. PCNSL lesions are typically isodense to hyperdense on CT scan and isointense to hypointense on T2-weighted MRI. Highly packed abnormal cells are thought to be responsible for the increased attenuation. Internal calcification is unusual in CNS lymphomas unless the patient has undergone prior chemotherapy or radiation treatment (Erdag et al., 2001). The enhancement pattern is usually homogeneous. Ring-like enhancement is rare in immunocompetent patients but commonly seen in immunodeficient patients. In the largest MRI series of 100 immunocompetent patients with PCNSL, a single lesion was seen in 65% and multiple lesions were seen in 35%. Lesions are located in a cerebral hemisphere (38%), deep gray matter (16%), corpus callosum (14%), ventricle wall and choroid plexus (12%), and cerebellum (9%). The contrast enhancement of the cerebral or spinal lesions was rated as strong in 85%and moderate in 10%. Absence of enhancement was seen in 1% (Kuker et al., 2005). Restricted diffusion of protons, although rare, has been reported and might be useful in non-enhancing PCNSL patients (Barajas et al., 2010; Fischer et al., 2010; Zacharia et al., 2008). A more recent study of MRI findings in 26 patients with PCNSL reported findings of open-ring enhancement in 2 patients. The open-ring enhancement is considered highly specific for brain demyelination, but it was noted that the ring is thick and not uniform in PCNSL compared with a thin and uniform open-ring pattern in brain demyelination. A newly described "notch sign", which is an abnormally deep depression at the tumor margin, was found in 3 patients (Zhang et al., 2010). The sensitivity and specificity of these findings need further validation.

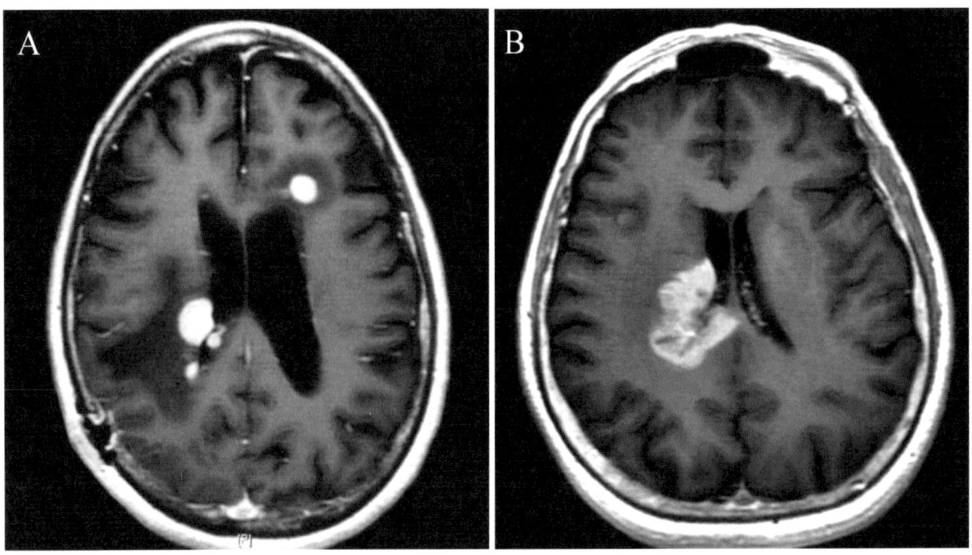

a. Typical MRI appearance of PCNSL shows homogeneous enhancement. Stereotactic biopsy confirmed PCNSL

b. Patient with suspected PCNSL. Pathology showed glioblastoma.

Fig. 1. MRI of patients with suspected PCNSL

6. Diagnostic evaluation

In 2005, the International PCNSL Collaborative Group (IPCG) published a guideline to standardize baseline evaluation, response criteria and outcome measures for patients enrolled onto clinical trials for PCNSL (Abrey et al., 2005). The recommendation has increasingly become accepted as a standard baseline evaluation for all immunocompetent patients with suspected PCNSL.

6.1 Pathologic evaluation

Histopathology is mandatory because other intracranial processes may also have similar appearance on imaging and transient response to corticosteroids (Zaki et al., 2004). A stereotactic needle biopsy is the procedure of choice due its low risk and no survival benefit of surgical resection. However, the diagnosis can also be established by positive CSF cytology or a vitrectomy specimen. Establishing immunophenotype characteristics of the tumors is recommended as the information may be useful for future development and application of targeted therapies. Corticosteroids significantly increase false negative biopsy results and should not be given to any patients suspected of having PCNSL before biopsy. Osmotic agents should be the first choice if patients need urgent treatment for increased intracranial pressure (Weller, 1999). Recently, CSF biomarkers of PCNSL such as MicroRNAs (Baraniskin et al., 2011) and antithrombin III (Roy et al., 2008), were discovered in order to facilitate early and noninvasive diagnosis. Further investigations are needed to validate the use of these biomarkers in clinical practice.

6.2 Clinical evaluation

A complete physical and neurologic examination should be recorded. Special attention should be given to peripheral lymph nodes, the liver and spleen. Testicular examination should be performed in older men as testicular lymphoma is the most common lymphoma in men over age sixty and has a higher risk of CNS metastasis (Hill & Owen, 2006). Age and performance status are widely used in prognostic models for PCNSL and should be recorded in every patient. Baseline cognitive function should be evaluated by using the Mini-Mental Status Examination (MMSE) as treatment-related neurocognitive complications are common.

6.3 Laboratory evaluation

In addition to routine hematologic function, hepatic and renal functions are important to ensure the safety of using high-dose methotrexate. The level of creatinine clearance above 50 to 60 mL/min is adequate. Serum LDH was found to be one of the prognostic variables. HIV infection should be tested in every patient with PCNSL.

6.4 Extent-of-disease evaluation

Choice of therapy depends on the extent of lesions. This should include evaluation of CNS, body and bone marrow. Gadolinium-enhanced MRI of the brain is recommended unless there is a contraindication; contrast-enhanced CT scan can be used. CSF examination with documented opening pressure should be performed in every patient unless contraindicated. CSF should be collected before surgical biopsy or 1 week after to avoid a false positive result. A minimum of 3 mL and ideally 10 mL should be sent for cytology. CSF total protein is mandatory as an important prognostic factor. CSF obtained from ventricles via Ommaya reservoir usually shows a much lower total protein level than CSF from lumbar puncture and the result should be interpreted with caution. The following studies are optional: cell count, beta2-microglobulin, immunoglobulin H gene rearrangement, and flow cytometry. Although cytopathology is a gold standard, flow cytometry was recently found to have better sensitivity and specificity in detection of leptomeningeal involvement in PCNSL and systemic lymphoma (Hegde et al., 2005; Schroers et al., 2010). Gadolinium-enhanced MRI of the spinal cord is required for those who have symptoms or signs of spinal cord involvement. A detailed ophthalmologic work up with slit-lamp examination should be performed to exclude vitreous, retinal, or optic nerve involvement. CT scan of the chest, abdomen, and pelvis and bone marrow biopsy with aspirate are minimum staging procedures. Body positron emission tomography (PET) imaging is commonly used as an additional tool for staging of PCNSL and a recent study showed that 18F-Fluorodeoxyglucose (FDG) PET may be more sensitive than conventional body staging (Mohile et al., 2008). Some patients in this study were found to have FDG-avid foci outside the thoracic, abdominal, and pelvic cavities, underscoring a major limitation of the conventional scan. Testicular ultrasound should be performed to rule out testicular lymphoma in older men.

7. Prognosis and prognostic factors

Overall, PCNSL carries a worse prognosis compared with non-CNS extranodal DLBCL. With supportive care alone, the averaged survival is 3.3 months from diagnosis (Henry et al., 1974). With active chemotherapy/radiotherapy treatment, median survival up to 51 months has been reported (Gavrilovic et al., 2006). Prognosis of AIDS-related PCNSL is particularly poor with the median survival of untreated patients measured in weeks (Kasamon et al., 2005). Attempts to prognosticate individual patients have been focused on a clinical scoring system and phenotypic/genetic features. As mentioned above, BCL-6 expression is associated with a favorable prognosis in systemic DLBCL but its role as a prognostic marker in PCNSL will need further validation. In addition, STAT6 and co-expression of p53 and c-Myc may correlate with poor survival outcome (Camilleri-Broet et al., 2006; Chang et al., 2003). Three clinical prognostic scoring systems have been proposed.

The Memorial Sloan-Kettering Cancer Center (MSKCC) prognostic score, published in 2006, uses age and Karnofsky performance score (KPS) to identify patients into 3 classes; Class 1: age ≤ 50, Class 2: age >50 and KPS ≥70, and Class 3: age >50 and KPS <70. Based on MSKCC and RTOG data set, a median overall survival (OS) was 5-8 years, 2-3 years and 1 year or less for class 1, 2, and 3, respectively. This system was developed from retrospective analysis of data from 282 patients and was validated using an external data set of 152 patients treated on RTOG PCNSL trials. This system has the advantage of simplicity and widespread applicability. Its limitation is the possible selection bias from using data from a single institution (Abrey et al., 2006).

The International Extranodal Lymphoma Study Group (IELSG), published in 2003, uses a 5-point scoring system which consists of age > 60, Eastern Cooperative Oncology Group (ECOG) performance status >1, elevated serum lactate dehydrogenase (LDH) level, elevated CSF total protein (>45 mg/dL if <60 years old, >60 mg/dL if >60 years old), and involvement of deep brain structures. This score was developed from a retrospective analysis of data from 48 treating centers which identified 105 patients who had complete data from a total cohort of 378 patients. This system identifies patients into three risk groups based on a number of unfavorable features; 0-1, 2-3 and 4-5. A 2-year OS was 80%, 48%, and 15% for patients with scores of 0-1, 2-3 and 4-5, respectively. Its limitation is that less than one-third of the total cohort had complete data. This emphasizes the complexity of the system; the median follow-up was relatively short, only 24 months (Ferreri et al., 2003).

The four point Nottingham/Barcelona score, published in 2004, uses a prediction score giving 1 point for each adverse prognostic factor; age ≥ 60, performance status ≥ 2, and multifocal and/or meningeal disease (advanced stage). This scoring system was derived from 77 consecutive patients treated on one of two clinical trials. A median survival of 55 months, 41 months, 32 months and 1 month was associated with a score of 0, 1, 2 and 3, respectively. Its limitation is a small number of patients included in this score. It also failed to discriminate prognosis for those patients who fell into the two middle categories and was only significant for differentiating the patients with the best and worst prognostic factors (Bessell et al., 2004).

8. Follow-up assessment and response criteria

In addition to clinical evaluation, a follow-up gadolinium-enhanced MRI scan every two months or at the time of treatment change is recommended. A detailed ophthalmologic examination and CSF cytology are required only if the initial studies are positive or clinically indicated.

The IPCG response criteria (Abrey et al., 2005), proposed in 2005, identifies patients based on their response to therapy as follow:

Complete response (CR): This requires complete disappearance of all enhancing abnormalities on gadolinium-enhanced MRI while the patients have not been on corticosteroid treatment for at least 2 weeks. Negative CSF cytology and/or negative ophthalmologic examination are required if these studies were initially positive.

Unconfirmed complete response (Cru): This includes patients who meet the CR criteria but are currently on corticosteroids which may decrease the enhancement seen on MRI as well as patients who continue to have persistent minor abnormalities on MRI or ophthalmologic examination which are not consistent with tumor infiltration.

Partial response (PR): This includes patients who have >50% decrease in the contrast-enhancing lesion seen on MRI as compared with baseline imaging while corticosteroid treatment does not affect the determination of response. Ophthalmologic examination should show a decrease in the vitreous cell count or retinal/optic nerve cellular infiltrate but may continue to show persistent malignant or suspicious cells. CSF examination may be negative or continue to show persistent malignant or suspicious cells.

Stable disease: This is defined as less than a PR but is not progressive disease.

Progressive disease: This includes patients who have >25% increase in the contrast-enhancing lesion seen on MRI as compared with baseline, or develop any new site of disease, or have an increase in the vitreous cell count or retinal/optic nerve cellular infiltrate.

Relapse disease: Patients with prior CR or CRu who develop any new site of disease will qualify for relapsed disease.

9. Therapy of newly diagnosed PCNSL

In contrast to other CNS metastases, PCNSL cells spread diffusely into the CNS parenchyma (Aho et al., 1993). Thus, therapies targeted to the tumor site alone are never curative. For this reason, surgical resection has no survival benefit. Corticosteroids, systemic chemotherapy and whole-brain radiation therapy (WBRT) are the mainstay of PCNSL therapy. Involvement of organs outside of the CNS is very rare, making systemic prophylaxis a less important consideration. The eye, however, is an important site for tumor spread at presentation and relapse. Dedicated therapy to the orbits is required since most chemotherapeutic agents do not achieve cytotoxic concentrations within the eye and standard whole-brain radiation fields do not involve the orbits.

9.1 Corticosteroids

The effects of corticosteroids in PCNSL are not solely mediated by a reduction of cerebral edema but also involve cytotoxic activity. Corticosteroids trigger the apoptosis cascade and an oncolytic response in malignant lymphocytes via the endogenous steroid receptor. The initial response rate up to 40% has been reported with 15% complete remission and 25% partial remissions (DeAngelis et al., 1990). Relapse after the initial corticosteroid-responsive period is common. The mechanism which underlies corticosteroid resistance during chronic treatment and the withdrawal period is still poorly understood. Long-term use of corticosteroids should be avoided to minimize their secondary complications.

9.2 Radiation therapy

Historically, conventional treatment of PCNSL had been WBRT and corticosteroids up until the use of effective chemotherapy over the past 20 years. The concerning issues of radiation therapy are its short-lived benefit and delayed neurotoxicity. The role of WBRT as the only mainstay of treatment was established in the prospective trial of cranial irradiation alone, Radiation Therapy Oncology Group (RTOG) 83-15, which was published in 1992. This trial demonstrated a dramatic CT scan response to WBRT with CR in 62% and partial CR in 19% of patients. However, this finding did not translate into improved long-term control or survival with a median survival of only 12 to 18 months and a 5-year survival rate of less than 5%in the trial (Nelson et al., 1992). A secondary analysis of this trial along with another RTOG trial showed that RT dose escalation by incorporating a boost to areas of bulky disease did not improve disease control or survival (Corn et al., 2000). Since then, WBRT has been incorporated into various chemotherapy regimens during consolidation after induction with methotrexate (MTX) alone or with other chemotherapeutic drugs. The optimal dose of WBRT in the setting of combined-modality treatment of PCNSL is not established.. The usual dose used in combined-modality therapy trials is 4000-4500 cGy. The combined-modality approaches followed by WBRT is associated with a 2-year OS of 43% to 73% (Ferreri et al., 2003). However, treatment-related toxicity was reported in 25%-49% of patients (Gavrilovic et al., 2006; Omuro et al., 2005; Thiel et al., 2010). Neurotoxicity is especially common in patients older than 60. For this reason, two strategies have been proposed to decrease the risk of neurotoxicity.

One strategy is to defer WBRT in patients who achieve a complete response with initial chemotherapy and are older than 50-60 years old. The major concern with this approach is that eliminating the use of whole-brain radiotherapy could compromise disease control. This strategy is supported by the findings from 2 large retrospective analyses which showed that the addition of WBRT to combination chemotherapy did not improve survival in patients treated with high-dose methotrexate (MTX), but was associated with improvements in long-term disease control (Ekenel et al., 2008; Ferreri et al., 2002). Recently, a large prospective randomized phase 3 trial, aiming to address this issue, was published in 2010 (Thiel et al., 2010). This trial randomized 551 patients to receive six cycles of MTX--based chemotherapy alone versus MTX-based chemotherapy with consolidation WBRT (4500 cGy), but only 318 patients treated per protocol were included in the primary analysis of noninferiority. The primary end point was noninferiority comparison of OS and the planned secondary end point was progression-free survival (PFS). There was no significant difference in OS between the two groups, but analysis of PFS suggested a trend for improved disease control in patients assigned to WBRT. There are many issues which interfere with the interpretation of this trial such as high number of protocol violations and the fact that this study failed to meet the predetermined criteria for noninferiority; thus, drawing any conclusions should not be appropriate for a noninferiority trial. Despite absence of flawless evidence, many experts agree that patients who have a CR and are older than 50-60 years, should not receive WBRT because data suggest that any improvement in outcome is outweighed by the consequences of neurotoxicity (Abrey, 2011; Deangelis, 2011). Whether WBRT in the setting of combined-modality therapy is safe in younger patients, and the risk-benefit balance between chances of cure versus long-term toxicity, have to be further studied.

The other strategy is to use reduced-dose WBRT. This strategy was first explored in a subset of patients in the RTOG 93-10 trial which studied combined-modality therapy with full dose WBRT (4500 cGy). In this subset, patients who achieved a CR after induction chemotherapy were treated with a hyperfractionated regimen of 3600 cGy delivered at 1200 cGy twice a day. There was no statistical difference in PFS and OS for this group despite the dose reduction. However, this regimen also did not eliminate the development of severe neurotoxicity (Fisher et al., 2005). The Nottingham and Barcelona group reported that young patients who received a low total dose (3060 cGy) of WBRT after achieving a CR had a significantly higher risk of relapse and shorter OS than patients who received standard (4500 cGy) radiotherapy (Bessell et al., 2002). In contrast to previous findings, a trial using a reduced-dose WBRT of 2340 cGy in 17 patients who achieved a CR following combined immunochemotherapy showed that reduced-dose WBRT did not compromise disease control and was not associated with neurocognitive decline (Shah et al., 2007). The strategy of using reduced-dose WBRT will need to be further studied in a large prospective multicenter trial.

9.3 Chemotherapy

Due to the poor outcome from WBRT alone, the use of chemotherapy for newly diagnosed PCNSL, either alone or as induction before WBRT, is widely accepted. The commonly used regimen for treatment of systemic NHL is the four-drug combination of cyclophosphamide, doxorubicin, vincristine, and prednisone (CHOP). Although CHOP can induce an initial response in PCNSL, the responses were not durable and relapses occurred rapidly. Inability to cross the blood-brain barrier (BBB) is the main limitation of most chemotherapy drugs. There is no doubt that MTX at a higher dose than that used for NHL is the most active single agent against PCNSL. Its efficacy has been confirmed in several phase 2 trials. However, controversies have involved the dosing strategy of MTX, the choice between MTX monotherapy and MTX-based multi-drug regimens, what multi-drug chemotherapy regimens should be used and the use of intrathecal/intraventricular chemotherapy. An alternative method of MTX delivery is BBB disruption (BBBD) in conjunction with intra-arterial (IA) MTX. This approach, in combination with intravenous etoposide and cyclophosphamide, was evaluated in the pooled analysis of 149 newly diagnosed PCNSL patients. The overall response rate (ORR) was 81.9% and median OS was 3.1 years. Although this approach gives a comparable result to conventional intravenous high-dose MTX, it requires an experienced team and invasive procedures (Angelov et al., 2009).

9.3.1 MTX dosing strategy

Three different doses have been studied in the clinical trials assessing activity of single-agent high-dose MTX: MTX 8 g/m^2 every 2 weeks deferring WBRT until failure (Batchelor et al., 2003; Herrlinger et al., 2005); MTX 3.5 g/m^2 every 3 weeks followed by WBRT(Glass et al., 1994; Ferreri et al., 2009); and MTX 1 g/m^2 immediately before WBRT(Abrey et al., 1998;

O'Brien et al., 2006). The dose of 8 g/m^2 yielded an apparently different ORR in Europe compared to the United States (51% for the German trial and 68% for the American trial). It should be noted that dose reduction due to impaired creatinine clearance was indicated in 45% of patients in the trials using the dose of 8 g/m^2, whereas in the 3.5 g/m^2 trials only a few patients needed a reduction in MTX dose. Both 8 g/m^2 trials and 3.5 g/m^2 trials resulted in a comparable 3-year OS rate of 30%-45%. The response rate has not been assessed in trials using MTX 1 g/m^2 but a reported 3-year OS rate was 45%-50%.

It was suggested in one study that a dose of MTX of 3 g/m^2 is considered the lowest dose to obtain the minimum CSF-steady-state concentration of MTX required to treat acute lymphocytic leukemia (>5 X 10^{-7} mol/L) (Lippens & Winograd, 1988). This study also showed that the MTX concentration in the CSF cannot be predicted by determining the plasma concentration. The rate of infusion also plays a major role in delivering MTX through the BBB. Rapid infusion of 3 g/m^2 of MTX over 3 h will consistently achieve therapeutic concentrations in the CSF, whereas this concentration is not reliably obtained with a 24-h continuous infusion of 8 g/m^2 (Vassal et al., 1990; Tetef et al., 2000). Currently, there is no clear evidence of difference in outcome of various doses of MTX above 3 g/m^2. In the absence of intrathecal treatment, the available data lend support to a recommendation for a MTX dose of at least 3 g/m^2 given over 3 h in all patients (Morris & Abrey, 2009).

9.3.2 MTX monotherapy versus MTX-based multi-drug regimens

The efficacy of single agent MTX and multi-drug MTX-based regimens (with or without WBRT) has been proven in several phase 2 trials. Recently, a prospective randomized multi-center phase 2 trial with a primary end point of CR, studied the use of four cycles of MTX (3.5 g/m^2) alone or in combination with cytarabine (2 g/m^2 every 12 h on days 2 and 3 of each cycle) followed by WBRT. Despite the expected increase in the toxicity, the combination arm was associated with an increased complete remission rate from 18% to 46%. The estimated 3-year failure-free survival was 21% following MTX alone and 38% following combined treatment. The estimated 3-year OS was 32% following MTX alone and 46% following combined treatment. This trial clearly showed the advantage to multi-drug MTX-based regimens over single agent MTX (Ferreri et al., 2009).

9.3.3 What multi-drug chemotherapy regimens should be used?

A combination of MTX, procarbazine and vincristine (MPV), given in 5 cycles followed by consolidation cytarabine (with or without WBRT), has been proposed based on their different mechanisms of action and different toxicity profiles. Although vincristine usually does not cross the BBB it may be able to reach the tumor where the BBB is disrupted. Procarbazine is an oral lipophilic alkylating drug that can cross the normal BBB. This regimen was studied in the RTOG 93-10 trial along with intraventricular MTX, WBRT and two cycles of cytarabine with a median OS of 37 months. The 2-year OS was 64% and 5-year OS was 32%(DeAngelis et al., 2002). Another study used this regimen along with Rituximab, a monoclonal antibody that targets the CD20 antigen, and WBRT, showed a 2-year OS of 67%. The ORR was 93% (Shah et al., 2007).

A combination of MTX and cytarabine was proposed and its efficacy established in a recent trial (Ferreri et al., 2009). The rationale of using cytarabine after MTX is the continuance of the exposure of proliferating cells to S-phase cytostatics and the increase of cytarabine cytidine triphosphate formation and DNA incorporation, with a consequent increased cytotoxicity (Carrabba et al., 2010).

A regimen consisting of MTX, teniposide, carmustine and methylprednisolone plus intrathecal chemotherapy and subsequent WBRT was used in the European Organization for Research and Treatment of Cancer (EORTC) Lymphoma Group phase II trial 20962. A 2-year OS was 69% and 3-year OS was 58%. It should be noted that 10% of patients died, probably because of infectious complications (Poortmans et al., 2003).
The MATILDE regimen consists of MTX, cytarabine, idarubicin and thiotepa. This regimen followed by WBRT resulted in an ORR of 83% and a 5-year OS of 41%(Ferreri et al., 2006).
A combination of MTX and temozolomide without radiotherapy or intrathecal chemotherapy was evaluated in one study of 23 elderly (age >60) patients. This regimen resulted in a favorable toxicity profile and comparable results to other regimens with a CR in 55% and a median OS of 35 months (Omuro et al., 2007).

9.3.4 Intrathecal / Intraventricular chemotherapy

The benefit of routine use of intrathecal MTX (12 mg x 5 doses, alternating with high-dose MTX) in newly diagnosed PCNSL patients was evaluated in a case-controlled retrospective study. Patients who already received high-dose MTX ($\geq$ 3.5 g/m^2) did not benefit from additional intrathecal/intraventricular MTX treatment (Khan et al., 2002). Another large multicenter retrospective study of 370 patients also failed to demonstrate any survival benefit of adjunct intrathecal MTX to a conventional high-dose MTX-based regimen (Ferreri et al., 2002). Currently, there is no evidence to support the routine use if intrathecal MTX in patients who receive high-dose MTX and have negative CSF cytology. Despite lack of information supporting this approach, intrathecal chemotherapy is being used in clinical practice as a supplement to systemic chemotherapy but restricted to patients who have positive CSF or receive MTX less than 3 g/m^2 (Morris & Abrey, 2009).

9.4 Immunotherapy

The survival benefit of adding rituximab to the standard treatment of systemic NHL has been established (Coiffier et al., 2010). Although rituximab has been incorporated into some treatment regimens for PCNSL (Shah et al., 2007), the benefit of using this approach is unclear. Recently, the largest series of patients with PCNSL treated with IV rituximab monotherapy has been published. Twelve patients were enrolled in the series. Confirmed radiographic responses were seen in 36% of patients (3 CR, 1 PR) (Batchelor et al., 2011). The benefit of rituximab in PCNSL, optimal dose, and treatment schedule will need to be further studied in larger multi-center trials.

9.5 High-dose chemotherapy with stem-cell transplant

High-dose chemotherapy supported by autologous stem cells transplant (HDC/ASCT) has been used as salvage therapy in patients who fail conventional chemo-radiotherapy or as upfront during consolidation phase. The strategy is to increase drug delivery through the BBB with high-dose chemotherapy which may eliminate the need for WBRT. The combinations used in the treatment of PCNSL can be carmustine, etoposide, cytarabine, and melphalan (BEAM) or thiotepa-based conditioning regimens. Two recent Phase II multi-institutional trials have established its feasibility. The OSHO-53 phase II study trial studied 16 patients (out of 23) who achieved CR/PR after induction chemotherapy and were treated with high-dose busulfan and thiotepa with ASCT followed by response-adapted WBRT. In the transplanted group, estimated 2-year EFS and OS were 56% and 61%, respectively

(Montemurro et al., 2007). The multicenter phase II study of the GOELAMS group studied 17 patients (out of 25) who responded to initial chemotherapy and were treated with a BEAM regimen with ASCT followed by WBRT. One patient died. With a median follow-up of 34 months, 16 patients were in CR at the time of the analysis (Colombat et al., 2006). Direct comparison between trials is difficult, but thiotepa-based regimens seem to be associated with better results than BEAM-based regimens. It should be noted that 3 patients in the OSHO trial and all patients in the GOELAMS trial still required WBRT after HDC/ASCT. These results, although encouraging, should be interpreted with caution because of the possibility of selection biases in which patients in these trials tended to be younger than patients in other studies and all chemotherapy resistant patients were excluded.

10. Salvage therapy for relapse and refractory PCNSL

Relapse after initial therapy has been reported in 30%-60% of patients (Gavrilovic et al., 2006; Glass et al., 1994). Approximately10%-15% of immunocompetent patients have primary refractory PCNSL (Reni et al., 2001). Prognosis for patients with relapsed PCNSL is poor, with a median survival of approximately 4.5 months. Choices of therapy includingWBRT (Hottinger et al., 2007), repeated high-dose MTX (Plotkin et al., 2004), temozolomide (Reni et al., 2004), rituximab (Batchelor et al., 2011), intraventricular rituximab (Rubenstein et al., 2007), topotecan (Fischer et al., 2006; Voloschin et al., 2008), other combinations such as the PCV regimen (procarbazine, lomustine, and vincristine) (Herrlinger et al., 2000), temozolomide plus rituximab (Enting et al., 2004), ifosfamide plus etoposide and cytarabine (Arellano-Rodrigo et al., 2003), and HDC/ASCT (Soussain et al., 2008) have been studied with median OS ranging from 3.5-62 months. Currently, there is no consensus regarding which salvage regimen to use in this setting. Therapeutic decisions should be based on individual patient characteristics.

11. Primary intraocular lymphoma

Primary intraocular lymphoma (PIOL) is a subset of PCNSL, which initially presents in the eye with or without simultaneous CNS involvement (Chan et al., 2002). It is distinct from secondary intraocular lymphoma which arises outside the CNS and later involves the eye. Metastatic lymphoma commonly involves the uveal tract, whereas PIOL typically involves the vitreous, subretinal pigment epithelial space and optic nerve head. The disease is bilateral in 80% of patients. Approximately 20% of PCNSL patients have ocular involvement at diagnosis (Davis, 2004). The diagnosis is based on positive CSF cytology, diagnostic vitrectomy, vitreous aspiration, or brain biopsy. When PIOL is suspected, CSF cytology should be performed before diagnostic vitrectomy as it is less invasive. The processing and examination of CSF and vitreous are the same and include cytology, immunocytochemistry, flow cytometry, cytokine, and molecular analyses (Sen et al., 2009). Optimal management of PIOL is not clearly defined. The goal of treatment is to eradicate tumor cells in the eyes and prevent subsequent CNS relapse. Historically, the primary focus has been on local therapy with ocular radiation and intraocular MTX. Ocular radiation has long been used with doses of 3500 to 4000 cGy and was found to have a 58% disease-free survival at 2 years in one small series (Margolis et al., 1980). Because bilateral disease is very common (>80%), radiation has to be given to both eyes. However, ocular radiotherapy can cause radiation keratopathy, dry eyes, cataracts, radiation retinopathy, and papillopathy (Gunduz et al., 2006). Intravitreal MTX was also reported to have excellent local disease control (Frenkel et al., 2008). However, in a large retrospective series of an international PCNSL collaborative group, 102 patients who had additional local ocular therapy (ocular radiotherapy, intravitreal MTX, or both) in addition to their therapy for PCNSL did not have a statistically significant decreased risk of failing in the eyes, and OS was not impacted (Grimm et al., 2008). Recently, there have been efforts to use HD-MTX for the treatment of POL. Systemic high-dose MTX of 8 g/m^2 was found to achieve a therapeutic concentration in the aqueous humor and vitreous (Batchelor et al., 2003). There has been concern regarding the efficacy of systemic chemotherapy as the sole therapy in patients with PIOL. Although CR may be achieved, relapse is common. In one report of 14 patients with ocular lymphoma and concurrent PCNSL treated with high-dose MTX, thiotepa, vincristine and intrathecal cytarabine/MTX, CR was achieved in 79% but relapse occurred a median of 16.5 months following diagnosis (Sandor et al., 1998). In another retrospective study, all patients who were treated with chemotherapy alone had CNS or ocular relapse. Despite unclear information, directed ocular treatment is still being used commonly with or without systemic chemotherapy (Frenkel et al., 2008). Recently, intraocular rituximab has been studied as CD20 is found in over 90% of tumors and is absent in normal intraocular tissues. Initial case series of intravitreal rituximab showed that it is tolerated in human eyes without reduction in visual acuity (Kitzmann et al., 2007). Futures studies are needed to confirm these findings.

12. References

Abrey, L. E. (2011). Advances in primary cns lymphoma: randomized clinical trials of chemotherapy and whole-brain radiotherapy. *Curr Neurol Neurosci Rep* [epub ahead of print]. ISSN 1528-4042

Abrey, L. E., Batchelor, T. T., Ferreri, A. J., Gospodarowicz, M., Pulczynski, E. J., Zucca, E., Smith, J. R., Korfel, A., Soussain, C., DeAngelis, L. M., Neuwelt, E. A., O'Neill, B. P., Thiel, E., Shenkier, T., Graus, F., van den Bent, M., Seymour, J. F., Poortmans, P., Armitage, J. O.& Cavalli, F. (2005). Report of an international workshop to standardize baseline evaluation and response criteria for primary CNS lymphoma. *J Clin Oncol*, Vol.23, No.22, (August 2005), pp. 5034-5043. ISSN:0732-183X

Abrey, L. E., Ben-Porat, L., Panageas, K. S., Yahalom, J., Berkey, B., Curran, W., Schultz, C., Leibel, S., Nelson, D., Mehta, M.& DeAngelis, L. M. (2006). Primary central nervous system lymphoma: the Memorial Sloan-Kettering Cancer Center prognostic model. *J Clin Oncol*, Vol.24, No.36, (December 2006), pp. 5711-5715. ISSN:0732-183X

Abrey, L. E., DeAngelis, L. M.& Yahalom, J. (1998). Long-term survival in primary CNS lymphoma. *J Clin Oncol*, Vol.16, No.3, (March 1998), pp. 859-863. ISSN:0732-183X

Aho, R., Ekfors, T., Haltia, M.& Kalimo, H. (1993). Pathogenesis of primary central nervous system lymphoma: invasion of malignant lymphoid cells into and within the brain parenchyme. *Acta Neuropathol*, Vol.86, No.1, (1993) pp. 71-76. ISSN:0001-6322

Alderson, L., Fetell, M. R., Sisti, M., Hochberg, F., Cohen, M.& Louis, D. N. (1996). Sentinel lesions of primary CNS lymphoma. *J Neurol Neurosurg Psychiatry*, Vol.60, No.1,(January 1996), pp. 102-105. ISSN: 022-3050

Angelov, L., Doolittle, N. D., Kraemer, D. F., Siegal, T., Barnett, G. H., Peereboom, D. M., Stevens, G., McGregor, J., Jahnke, K., Lacy, C. A., Hedrick, N. A., Shalom, E., Ference, S., Bell, S., Sorenson, L., Tyson, R. M., Haluska, M.& Neuwelt, E. A. (2009). Blood-brain barrier disruption and intra-arterial methotrexate-based therapy for newly diagnosed primary CNS lymphoma: a multi-institutional experience. *J Clin Oncol*, Vol.27, No.21, (July 2009), pp. 3503-3509. ISSN:0732-183X

Arellano-Rodrigo, E., Lopez-Guillermo, A., Bessell, E. M., Nomdedeu, B., Montserrat, E.& Graus, F. (2003). Salvage treatment with etoposide (VP-16), ifosfamide and cytarabine (Ara-C) for patients with recurrent primary central nervous system lymphoma. *Eur J Haematol*, Vol.70, No.4, (April 2003), pp. 219-224. ISSN:0902-4441

Barajas, R. F., Jr., Rubenstein, J. L., Chang, J. S., Hwang, J.& Cha, S. (2010). Diffusion-weighted MR imaging derived apparent diffusion coefficient is predictive of clinical outcome in primary central nervous system lymphoma. *AJNR Am J Neuroradiol*, Vol.31, No.1, [epub January 2009), pp. 60-66. ISSN: 0195-6108

Baraniskin, A., Kuhnhenn, J., Schlegel, U., Chan, A., Deckert, M., Gold, R., Maghnouj, A., Zollner, H., Reinacher-Schick, A., Schmiegel, W., Hahn, S. A.& Schroers, R. (2011). Identification of microRNAs in the cerebrospinal fluid as marker for primary diffuse large B-cell lymphoma of the central nervous system. *Blood* [epub ahead of print 2011]. ISSN:0006-4971

Bataille, B., Delwail, V., Menet, E., Vandermarcq, P., Ingrand, P., Wager, M., Guy, G.& Lapierre, F. (2000). Primary intracerebral malignant lymphoma: report of 248 cases. *J Neurosurg*, Vol.92, No.2, (February 2000), pp. 261-266. ISSN: 0022-3085

Batchelor, T., Carson, K., O'Neill, A., Grossman, S. A., Alavi, J., New, P., Hochberg, F.& Priet, R. (2003). Treatment of primary CNS lymphoma with methotrexate and deferred radiotherapy: a report of NABTT 96-07. *J Clin Oncol*, Vol.21, No.6, (March 2003), pp. 1044-1049. ISSN:0732-183X

Batchelor, T.& Loeffler, J. S. (2006). Primary CNS lymphoma. *J Clin Oncol*, Vol.24, No.8, (March 2006), pp. 1281-1288. ISSN:0732-183X.

Batchelor, T. T., Grossman, S. A., Mikkelsen, T., Ye, X., Desideri, S.& Lesser, G. J. (2011). Rituximab monotherapy for patients with recurrent primary CNS lymphoma. *Neurology*, Vol.76, No.10, (March 2011), pp. 929-930. ISSN:0028-3878

Batchelor, T. T., Kolak, G., Ciordia, R., Foster, C. S.& Henson, J. W. (2003). High-dose methotrexate for intraocular lymphoma. *Clin Cancer Res*, Vol.9, No.2, (February 2003), pp. 711-715. ISSN:1078-0432

Bessell, E. M., Graus, F., Lopez-Guillermo, A., Lewis, S. A., Villa, S., Verger, E.& Petit, J. (2004). Primary non-Hodgkin's lymphoma of the CNS treated with CHOD/BVAM or BVAM chemotherapy before radiotherapy: long-term survival and prognostic factors. *Int J Radiat Oncol Biol Phys*, Vol.59, No.2, (June 2004), pp. 501-508. ISSN: 0360-3016

Bessell, E. M., Lopez-Guillermo, A., Villa, S., Verger, E., Nomdedeu, B., Petit, J., Byrne, P., Montserrat, E.& Graus, F. (2002). Importance of radiotherapy in the outcome of patients with primary CNS lymphoma: an analysis of the CHOD/BVAM regimen followed by two different radiotherapy treatments. *J Clin Oncol*, Vol.20, No.1, (January 2002), pp. 231-236. ISSN:0732-183X

Bhagavathi, S.& Wilson, J. D. (2008). Primary central nervous system lymphoma. *Arch Pathol Lab Med*, Vol.132, No.11, (November 2008), pp. 1830-1834. ISSN: 0003-9985

Braaten, K. M., Betensky, R. A., de Leval, L., Okada, Y., Hochberg, F. H., Louis, D. N., Harris, N. L.& Batchelor, T. T. (2003). BCL-6 expression predicts improved survival in patients with primary central nervous system lymphoma. *Clin Cancer Res*, Vol.9, No.3, (March 2003), pp. 1063-1069. ISSN:1078-0432

Camilleri-Broet, S., Criniere, E., Broet, P., Delwail, V., Mokhtari, K., Moreau, A., Kujas, M., Raphael, M., Iraqi, W., Sautes-Fridman, C., Colombat, P., Hoang-Xuan, K.& Martin, A. (2006). A uniform activated B-cell-like immunophenotype might explain the poor prognosis of primary central nervous system lymphomas: analysis of 83 cases. *Blood*, Vol.107, No.1, (January 2006), pp. 190-196. ISSN:0006-4971

Carrabba, M. G., Reni, M., Foppoli, M., Chiara, A., Franzin, A., Politi, L. S., Villa, E., Ciceri, F.& Ferreri, A. J. (2010). Treatment approaches for primary CNS lymphomas. *Expert Opin Pharmacother*, Vol.11, No.8,(June 2010), pp. 1263-1276. ISSN: 1465-6566

Chan, C. C., Buggage, R. R.& Nussenblatt, R. B. (2002). Intraocular lymphoma. *Curr Opin Ophthalmol*, Vol.13, No.6, (December 2002), pp. 411-418. ISSN:1040-8738

Chang, C. C., Kampalath, B., Schultz, C., Bunyi-Teopengco, E., Logan, B., Eshoa, C., Dincer, A. P.& Perkins, S. L. (2003). Expression of p53, c-Myc, or Bcl-6 suggests a poor prognosis in primary central nervous system diffuse large B-cell lymphoma among immunocompetent individuals. *Arch Pathol Lab Med*, Vol.127, No.2, (February 2003), pp. 208-212. ISSN: 0003-9985

Coiffier, B., Thieblemont, C., Van Den Neste, E., Lepeu, G., Plantier, I., Castaigne, S., Lefort, S., Marit, G., Macro, M., Sebban, C., Belhadj, K., Bordessoule, D., Ferme, C.& Tilly, H. (2010). Long-term outcome of patients in the LNH-98.5 trial, the first randomized study comparing rituximab-CHOP to standard CHOP chemotherapy in DLBCL patients: a study by the Groupe d'Etudes des Lymphomes de l'Adulte. *Blood*, Vol.116, No.12, (September 2010), pp. 2040-2045. ISSN:0006-4971

Colombat, P., Lemevel, A., Bertrand, P., Delwail, V., Rachieru, P., Brion, A., Berthou, C., Bay, J. O., Delepine, R., Desablens, B., Camilleri-Broet, S., Linassier, C.& Lamy, T. (2006). High-dose chemotherapy with autologous stem cell transplantation as first-line therapy for primary CNS lymphoma in patients younger than 60 years: a multicenter phase II study of the GOELAMS group. *Bone Marrow Transplant*, Vol.38, No.6, (September 2006), pp. 417-420. ISSN: 0268-3369

Corn, B. W., Dolinskas, C., Scott, C., Donahue, B., Schultz, C., Nelson, D. F.& Fisher, B. (2000). Strong correlation between imaging response and survival among patients with primary central nervous system lymphoma: a secondary analysis of RTOG studies 83-15 and 88-06. *Int J Radiat Oncol Biol Phys*, Vol.47, No.2, (May 2000), pp. 299-303. ISSN: 0360-3016Davis, J. L. (2004). Diagnosis of intraocular lymphoma. *Ocul Immunol Inflamm*, Vol.12, No.1, (March 2004), pp. 7-16. ISSN: 0927-3948

Deangelis, L. M. (2011). Radiotherapy: Has the role of WBRT in primary CNS lymphoma been settled? *Nat Rev Clin Oncol.* ISSN: 1759-4774.

DeAngelis, L. M., Seiferheld, W., Schold, S. C., Fisher, B.& Schultz, C. J. (2002). Combination chemotherapy and radiotherapy for primary central nervous system lymphoma: Radiation Therapy Oncology Group Study 93-10. *J Clin Oncol*, Vol.20, No.24,(December 2002), pp. 4643-4648. ISSN:0732-183X

DeAngelis, L. M., Yahalom, J., Heinemann, M. H., Cirrincione, C., Thaler, H. T.& Krol, G. (1990). Primary CNS lymphoma: combined treatment with chemotherapy and radiotherapy. *Neurology*, Vol.40, No.1, (January 1990), pp. 80-86. ISSN:0028-3878

Deckert, M.& Paulus, W. (2007). Tumours of the Haematopoietic System, Malignant lymphoma, In: *WHO Classification of Tumours of the Central Nervous System,* Louis, D. N., Ohgaki, H., Wiestler, O. D.& Cavenee, W. K., pp. 187-192, the International Agency of Research on Cancer (IARC), Lyon Cedex, France

Ekenel, M., Iwamoto, F. M., Ben-Porat, L. S., Panageas, K. S., Yahalom, J., DeAngelis, L. M.& Abrey, L. E. (2008). Primary central nervous system lymphoma: the role of consolidation treatment after a complete response to high-dose methotrexate-based chemotherapy. *Cancer,* Vol.113, No.5, (September 2008), pp. 1025-1031. ISSN:0008-543X

Enting, R. H., Demopoulos, A., DeAngelis, L. M.& Abrey, L. E. (2004). Salvage therapy for primary CNS lymphoma with a combination of rituximab and temozolomide. *Neurology,* Vol.63, No.5, (September 2004), pp. 901-903. ISSN:0028-3878

Erdag, N., Bhorade, R. M., Alberico, R. A., Yousuf, N.& Patel, M. R. (2001). Primary lymphoma of the central nervous system: typical and atypical CT and MR imaging appearances. *AJR Am J Roentgenol,* Vol.176, No.5, (May 2001), pp. 1319-1326. ISSN:0361-803X

Ferreri, A. J., Abrey, L. E., Blay, J. Y., Borisch, B., Hochman, J., Neuwelt, E. A., Yahalom, J., Zucca, E., Cavalli, F., Armitage, J.& Batchelor, T. (2003). Summary statement on primary central nervous system lymphomas from the Eighth International Conference on Malignant Lymphoma, Lugano, Switzerland, June 12 to 15, 2002. *J Clin Oncol,* Vol.21, No.12, (June 2003), pp. 2407-2414. ISSN:0732-183X

Ferreri, A. J., Blay, J. Y., Reni, M., Pasini, F., Spina, M., Ambrosetti, A., Calderoni, A., Rossi, A., Vavassori, V., Conconi, A., Devizzi, L., Berger, F., Ponzoni, M., Borisch, B., Tinguely, M., Cerati, M., Milani, M., Orvieto, E., Sanchez, J., Chevreau, C., Dell'Oro, S., Zucca, E.& Cavalli, F. (2003). Prognostic scoring system for primary CNS lymphomas: the International Extranodal Lymphoma Study Group experience. *J Clin Oncol,* Vol.21, No.2, (January 2003), pp. 266-272. ISSN:0732-183X

Ferreri, A. J., Dell'Oro, S., Foppoli, M., Bernardi, M., Brandes, A. A., Tosoni, A., Montanari, M., Balzarotti, M., Spina, M., Ilariucci, F., Zaja, F., Stelitano, C., Bobbio, F., Corazzelli, G., Baldini, L., Ponzoni, M., Picozzi, P., Caligaris Cappio, F.& Reni, M. (2006). MATILDE regimen followed by radiotherapy is an active strategy against primary CNS lymphomas. *Neurology,* Vol.66, No.9, (May 2006), pp. 1435-1438. ISSN:0028-3878

Ferreri, A. J., Reni, M., Foppoli, M., Martelli, M., Pangalis, G. A., Frezzato, M., Cabras, M. G., Fabbri, A., Corazzelli, G., Ilariucci, F., Rossi, G., Soffietti, R., Stelitano, C., Vallisa, D., Zaja, F., Zoppegno, L., Aondio, G. M., Avvisati, G., Balzarotti, M., Brandes, A. A., Fajardo, J., Gomez, H., Guarini, A., Pinotti, G., Rigacci, L., Uhlmann, C., Picozzi, P., Vezzulli, P., Ponzoni, M., Zucca, E., Caligaris-Cappio, F.& Cavalli, F. (2009). High-dose cytarabine plus high-dose methotrexate versus high-dose methotrexate alone in patients with primary CNS lymphoma: a randomised phase 2 trial. *Lancet,* Vol.374, No.9700, (October 2009), pp. 1512-1520. ISSN:0140-6736

Ferreri, A. J., Reni, M., Pasini, F., Calderoni, A., Tirelli, U., Pivnik, A., Aondio, G. M., Ferrarese, F., Gomez, H., Ponzoni, M., Borisch, B., Berger, F., Chassagne, C., Iuzzolino, P., Carbone, A., Weis, J., Pedrinis, E., Motta, T., Jouvet, A., Barbui, T., Cavalli, F.& Blay, J. Y. (2002). A multicenter study of treatment of primary CNS lymphoma. *Neurology,* Vol.58, No.10, (May 2002), pp. 1513-1520. ISSN:0028-3878

Fine, H. A.& Mayer, R. J. (1993). Primary central nervous system lymphoma. *Ann Intern Med*, Vol.119, No.11, (December 1993), pp. 1093-1104. ISSN:0028-3878

Fischer, L., Koch, A., Schlegel, U., Koch, H. C., Wenzel, R., Schroder, N., Thiel, E.& Korfel, A. (2010). Non-enhancing relapse of a primary CNS lymphoma with multiple diffusion-restricted lesions. *J Neurooncol*, Vol. 102, No.1, (March 2011), pp. 163-166

Fischer, L., Thiel, E., Klasen, H. A., Birkmann, J., Jahnke, K., Martus, P.& Korfel, A. (2006). Prospective trial on topotecan salvage therapy in primary CNS lymphoma. *Ann Oncol*, Vol.17, No.7, (July 2006), pp. 1141-1145. ISSN:0923-7534

Fisher, B., Seiferheld, W., Schultz, C., DeAngelis, L., Nelson, D., Schold, S. C., Curran, W.& Mehta, M. (2005). Secondary analysis of Radiation Therapy Oncology Group study (RTOG) 9310: an intergroup phase II combined modality treatment of primary central nervous system lymphoma. *J Neurooncol*, Vol.74, No.2, (September 2005), pp. 201-205. ISSN:0167-594X

Frenkel, S., Hendler, K., Siegal, T., Shalom, E.& Pe'er, J. (2008). Intravitreal methotrexate for treating vitreoretinal lymphoma: 10 years of experience. *Br J Ophthalmol*, Vol.92, No.3, (March 2008), pp. 383-388. ISSN: 0007-1161

Gavrilovic, I. T., Hormigo, A., Yahalom, J., DeAngelis, L. M.& Abrey, L. E. (2006). Long-term follow-up of high-dose methotrexate-based therapy with and without whole brain irradiation for newly diagnosed primary CNS lymphoma. *J Clin Oncol*, Vol.24, No.28, (October 2006), pp. 4570-4574. ISSN:0732-183X

Glass, J., Gruber, M. L., Cher, L.& Hochberg, F. H. (1994). Preirradiation methotrexate chemotherapy of primary central nervous system lymphoma: long-term outcome. *J Neurosurg*, Vol.81, No.2, (August 1994), pp. 188-195. ISSN: 0022-3085

Grimm, S. A., McCannel, C. A., Omuro, A. M., Ferreri, A. J., Blay, J. Y., Neuwelt, E. A., Siegal, T., Batchelor, T., Jahnke, K., Shenkier, T. N., Hall, A. J., Graus, F., Herrlinger, U., Schiff, D., Raizer, J., Rubenstein, J., Laperriere, N., Thiel, E., Doolittle, N., Iwamoto, F. M.& Abrey, L. E. (2008). Primary CNS lymphoma with intraocular involvement: International PCNSL Collaborative Group Report. *Neurology*, Vol.71, No.17, (October 2008), pp. 1355-1360. ISSN:0028-3878

Gunduz, K., Pulido, J. S., McCannel, C. A.& O'Neill, B. P. (2006). Ocular manifestations and treatment of central nervous system lymphomas. *Neurosurg Focus*, Vol.21, No.5, (November 2006), pp. E9, ISSN:1092-0684

Habek, M., Brinar, V. V., Zarkovic, K.& Ozretic, D. (2008). Is there sentinel demyelination before development of primary CNS lymphoma? *J Clin Neurosci*, Vol.15, No.9, (September 2008), pp. 1069-1070; author reply 1071. ISSN:0967-5868

Harris, N. L., Jaffe, E. S., Stein, H., Banks, P. M., Chan, J. K., Cleary, M. L., Delsol, G., De Wolf-Peeters, C., Falini, B., Gatter, K. C.& et al. (1994). A revised European-American classification of lymphoid neoplasms: a proposal from the International Lymphoma Study Group. *Blood*, Vol.84, No.5, (September 1994), pp. 1361-1392. ISSN:0006-4971

Hegde, U., Filie, A., Little, R. F., Janik, J. E., Grant, N., Steinberg, S. M., Dunleavy, K., Jaffe, E. S., Abati, A., Stetler-Stevenson, M.& Wilson, W. H. (2005). High incidence of occult leptomeningeal disease detected by flow cytometry in newly diagnosed aggressive B-cell lymphomas at risk for central nervous system involvement: the role of flow cytometry versus cytology. *Blood*, Vol.105, No.2, (January 2005), pp. 496-502. ISSN:0006-4971

Henry, J. M., Heffner, R. R., Jr., Dillard, S. H., Earle, K. M.& Davis, R. L. (1974). Primary malignant lymphomas of the central nervous system. *Cancer*, Vol.34, No.4, (October 1974), pp. 1293-1302. ISSN:0008-543X

Herrlinger, U., Brugger, W., Bamberg, M., Kuker, W., Dichgans, J.& Weller, M. (2000). PCV salvage chemotherapy for recurrent primary CNS lymphoma. *Neurology*, Vol.54, No.8, (April 2000), pp. 1707-1708. ISSN:0028-3878

Herrlinger, U., Kuker, W., Uhl, M., Blaicher, H. P., Karnath, H. O., Kanz, L., Bamberg, M.& Weller, M. (2005). NOA-03 trial of high-dose methotrexate in primary central nervous system lymphoma: final report. *Ann Neurol*, Vol.57, No.6(June 2005),pp. 843-847. ISSN:0364-5134

Hill, Q. A.& Owen, R. G. (2006). CNS prophylaxis in lymphoma: who to target and what therapy to use. *Blood Rev*, Vol.20, No.6, (November 2006), pp. 319-332. ISSN:0268-960X

Hottinger, A. F., DeAngelis, L. M., Yahalom, J.& Abrey, L. E. (2007). Salvage whole brain radiotherapy for recurrent or refractory primary CNS lymphoma. *Neurology*, Vol.69, No.11, (September 2006), pp. 1178-1182. ISSN:0028-3878

Jaffe, E. S. (2009). The 2008 WHO classification of lymphomas: implications for clinical practice and translational research. *Hematology Am Soc Hematol Educ Program*, (2009), pp. 523-531

Jiang, L., Marlow, L. A., Cooper, S. J., Roemeling, C. V., Menke, D. M., Copland, J. A.& Tun, H. W. (2010). Selective central nervous system tropism of primary central nervous system lymphoma. *Int J Clin Exp Pathol*, Vol.3, No.8, (October 2010), pp. 763-767. ISSN: 1936-2625

Kasamon, Y. L.& Ambinder, R. F. (2005). AIDS-related primary central nervous system lymphoma. *Hematol Oncol Clin North Am*, Vol.19, No.4, (August 2005), pp. 665-687, vi-vii. ISSN:0889-8588

Khan, R. B., Shi, W., Thaler, H. T., DeAngelis, L. M.& Abrey, L. E. (2002). Is intrathecal methotrexate necessary in the treatment of primary CNS lymphoma? *J Neurooncol*, Vol.58, No.2, (June 2002), pp. 175-178. ISSN: 0167-594X

Kitzmann, A. S., Pulido, J. S., Mohney, B. G., Baratz, K. H., Grube, T., Marler, R. J., Donaldson, M. J., O'Neill, B. P., Johnston, P. B., Johnson, K. M., Dixon, L. E., Salomao, D. R.& Cameron, J. D. (2007). Intraocular use of rituximab. *Eye (Lond)*, Vol.21, No.12,(December 2007), pp. 1524-1527. ISSN:0950-222X

Knowles, D. M. (2003). Etiology and pathogenesis of AIDS-related non-Hodgkin's lymphoma. *Hematol Oncol Clin North Am*, Vol.17, No.3, (June 2003), pp. 785-820. ISSN:0889-8588

Krumbholz, M., Theil, D., Derfuss, T., Rosenwald, A., Schrader, F., Monoranu, C. M., Kalled, S. L., Hess, D. M., Serafini, B., Aloisi, F., Wekerle, H., Hohlfeld, R.& Meinl, E. (2005). BAFF is produced by astrocytes and up-regulated in multiple sclerosis lesions and primary central nervous system lymphoma. *J Exp Med*, Vol.201, No.2,(December 2005), pp. 195-200. ISSN:0022-1007

Kuker, W., Nagele, T., Korfel, A., Heckl, S., Thiel, E., Bamberg, M., Weller, M.& Herrlinger, U. (2005). Primary central nervous system lymphomas (PCNSL): MRI features at presentation in 100 patients. *J Neurooncol*, Vol.72, No.2, (October 2005), pp. 169-177. ISSN: 0167-594X

Larocca, L. M., Capello, D., Rinelli, A., Nori, S., Antinori, A., Gloghini, A., Cingolani, A., Migliazza, A., Saglio, G., Cammilleri-Broet, S., Raphael, M., Carbone, A.& Gaidano, G. (1998). The molecular and phenotypic profile of primary central nervous system lymphoma identifies distinct categories of the disease and is consistent with histogenetic derivation from germinal center-related B cells. *Blood*, Vol.92, No.3, (August 1998), pp. 1011-1019. ISSN:0006-4971

Lippens, R. J.& Winograd, B. (1988). Methotrexate concentration levels in the cerebrospinal fluid during high-dose methotrexate infusions: an unreliable prediction. *Pediatr Hematol Oncol*, Vol.5, No.2, (1988), pp. 115-124. ISSN:0278-0232

Margolis, L., Fraser, R., Lichter, A.& Char, D. H. (1980). The role of radiation therapy in the management of ocular reticulum cell sarcoma. *Cancer*, Vol.45, No.4, (February 1980), pp. 688-692

Mohile, N. A., Deangelis, L. M.& Abrey, L. E. (2008). The utility of body FDG PET in staging primary central nervous system lymphoma. *Neuro Oncol*, Vol.10, No.2, (November 2008), pp. 223-228. ISSN:0008-543X

Montemurro, M., Kiefer, T., Schuler, F., Al-Ali, H. K., Wolf, H. H., Herbst, R., Haas, A., Helke, K., Theilig, A., Lotze, C., Hirt, C., Niederwieser, D., Schwenke, M., Kruger, W. H.& Dolken, G. (2007). Primary central nervous system lymphoma treated with high-dose methotrexate, high-dose busulfan/thiotepa, autologous stem-cell transplantation and response-adapted whole-brain radiotherapy: results of the multicenter Ostdeutsche Studiengruppe Hamato-Onkologie OSHO-53 phase II study. *Ann Oncol*, Vol.18, No.4, (April 2007), pp. 665-671. ISSN:0923-7534

Morris, P. G.& Abrey, L. E. (2009). Therapeutic challenges in primary CNS lymphoma. *Lancet Neurol*, Vol.8, No.6, (June 2009), pp. 581-592. ISSN: 1474-4422

Nelson, D. F., Martz, K. L., Bonner, H., Nelson, J. S., Newall, J., Kerman, H. D., Thomson, J. W.& Murray, K. J. (1992). Non-Hodgkin's lymphoma of the brain: can high dose, large volume radiation therapy improve survival? Report on a prospective trial by the Radiation Therapy Oncology Group (RTOG): RTOG 8315. *Int J Radiat Oncol Biol Phys*, Vol.23, No.1, pp. 9-17. ISSN: 0360-3016

Ng, S., Butzkueven, H., Kalnins, R.& Rowe, C. (2007). Prolonged interval between sentinel pseudotumoral demyelination and development of primary CNS lymphoma. *J Clin Neurosci*, Vol.14, No.11, (November 2007), pp. 1126-1129. ISSN:0967-5868

O'Brien, P. C., Roos, D. E., Pratt, G., Liew, K. H., Barton, M. B., Poulsen, M. G., Olver, I. N.& Trotter, G. E. (2006). Combined-modality therapy for primary central nervous system lymphoma: long-term data from a Phase II multicenter study (Trans-Tasman Radiation Oncology Group). *Int J Radiat Oncol Biol Phys*, Vol.64, No.2, (February 2006), pp. 408-413. ISSN: 0360-3016

Olson, J. E., Janney, C. A., Rao, R. D., Cerhan, J. R., Kurtin, P. J., Schiff, D., Kaplan, R. S.& O'Neill, B. P. (2002). The continuing increase in the incidence of primary central nervous system non-Hodgkin lymphoma: a surveillance, epidemiology, and end results analysis. *Cancer*, Vol.95, No.7, (October 2002), pp. 1504-1510. ISSN:0008-543X

Omuro, A. M., Ben-Porat, L. S., Panageas, K. S., Kim, A. K., Correa, D. D., Yahalom, J., Deangelis, L. M.& Abrey, L. E. (2005). Delayed neurotoxicity in primary central nervous system lymphoma. *Arch Neurol*, Vol.62, No.10, (October 2005), pp. 1595-1600. ISSN:0003-9942

Omuro, A. M., Taillandier, L., Chinot, O., Carnin, C., Barrie, M.& Hoang-Xuan, K. (2007). Temozolomide and methotrexate for primary central nervous system lymphoma in the elderly. *J Neurooncol*, Vol.85, No.2, (November 2007), pp. 207-211. ISSN: 0167-594X

Paulus, W. (1999). Classification, pathogenesis and molecular pathology of primary CNS lymphomas. *J Neurooncol*, Vol.43, No.3, (July 1999), pp. 203-208. ISSN: 0167-594X

Plotkin, S. R., Betensky, R. A., Hochberg, F. H., Grossman, S. A., Lesser, G. J., Nabors, L. B., Chon, B.& Batchelor, T. T. (2004). Treatment of relapsed central nervous system lymphoma with high-dose methotrexate. *Clin Cancer Res*, Vol.10, No.17, (September 2004), pp. 5643-5646. ISSN:1078-0432

Poortmans, P. M., Kluin-Nelemans, H. C., Haaxma-Reiche, H., Van't Veer, M., Hansen, M., Soubeyran, P., Taphoorn, M., Thomas, J., Van den Bent, M., Fickers, M., Van Imhoff, G., Rozewicz, C., Teodorovic, I.& van Glabbeke, M. (2003). High-dose methotrexate-based chemotherapy followed by consolidating radiotherapy in non-AIDS-related primary central nervous system lymphoma: European Organization for Research and Treatment of Cancer Lymphoma Group Phase II Trial 20962. *J Clin Oncol*, Vol.21, No.24, (December 2003), pp. 4483-4488. ISSN:0732-183X

Reni, M.& Ferreri, A. J. (2001). Therapeutic management of refractory or relapsed primary central nervous system lymphomas. *Ann Hematol*, Vol.80 Suppl 3, (October 2001), pp. B113-117. ISSN: 0939-5555

Reni, M., Mason, W., Zaja, F., Perry, J., Franceschi, E., Bernardi, D., Dell'Oro, S., Stelitano, C., Candela, M., Abbadessa, A., Pace, A., Bordonaro, R., Latte, G., Villa, E.& Ferreri, A. J. (2004). Salvage chemotherapy with temozolomide in primary CNS lymphomas: preliminary results of a phase II trial. *Eur J Cancer*, Vol.40, No.11, (July 2004), pp. 1682-1688. ISSN: 0959-8049

Rosenwald, A., Wright, G., Chan, W. C., Connors, J. M., Campo, E., Fisher, R. I., Gascoyne, R. D., Muller-Hermelink, H. K., Smeland, E. B., Giltnane, J. M., Hurt, E. M., Zhao, H., Averett, L., Yang, L., Wilson, W. H., Jaffe, E. S., Simon, R., Klausner, R. D., Powell, J., Duffey, P. L., Longo, D. L., Greiner, T. C., Weisenburger, D. D., Sanger, W. G., Dave, B. J., Lynch, J. C., Vose, J., Armitage, J. O., Montserrat, E., Lopez-Guillermo, A., Grogan, T. M., Miller, T. P., LeBlanc, M., Ott, G., Kvaloy, S., Delabie, J., Holte, H., Krajci, P., Stokke, T.& Staudt, L. M. (2002). The use of molecular profiling to predict survival after chemotherapy for diffuse large-B-cell lymphoma. *N Engl J Med*, Vol.346, No.25, (June 2002), pp. 1937-1947. ISSN: 0959-8049

Roy, S., Josephson, S. A., Fridlyand, J., Karch, J., Kadoch, C., Karrim, J., Damon, L., Treseler, P., Kunwar, S., Shuman, M. A., Jones, T., Becker, C. H., Schulman, H.& Rubenstein, J. L. (2008). Protein biomarker identification in the CSF of patients with CNS lymphoma. *J Clin Oncol*, Vol.26, No.1, (January 2008), pp. 96-105. ISSN:0732-183X

Rubenstein, J. L., Fridlyand, J., Abrey, L., Shen, A., Karch, J., Wang, E., Issa, S., Damon, L., Prados, M., McDermott, M., O'Brien, J., Haqq, C.& Shuman, M. (2007). Phase I study of intraventricular administration of rituximab in patients with recurrent CNS and intraocular lymphoma. *J Clin Oncol*, Vol.25, No.11, (April 2007), pp. 1350-1356. ISSN:0732-183X

Rubenstein, J. L., Fridlyand, J., Shen, A., Aldape, K., Ginzinger, D., Batchelor, T., Treseler, P., Berger, M., McDermott, M., Prados, M., Karch, J., Okada, C., Hyun, W., Parikh, S.,

Haqq, C.& Shuman, M. (2006). Gene expression and angiotropism in primary CNS lymphoma. *Blood*, Vol.107, No.9, (May 2006), pp. 3716-3723. ISSN:0006-4971

Sandor, V., Stark-Vancs, V., Pearson, D., Nussenblat, R., Whitcup, S. M., Brouwers, P., Patronas, N., Heiss, J., Jaffe, E., deSmet, M., Kohler, D., Simon, R.& Wittes, R. (1998). Phase II trial of chemotherapy alone for primary CNS and intraocular lymphoma. *J Clin Oncol*, Vol.16, No.9, (September 1998), pp. 3000-3006. ISSN:0732-183X

Schabet, M. (1999). Epidemiology of primary CNS lymphoma. *J Neurooncol*, Vol.43, No.3, (July 1999), pp. 199-201. ISSN: 0167-594X

Schlegel, U., Schmidt-Wolf, I. G.& Deckert, M. (2000). Primary CNS lymphoma: clinical presentation, pathological classification, molecular pathogenesis and treatment. *J Neurol Sci*, Vol.181, No.1-2, (December 2000), pp. 1-12. ISSN:1590-1874

Schroers, R., Baraniskin, A., Heute, C., Vorgerd, M., Brunn, A., Kuhnhenn, J., Kowoll, A., Alekseyev, A., Schmiegel, W., Schlegel, U., Deckert, M.& Pels, H. (2010). Diagnosis of leptomeningeal disease in diffuse large B-cell lymphomas of the central nervous system by flow cytometry and cytopathology. *Eur J Haematol*, Vol.85, No.6, (December 2010), pp. 520-528. ISSN:0902-4441

Sen, H. N., Bodaghi, B., Hoang, P. L.& Nussenblatt, R. (2009). Primary intraocular lymphoma: diagnosis and differential diagnosis. *Ocul Immunol Inflamm*, Vol.17, No.3, (May-June 2009) pp. 133-141. ISSN: 0927-3948

Shah, G. D., Yahalom, J., Correa, D. D., Lai, R. K., Raizer, J. J., Schiff, D., LaRocca, R., Grant, B., DeAngelis, L. M.& Abrey, L. E. (2007). Combined immunochemotherapy with reduced whole-brain radiotherapy for newly diagnosed primary CNS lymphoma. *J Clin Oncol*, Vol.25, No.30, (October 2007), pp. 4730-4735. ISSN:0732-183X

Song, M. K., Chung, J. S., Joo, Y. D., Lee, S. M., Oh, S. Y., Shin, D. H., Yun, E. Y., Kim, S. G., Seol, Y. M., Shin, H. J., Choi, Y. J.& Cho, G. J. (2011). Clinical importance of Bcl-6-positive non-deep-site involvement in non-HIV-related primary central nervous system diffuse large B-cell lymphoma. *J Neurooncol*, March [Epub ahead of print] ISSN: 0167-594X

Soussain, C., Hoang-Xuan, K., Taillandier, L., Fourme, E., Choquet, S., Witz, F., Casasnovas, O., Dupriez, B., Souleau, B., Taksin, A. L., Gisselbrecht, C., Jaccard, A., Omuro, A., Sanson, M., Janvier, M., Kolb, B., Zini, J. M.& Leblond, V. (2008). Intensive chemotherapy followed by hematopoietic stem-cell rescue for refractory and recurrent primary CNS and intraocular lymphoma: Societe Francaise de Greffe de Moelle Osseuse-Therapie Cellulaire. *J Clin Oncol*, Vol.26, No.15, (May 2008), pp. 2512-2518. ISSN:0732-183X

Tetef, M. L., Margolin, K. A., Doroshow, J. H., Akman, S., Leong, L. A., Morgan, R. J., Jr., Raschko, J. W., Slatkin, N., Somlo, G., Longmate, J. A., Carroll, M. I.& Newman, E. M. (2000). Pharmacokinetics and toxicity of high-dose intravenous methotrexate in the treatment of leptomeningeal carcinomatosis. *Cancer Chemother Pharmacol*, Vol.46, No.1, pp. 19-26. ISSN: 0344-5704

Thiel, E., Korfel, A., Martus, P., Kanz, L., Griesinger, F., Rauch, M., Roth, A., Hertenstein, B., von Toll, T., Hundsberger, T., Mergenthaler, H. G., Leithauser, M., Birnbaum, T., Fischer, L., Jahnke, K., Herrlinger, U., Plasswilm, L., Nagele, T., Pietsch, T., Bamberg, M.& Weller, M. (2010). High-dose methotrexate with or without whole brain radiotherapy for primary CNS lymphoma (G-PCNSL-SG-1): a phase 3, randomised, non-inferiority trial. *Lancet Oncol*, Vol.11, No.11, (November 2010), pp. 1036-1047. ISSN:1470-2045

Thompsett, A. R., Ellison, D. W., Stevenson, F. K.& Zhu, D. (1999). V(H) gene sequences from primary central nervous system lymphomas indicate derivation from highly mutated germinal center B cells with ongoing mutational activity. *Blood*, Vol.94, No.5, (October 1999), pp. 1738-1746. ISSN:0006-4971

Tun, H. W., Personett, D., Baskerville, K. A., Menke, D. M., Jaeckle, K. A., Kreinest, P., Edenfield, B., Zubair, A. C., O'Neill, B. P., Lai, W. R., Park, P. J.& McKinney, M. (2008). Pathway analysis of primary central nervous system lymphoma. *Blood*, Vol.111, No.6, (March 2008), pp. 3200-3210. ISSN:0006-4971

Vassal, G., Valteau, D., Bonnay, M., Patte, C., Aubier, F.& Lemerle, J. (1990). Cerebrospinal fluid and plasma methotrexate levels following high-dose regimen given as a 3-hour intravenous infusion in children with non Hodgkin's lymphoma. *Pediatr Hematol Oncol*, Vol.7, No.1, pp. 71-77. ISSN:0888-0018

Voloschin, A. D., Betensky, R., Wen, P. Y., Hochberg, F.& Batchelor, T. (2008). Topotecan as salvage therapy for relapsed or refractory primary central nervous system lymphoma. *J Neurooncol*, Vol.86, No.2, (January 2008), pp. 211-215. ISSN: 0167-594X

Weller, M. (1999). Glucocorticoid treatment of primary CNS lymphoma. *J Neurooncol*, Vol.43, No.3, (July 1999), pp. 237-239. ISSN: 0167-594X

Yang, J. H.& Wu, S. L. (2007). Multiple sclerosis preceding CNS lymphoma: a case report. *Acta Neurol Taiwan*, Vol.16, No.2, (June 2007), pp. 92-97. ISSN: 1028-768X

Zacharia, T. T., Law, M., Naidich, T. P.& Leeds, N. E. (2008). Central nervous system lymphoma characterization by diffusion-weighted imaging and MR spectroscopy. *J Neuroimaging*, Vol.18, No.4, (October 2008), pp. 411-417. ISSN:1051-2284

Zaki, H. S., Jenkinson, M. D., Du Plessis, D. G., Smith, T.& Rainov, N. G. (2004). Vanishing contrast enhancement in malignant glioma after corticosteroid treatment. *Acta Neurochir (Wien)*, Vol.146, No.8, (August 2004), pp. 841-845. ISSN:0001-6268

Zhang, D., Hu, L. B., Henning, T. D., Ravarani, E. M., Zou, L. G., Feng, X. Y., Wang, W. X.& Wen, L. (2010). MRI findings of primary CNS lymphoma in 26 immunocompetent patients. *Korean J Radiol*, Vol.11, No.3, (May 2010), pp. 269-277. ISSN: 1229-6929

CBTRUS Statistical Report: Primary Brain and Central Nervous System Tumors Diagnosed in the United States in 2004-2007, In: *CBTRUS Statistical Report*, 31.03.2011, Available from http://www.cbtrus.org/reports/reports.html

17

Reversible Posterior Leukoencephalopathy Syndrome

Željka Petelin Gadže[1], Davorka Milat[2], Sanja Hajnšek[1], Branka Ribarić[1], Jasna Franjić[1] and Damir Petravić[1]
[1]*University of Zagreb, School of Medicine and University Hospital Centre Zagreb, Department of Neurology, Zagreb, Referral Centre of the Ministry of Health and Social Welfare of the Republic of Croatia for Epilepsy*
[2]*Polyclinic "Nemetova", Zagreb, Croatia*

1. Introduction

Hinchey et al used the term „reversible posterior leukoencephalopathy syndrome" in 1996 to describe a syndrome characterized by headache, confusion, seizures and vision disturbances, including cortical blindness, connected with reversible changes on brain magnetic resonance imaging (MRI) which pointed to the white matter eodema, predominantly in the posterior brain regions (1). Initially, this syndrome was believed to be secondary to arterial hypertension, with or without hypertensive encephalopathy, renal disease, or immunosuppressive therapy, such as *cyclosporin A*, tacrolimus and interferon-α. However, it has recently been identified in a wide variety of conditions, including eclampsia, hemolytic-uremic syndrome, connective tissue diseases, vasculitis, malignancies, chemotherapy, transfusions, intravenous immunoglobulin (IVIG) therapy, therapy with erythropoietin, thrombotic thrombocytopenic purpura, porphyria, etc. (2-14).
The normal response of the cerebral arterioles to acute rising blood pressure is sympathetic nerve-mediated vascular constriction to prevent increasing blood flow (autoregulation). But in the case of reversible posterior leukoencephalopathy syndrome, the response does not work well when there is excess high pressure or recent onset of a modest increase in blood pressure, and excess dilatation of the arterioles following disruption of cerebral small vessel endothelial cells (i.e., the blood-brain barrier) can occur, resulting in vasogenic brain edema. Therefore, disruption of cerebral vascular endothelial cells plays a critical role in the pathogenesis of reversible posterior leukoencephalopathy syndrome
In this article we describe a case of a patient with clinical signs and neuroradiological presentation typicial for reversible posterior leukoencephalopathy syndrome.

2. Case report

A 72-year-old woman with a history of arterial hypertension in June 2009 suddenly developed headache, confusion, left homonymous hemianopsia, and left hemiparesis, associated with high blood pressure (220/110 mm Hg). From her case history we have revealed that she was treated for pulmonary tuberculosis in the youth. Brain MRI performed in another institution revealed extensive white matter lesion in the right parietal and occipital lobe, splenium corpus callosum and left occipital lobe, suggestive of expansive process (Figure 1a and 1b). There were also bilateral chronic vascular lesions in the

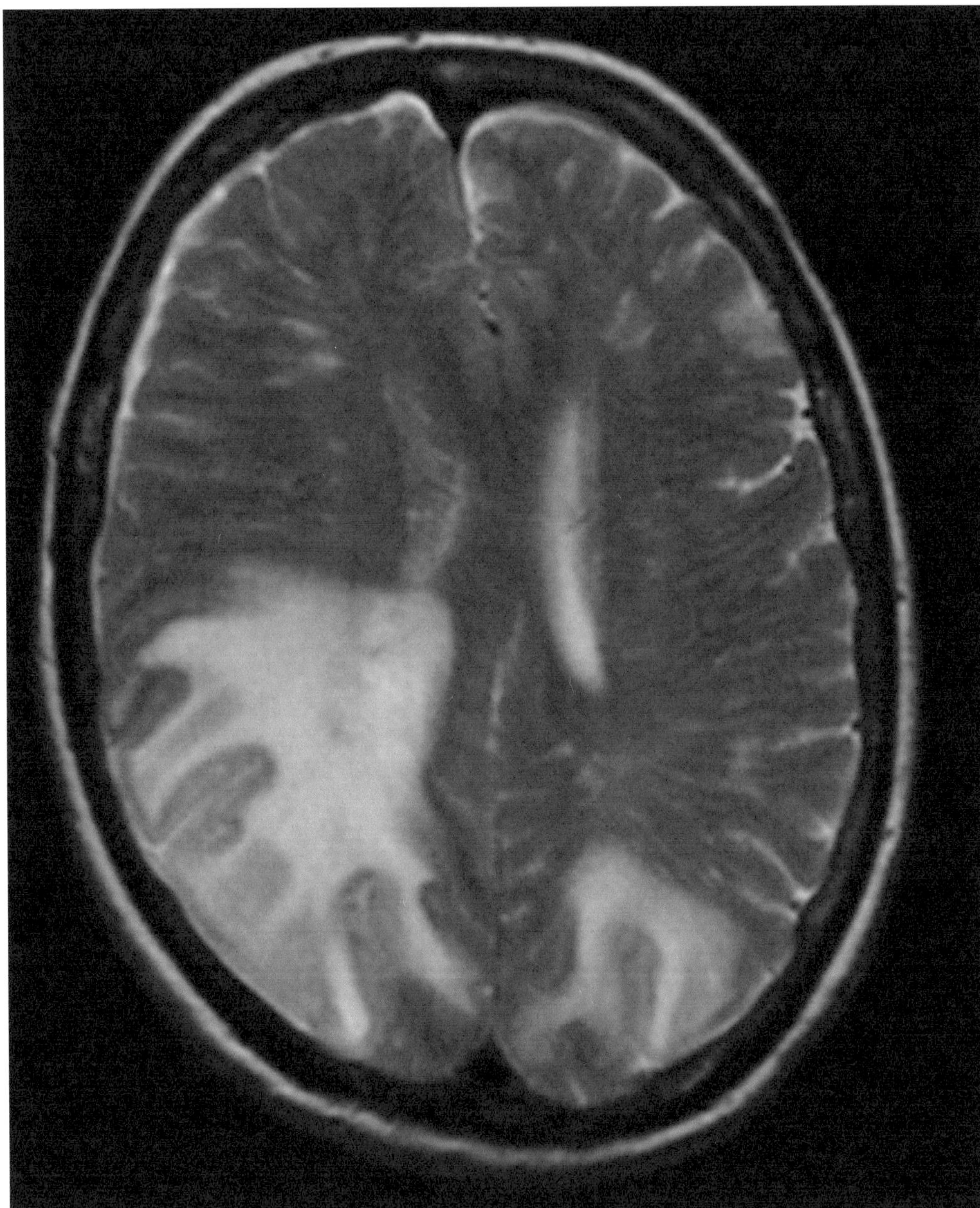

Fig. 1. Brain MRI in 72-year-old woman performed in June 2009 reveals extensive white matter lesion in the right parietal and occipital lobe, splenium corpus callosum and left occipital lobe. Figure 1a – transversal MRI section, hyperintense lesion on T2 – weighted image.

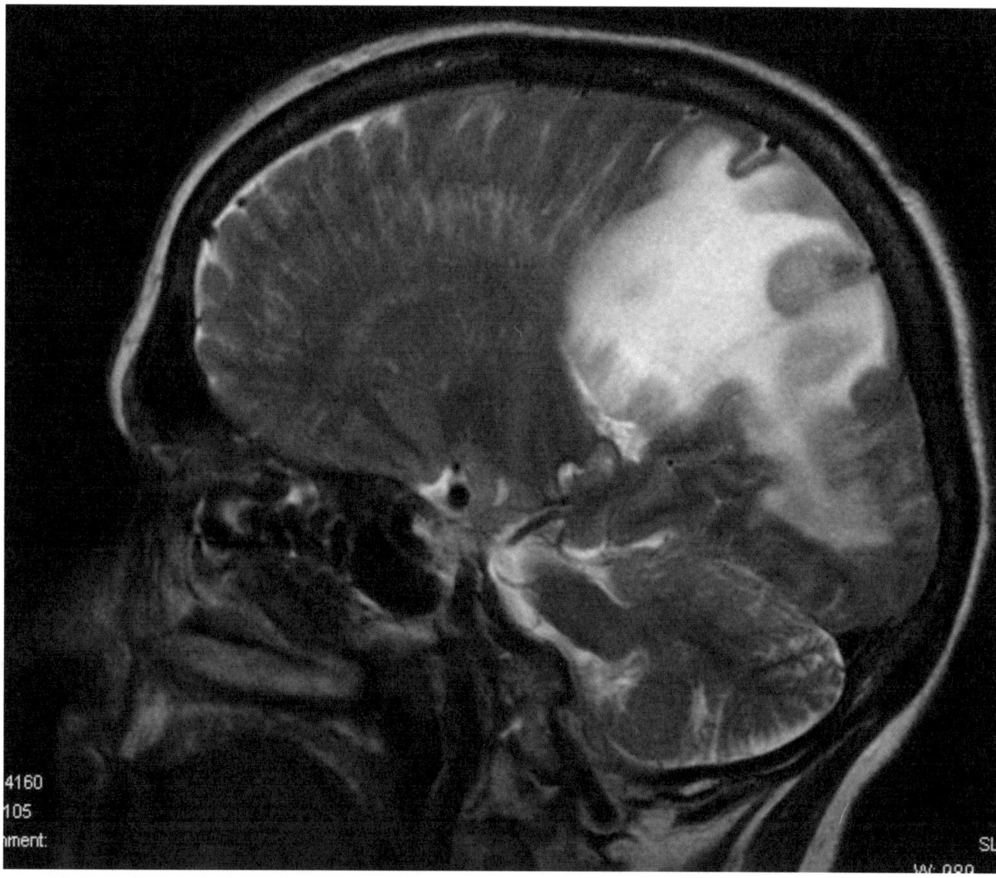

Fig. 1b. Sagittal MRI section, hyperintense lesion on T2 - weighted image.

subcortical white matter. Electroencephalogram (EEG) was diffuse paroxysmal dysrhythmic with focus of slow waves (frequency 2-3 Hz) above the parieto-occipital regions. Laboratory tests revealed hypercholesterolaemia and sideropenic anemia, as well as increased erythrocyte *sedimentation rate* (ESR) and fibrinogen levels, while complete blood cells count, electrolites, tests of liver and renal function, as well as other biochemical tests were within normal levels. After one month patient was transferred to our institution in order to perform stereotactic biopsy and pathohistological verification. In the meantime antihypertensive and antiedematous therapy was introduced with gradual normalization of blood pressure levels (130/80 mm Hg) and significant improvement of neurological status, with only discrete residual left hemiparesis. Control brain MRI revealed unexpected regression of the formerly described white matter lesion. MR spectroscopy verified increased levels of choline in the described area, with the inversion of the choline/creatine ratio, but with preserved values of *N-acetylaspartate* (NAA), and preserved NAA/choline ratio. In cerebrospinal fluid there were 5 lymphocytes/mm3, 0.29 g/L of total proteins, oligoclonal bands were negative. Immunological blood tests were normal, as well as analysis of serum and cerebrospinal fluid on Borrelia burgdorferi, neurotropic viruses including HIV, syphilis, tuberculosis, mycosis, and serum on hepatitis.

Carcinoembryonic antigen (CEA), Ca 19.9, Ca 15.3, Ca 125, neuron specific enolase (NSE), CYFRA 21-1 were also negative, as well as findings of paraneoplastic antibodies (anti-Hu, anti-Yo and anti-Ri). Finding of visual evoked potentials pointed to neuronal lesion of the both optic pathways. Control EEG was diffuse paroxysmal dysrhythmic. Considering all mentioned findings, especially finding of the brain MRI and MR spectroscopy, which points to the leukoencephalopathy of vascular genesis (arterial hypertension), and improvement in neurological status, initially diagnosis of brain tumour was rejected and we did not proceed with the planned stereotactic brain biopsy.

Control brain MRI performed after three months pointed to further regression of the described white matter lesion. At the moment patient is clinically stable and has normal neurological status. Brain MRI performed in October 2010 pointed to complete regression of the white matter lesion.

3. Discussion

Diagnostic criteria of the reversible posterior leukoencephalopathy syndrome include clinical and neuroradiological findings. Very often clinical manifestations are altered consciousness, headache, seizures and vision disturbances (1). According to the literature data, all patients do not develop all mentioned clinical symptoms. Our patient developed all mentioned clinical symptoms except seizures, however, she also had motorical weakness - left hemiparesis.

Neuroradiological findings include reversible abnormalities of the white matter of the brain which present as hypodense areas on the brain CT, or hypointense areas on the T1-weighted images, hyperintense areas on the T2-weighted and FLAIR ("fluid-attenuated inversion recovery") brain MR images, and isointense areas on the DWI ("diffusion-weighted imaging") sequences, which all points to vasogenic edema (15, 16). Neuroradiological findings of the patient described in this paper correspond with the findings in the literature - edema was localized predominantly in the parieto-occipital brain regions. Although in most of the cases distribution of edema is symmetrical, there are cases with asymmetrical lesion localisation, as it was in the case of our patient.

Involvement of grey matter and other brain regions including brainstem, cerebellum, basal ganglia and frontal lobes has also been described in the literature (17).

The pathophysiology of RPLS appears to be multifactorial. The mechanism of the syndrome is a brain-capillary leak syndrome related to hypertension, fluid retention, and possibly the cytotoxic effects of immunosuppressive agents on the vascular endothelium. Severe hypertension per se is perhaps the most common cause. The sudden elevation in blood pressure exceeds the auto-regulatory capacity of the brain vasculature. A region of vasodilatation and vasoconstriction develops, especially in the arterial boundary zone, and there is breakdown of the blood-brain barrier with transudation of fluid and petechial hemorrhage. In experimental rats that were made suddenly hypertensive, these signs appeared and disappeared suddenly, within hours after relieving hypertension, suggesting the functional vascular changes and vasogenic edema. There is rapid resolution of clinical signs and symptoms and imaging abnormalities of reversible posterior leukoencephalopathy when blood pressure is lowered in such patients. While the reversibility of such vasogenic edema is most characteristic, it should be noted that it might result in permanent neurological deficit and cerebral infarct. Uremic encephalopathies represent additional etiologies of RPLS that have a greater tendency for central distribution for unknown reason.

The predilection for the more posterior involvement in leukoencephalopathy may be due to relatively fewer sympathetic innervations in the posterior cerebral vasculature, which helps auto-regulate the cerebral vessels during an acute rise in blood pressure. The calcarine and paramedian occipital lobe structures are usually spared. This distinguishes RPLS from bilateral infarction of the posterior cerebral artery territory. Simultaneous bilateral infarction of the posterior cerebral artery territory occurs in patients with embolism to the rostral basilar artery, but with "top of the basilar embolism" the calcarine regions are invariably involved and often there are accompanying thalamic and midbrain infarcts. It has been observed that an incorrect diagnosis of gliomatosis cerebri, progressive multifocal leukoencephalopathy, demyelinating disease, or infarction may be advanced on the basis of MRI, if all aspects of the clinical presentation are not mentioned to the radiologist. This may result in unnecessary invasive therapy and biopsies. In most cases the leukoencephalopathy is reversible within 1-2 weeks. However, prolonged seizure, hypertension, or both may result in permanent neurological deficit and cerebral infarction. The multiple cerebral infarctions may result in early dementia. A few patients may not recover completely or may have neurodevelopmental sequelae (18, 19).

The role of the immunosuppressive therapy in the etiology of this syndrome is not so clear. According to the literature data, immunosuppressive or cytotoxic agents can cause this syndrome by toxic effect on the vascular endothelial cells or directly causing axonal damage (6,7,19,20).

After extensive diagnostic evaluation that excluded brain tumour that was initially suspected, as well as other factors that could cause leukoencephalopathy such as systemic tissue diseases, renal diseases, inflammatory diseases and malignant diseases, we believe that the main cause of development of reversible posterior leukoencephalopathy syndrome in our patient was arterial hypertension, respectively abrupt and severe increase of arterial blood pressure. That supports improvement of clinical symptoms after correction of blood pressure, as well as finding of MR spectroscopy.

4. Conclusion

Early recognizing of the reversible posterior leukoencephalopathy syndrome is of great importance, because prompt regulation of elevated blood pressure, or in certain cases decreasing of dose or discontinuing immunosuppressive therapy , that is treatment of specific causes, can improve clinical condition of the patient and cause complete regression of the lesion of the brain white matter. Great importance has the fact that the proper diagnosis, and distinction from expansive process, can stop invasive diagnostic procedures. If in some cases we suspect that patient could have reversible posterior leukoencephalopathy, it is better to wait few weeks and then repeat brain MRI before the patient undergoes to the invasive diagnostic procedure such as stereotactic brain biopsy.

5. References

[1] Hinchey J, Chaves C, Appignani B et al. A reversible posterior leukoencephalopathy syndrome. *N Engl J Med* 1996; 334: 494–500.

[2] Delanty N, Vaughan C, Frucht S, Stubgen P. Erythropoietin associated hypertensive posterior leukoencephalopathy. *Neurology* 1997;49:686–9.
[3] Ito Y, Niwa H, Iida T et al. Post-transfusion reversible posterior leukoencephalopathy syndrome with cerebral vasoconstriction. *Neurology* 1997;49:1174–5.
[4] Laguna P, Martin T, Marchena MJ, Moya M. Posterior leukoencephalopathy reversible syndrome secondary to panarteritis nodosa. *Med Clin (Barc)* 1997;109:397–8.
[5] Mathy I, Gille M, van Raemdonck F et al. Neurological complications of intravenous immunoglobulin (IVIG) therapy: An illustrative case of acute encephalopathy following IVIG therapy and a review of the literature. *Acta Neurol Belg* 1998;98:347-51.
[6] Edwards MJ, Walker R, Vinnicombe S et al. Reversible posterior leukoencephalopathy syndrome following CHOP chemotherapy for diffuse large B- cell lymphoma. *Ann Oncol* 2001;12:1327–9.
[7] Gimenez-Mesa E, Martinez-Salio A, Porta-Etessam J et al. Reversible posterior leukoencephalopathy in a patient with non-Hodgkin's lymphoma after treatment with CHOP. *An Med Interna* 2001;18:591–3.
[8] Utz N, Kinkel B, Hedde JP, Bewermeyer H. MR imaging of acute intermittent porphyria mimicking reversible posterior leukoencephalopathy syndrome. N*euroradiology* 2001;43:1059-62.
[9] Ozyurek H, Oguz G, Ozen S et al. Reversible posterior leukoencephalopathy syndrome: report of three cases. *J Child Neurol* 2005;20:990-3.
[10] Cassano G, Góngora V, Zunino A, Roverano S, Paira S. Reversible posterior leukoencephalopathy in systemic lupus erythematosus with thrombotic thrombocytopenic purpura. *J Clin Rheumatol* 2007;13:55-7.
[11] Bas DF, Oguz KK, Topcuoglu MA. Atypical reversible posterior leukoencephalopathy syndrome in thrombotic thrombocytopenic purpura. *Intern Med* 2008; 47:1931-4.
[12] El Karoui K, Le Quintrec M, Dekeyser E, Et al. Posterior reversible encephalopathy syndrome in systemic lupus erythematosus. *Nephrol Dial Transplant* 2008; 23: 757-63.
[13] Ergün T, Lakadamyalı H, Yılmaz A. Recurrent posterior reversible encephalopathy syndrome in a hypertensive patient with end-stage renal disease. *Diagn Interv Radiol* 2008; 14:182–5.
[14] Ahn KJ, You WJ, Jeong SL, et al. Atypical manifestations of reversible posterior leukoencephalopathy syndrome: findings on diffusion imaging and ADC mapping. *Neuroradiology* 2004; 46:978–83.
[15] Lee VH, Wijdicks EF, Manno EM, Rabinstein AA. Clinical spectrum of reversible posterior leukoencephalopathy syndrome. *Arch Neurol* 2008;65:205-10.
[16] Ay H, Buonanno FS, Schaefer PW, et al. Posterior leukoencephalopathy without severe hypertension: Utility of diffusion weighted MRI. *Neurology* 1998;51:1369–76.
[17] Schwartz RB, Jones KM, Kalina P, et al. Hypertensive encephalopathy: Findings on CT, MR imaging and SPECT imaging in 14 cases. *AJR Am J Roentgenol* 1992;159:379–83.
[18] Sundt T. The cerebral autonomic nervous system: A proposed physiologic function and pathophysiologic response in subarachnoid hemorrhage and in focal cerebral ischemia. *Mayo Clin Proc* 1973;48:127–37.
[19] Garg RK. Posterior leukoencephalopathy syndrome. *Postgrad Med J* 2001; 77: 24-8.
[20] Noda K, Fukae J, Fujishima K, Mori K, Urabe T, Hattori N, Okuma Y. Reversible cerebral vasoconstriction syndrome presenting as subarachnoid hemorrhage, reversible posterior leukoencephalopathy, and cerebral infarction. *Intern Med.* 2011;50(11):1227-33.

18

Brain Tumor and Seizures: Incidence, Pathophysiology, Diagnosis and Treatment

Elysia James and Panayiotis N. Varelas
Henry Ford Hospital, Detroit
United States

1. Introduction

Seizures can arise as a complication of a number of disease states such as metabolic abnormalities, intoxication or withdrawal from drugs, acute trauma, infection; the list is exhaustive (Delanty, Vaughan et al. 1998). One of the most common causes of seizures is indeed the presence of a brain tumor. Seizures present a preventative, diagnostic and management challenge for a number of reasons in this situation. The drugs used for treatment may interfere with chemotherapy, may produce untoward cognitive or medical side effects, and may not even reach the intended target since the blood brain barrier may be pathologic in the abnormal environment of the tumor. The many genetic and pathological variations in tumor type may further impact therapies aimed at treating seizures in this setting. Further complicating this scenario is the post-operative management of these patients, which may occur in an ICU most complex environment. This chapter will review contemporary issues in pathophysiology, clinical presentation, complications, treatment, and outcomes of seizures associated with brain tumors.

2. Incidence

Overall, the incidence of brain tumors is 4% in patients with epilepsy (van Breemen, Wilms et al. 2007). On the other hand, seizures complicate the natural history in 30-70% of patients with a primary tumor. (LeBlanc 1974; McKeran 1980; Cascino 1990; Bartolomei 1997). About 40% of all the patients with metastatic brain tumors will have a seizure during their disease (Simonescu 1960; Cohen 1988). Half of these seizures will be simple or partial complex seizures and the other half secondary generalized seizures (Ketz 1974; Moots 1995). Some tumors, like DNETs and gangliogliomas, with significantly higher seizure frequencies, have been associated with intrinsic epileptogenic properties. Among the primary brain tumors, the higher incidence of seizures is found in patients with oligodendroglioma (92%) and dysembryoplastic neuroectodermal tumors (DNET, 100%) (van Breemen, Wilms et al. 2007). Melanoma, choriocarcinoma, lung cancer and breast cancer are tumors frequently metastasizing to the brain and associated with hemorrhage and seizures. Among metastatic tumors, melanoma seems to have the highest incidence of seizures. Conversely, based on a study from the Cleveland Clinic, among patients with intractable chronic epilepsy the most common types of tumors discovered are ganglioglioma [in 49/127 (39%) of cases] and low grade astrocytoma [in 48/127 (38%) of cases] (Morris 1996). Pleomorphic xanthoastrocytoma, dysembryoplastic neuroectodermal tumors, and oligodendroglioma are also tumors frequently associated with chronic epilepsy. Overall, it seems likely that low grade, well-differentiated gliomas have higher incidence of seizures than more aggressive glioblastomas or anaplastic astrocytomas (Beaumont 2000; van Breemen, Wilms et al. 2007). The location of the brain tumor also plays a role in the incidence of seizures, because different brain areas are characterized by varying susceptibility to seizures. For example, among patients with gliomas, seizures occur in 59% of frontal tumors, 42% of parietal tumors, 35% of temporal tumors and 33% of occipital tumors (Scott 1980). Similar observations suggest that the limbic and temporal lobe, primary and supplementary motor (M-I, M-II) areas, primary and secondary somatosensory (S-I, S-II opercula and insula) areas have the lowest thresholds for seizures (Beaumont 2000). In contrast to the other lobes, the occipital lobe has a much higher threshold and lower incidence of seizures (Mahaley 1981). Tumors in the subcortical areas, such as thalamus and posterior fossa, are much less epileptogenic as well.

3. Pathophysiology of seizures in the context of a brain tumor

Although the pathogenic mechanism of epileptogenesis in patients with brain tumors has not been fully elucidated (Beaumont 2000), it can be traced to the cellular workings and intercellular connections within the nervous system. A better understanding of these processes may provide new therapeutic targets not just for tumors, but for improved seizure control. There are many theories behind the cause of seizures in patients with brain tumors. To complicate the matter, different types of tumors may cause seizures through different mechanisms. In the late 1950's Echlin proposed that brain tumors are cause partial isolation and deafferentation of the cerebral cortex, resulting in denervation hypersensitivity (Echlin 1959). More recent studies have focused on molecular pathobiology and pathophysiology that underlie these lesions and differentiate them from normal tissue. There are differences in the ion channel profile between normal glial cell types (Patt 1996). Patt et.al used these differences in their study in order to further categorize the properties of oligiodendrogliomas and mixed oligiodendrogliomas in eight patients. Using patch clamp techniques, he postulated that oligiodendrogliomas are dominated by action potential generating cells (Patt 1996). Sodium channels in tumor cells may play a role in epileptogenesis, since these channels are responsible for generating action potentials more frequently than others (Patt 1996; Labrakakis 1997). Normal glial cells have a limited number of sodium channels. It is not difficult to imagine that a tumor with a mixed cellular profile would produce enough sodium channels to allow excitatory circuitry to become the dominant player (Beaumont 2000). There are differences in the pathophysiology between temporal epilepsy and epilepsy in the temporal lobe secondary to seizure kindling (Beaumont 2000). Changes in the extracellular environment, changes in the regulation of inhibitory and excitatory amino acids, responses to amino acids, alterations in glial gap junctions have all been implicated in epileptogenesis (Beaumont 2000). Tumors that tend to cause hemorrhage, necrosis, inflammation and ischemia have a higher incidence of seizures. Focal hypoxia, mass effect and edema, altered levels of excitatory amino acids, all have been postulated to play a role in epileptogenesis. Derangements in the blood-brain barrier (BBB) and its constituents may be another factor that impacts the development and treatment of seizures in brain tumors. Although Marchi et. al in their study using acute disruption of the blood brain barrier(Marchi, Angelov et al. 2007) did not find that the presence of tumor determined the onset of the seizure in their cohort, BBB disruption may be another contribution to an already unstable and pathologic state. The multidrug-resistance gene MDR1 (ABCB1, P-glycoprotein) and multidrug-resistance-related protein (MRP, ABCC1) are expressed in the cells forming many blood-brain and blood-CSF barriers. These genes and proteins contribute to decreased entry of multiple AEDs to the brain parenchyma such as phenytoin, carbamazepine, phenobarbital, lamotrigine and felbamate. These proteins are over-expressed in the cells of patients with glioma (Calatozzolo, Gelati et al. 2005), focal cortical dysplasia and ganglioglioma (Aronica, Gorter et al. 2003). The genetic characteristics of the tumor play a substantial role in their treatment, thereby impacting the treatment of seizures too. Loci 1p and 19q have been implicated in the prognosis of oligiodendrogliomas in a number of studies. (Hata, Shono et al. 2007; Ramirez, Bowman et al. 2010). Despite the advances in research in these key areas of molecular biology, genetics and ion channel function, estimating the individual's susceptibility to the above alterations is still an elusive target.

In addition to primary brain neoplasms, systemic cancer can metastasize to the brain and produce seizures as their first manifestation. The intracranial metastases usually originate from embolization of neoplastic cells to the brain, commonly in terminal arterial supply territories, such as the gray white matter junction. Systemic cancer may induce seizures through additional non-invasive mechanisms: coagulopathy and stroke (sinus thrombosis), non-bacterial thrombotic endocarditis with cerebral emboli, systemic metabolic derangements, such as hypomagnesemia (van de Loosdrecht, Gietema et al. 2000) or hyponatremia (McDonald and Dubose 1993), opportunistic infections after chemotherapy or direct toxicity of chemotherapeutic agents to the brain (Meropol, Creaven et al. 1995; Delanty, Vaughan et al. 1998). Paraneoplastic syndromes, such as limbic encephalopathy with anti Hu antibodies can be associated with seizures preceding the diagnosis of cancer (Dalmau, Graus et al. 1992). EEG or continuous video-EEG may be necessary to evaluate these patients and reach the correct diagnosis (Figure 1).

4. Clinical presentation

Seizures are one of the most common presentations in patients with brain tumors. A first, unprovoked seizure in an adult is always suggestive of an intracranial tumor, until proven otherwise (Ropper 2009). As a sign, seizures may accompany other vague, non-localizing symptoms such as apathy, irritability, altered mental status, dizziness (Ropper 2009), as well as signs of increased intracranial pressure, such as diplopia, nausea, headache and decreased visual acuity.

Several seizure types have been reported and mainly reflect the location of the lesion. Parasagittal meningiomas may present with generalized seizures when located in the anterior one third of the sagittal sinus, whereas meningiomas of the middle third usually present with focal seizures, at times following a Jacksonian marching pattern. Simple or partial seizures characterized by olfactory, gustatory and epigastric auras, depersonalization, feelings of fear or pleasure, are usually an indication of temporal lobe pathology. Complex partial seizures with repetitive psychomotor movements, impairment of consciousness or déjà-vu phenomena are also associated with the temporal lobe. Delusions and psychotic behaviour have been reported with frontal lobe tumors (Sato, Takeichi et al. 1993). Lesions involving the frontal eye fields are associated with turning of the eyes and head to one side (contraversive or ipsiversive, depending on the side of turning compared to the lesion and the timing of the observation, ie ictal vs interictal). Parietal lobe tumors are associated with sensory seizures and occipital lobe tumors can cause seizures with lights, colors, and geometric patterns (Ropper 2009). Even non-neoplastic mass lesions may have seizures as a part of their clinical presentation. The classic example is gelastic seizures in hypothalamic hamartomas (Addas, Sherman et al. 2008; Striano, Striano et al. 2009).

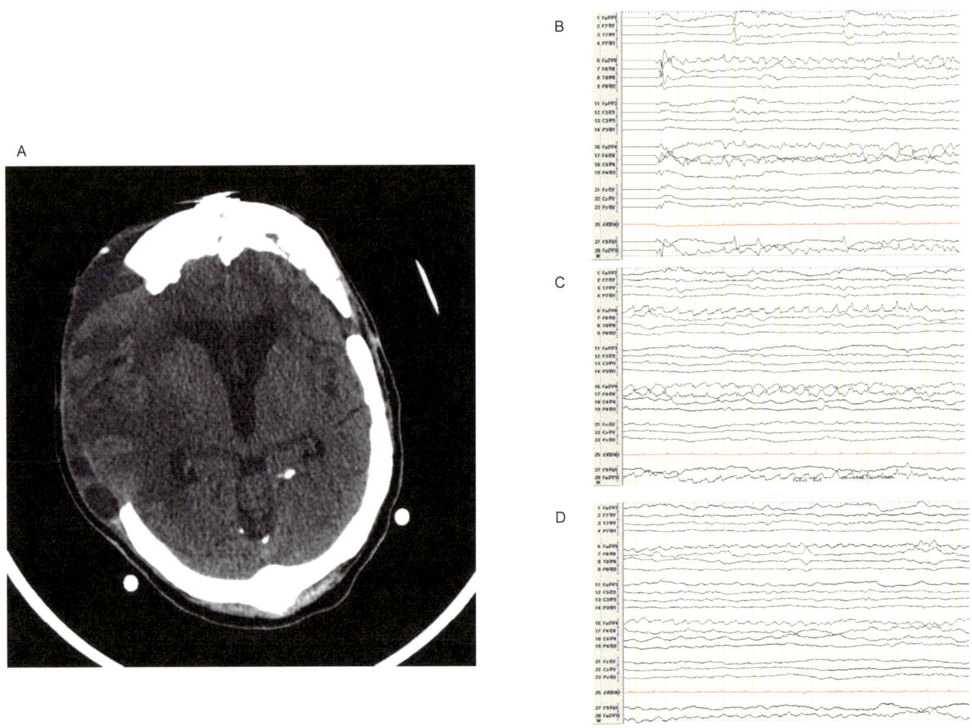

Fig. 1. 57 year old woman, history of multiple resections of reccuren right frontal meningioma, with altered mental status, in non-convulsive status epilepticus. The seizures were treated successfully with multiple anti-epileptic medications including a midazolam drip. (a) CT brain without contrast, evidence of encephalomalacia in the resection cavity with increased edema. (b) start of ictal activity in the frontal derivations (F2, F4, F8) consistent with the region of the prior meningioma resection (c) evolution of the ictal activity into non-convulsive status epilepticus (d) end of ictal activity.

4.1 Status epilepticus

Status epilepticus (SE) can also occur in patients with brain tumors, either convulsive or non-convulsive. In a recent study from the University of Virginia, 555 patients were admitted with a diagnosis of SE over a 7-year period. Fifty patients had a concurrent diagnosis of cancer, 28 (5%) of whom had SE related to the tumor or its treatment (Cavaliere, Farace et al. 2006). SE occurs either at the time of tumor diagnosis (29%) or during tumor progression (23%). However, an almost equal percentage of SE occurred while the tumor was stable (23%) in a recent study (Cavaliere, Farace et al. 2006). Because some tumors present with non-convulsive seizures or non-convulsive status epilepticus (NCSE), a clinical presentation of decreased or altered mental status, should not be primarily attributed to the tumor. An evaluation with EEG should be undertaken to exclude NCSE, that may be amenable to treatment. Drislane reported 6 patients with systemic cancer, whose EEGs showed NCSE. Three patients were confused, and the other three were stuporous or comatose. The possibility of paraneoplastic encephalopathy was raised in 3 of them. Antiepileptic treatment led to an improved mental status in four of these patients (Drislane 1994). Five patients out of 84 (6%) with cancer and altered mental status (coma or delirium) were found to be on NCSE by EEG in another study from Italy. None of these patients had brain metastases: one was aphasic, 2 patients treated with ifosfamide had absence and 2 patients treated with cisplatin complex partial status epilepticus. All had rapid recovery after antiepileptic treatment (Cocito, Audenino et al. 2001). In a recent study, four patients never diagnosed before with metastatic CNS disease presented with altered mental status. All patients had abnormal neuroimaging of the brain, were in NCSE by EEG and were treated with fosphenytoin IV. In 2 patients the NCSE resolved, but in the other two, despite an initial mental status improvement, status recurred and both eventually died after 5 and 20 days, respectively (Blitshteyn and Jaeckle 2006).

5. Diagnosis

In most cases, seizures can be easily diagnosed, if they present as convulsions. However, other paroxysmal or repetitive movements can occur in patients with intracranial pathology, such as extrapyramidal tremor, clonus, blepharospasm, fasciculations, shivering or posturing and occasionally this may lead to confusion, especially if a physician or nurse is not present during their occurrence. On the other hand, many epileptic phenomena are non-convulsive and can present with a pleiade of symptoms and signs, including confusion, blank starring, fugue, subtle (and frequently unnoticeable) twitching of the face or eyelids or nystagmus. The routine electroencephalogram may not catch any of these events or may be compromised by movement artifacts. In this case of uncertainty, we recommend a continuous video-EEG monitoring lasting for few hours to a day. If the events are recorded and are not epileptic in nature, then the test should be discontinued, otherwise should be extended until a conclusion is reached.

Neuroimaging is also paramount, especially in cases of refractory seizures, to exclude additional pathology than the tumor per se (new bleed, infarction, sinus thrombosis or infection, which can occur in patients undergoing chemotherapy or radiation). A magnetic resonance imaging is considered a better test than computed tomography, since it can reveal smaller anatomical details and differentiate faster between a new stroke vs paralysis due to

Todd's phenomenon. If the patient is actively having seizures or SE, the diffusion-weighted imaging sequence can reveal restricted diffusion in the cortical mantle, where the seizures emanate from. Lastly, a lumbar puncture, performed if there are no signs of hydrocephalus or midline shift, can also infrequently contribute to the diagnosis, by revealing leptomeningeal extension of the tumor, measuring the opening pressure or identifying an infectious agent.

6. Treatment - Issues in management

6.1 Use of anti-epileptic medications

There are several important details regarding the management of these complex patients. One main theme is the understanding that surgical management supersedes medical management. Studies have shown that resection of the epileptogenic zone due to brain tumors may lead to seizure freedom or significant control of seizures in 70-90% of patients (Britton, Cascino et al. 1994; Zentner, Hufnagel et al. 1997).

Medication interactions are a very important problem and can lead to difficulties in compliance, tolerance and side effects. Most patients are on a regimen of antiepileptic drugs (AEDs), radiation therapy and chemotherapy. Antiepileptics, especially those affecting the cytochrome P450 system, may affect the metabolism of chemotherapeutic agents. These agents have a narrow therapeutic window and real potential for toxicity or lethal side effects. Usually, the addition of phenytoin, carbamazepine, phenobarbital and other inducers, reduces the levels or efficacy of cyclophosphamide, methotrexate, adriamycin, nitrosoureas, paclitaxel, etoposide, topotecan, irinotecan, thiotepa and corticosteroids (Glantz, Cole et al. 2000; Patsalos, Froscher et al. 2002). Valproic acid, being an inhibitor, can have the opposite effect and increase the chemotherapeutic agents' levels. In addition, competition for binding to plasma proteins may be important with several of those medications. Choosing an appropriate anti-epileptic for patients with brain tumors involves more than adequate control of seizures. The appropriate use of certain AEDs can alleviate other symptoms of brain neoplasm, including pain, depression, anxiety, and weight gain. Because of their intrinsic mechanism of action, AED may be uniquely qualified to address these additional symptoms. There are multiple studies in both the Psychiatric and Neuroncology literature to support the use of AEDs for symptoms related to depression, anxiety, and pain (Thompson, Takeshita et al. 2006).

An interesting aspect of the antiepileptic drug use in patients with cancer is their potential for antineoplastic or immunosuppressive effect (Bardana, Gabourel et al. 1983; Kikuchi, McCormick et al. 1984; Blaheta and Cinatl 2002). Valproate exhibits inherent antitumor activity through inhibition of histone deacetylase. In the treatment of medulloblastoma in children, Li et. al concluded that valproic acid possesses potent in vitro and in vivo antimedulloblastoma activities correlating with induction of histone hyperacetylation and regulation of pathways critical for maintaining growth inhibition and cell cycle arrest (Li, Shu et al. 2005). Pregabalin, a newer agent was found in a small study to be effective as monotherapy, encouraging the study authors to do a larger prospective study (Novy, Stupp et al. 2009). Gabapentin in another small study was postulated to interact with a leucine binding site to reduce seizures in a group of 14 patients (Perry and Sawka 1996).Anti-epileptic medications, and their many applications, are a unique area of further research in the world of brain tumors. This is an area where individualized treatment is of paramount importance. One should take into account the histopathology of the tumor, the location of the mass, the presence of pre-existing epilepsy, the extent of additional injury incurred by craniotomy, the involvement of other important organs metabolizing the drugs, the nutritional state of the patient, the pharmacological interactions between the agents and the ability of the patient to tolerate side effects of the treatment.

6.2 Side effects of antiepileptic medications

The adverse interactions between AEDs and chemotherapy are often related to enzyme induction by the former (Pursche, Schleyer et al. 2008). Major offenders include carbamazepine, phenytoin, phenobarbital, primidone, and valproic acid (Ruggiero, Rizzo et al. 2010). Interaction between antiepileptics and irradiation treatment offered to the brain or spine may lead to dermatologic complications. Skin rash in patients treated with phenytoin and brain irradiation may herald Stevens-Johnson syndrome (Cockey, Amann et al. 1996; Eralp, Aydiner et al. 2001). One retrospective study, however, of 289 patients with brain tumors treated with antiepileptics and radiation found only one (0.3%) patient who developed erythema multiforme. Phenytoin was associated with milder rashes in 22% of patients, a higher incidence than the usual 5-10%. These rashes did not appear to have a temporal relation to radiation, because they usually occurred before its initiation (Mamon, Wen et al. 1999). Valproic acid has been implicated in Rowell's syndrome - lupus erythematosus associated with erythema multiforme-like lesions (Esteve, Favre et al. 2002).

6.3 Prophylactic treatment with antiepileptic medications

The issue of prophylactic treatment of patients with brain tumors is very complex. If a seizure has already occurred, there is little doubt for the value of antiepileptics (Glantz, Cole et al. 2000), but when the patient has never exhibited epileptic phenomena, such a treatment becomes more controversial. Efficacy of the treatment has to be balanced with adverse events associated with the chosen drugs. Despite the best efforts, a significant percentage of patients still have breakthrough seizures and the response to the treatment is very unpredictable. Several reasons have to be considered: (1) inability of the AED to address or correct the vast range of physiologic derangements induced by brain tumors, (2) difficulty maintaining appropriate antiepileptic levels and (Lee, Wen et al.) tumor progression or recurrence (Beaumont 2000; Schaller and Ruegg 2003). Therefore, it is not surprising that there is conflicting literature regarding the use of anticonvulsants in this clinical setting. The design of the study (prospective or retrospective, randomized and blinded or not), the uniformity of the tumors studied (AEDs against a certain type of tumor or against tumors of various pathologies and locations), the drugs used (older or newer AEDs), the comparison arm (placebo vs another AED), the dose utilized (with or without a loading dose, based on ideal or unadjusted patient weight), the timing of the administration (pre-, intra- or postoperatively), the adjustment of the dose based on AED levels (total or free, depending on levels of albumin and their binding to it), the concurrent administration of other medications that can affect the AED levels (such as chemotherapy or steroids), all these are factors that play a role in the results and conclusions and contribute to the confusion. Early studies were in agreement that prophylaxis against seizure was very important. In the 80's, Kvam et al. from Columbia Presbyterian Hospital in New York, reported only 5 patients having preoperative seizures out of 538 who underwent craniotomy. The authors suggested a preoperative loading dose of 10mg/kg of phenytoin, followed by a postoperative dose of 5mg/kg/day (Kvam 1983). In a double-blind, randomized study of phenytoin (100 mg tid) vs placebo in 281 post-craniotomy patients, the phenytoin group had significantly less seizures (12.9% vs 18.4%) and highest protection was present between days 7 and 72. Routine prophylaxis with phenytoin (in a dosage of 5 to 6 mg/kg/day) was recommended by the authors in high-risk patients post craniotomy. They also recommended that treatment should be started 1 week preoperatively and therapeutic levels of phenytoin should be maintained (North, Penhall et al. 1983). In another study, 374 patients post-craniotomy were randomized to receive phenytoin (15 mg/kg IV during surgery, followed by 3-6 mg/kg/day for 3 days) or placebo (Lee 1989). The group receiving phenytoin had two early postoperative seizures and the placebo nine, but the difference was not statistically significant. Eighty percent of the seizures occurred within twenty minutes after surgery. Thus, the authors recommended that prophylactic anticonvulsant medication be given at least 20 minutes before completion of wound closure. In a subsequent Italian study, 65/128 (51%) patients with supratentorial brain tumors had preoperative seizures and were treated with antiepileptic drugs. Those without preoperative seizures, were randomized to receive phenobarbital or phenytoin as prophylactic treatment or no treatment. No significant difference in seizure incidence was found between patients treated (7%) and those not treated (18%). The authors suggested short-term preventive antiepileptic treatment after surgery in patients without preoperative seizures and continuation of postoperative treatment in patients with preoperative epilepsy (Franceschetti, Binelli et al. 1990). This view was not shared by the authors of a subsequent large study, who did not recommend prophylactic antiepileptics after supratentorial craniotomy. In this study, 276 post-craniotomy patients were randomized to receive carbamazepine or phenytoin for six or 24 months, or no treatment (Foy, Chadwick et al. 1992). The three treatment groups did not overall differ in the risk of seizures, but there was a non-significant 10% reduction of seizures in the two groups which received antiepileptic medications. Meningiomas had the highest risk for seizures (75% by 4 years) and pituitary tumors the lowest (21% by 4 years). Longer operations, those associated with dissection of the lesion away from the surface of the brain and left-sided or bilateral lesions also carried a higher risk. Early seizures (within one week) after craniotomy did not increase the likelihood of late epilepsy. Based on these data, prophylactic anticonvulsants could not be recommended by the authors routinely following supratentorial craniotomy. Additional conflicting data comes from the results of a prospective, stratified, randomised, double-blind Dutch study, comparing 300 mg phenytoin/day to 1500 mg valproate/day given for 1 year in one hundred post craniotomy patients. Fourteen patients had postoperative seizures, but there was no difference in seizure incidence between the two groups (Beenen, Lindeboom et al. 1999). Finally, a meta-analysis of six controlled studies addressing the issue showed a tendency of prophylactic antiepileptics to prevent postoperative convulsions in patients without pre-existing seizures, but this effect did not reach statistical significance.(Kuijlen, Teernstra et al. 1996).

There are also studies looking at anti-epileptics other than phenytoin. Glantz et al. conducted a well designed randomized, double-blind, placebo-controlled study comparing the incidence of first seizures in 74 valproate and placebo-treated patients with newly diagnosed supratentorial brain tumors. The drug and placebo groups did not differ significantly in the incidence of seizures [35% in the valproate and 24% in the placebo treated group (odds ratio 1.7, 95% CI 0.6-4.6, p = 0.3)]. Based on these results no prophylactic treatment with valproate could be recommended (Glantz, Cole et al. 1996). In a large retrospective analysis of 195 patients with metastatic brain tumors, Cohen et al. reported that 18% of patients presented with seizures. Of the remaining seizure-free patients, 40% were treated prophylactically with antiepileptics (phenytoin in > 90%). In a follow-up period of up to 59 weeks, 10% of patients developed late seizures. The incidence of seizures did not differ between treated (13.1%) and untreated (11.1%) groups. However, this study is flawed by the fact that two third of patients with seizures had sub-therapeutic antiepileptic levels. The authors did not advocate antiepileptic use, unless the patient has the first seizure (Cohen 1988). More recently, a meta-analysis evaluated 5 trials with the following inclusion criteria: (1) patients with a neoplasm, (2) either primary glial tumors, cerebral metastases or meningiomas, (3) no history of epilepsy. These patients were randomized to either an antiepileptic drug or placebo. The three antiepileptics studied were phenobarbital, phenytoin, and valproic acid. This meta-analysis confirmed the lack of antiepileptic benefit at one week and at six months of follow-up. In addition, the antiepileptics had no effect on seizure prevention for specific tumor pathology (Sirven, 2004 #83). Moreover, there is growing evidence supporting increased frequency and severity of side effects from antiepileptics in this population: in a meta-analysis of studies examining prophylactic treatment in patients with newly diagnosed brain tumors, 23.8% (range 5-38%) of treated patients experienced side-effects that were severe enough to lead to change or discontinuation of the medications. This incidence is higher than that in the general population and should make physicians skeptical regarding use in this setting (Glantz, Cole et al. 2000).

Other important factors frequently playing a role are personal preference, previous training or experience in the decision to prescribe anti-epileptic medications. According to a study conducted in Rhode Island, 55% of participating physicians gave antiepileptic prophylaxis, but the percentage differed according to the subspecialty: 33% of radiation oncologists, 50% of oncologists, 53% of neurologists and 81% of neurosurgeons (Glantz, Cole et al. 1996; Glantz, Cole et al. 2000). One of the most authoritative reports on this subject is the Quality Standards Subcommittee of the American Academy of Neurology, who published a meta-analysis of 12 studies, which had addressed the issue of prophylactic antiepileptic treatment for newly diagnosed brain tumor patients. Four were randomized and 8 were cohorts. Only one study showed significant difference between treated and untreated groups and, actually, favored the untreated. The overall odds ratio from the randomized trials was 1.09, 95% CI 0.63–1.89 ($P = 0.8$) for seizure incidence and 1.03, 0.74-1.44 ($P = 0.9$) for seizure-free survival. Therefore, the Subcommittee recommended no prophylactic use of antiepileptics on patients with newly diagnosed brain tumors. Although not excluding the possibility that some subgroups of brain tumor patients may be at a higher risk for seizures (melanoma, hemorrhagic or multiple metastatic lesions, tumors located near the Rolandic fissure, slow-growing primary CNS tumors), the Subcommittee did not find any reason for prophylaxis in those patients (Glantz, Cole et al. 2000). In the contemporary literature, there are still no concrete answers. A recent review(Kargiotis, Markoula et al. 2011) recommend that short-term anticonvulsant prophylaxis after surgical excision since they found that up to 13% of the patients may experience seizures within the first postoperative week, irrespective of the presence of preoperative seizure history or not. Alternatively guidelines from the American Association of Neurological Surgeons (AANS) and the Congress of Neurological Surgeons (CNS) do not recommend the prophylactic use of antiepileptic drugs to prevent seizures in brain metastases (Mikkelsen, Paleologos et al. 2010).

7. Post-operative complications

Seizures may present at two distinct periods of time in the course of the disease. They can present as one of the initial symptoms or later in the course of the disease during chemotherapy or after surgical intervention (Kargiotis, Markoula et al. 2011). What is the current risk of postoperative seizures in patients with neoplasm? There are no current prospective trials looking at this issue. In the aforementioned study by Kvam et al., 538 patients underwent elective craniotomy. Only 23 of these patients had a post operative seizure. They concluded that in this case-series, the most common risk factor for post-operative seizure was inadequate anticonvulsant prophylaxis. Patients in this series were also noted to have serum sodium level less than 130, which may have played a role in reducing the seizure threshold and is not uncommon in postoperative neurosurgical patients (Kvam 1983). In a case series by Fukamachi, risk factors for post-operative seizures included pre-operative seizures, sites of the lesion, and subtherapeutic anti-convulsants (Fukamachi 1985). In more contemporary studies post-operative seizures are reported in complications for new techniques (Kassam, Engh et al. 2009), and seizure rates retrospectively in specific tumor types (Lwu, Hamilton et al. 2010). Surgical approaches can also determine the risk of post-operative seizures. In a study conducted in Mayo clinic, Milligan et. al, retrospectively analyzed 197 patients comparing transcallosal approach to a transcortical approach for resection of an intraventricular lesion. They found that patients undergoing the transcallosal approach had a 4.4 fold increase in the risk of seizure (Milligan and Meyer 2010).

Seizures may also compromise the airway, cause limb injuries or structural brain injury, possibly predisposing the patient to more seizures or even status epilepticus (Deutschman 1985). Seizures can also cause cerebral acidosis, cerebral edema and further elevations of the intracranial pressure (which may already be elevated), all of them challenging the compensatory mechanisms of the brain (Lee 1989). Metabolic disturbances, such as hyponatremia or hypernatremia, hypoxia, pain-induced hyperventilation and hyperglycemia that are frequently noted postoperatively may also contribute to increased seizure frequency and should be treated aggressively.

8. Outcomes

Against easy assumptions, there is data supporting a better outcome in patients with brain tumors and seizures (Beaumont 2000). Despite complicating the course of the disease process in a brain neoplasm, seizures are actually among the factors that may improve patient outcome (Chandana, Movva et al. 2008), although this view may not be shared by all experts. In a retrospective analysis of 560 patients with primary supratentorial tumors, the median survival of the 164 (29%) patients presenting with epilepsy was 37 months compared to 6 months of those presenting with other symptoms ($P < 0.0001$) (Smith, Hutton et al. 1991). In the study by Whittle and Beaumont of 34 supratentorial oligodendrogliomas, 17% of patients who presented with seizures and 67% of those who presented with other symptoms had died in the follow-up. However, in a multivariate model, young age and not epilepsy was a favorable independent predictor (Whittle 1995). In a recent study of 35 patients with SE, 8 (23%) died within 30 days after the status. More patients with systemic cancer (50%) than with primary brain tumors (14%) died within 30 days, implying that the tumor histology is a more important factor for mortality than SE (Cavaliere, Farace et al. 2006).

9. Conclusions

Anti-epileptic medications, and their many applications, are a unique area of further research in the world of brain tumors. This is an area where individualized treatment is of paramount importance. One should take into account the histopathology of the tumor, the location of the mass, the presence of pre-existing epilepsy, the extent of additional injury incurred by craniotomy, the involvement of other important organs metabolizing the drugs, the nutritional state of the patient, the pharmacological interactions between the agents and the ability of the patient to tolerate side effects of the treatment. Future areas of research include pain control, synergistic interplay between anti-epileptics and chemotherapeutic agents, and mood stabilization.

10. Abbreviations

DNET - dysembryoplastic neuroepithelial/neuroectodermal Tumor
MDR – multi-drug resistant
AED – anti-epileptic drug
EEG - Electroencephalogram
SE – status epilepticus
NCSE – non-convulsive status epilepticus
CNS – central nervous system

11. References

Addas, B., E. M. Sherman, et al. (2008). Surgical management of hypothalamic hamartomas in patients with gelastic epilepsy. *Neurosurg Focus* 25(3): E8.

Aronica, E., J. A. Gorter, et al. (2003). Expression and cellular distribution of multidrug transporter proteins in two major causes of medically intractable epilepsy: focal cortical dysplasia and glioneuronal tumors. *Neuroscience* 118(2): 417-429.

Bardana, E. J., Jr., J. D. Gabourel, et al. (1983). Effects of phenytoin on man's immunity. Evaluation of changes in serum immunoglobulins, complement, and antinuclear antibody. *Am J Med* 74(2): 289-296.

Bartolomei, J., Christopher, S, Vives, K, Spencer, DD, Piepmeier, JM (1997). Low grade gliomas of chronic epilepsy: a distinct clinical and pathological entity. *J Neurooncol* 34: 79-84.

Beaumont, A., Whittle,IR (2000). The pathogenesis of tumor associated epilepsy. *Acta Neurochir* 142: 1-15.

Beenen, L. F., J. Lindeboom, et al. (1999). Comparative double blind clinical trial of phenytoin and sodium valproate as anticonvulsant prophylaxis after craniotomy: efficacy, tolerability, and cognitive effects. *J Neurol Neurosurg Psychiatry* 67(4): 474-480.

Blaheta, R. A. and J. Cinatl, Jr. (2002). Anti-tumor mechanisms of valproate: a novel role for an old drug. *Med Res Rev* 22(5): 492-511.

Blitshteyn, S. and K. A. Jaeckle (2006). Nonconvulsive status epilepticus in metastatic CNS disease. *Neurology* 66(8): 1261-1263.

Britton, J. W., G. D. Cascino, et al. (1994). Low-grade glial neoplasms and intractable partial epilepsy: efficacy of surgical treatment. *Epilepsia* 35(6): 1130-1135.

Calatozzolo, C., M. Gelati, et al. (2005). Expression of drug resistance proteins Pgp, MRP1, MRP3, MRP5 and GST-pi in human glioma. *J Neurooncol* 74(2): 113-121.

Cascino , G. (1990). Epilepsy and Brain Tumors: implications to treatment. *Epilepsia* 31(Suppl 3): S37-44.

Cavaliere, R., E. Farace, et al. (2006). Clinical implications of status epilepticus in patients with neoplasms. *Arch Neurol* 63(12): 1746-1749.

Chandana, S. R., S. Movva, et al. (2008). Primary brain tumors in adults. *Am Fam Physician* 77(10): 1423-1430.

Cocito, L., D. Audenino, et al. (2001). Altered mental state and nonconvulsive status epilepticus in patients with cancer. *Arch Neurol* 58(8): 1310.

Cockey, G. H., S. T. Amann, et al. (1996). Stevens-Johnson syndrome resulting from whole-brain radiation and phenytoin. *Am J Clin Oncol* 19(1): 32-34.

Cohen, N., Strauss,G, Lew,R, Silver,R, Recht, L (1988). Should prophylactic anticolvusants be administered to patients with newly diagnosed cerebral metastases? A retrospective analysis. *J Clin Oncol* 6: 1621-1624.

Dalmau, J., F. Graus, et al. (1992). Anti-Hu--associated paraneoplastic encephalomyelitis/sensory neuronopathy. A clinical study of 71 patients. *Medicine (Baltimore)* 71(2): 59-72.

Delanty, N., C. J. Vaughan, et al. (1998). Medical causes of seizures. *Lancet* 352(9125): 383-390.

Deutschman, C., Haines,SJ (1985). Anticonvulsant prophylaxis in neurological surgery. *Neurosurgery* 17: 510-516.

Drislane, F. W. (1994). Nonconvulsive status epilepticus in patients with cancer. *Clin Neurol Neurosurg* 96(4): 314-318.

Echlin, F. (1959). The supersensitivity of chronically isolated cerebral cortex as a mechanism in focal epilepsy. *Electroencephalog Clin Neurophysiol* 11: 697-732.

Eralp, Y., A. Aydiner, et al. (2001). Stevens-Johnson syndrome in a patient receiving anticonvulsant therapy during cranial irradiation. *Am J Clin Oncol* 24(4): 347-350.

Esteve, E., A. Favre, et al. (2002). [Post-radiotherapy eruption in a patient treated with valproic acid. Rowell's syndrome?]. *Ann Dermatol Venereol* 129(6-7): 901-903.

Foy, P. M., D. W. Chadwick, et al. (1992). Do prophylactic anticonvulsant drugs alter the pattern of seizures after craniotomy? *J Neurol Neurosurg Psychiatry* 55(9): 753-757.

Franceschetti, S., S. Binelli, et al. (1990). Influence of surgery and antiepileptic drugs on seizures symptomatic of cerebral tumors. *Acta Neurochir (Wien)* 103(1-2): 47-51.

Fukamachi, A., Koizumi,H, Nukui,H (1985). Immediate postoperative seizures - incidence and computed tomographic findings. *Surg Neurol* 24: 671-676.

Glantz, M. J., B. F. Cole, et al. (2000). Practice parameter: anticonvulsant prophylaxis in patients with newly diagnosed brain tumors. Report of the Quality Standards Subcommittee of the American Academy of Neurology. *Neurology* 54(10): 1886-1893.

Glantz, M. J., B. F. Cole, et al. (1996). A randomized, blinded, placebo-controlled trial of divalproex sodium prophylaxis in adults with newly diagnosed brain tumors. *Neurology* 46(4): 985-991.

Hata, N., T. Shono, et al. (2007). Loss of heterozygosity analysis in an anaplastic oligodendroglioma arising after radiation therapy. *Neurol Res* 29(7): 723-726.

Kargiotis, O., S. Markoula, et al. (2011). Epilepsy in the cancer patient. *Cancer Chemother Pharmacol* 67(3): 489-501.

Kassam, A. B., J. A. Engh, et al. (2009). Completely endoscopic resection of intraparenchymal brain tumors. *J Neurosurg* 110(1): 116-123.

Ketz, E. (1974). Brain tumors and Epilepsy. *Handbook of Clinical Neurology*. P. Vinken, Bruyn, GW. Amsterdam: 254-269.

Kikuchi, K., C. I. McCormick, et al. (1984). Immunosuppression by phenytoin: implication for altered immune competence in brain-tumor patients. J *Neurosurg* 61(6): 1085-1090.

Kuijlen, J. M., O. P. Teernstra, et al. (1996). Effectiveness of antiepileptic prophylaxis used with supratentorial craniotomies: a meta-analysis. *Seizure* 5(4): 291-298.

Kvam, D., Loftus,CM, Copeland,B, Quest, DO (1983). Seizures during the immediate postoperative period. *Neurosurgery* 12: 14-17.

Labrakakis, C., Patt,S, Weydt,P, et al (1997). Action potential generating cells in human glioblastoma. *J Neuropath Exp Neurol* 56: 243-254.

LeBlanc, F., Rasmussen,T (1974). Cerebral Seizures and Brain Tumors. *Handbook of Clinical Neurology*. B. G. Vinken PJ. Amsterdam: 295-301.

Lee, J. W., P. Y. Wen, et al. (2010). Morphological characteristics of brain tumors causing seizures. *Arch Neurol* 67(3): 336-342.

Lee, S., Lui,TN, Chang,CN, Cheng,WC, Wang,DJ, Heimbarger,RF, Lin,CG (1989). Prophylactic anticonvulsants for prevention of immediate and early postcraniotomy seizures. *Surg Neurol* 31: 361-364.

Li, X. N., Q. Shu, et al. (2005). Valproic acid induces growth arrest, apoptosis, and senescence in medulloblastomas by increasing histone hyperacetylation and regulating expression of p21Cip1, CDK4, and CMYC. *Mol Cancer Ther* 4(12): 1912-1922.

Lwu, S., M. G. Hamilton, et al. (2010). Use of peri-operative anti-epileptic drugs in patients with newly diagnosed high grade malignant glioma: a single center experience. *J Neurooncol* 96(3): 403-408.

Mahaley, M. J., Dudka,L (1981). The role of anticonvulsant medications in the management of patients with anaplastic gliomas. *Surg Neurol* 16: 399-401.

Mamon, H. J., P. Y. Wen, et al. (1999). Allergic skin reactions to anticonvulsant medications in patients receiving cranial radiation therapy. *Epilepsia* 40(3): 341-344.

Marchi, N., L. Angelov, et al. (2007). Seizure-promoting effect of blood-brain barrier disruption. *Epilepsia* 48(4): 732-742.

McDonald, G. A. and T. D. Dubose, Jr. (1993). Hyponatremia in the cancer patient. *Oncology (Huntingt)* 7(9): 55-64; discussion 67-58; 70-51.

McKeran, R., Thomas, DGT (1980). The clinical study of gliomas. *Brain tumors: scientific basis, clinical investigation and current therapy*. D. Thomas, Graham, DL. Baltimore: 194-230.

Meropol, N. J., P. J. Creaven, et al. (1995). Seizures associated with leucovorin administration in cancer patients. *J Natl Cancer Inst* 87(1): 56-58.

Mikkelsen, T., N. A. Paleologos, et al. (2010). The role of prophylactic anticonvulsants in the management of brain metastases: a systematic review and evidence-based clinical practice guideline. *J Neurooncol* 96(1): 97-102.

Milligan, B. D. and F. B. Meyer (2010). Morbidity of transcallosal and transcortical approaches to lesions in and around the lateral and third ventricles: a single-institution experience. *Neurosurgery* 67(6): 1483-1496; discussion 1496.

Moots, P., Maciunas,RJ, Eisert,DR, Parker,RA, Laporte,K, Abou-Khalil,B (1995). The course of seizure disorders in patients with malignant gliomas. *Arch Neurol* 52: 717-724.

Morris, H., Estes,ML, Prayson,RA, et al (1996). Frequency of different tumor types encountered in the Cleveland Clinic epilepsy surgery program. *Epilepsia* 37(suppl.5): 96.

North, J. B., R. K. Penhall, et al. (1983). Phenytoin and postoperative epilepsy- a double blind study. *J Neurosurg* 58: 672-677.

Novy, J., R. Stupp, et al. (2009). Pregabalin in patients with primary brain tumors and seizures: a preliminary observation. *Clin Neurol Neurosurg* 111(2): 171-173.

Patsalos, P. N., W. Froscher, et al. (2002). The importance of drug interactions in epilepsy therapy. *Epilepsia* 43(4): 365-385.

Patt, S., Labrakakis,C, Bernstein,M, et al (1996). Neuron-like physiological properties of cells from human oligodendroglial tumors. *Neuroscience* 71: 601-611.

Perry, J. R. and C. Sawka (1996). Add-on gabapentin for refractory seizures in patients with brain tumors. *Can J Neurol Sci* 23(2): 128-131.

Pursche, S., E. Schleyer, et al. (2008). Influence of enzyme-inducing antiepileptic drugs on trough level of imatinib in glioblastoma patients. *Curr Clin Pharmacol* 3(3): 198-203.

Ramirez, C., C. Bowman, et al. (2010). Loss of 1p, 19q, and 10q heterozygosity prospectively predicts prognosis of oligodendroglial tumors--towards individualized tumor treatment? *Neuro Oncol* 12(5): 490-499.

Ropper, A. H. (2009). *Adams and Victor's Prinicples of Neurology*, The McGraw-Hill Companies, Inc.

Ruggiero, A., D. Rizzo, et al. (2010). Interactions between antiepileptic and chemotherapeutic drugs in children with brain tumors: is it time to change treatment? *Pediatr Blood Cancer* 54(2): 193-198.

Sato, T., M. Takeichi, et al. (1993). Frontal lobe tumor associated with late-onset seizure and psychosis: a case report. *Jpn J Psychiatry Neurol* 47(3): 541-544.

Schaller, B. and S. J. Ruegg (2003). Brain tumor and seizures: pathophysiology and its implications for treatment revisited. *Epilepsia* 44(9): 1223-1232.

Scott, G., Gibberd, FB (1980). Epilepsy and other factors in the prognosis of gliomas. *Acta Neurologica Scandinavia* 61: 227-239.

Simonescu, M. (1960). Metastatic tumors of the brain. A follow-up study of 195 patients with neurosurgical considerations. *J Neurosurg* 17: 361-373.

Smith, D. F., J. L. Hutton, et al. (1991). The prognosis of primary intracerebral tumors presenting with epilepsy: the outcome of medical and surgical management. *J Neurol Neurosurg Psychiatry* 54(10): 915-920.

Striano, S., P. Striano, et al. (2009). The syndrome gelastic seizures-hypothalamic hamartoma: severe, potentially reversible encephalopathy. *Epilepsia* 50 Suppl 5: 62-65.

Thompson, D., J. Takeshita, et al. (2006). Selecting antiepileptic drugs for symptomatic patients with brain tumors. *J Support Oncol* 4(8): 411-416.

van Breemen, M. S., E. B. Wilms, et al. (2007). Epilepsy in patients with brain tumors: epidemiology, mechanisms, and management. *Lancet Neurol* 6(5): 421-430.

van de Loosdrecht, A. A., J. A. Gietema, et al. (2000). Seizures in a patient with disseminated testicular cancer due to cisplatin-induced hypomagnesaemia. *Acta Oncol* 39(2): 239-240.

Whittle, I., Beaumont,A (1995). Seizures in patients with supratentorial oligodendroglial tumors; clinicopahtological features and management considerations. *Acta Neurochir* 135: 19-24.

Zentner, J., A. Hufnagel, et al. (1997). Surgical treatment of neoplasms associated with medically intractable epilepsy. *Neurosurgery* 41(2): 378-386; discussion 386-377.

19

Brain Tumors at the Department of Neurology in Sarajevo: Retrospecitve Analysis

A. Alajbegović[1] and A. Gutošić[2]
[1]*Clinical Center University of Sarajevo, Department of Neurology*
[2]*Regional Medical Centre Dr. Safet Mujic, Mostar*
Bosnia and Herzegovina

1. Introduction

Brain tumors are unique and heterogeneous group of tumors which face a variety of specialty, most oncologists, neurologists, and neurosurgeons. Due to its specific location, all brain tumors are malignant, regardless of their malignant potential, because any expansion process inside the skull, increasing intracranial pressure and the destruction of surrounding structures, which may cause neurological injuries, quantitative disturbances of consciousness or death.

1.1 The incidence of brain tumors

In the United States are diagnosed annually 17 000 new cases of brain tumors. In Croatia, their average frequency is 18 per 100 000 inhabitants. The incidence of brain tumors in B&H is not known. Brain tumors are more common in older people. The most common are at the age from 65 to 74 years. The incidence of brain tumors in persons older than 70 years is 70 per 100 000 inhabitants. Some authors suggest that brain tumors are more common in men, while others argue that there is no difference in incidence according to sex, except for neuromas, which occur twice as frequently in women (1).

1.2 Etiopathogenesis

Genetic determination of neoplastic growth exists also in intracranial tumors and is related to a disorder of neuroectoderm and mesoderm development. Here belongs certain number of hereditary diseases which are due to the association with intracranial tumors and changes in the skin called facomatoses (neurofibromatosis, tuberous sclerosis).
Tumors arise from congenital malformations where the abnormal development creates conditions for the development of neoplastic tissue (angioblasts, ganglioneuroma).
It has been shown that exposure to radiation may be the cause of brain tumors while the role of trauma and infection was not significant.
Under experimental conditions it was shown that injection of oncogenic virus can cause brain tumors.

1.3 Pathophysiology

The inability of the skull of adults to spread if the internal pressure increases causes disorders that bear a common name as the symptoms of increased intracranial pressure. The increase in intracranial pressure is due to increase in tumors mass, due to edema that accompanies the tumor, and because of obstacles in the flow of cerebrospinal fluid. Since the brain is virtually incompressible, the tumor will grow with no signs of increased intracranial pressure only until it reaches a size of about 150 cc, for as long as the brain volume is smaller than the volume of the skull. As a rule increasing intracranial pressure is proportional to the growth speed of expansive processes. The brain can adapt to large tumor if it grows slowly, whereas smaller tumors that grow rapidly may give severe symptoms.

One of the consequences of the expansive process of the brain is edema. Edema principally affects the white mass of the hemispheres (centrum semiovale), is less pronounced in the internal capsule, corpus callosum and optic radiation, it almost does not use at all the large brain. Even edema acts as a mass that increases the volume of the brain, causing the above flattened gyrus, a brain ventricle can be suppressed. It is believed that the edema is caused by abnormal capillary permeability, which is a consequence of venous stasis and anoxia.

Since the cranial cavity from the outside is limited by bony shell and internal partitioned into three sections (falx into two supratentorial and by tentorium into the third, infratentorially cavity), the tumor will cause the clamp of the parts of the brain as follows:

a. Subfalx
b. Tentorially (up and down)
c. Occipitaly trough foramen magnum protrudes the cerebellar tonsils.

This increase in volume of the frontal parts of one hemisphere leads to pressure on the corpus callosum and gyrus subcalloosusa prolapse below the falx free edge. Because of this and move to the side chambers to the opposite side.

Similarly, the increase in the volume of the brain above tentorium causes a protrusion of part or all gyrus hippocampus through tentorium incision. If this protrusion is one-sided, opposite pedunculus is being pressed to the tentorium edge. The midbrain also protrudes. Due to pressure on aqueducts hydrocephalus occurs.

1.4 Symptoms of tumors

Symptoms of brain tumors can be divided into two groups: general and focal or focal. Common symptoms in most cases are preceded by focal symptoms and occur in 60% of patients with brain tumor. General symptoms are:

1.4.1 Symptoms of increased intracranial pressure (headache, vomiting, trail papilla optic nerve)

Headaches are initially reported in seizures. By further tumor growth they become longer and remain constant. They are more frequent in the morning and during the night. Localization importance of headache is a small place and the pain rarely coincides with the localization of tumors. Sometimes a headache may be on the opposite side of tumors but are usually in the frontal and occipital lobe. They occur in 49% of cases.

Vomiting usually occurs suddenly and without any connection with food intake. More often in the evening and morning.

Route of optic nerve papilla is most often seen in tumors of the cerebellum and temporal lobes, rarely in tumors of the brain hemispheres and the pons.

1.4.2 Pulse and respiration

Because of the pressure on the brain stem and nucleus vagus pulse is first slowed to below 60 per minute. Later, when intracranial pressure increases, the pulse becomes rapid and is more severe the sign than bradycardia.

1.4.3 Epileptic seizures

Focal epilepsy may be one of the signs of a brain tumor. Generalized seizures occur in many cases of brain tumors. It was observed that the same tumor size and localization in one patient caused epileptic seizure, while in the other does not.

The most common is epilepsy in case of astrocytoma, meningioma and glioblastoma of the brain. More often is the localization of tumors in the anterior parts of the brain than in posterior. They occur in 20-50% of cases, depending on the author.

1.4.4 Mental disorders

Psychological symptoms may be the first signs of a brain tumor, sometimes for months and years preceding the neurologic signs. The first symptoms of brain tumors occur in approximately 15-20% of cases. Psychic symptoms in brain tumors are classified into three groups: general symptoms (mild personality changes, anxiety, confusion, and neurasthenic catatonic states), specific symptoms (changes in affect, memory and attention disorders), and associated psychological changes (hysterical state).

Focal neurological deficit is manifested by sensibility problems, dysphasia, visual field problems, hemiparesis, etc., and are depend on the tumor location (13).

1.5 Classification of brain tumors

The basic division of a brain tumor is on the primary and secondary. Primary tumors are those arising from the brain parenchyma in the skull while secondary tumors of the brain are metastases, which occur by joining of malignant tumor cells of distant organs at their arrival into the brain. Primary tumors are most commonly seen in children (first decade of life). In adults, incidence increases with age and for persons over 65 years of age is 18 per 100 000. Primary tumors can be divided into malignant and benign, although essentially all brain tumors are malignant due to their specific location. The difference between benign and malignant brain tumors is in their growth rate, partly in the way of growth and the percentage of recovery. Benign brain tumors grow slowly, putting pressure on the surrounding parts of the brain, while malignant tumors grow rapidly and permeate (infiltrate) the brain.

From the histological aspect and by the **World Health Organization (WHO)** brain tumors are:

a. **NEUROEPITHELIAL**

1. Astrocytoma
2. Oligodendroglioma
3. Ependymoma
4. Pinealoma
5. Gangliocitoma
6. Medulloblastoma
7. Glioblastoma

b. **TUMORS OF THE NERVE SHEATHS**

c. **TUMORS MENING**

d. **PITUITARY TUMORS**

e. **VASCULAR TUMOR**

f. **CONGENITAL TUMORS:**

1. Craniofaringioma

2. Dermoids
3. Lipomas

g. **METASTATIC TUMORS**

There are over 80 types of tumors that can grow inside the skull and cause brain damage. However, in adults 5 types of tumors is encountered in over 90% of cases. These are:

1. Gliomas - this includes astrocytoma, oligodendroglioma, anaplastic astrocytoma and glioblastoma
2. Meningioma
3. Neuroma
4. Pituitary adenoma
5. Brain metastases from distant malignant tumors.

1.6 Specificity of tumor types

1.6.1 Gliomas

These are the most common brain tumors. They make up 50% of the total number of brain tumors. Annually in the United States they affect 7 people per 100 000. More frequent in men than women. Most often when grow permeate the surrounding brain structures. They have great potential to become malignant. According to the degree of malignancy have three or four stages. In the first stage healing is likely. Already in the second stage the survival for more than 5 years is 50-75%. In 3rd and 4th stage survival is even shorter. After the surgery is always indicated radiation and is often used is chemotherapy.

1.6.2 Meningiomas

Meningiomas are mostly benign tumors. 1-2% is malignant ones. Make up 15% to 20% of all tumors and 25% of brain tumors. Annually in the United States are affected 2 per 100 000 people. They are more often in women than men. Increase with the depletion of brain pressing the surrounding parts of the brain, nerves and blood vessels.

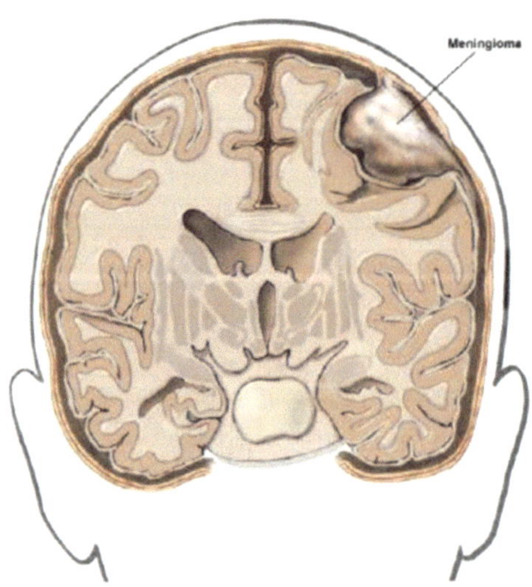

Fig. 1. Meningioma

The treatment is usually radical, surgical excision.

1.6.3 Neuroma

Arise from cells that are found in nerves. Constitute 5-10% of all brain tumors. Every year in United States 3000 new cases is diagnosed. The incidence is 1 in 100 000 people. The most common sites are the nerves of hearing and balance (neurinoma, schwanoma vestibullaris nerves, tumor of angulo pontocerebellaris). Because of that usually start with hearing impairment and dizziness. This symptom may remain for years. Later it can cause numbness and facial pain (symptomatic trigeminal neuralgia), bending of the face due to facial nerve damage, weakness of limbs due to pressure on the brain stem, hydrocephalus, etc.

It is usually possible to remove completely these tumors. Alternative therapy, particularly in case of small neuromas, is the stereotaxic radiation.

1.6.4 Pituitary adenoma

These are tumors that arise from the pituitary gland, glands of internal secretion. Make 14% of all brain tumors. Can secrete excessive hormones and then are usually diagnosed earlier, while still small. Depending on the hormone secreted by the patient will develop hyperprolactinemia, Cushing's disease, etc. If they secrete hormones in the gland tumor can rather grow until the first symptoms. Large adenomas are first manifested by visual disturbances. Later it can occur: reduced secretion of pituitary hormones, strabismus, double vision, frequent urination, difficulty in walking and mental symptoms and signs of hydrocephalus.

1.6.5 Brain metastases

Brain metastases are the complications of systemic dissemination of primary tumors. Malignant primary tumors of the blood and lymphoma reach distant organs (usually the lungs, liver and brain), multiply and produce a new tumor.

Brain metastases are the most common intracranial neoplasm in adults. Constitute about 12-27% of total CNS neoplasms. They occur in about 20-40% of cancer patients.

The incidence of brain metastases is increasing. Every year in the U.S. are diagnosed between 98 000 and 170 000 new cases of brain metastases.

In brain usually metastasize the tumors of the lungs (50%), breast cancer (15%), and malignant melanoma (10%).

Eighty percent of brain metastases were located in the cerebral hemispheres, 15% in the cerebellum, and 5% in the brain stem.

Survival of patients with brain metastases are treated only symptomatic therapy for 1-2 months, whole brain irradiation 3-6 months, a surgical procedure, and whole brain irradiation for 8-9 months.

1.7 Diagnosis of brain tumors

1. Physical examination: reveals the excesses of motion and sensitivity, impaired vision and hearing, and the spade in the field of cranial nerves, edema of the pupil and paralysis of n. abducens with elevated intracranial pressure, cognitive problems, etc.
2. CT of the brain: on computer assisted tomography images brain tumors are showed as isodens, hypo or hiper dens lesions, and sometimes can be seen areas of hemorrhage, necrotic foci and areas of calcification.
3. MRI is much more sensitive method and is able to clearly distinguish tumor from perifocal edema

4. X-ray of the skull
5. EEG
6. Lumbar puncture
7. 7th Angiography
8. PET (positron emission tomography) is based on isotopes that emit positrons, which in a collision with free electrons lead to a photon that was detected on PET. Used to differentiate tumor from scar tissue formed after the therapy.
9. Stereotaxic biopsy

1.8 Therapy of brain tumors

Therapy of brain tumors may be:
1. Symptomatic
2. Surgical
3. Radiation and chemotherapy.

Symptomatic treatment involves the inclusion of corticosteroids (dexason, dexamethasone) if there is brain edema. Administered are also anticonvulsants, and hypermolar analgesics solutions as needed.

Brain tumor surgery involves craniotomy (opening of the skull), reaching the tumors and its complete (ablation) or partially (reduction) removal. The tumor must be separated from the surrounding structures. This is impossible if the tumor grows by infiltration (malignant tumors). In as much as a benign tumor growth in a long time and become big, it really press, and want to stick to surrounding structures. Then is often impossible to separate them and preserve function. This is the main reason why it is important to diagnose the tumor as early as possible, while they have smaller sizes.

Mortality related to surgery is generally less than 1% and is usually caused by worsening of other diseases.

Neurological damage associated with surgery depends on the size and tumor location. In most cases is less than 1%. In difficult localizations and large tumors occurs in 20% of patients.

Accurate radiation can be achieved by using radio surgical methods, Gamma Knife and Linac. Thus precise radiation can stop tumor growth, if not already 2.5 cm in diameter and are very close to the structure of the brain that cannot tolerate radiation. Also they can stop the growth of small parts of tumors that were left behind after surgery. This method has not yet begun to be applied in our country. In developed countries it is for a long time the standard treatment.

Chemotherapy usually today involves use of Tamodal. According to recent studies conducted in Australia, chemotherapy has helped in only 2% of cases suffering from cancer.

2. Problem formulation

This raises the question of the incidence of brain tumors at the Neurology Clinic Sarajevo from January 1st 2006 - December 31st 2009.

3. Problem definition

Brain tumors are neoplasms arising from nerve cells, supporting cells of the nervous tissues and cells of meninges and blood vessels of the brain. Like other tumors are divided into malignant and benign although because the specifics of their location it is difficult to talk about benign brain tumors. Its growth and pressure on surrounding structures causing increased intracranial pressure, headaches, vomiting, seizures and neurological disturbances. Brain tumors constitute 9-10% of all tumors. They are more common in men than in women. Are quite common in the child's age, where have second place in relation to other tumors. It is usually diagnosed at age of 5-10 years, mostly astrocytoma (40%) and medulloblastoma (20%). In older populations, the incidence of tumors increases with age and is highest after age of 60. The most common tumors are gliomas and make up 50% of brain tumors, and meningiomas, which represent 25% of brain tumors.

4. Goals

4.1 Primary goals

1. Prove that the incidence of brain tumors at the Neurology Clinic Sarajevo from January 1st 2006 - December 31st 2009 is less than 1%.
2. Prove that there is no statistically significant difference in the incidence of brain tumors at the Neurology Clinic Sarajevo by years of research.

4.2 Secondary goals

1. Conduct analysis of age and sex structure of patients with brain tumors.
2. To determine the incidence of tumors in relation to the type (histological structure).
3. To determine the incidence of tumors in relation to the localization.
4. To determine the prevalence of general and focal symptoms of brain tumors.
5. To determine the incidence of brain metastases.
6. To determine the incidence of brain tumors in relation to the total number of hospitalized patients.

5. Hypothesis

1st Working hypothesis: The incidence of brain tumors at the Clinic of Neurology CCUS from January 1st 2006 - December 31st 2009 is less than 1%.
Null Hypothesis: The incidence of brain tumors at the Clinic of Neurology CCUS from January 1st 2006 - December 31st 2009 is greater than 1%.
2nd Working hypothesis: There is no difference in the incidence of brain tumors at the Clinic of Neurology CCUS by years of research.
Null hypothesis: There is a difference in the incidence of brain tumors at the Clinic of Neurology CCUS by years of research.

6. Material and methods

6.1 Study design

The study was conducted at Clinic of Neurology, Clinical Centre of Sarajevo University.
Performed is a retrospective study that included 33 patients with brain cancer, aged between 28 and 79 years, who were treated at the Neurology Clinic Sarajevo from January 1st 2006 - December 31st 2009.

6.2 Methods of data collection

Was reviewed medical records and history of illness of patients treated at the aforementioned Clinic. All patients were processed in an identical manner using the following questionnaire:

- **General information about the patient:**

1. Name and surname
2. Age
3. Gender
4. Admission date
5. Discharge date

- **General information about the disease:**

1. Symptoms (headache, vomiting, seizures, hemiparesis, disorders of the cranial nerves, speech disorders)
2. Type of tumors (primary tumor or brain metastases; histological structure)
3. CT and MRI (localization)
4. Therapy

6.3 Statistical analysis

Data collection was done by examining the medical records, and then performed a data entry in MS Excel 2003. Data after sorting, control and grouping were exported into the statistical software package SPSS 16.0, where the definition of variables made statistical analysis of data using chi-square test and Student t test. The results are presented in the appropriate number of charts and tables, statistical analysis and descriptive statistics using the software package SPSS 16.0 and MS Excel 2003.

7. Results

7.1 Demographic analysis by gender

Of the total number of respondents (N = 33), 12 (36.4%) were male and 21 (63.6%) were female. It was found that there was a statistically significant difference in the higher risk of brain tumors for the female population.

	Gender	
	N	%
Male	12	36.4
Female	21	63.6
Total	33	100.0

Table 1. Presentation of gender structure of respondents with a brain tumor, CCUS, January 1st 2006 – December 31st 2009.

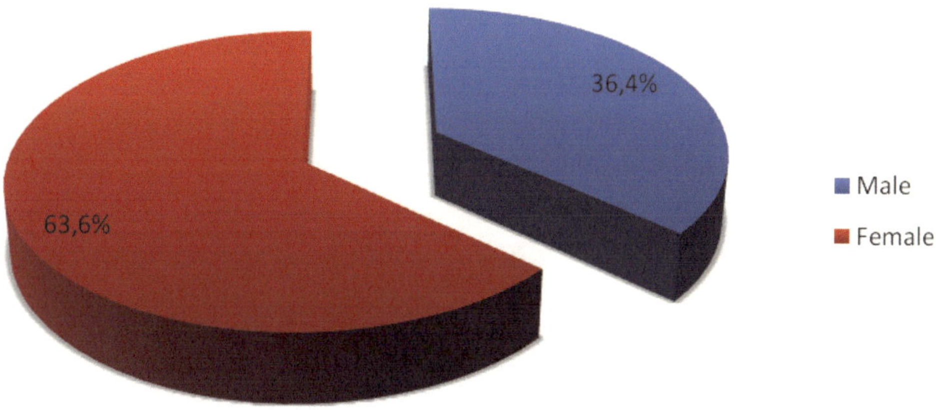

Fig. 2. Presentation of gender structure of respondents with a brain tumor, CCUS, January 1st 2006 – December 31st 2009.

		Year of the hospitalization				Total
		2006	2007	2008	2009	
Male	N	3	0	3	6	12
	%	37.5	.0	50.0	66.7	36,4
Female	N	5	10	3	3	21
	%	62.5	100.0	50.0	33.3	63,6
Total	N	8	10	6	9	33
	%	24,2	30.3	18.2	27.3	100.0

$\chi^2=9.772$, $p=0.021$

Table 2. Presentation of sex structure of respondents in CCUS by years of research.

Of the total number of respondents in 2006 (N=8), three of them (37.5%) were male and 5 (62.5%) female. Total number of respondents was in 2007 - 10 (N=10) and all were female. Of the total number of patients with brain tumors in 2008 (N=6), 3 (50%) were male and the remaining 3 (50%) female. In 2009 the total number of respondents was 9, of which 6 (66.7%) males and 3 (33.3%) female.

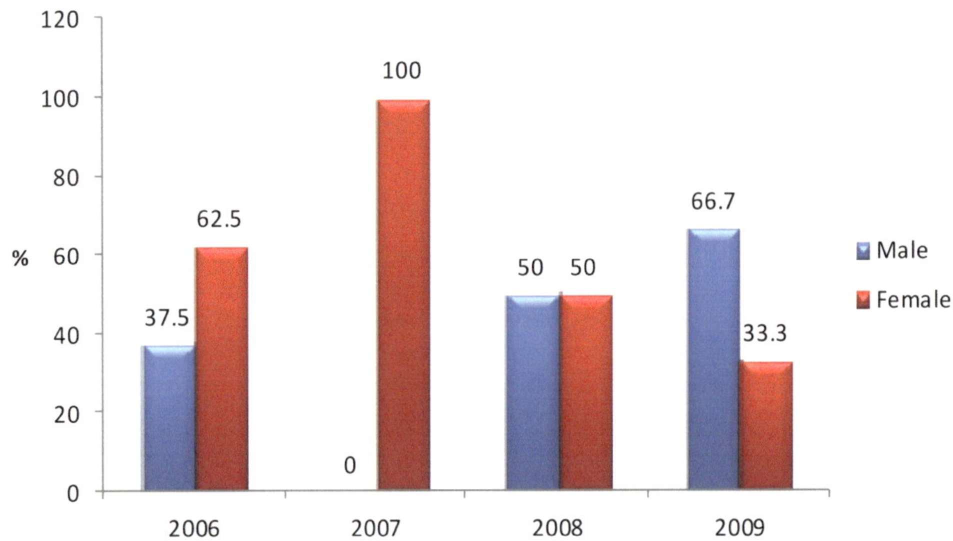

Fig. 3. Presentation of sex structure of respondents in CCUS by years of research.

Statistical analysis using chi-square test revealed statistically significant differences in gender distribution according to year of study ($p < 0.05$).

7.2 Demographic analysis according to age of respondents

A review of the age structure of respondents revealed that the average age of patients with brain tumors at the Clinic of Neurology CCUS from 2006-2009 was 53.6 years with the youngest patient aged 28 and the oldest aged 79 years.

Mean	53.6061
Std. error	2.53533
Std. deviation	14.56438
Minimum	28.00
Maximum	79.00

Table 3. Presentation of age structure of respondents with a brain tumor, CCUS, January 1st 2006 - December 31st 2009.

	N	Mean	Std. deviation	Std. error	Minimum	Maximum
2006	8	50.0000	14.55041	5.14435	28.00	71.00
2007	10	57.5000	14.50862	4.58803	29.00	77.00
2008	6	59.6667	18.09604	7.38768	33.00	79.00
2009	9	48.4444	11.50121	3.83374	30.00	67.00
Total	33	53.6061	14.56438	2.53533	28.00	79.00

$t=1.140$, $p=0.350$

Table 4. Presentation of age structure of respondents in CCUS by years of research.

Statistical analysis of the average age of the patient, by years of research, showed that in 2006 the average age of respondents was 50, for 2007 - 57.5 years, in 2008 - 59.6667 year and for 2009 of 48.4444 years, also shows no statistically significant difference ($p>0.05$). In the table is given the minimum and maximum age of respondents by years of research.

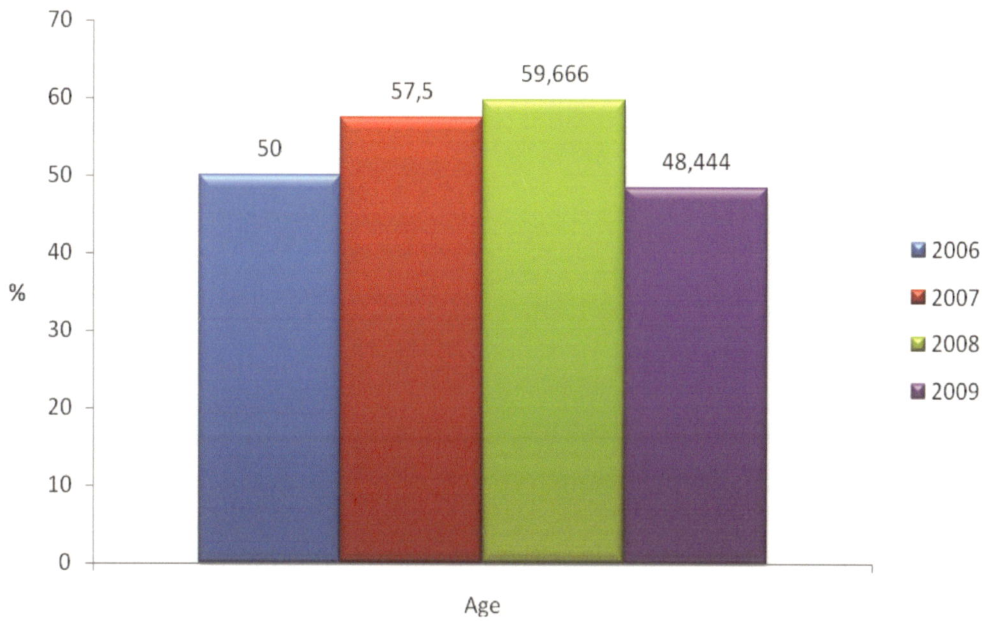

Fig. 4. Percentage display of the age structure of patients with brain tumors, CCUS, by years of research.

7.3 Statistical analysis of distribution by type of tumor

Statistical analysis of the incidence of tumors, according to the type of cancer, by years of research, is not showing statistically significant difference. The most common tumors in this period were meningiomas (23.3%). In 2006 meningiomas occur in two patients (30%). 2007 the meningioma is registered in 4 (40%) patients and in 2008 1 (16.7%) patient. Gliomas (6.7%) together with oligodendroglioma (6.7%) and astrocytoma (3.3%) specifically referred to as a group, constitute 16.7% of all tumors. Note that for the 10 tumors in the medical history of patients are not listed their histological structure, and type of tumor. From the other tumors, which are primarily originated from the brain, there are also pituitary micro adenoma in 2008 - 1 patient (16.7%) and 2009 also 1 (11.1%) patient, and cavernous angioma, in 2007 one patient (10%) and in 2009 - 1 (11.1%).

Since tumors that were primarily formed in another places in the body in relation to the total number of patients (N=33), are represented by adenocarcinoma of the lung with 2 (6.7%), and periurethral adenoma with 1 (3.3%), malignant melanoma with 1 (3.3%) and one patient with sarcoma (3.3%). In one case from 2007 unknown is the primary localization of the brain tumor.

			Year of the hospitalization 2006	2007	2008	2009	Total
Tumor type	Unknown	N	0	2	1	4	7
		%	.0	20.0	16.7	44.4	23.3
	Pituitary micro adenoma	N	0	0	1	1	2
		%	.0	.0	16.7	11.1	6.6
	Angioma cavernosum	N	0	1	0	1	2
		%	.0	10.0	.0	11.1	6.7
	Astrocytoma	N	0	0	0	1	1
		%	.0	.0	.0	11.1	3.3
	Glioma	N	1	0	1	0	2
		%	10.0	.0	16.7	.0	6,7
	Meningeoma	N	2	4	1	0	7
		%	30.0	40.0	16.7	.0	23,3
	Oligodendroglioma	N	1	0	1	0	2
		%	10.0	.0	16.7	.0	6,7
	Primary tumor -ca. mammae	N	0	1	0	0	1
		%	.0	10.0	.0	.0	3,3
	Primary tumor - unknown	N	3	1	0	0	4
		%	40.0	10.0	.0	.0	13,2
	Primary tumor -adenocarcinoma of the lungs	N	1	0	0	1	2
		%	10.0	.0	.0	11.1	6,7
	Primary tumor -adenoma periurthrale	N	0	0	1	0	1
		%	.0	.0	16.7	.0	3,3
	Primary tumor-melanoma malignum	N	0	0	0	1	1
		%	.0	.0	.0	11.1	3,3
	Primary tumor -SARCOMA sterni	N	0	1	0	0	1
		%	.0	10.0	.0	.0	3,3
Total		N	8	10	6	9	33
		%	16,7	33.3	20.0	30.0	100.0

χ^2=44.722 , p=0.358

Table 5. Type of tumor

			Year of the hospitalization 2006	2007	2008	2009	Total
Metastases	No	N	6	7	5	5	23
		%	75.0	70.0	83.3	55.6	69,7
	Meta cerebri	N	2	3	1	4	10
		%	25.0	30.0	16.7	44.4	30,3
Total		N	8	10	6	9	33
		%	24,2	30.3	18.2	27.3	100.0

χ^2=1.487, p=0.685

Table 6. Brain metastases

During the 2006 from the total of 8 patients, 2 (25%) patients had brain metastasis. In 2007 from the total of 10 patients 3 (30%) had brain metastasis. 1 (16.7%) of 6 patients in 2008 and four (44.4%) of the nine patients 2009 had brain metastases. The total number of patients with brain metastasis was 10 (30.3%). Statistical analysis of the incidence of brain metastases by years of research shows no statistically significant differences.

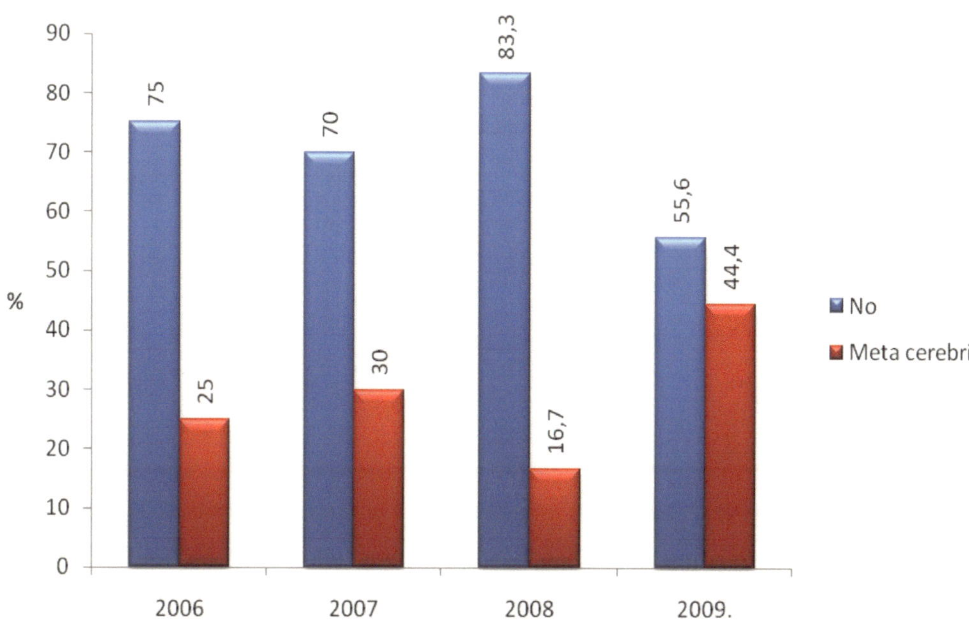

Fig. 5. Percentage representation of brain metastases, CCUS, by years of research

7.4 Analysis of the frequency of general and local symptoms by years of research

In 2006, 2 (25%) patients had a headache. In 2007, 4 (40%), 2008 two (33.3%), and in 2009, 1 (11.1%) patient had a headache. Statistical analysis of the frequency of headache in patients with brain tumors, by years of research shows no statistically significant difference. Total of 9 (27.3%) patients had headaches compared to 33 (100%) affected.

		Year of the hospitalization				Total
		2006	2007	2008	2009	
Present	N	2	4	2	1	9
	%	25.0	40.0	33.3	11.1	27,3
Not present	N	6	6	4	8	24
	%	75.0	60.0	66.7	88.9	72,7
Total	N	8	10	6	9	33
	%	24.2	30.3	18.2	27.3	100.0

χ^2=2.134, p=0.545

Table 7. Headache

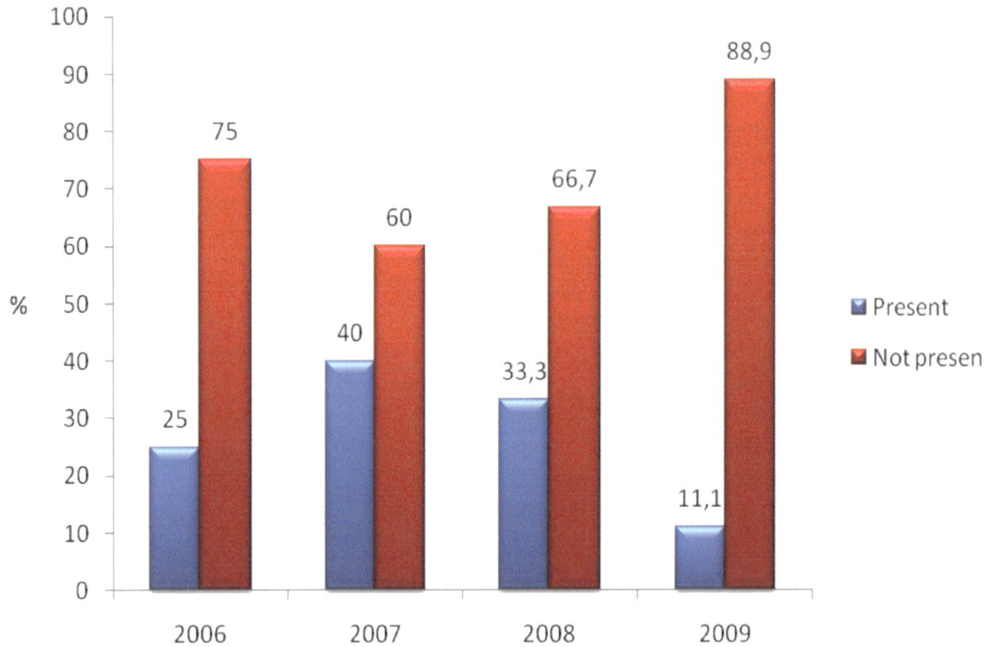

Fig. 6. Percentage representation of headache in patients with brain tumors, CCUS, by years of research.

		Year of the hospitalization				Total
		2006	2007	2008	2009	
Morning vomiting	N	1	1	0	1	3
	%	12.5	10.0	.0	11.1	9,1
No	N	7	9	6	8	30
	%	87.5	90.0	100.0	88.9	90,9
Total	N	8	10	6	9	33
	%	24.2	30.3	18.2	27.3	100.0

χ^2=0.767, p=0.857

Table 8. Vomiting

In 2006 is registered 1 (12.5%) patient, in 2007, 1 (10%) and in 2009, 1 (11.1%) patient had morning vomiting. In 2008 none of the participants had this symptom. Statistical analysis of the incidence of vomiting in patients with brain tumors, by study years, shows no statistically significant differences. Total of 3 (9.1%) patients out of 33 (100%) had vomiting as a symptom of a brain tumor.

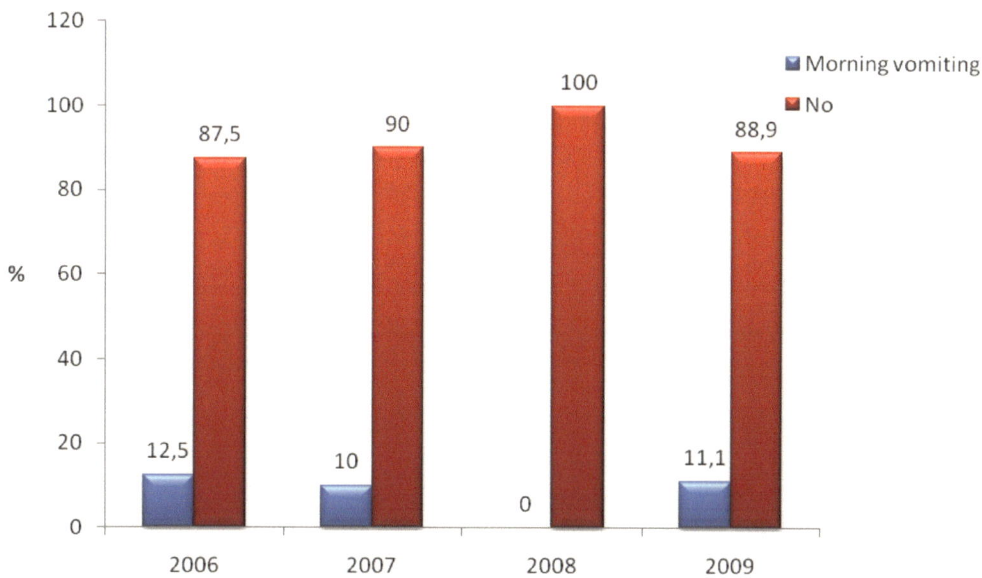

Fig. 7. Percentage representation of morning vomiting in patients with brain tumors, CCUS, by years of research.

		Year of the hospitalization				Total
		2006	2007	2008	2009	
Present	N	2	2	1	5	10
	%	25.0	20.0	16.7	55.6	30,3
Absent	N	6	8	5	4	23
	%	75.0	80.0	83.3	44.4	69,7
Total	N	8	10	6	9	33
	%	24.2	30.3	18.2	27.3	100.0

χ^2=3.855, p=0.278

Table 9. Epileptic seizures

In 2006 seizures had 2 (25%) patients, in 2007, 2 (20%), in 2008, 1 (16.7) and in 2009 five (55.6%). Statistical analysis of the frequency of seizures in patients with brain tumors, by years of research shows no statistically significant differences.
Ten (30%) patients compared to 33 (100%) had epileptic seizures.

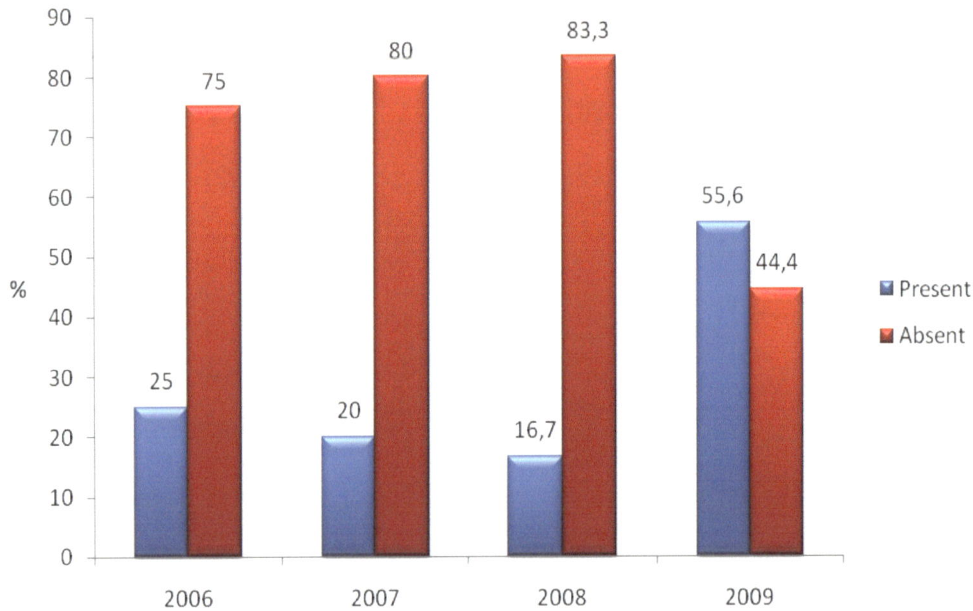

Fig. 8. Percentage representation of seizures in patients with brain tumors, CCUS, by years of research.

		Year of the hospitalization				Total
		2006	2007	2008	2009	
No	N	6	9	2	7	24
	%	75.0	90.0	33.3	77.8	72,7
Hemiparesis cerebralis lateris dextri	N	1	1	3	1	6
	%	12.5	10.0	50.0	11.1	18,2
Hemiparesis cerebralis lateris sinistri	N	1	0	1	1	3
	%	12.5	.0	16.7	11.1	9,1
Total	N	8	10	6	9	33
	%	24.2	30.3	18.2	27.3	100.0

χ^2=7.257, p=0.298

Table 10. Hemiparesis

In 2006 is registered one patient (12.5%), in 2007, 1 (10%), in 2008, 3 (50%), and in 2009, 1 (11.1%) patient had a right hemiparesis. Left hemiparesis in 2006 occurs in one patient (12.5%), in 2008. at 1 (16.5%) and 2009 at 1 (11.1%) patients. In 2007 there was no patient with left hemiparesis. Statistical analysis of the frequency of hemiparesis in patients with brain tumors, CCUS, by years of research showed no statistically significant differences.

Total of 9 (27.3%) patients at 33 (100%) had hemiparesis.

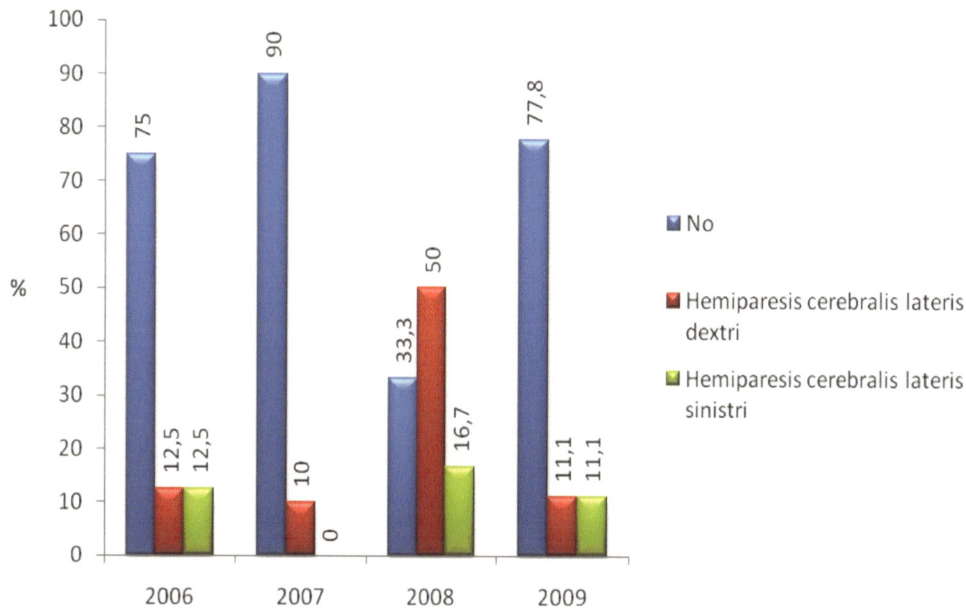

Fig. 9. Percentage representation of the right and left hemiparesis in patients with brain tumors, CCUS, by years of research.

		Year of the hospitalization				Total
		2006	**2007**	**2008**	**2009**	
Not present	N	6	8	5	8	27
	%	75	80.0	83.3	88.9	81,8
Motor dysphasia	N	0	1	0	1	2
	%	.0	10.0	.0	11.1	6,0
of dysartric type	N	0	1	0	0	1
	%	.0	10.0	.0	.0	3,0
Difficult speech	N	2	0	1	0	3
	%	25.0	.0	16.7	.0	9,1
Total	N	8	10	6	9	33
	%	24.2	30,3	18,2	27,3	100,0

χ^2=11.706, p=0.470

Table 11. Speech problems

In 2006 two (25%) patients had difficulties to speak. in 2007 one (10%) patient has a motor dysphasia, 1 (10%) patients have disturbances of speech of dysartric type, in 2008 one (16.7%) patients had difficulties to speak and in 2009 one (11.1%) patient has a motor dysphasia. 27 (81.8%) of patients with speech disorders. Statistical analysis of the incidence of speech disturbance in patients with brain tumors by years of research, showed no statistically significant differences.

Of the total number of respondents (N=33), 6 (18.2%) of them have speech problems.

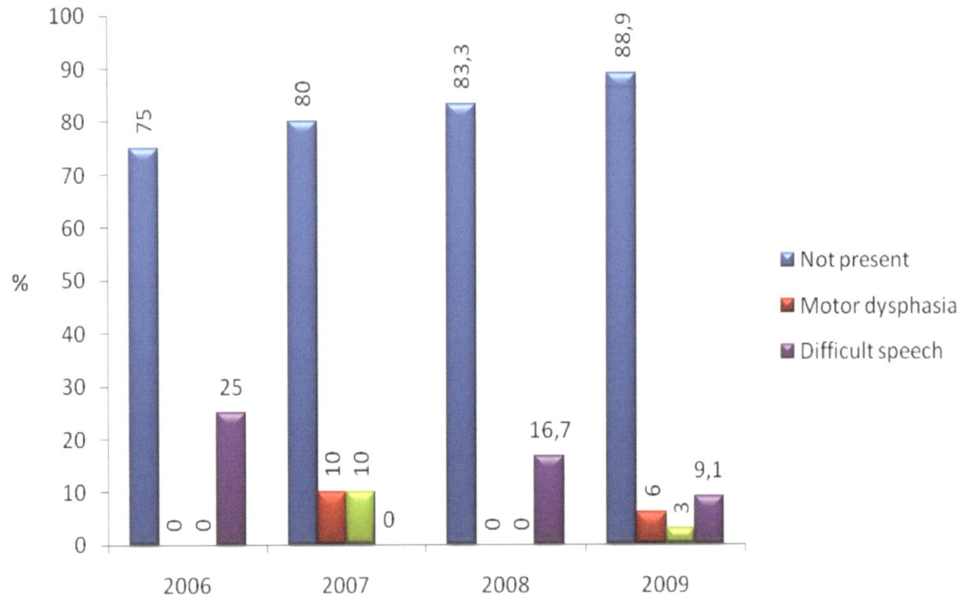

Fig. 10. Percentage representation of speech disorders in patients with brain tumors, CCUS, by years of research.

			Year of the hospitalization				Total
			2006	2007	2008	2009	
	No	N	7	10	4	8	29
		%	87.5	100.0	66.7	88.9	87,9
	depression	N	1	0	1	1	3
		%	12.5	.0	16.7	11.1	9,1
	Inadequate affect exploration	N	0	0	1	0	1
		%	.0	.0	16.7	.0	3,0
Total		N	8	10	6	9	33
		%	24.2	30.3	18.2	27.3	100.0

χ^2=6.406, p=0.379

Table 12. Mental disorders

Of the total number of respondents (N=33), 4 (12.1%) had mental disorders, and 29 (87.9%) no mental disorders. In 2006th one (12.5%) patient had depression. In 2007 there have been no patients with mental disorders caused by brain tumors. In 2008 one (16.7%) patient had depression, one (16.7%) showed inadequate affective exploration. In 2009 one (11.1%) patient was suffering from depression. Without statistically significant differences.

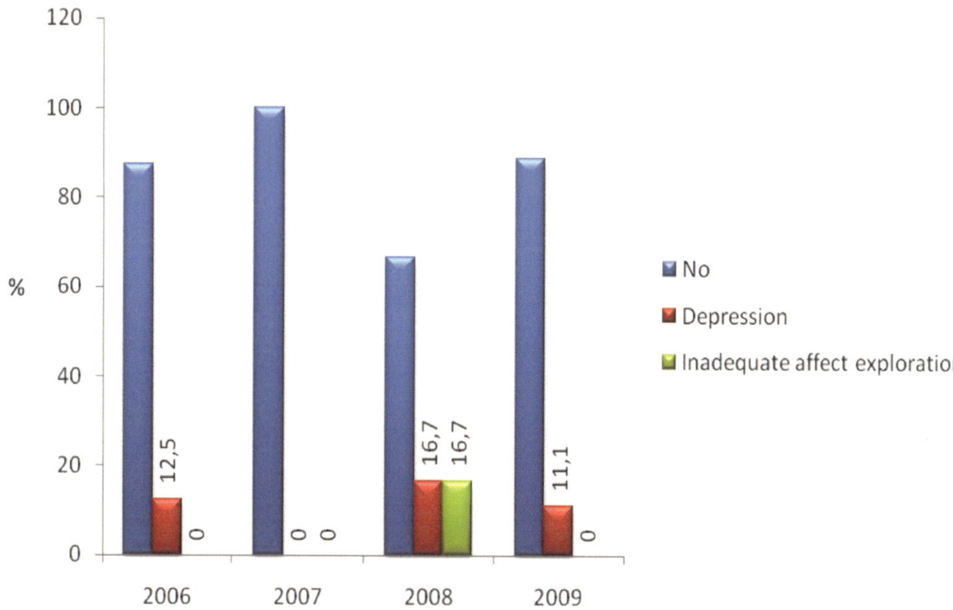

Fig. 11. Percentage display representation of mental disorders in patients with brain tumors, CCUS, by years of research.

		Year of the hospitalization				Total
		2006	2007	2008	2009	
No	N	7	8	5	9	29
	%	87.5	80.0	83.3	100.0	87,9
Paralysis 3, 4, & 5	N	0	1	0	0	1
	%	.0	10.0	.0	.0	3,0
Paresis 3	N	0	0	1	0	1
	%	.0	.0	16.7	.0	3,0
Paresis 6 left	N	0	1	0	0	1
	%	.0	10.0	.0	.0	3,0
Paresis 6 right	N	1	0	0	0	1
	%	12.5	.0	.0	.0	3,0
Total	N	8	10	6	9	33
	%	24.2	30.3	18.2	27.3	100.0

χ^2=12.460, p=0.409

Table 13. Excesses of cranial nerves

In 2006 from the total of 8 patients, one (12.5%) patient had paresis of 6 cranial nerve. In 2007 from the total of 10 patients, one (10.0%) had paralysis, 3, 4, and 5 cranial nerve, one (10.0%), paresis of the left sixth cranial nerve. In 2008 from a total of 6 patients, 1 (16.7%) patient has paresis of third cranial nerve. In 2009 the patients does not have any outbursts of cranial nerves. There is no statistically significant difference.

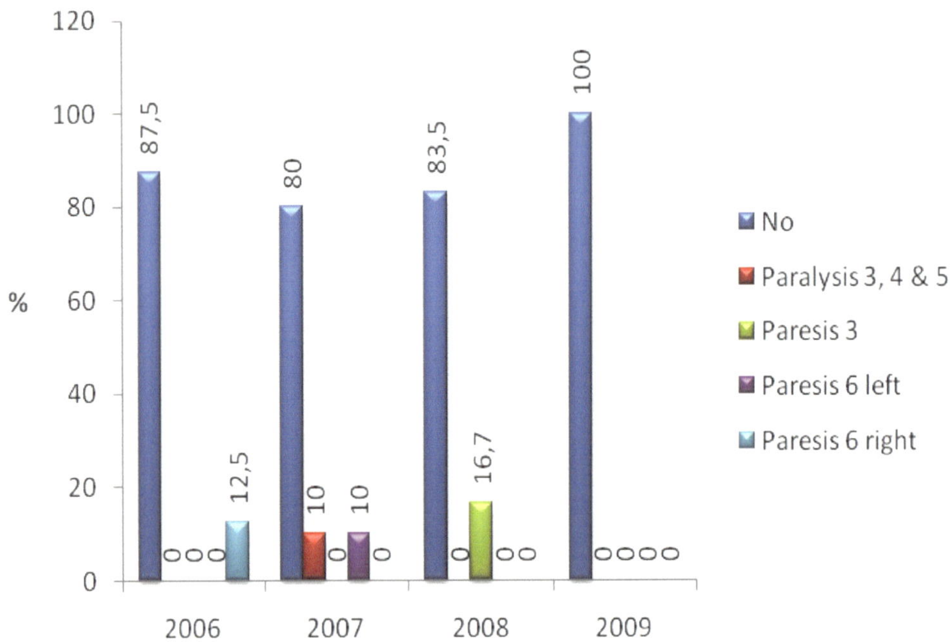

Fig. 12. Percentage representation of failure of the cranial nerves, CCUS, after years of research.

7.5 Analysis of the localization of brain tumors

From 33 analyzed patients showed that the brain tumors are located mostly in the cerebellum (21%), then frontoparietal (18.1%) in the brain stem (15.1%), parietal (12%). In sphenoid sinus are located 9.1% of tumors. The frontal, occipital, and parietoccipital in the cavernous sinus are located 6.1% of the tumors.

Statistical analysis of the incidence of tumors in relation to their location, by years of research, showed no statistically significant difference.

7.6 Analysis of the incidence of tumors in relation to the total number of hospitalized patients

A review of years of hospitalization, showed that most patients with brain tumors in relation to the total number of patients were hospitalized during 2009 (9 or 0.7%) where the total number of patients was 1731. Followed 2007 when from the 1699 hospitalized patients 10 or 0.6% was with brain tumors. In 2008 hospitalized was 1700 patients, of which 6 or 0.4 with brain tumors, and in 2006 from the 1731 patients hospitalized, of which 8 or 0.5% with brain tumors.

The frequency of brain tumors at Neurology Clinic CCUS, from January 1st 2006 - December 31st 2009 is 33 of 6358 patients, or 0.5%.

		Year of the hospitalization				Total
		2006	2007	2008	2009	
Frontal	N	1	.0	.0	1	2
	%	12.5	.0	.0	11.1	6.1
Parietal	N	2	0	0	2	4
	%	25.0	.0	.0	22.2	12.1
Occipital	N	1	0	1	0	2
	%	12.5	.0	16.7	.0	6,1
Frontoparietal	N	1	0	3	2	6
	%	12.5	.0	50.0	22.2	18.1
Parietoccipital	N	0	2	0	0	2
	%	.0	20.0	.0	.0	6,1
Brain stem	N	0	5	0	0	5
	%	.0	50.0	.0	.0	15,1
Sphenoid sinus	N	0	1	1	1	3
	%	.0	10.0	16.7	11.1	9,1
Cerebellum	N	2	1	1	3	7
	%	25.0	10.0	16.7	33.3	21,1
Cavernous sinus	N	1	1	0	0	2
	%	12.5	10.0	.0	.0	6,1
Total	N	8	10	6	9	33
	%	24.2	30.3	18.2	27.3	100.0

χ^2=65.519, p=0.389

Table 14. Tumor location

		Year of the hospitalization				Total
		2006	2007	2008	2009	
Brain tumor	N	8	10	6	9	33
	%	0.5	0.6	0.4	0.7	0,5
Other diseases	N	1723	1689	1694	1219	6325
	%	99.5	99.4	99.6	99.3	99,5
Total	N	1731	1699	1700	1228	6358
	%	27.2	26.7	26.7	19.3	100.0

Table 15. Tumors frequency

8. Discussion

In a study conducted at the Neurology Clinic Sarajevo from January 1st 2006 - December 31st 2009, it was found that the incidence of brain tumors is less than 1%, and there is no significant statistical difference in the incidence of tumors by years of research, except when it comes to the gender distribution of patients.

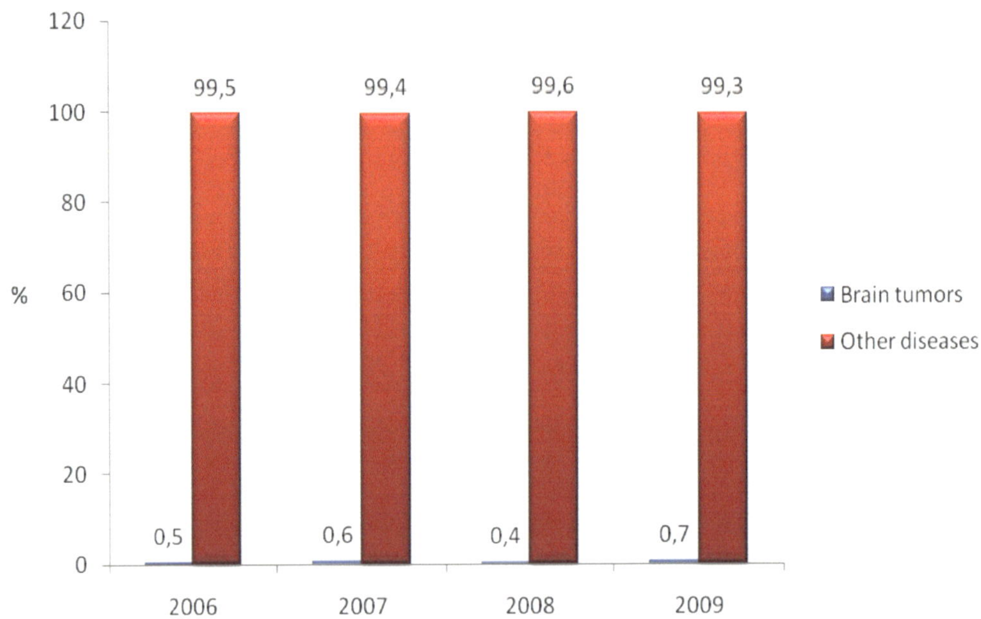

Fig. 13. Percentage representation of a brain tumor in relation to the total number of hospitalizations, by years of research.

There were 33 patients with brain tumor. From this number of patients, 36.4% were male and 63.6% women.

In 2006 from the total number of patients (N=8), 37.5% were male and 62.5% women. In 2007 all patients (N=10) were female (100%). During 2008 from a total of 6 patients, 50% were male and 50% female.

In 2009 from a total of 9 patients, 66.7% were male and 33.3% women.

The survey also showed that in the mentioned period of research (2006-2009), the most common tumors were meningiomas (23.3%). In 2006 the meningiomas occur in 2 patients (30%), 2007 in 4 (40%) patients, in 2008. in 1 patient (16.7%) and in 2009there were no patients with meningioma.

Gliomas accounted for 16.7% of the total number of tumors, and the frequency was at the second place. In 2006 there were 2 (20%) patients, 2008 also 2 (20%), and 2009 there was 1 (11.1%) patient with this malignant tumor.

Some authors argue that there is no difference in the incidence of brain tumors by sex (1), while others claim that brain tumors are more common in men, and also state that meningiomas are 2.3 times more common in women, gliomas 1.7 times more common in men (4).

The survey conducted by Monica Brown and Rudolph Schot and his associates in California, in the period since 2001 - 2005, on the sample of 24 923 patients with primary brain tumors, which obtained data using the California Cancer Registry, showed that the incidence of this disease is less than 1% (0.07%) and that 59.5% of patients were in age from 20 to 64 years, of which 56.5% were women.

56.4% of tumors were benign, malignant 37.1%, and for 6.5% tumors it was difficult to determine malignant potential. The most common benign tumors were meningiomas (51.6%), and malignant tumors, gliomas (52.5%).

Retrospective survey conducted by Srdjana and Sinisa Telarovic, in Istria (Croatia), in the period from January 1st 1986 to December 31st 2000 at the Neurological Department of the General Hospital in Pula, found the incidence of tumors less than 1%. Of the 364 patients, 213 (57.69%) were male and 151 patients (42.31%) female. The most common tumors were gliomas 47.7%.

The survey by Peter D. and associates in Cyprus in the period since 1998 - 2001, 56% of the total 150 patients were male and 44% were women. The most common cancers in the population aged 50-69 years were gliomas.

It should be noted that at the 2007 at the Clinic of Neurology was only female population, and that same year recorded four meningiomas from a total of 7 cancers.

Previous two studies and research at the Clinic of Neurology, which are included in this survey, confirming the dependence of the frequency of brain tumors by sex on the incidence of brain tumors in relation to the type of tumors.

The research at Clinic of Neurology, which is included in this study, has registered 10 (30%) of 33 patients with brain metastases. In four brain metastases was not found listed species or location of primary tumors in the patient's medical history. Primary brain tumors of the other 6 metastases were adenocarcinoma of the lung metastases (N=2), malignant melanoma (N=1), periurethral adenoma (N=1), sarcoma (N=1), and breast cancer (N=1).

According to world literature metastases make 12-25% of brain tumors (1).

The survey conducted by Teletovic and associates, in Istria (Croatia), at the Neurological Department of the General Hospital in Pula, in the period from 1986 to 2000, it was found that 56.87% were primary, mostly malignant tumors, 43.13% brain metastases. Thus a large number of brain metastases in Istria are explained by stress caused by war during nineties in Croatian territory, and weakening of immunity, and increased use of cigarettes and alcohol. According to a retrospective study, the incidence of brain tumors at the Department of Neurology CCUS, for the period from January 1st 1990 to December 31st 1999, which conducted Alajbegovic and Hrnjica with associates, 36% of patients (N=105) had brain metastasis.

Research at the Clinic of Neurology, which is included in this study showed that the average age of patients with brain tumor is 53.6 years with the youngest patient aged 28 and the oldest aged 79 years. According to a study conducted by Srdjan and Sinisa Telarovic with associates, found the illness mostly in the population aged 50-59 years. A study conducted by Peter D. and associates in Cyprus, confirmed that the brain tumors usually occur in the population of at age 50-69 years and in 40% of cases.

In 33 analyzed patients showed that the brain tumors are located in the cerebellum (21%), then frontal parietal (18.1%) in the brain stem (15.1%) and parietal (12%). In sfenoidal sinus was located 9.1%tumors. The frontal, occipital, and partial occipital in the cavernous sinus was located 6.1% tumors. In other words, most of the tumors was located in the cerebral hemispheres, and in the cerebellum, and then in the brain stem. This coincides with a study by Peter D. in Cyprus by which 34.8% tumors are located in the cerebral hemispheres, 4.7% in the cerebellum, 2% in the brain stem and 2% in the spinal cord. For the other 48% tumors location was not specified. According to a study by Sinisa and Srdjan Teletovic, 43% tumors were localized in the cerebral hemispheres, 15.2% in the cerebellum and the rest of the tumors were located in the brain stem and spinal cord.

The research at Department of Neurology is covered a general and focal symptomatology. Most were represented seizures (30.3%), followed by headache (27.3%), hemiparesis 27.3% (18.2% right, left 9.1%), speech disturbances 18.2%, mental disorders 12.0%, morning vomiting 9.1%, and the problems of the cranial nerves with 9.0%. These data correspond to the data given in world literature (1). According to a retrospective study conducted by Alajbegovic, Loga and associates at the Clinic of Neurology CCUS, from January 1st 2001 - December 31st 2005, 15-20% of patients had psychological disturbances. According to the already mentioned study, conducted by Alajbegovic and Hrnjica about 35% of patients had seizures.

9. Conclusions

1. The incidence of brain tumors at the Neurology Clinic Sarajevo from January 1st 2006 - December 31st 2009 was 0.5% (less than 1%).
2. There was no statistically significant difference in the incidence of tumors by years of research, except in the frequency of sex.
3. Of 33 patients, 36.4% were male and 63.6% women.
4. The mean age of patients with brain tumors was 53.6 years, with the youngest patient aged 29 and the oldest aged 79 years.
5. The most common tumors were meningiomas (23.3%), and gliomas (16.7%).
6. Brain metastases were confirmed in 10 (30%) patients.
7. The most common tumor site was the cerebral hemispheres, and in the cerebellum, and then in the brain stem.
8. The most common symptoms of brain tumors were seizures (30.3%) followed by headache and hemiparesis with 27.3%.

10. References

[1] Alajbegović Azra, Hrnjica Muhamed, Dimitrijević Jovan, Zukić Tarik, Subašić Nihada. Central nervous system neoplasms in clinical data from the Neurology CU Sarajevo, 1990-1999.

[2] Alajbegović Azra, Logo Nataša, Alajbegović Salem, Resić Halima. Psihičke promjene pacijenata sa moždanim tumorom, 2008.

[3] Aleksandar kostić, Milorad Radić, Goran Ignjatović, Miloš Janićijević. Odnos preoperativne veličine tumora I preživljavanja kod obolelih od astrocitoma mozga,2009.

[4] Chan TA, Weingart JD, ParisiM, et al. Treatment of recurrent glioblastoma multiforme with GliaSite brachytherapy. Int J Radiat Oncol Biol Phys 2005.

[5] Dr.sc. Lijerka Makulin- Grgić. Radioterapija i kemoterapija tumora živčanog sistema.

[6] Glantz MJ, Cole BF, Forsyth PA, et al. Parctice parameter : Anticonvulsant prophylaxis in patients with newly diagnosed brain tumors. Neurology, 2000; 54:1886 - 1893.

[7] Kondziolk D, Martin J J. Indication for resection and radiosurgery for brain metastases. Current Opinion in Oncology 2005.

[8] Monica Brown, Rudolf Schrot, Katrina Bauer, Deanna Le Tendre. Incidence of First Primary Central Nervous System Tumors in California, 2005.

[9] Nacional Cancer Institute of USA. Brain and Central Nervous systems cancer, 2005.

[10] Peter D., Elaine Row. Brain and Other Central Nervous System Cancer, 2001.

[11] Šamija M, Vrdoljak E, Krajina Z. Klinička onkologija, Medicinska naklada Zagreb 2006.

[12] Srđana Telarović, Siniša Telarović, Maja Relja. Impact of War on Central Nervous Sistem, 2000.

[13] Tosoni A, Ermani M, Brandes A A. the pathogenesis and treatment of brain metastases: a komprehesivereview, critical Reviews in Oncology/Hematology 2004.

20

Clinicopathological Diagnosis of Gliomatosis Cerebri

Jiro Akimoto
Department of Neurosurgery, Tokyo Medical University
Japan

1. Introduction

Regarding the definition of gliomatosis cerebri (hereinafter referred to as "GC"), the 3rd edition of the WHO Classification of Central Nervous System Tumors (hereinafter referred to as "3rd ed.") provides only a five-line description that GC is a diffuse, frequently bilateral, glioma that infiltrates the brain, involving more than two lobes. It often extends to the infratentorial structures and even to the spinal cord. Compared with this, the definition in its 4th edition (hereinafter referred to as "4th ed.") is described in 13 lines, stating that GC involves at least 3 lobes and is usually bilateral, extending from the cerebral white matter, including the deep and subcortical portions, and often infiltrating the brain stem and the spinal cord. In the 4th ed., GC is characterized by a widespread infiltration of the brain by tumor, occurring as bilateral lesions involving commissural fibers, and frequently infiltrating from the brain stem to the spinal cord. Moreover, the 4th ed. states that GC is mainly astrocytic tumor but, in some cases, mainly consists of oligodendroglial tumor cells (Akimoto, 2004; Balko, 1996; Levin, 2004; Sanson, 2004, Taillibert, 2006). Unlike the 3rd ed., which specifies the histological malignancy as Grade III, the 4th ed. rates it basically as Grade III, without specifying it, although recognizing the importance of the evaluation of histological malignancy, in consideration of the possibility that the grade may be underestimated in some cases due to tissue sampling problems (Akimoto, 2004; Nishioka, 1996). These changes in the description of the definition in the WHO Classification have reflected the findings of many clinicopathological researches on GC.

This situation requires us neuro-oncologists to diagnose GC before operation and to provide appropriate treatment. In that sense, it is important to evaluate the extent of tumor progression by imaging diagnosis, mainly using MRI, and to perform adequate tissue sampling to enable accurate histopathological diagnosis, in accordance with the 4th ed. (Akimoto et al., 2004). In addition, it is important to establish a treatment protocol mainly consisting of adjunctive therapy.

2. Clinical cases (Table 1)

We have encountered 8 cases in which GC was suspected based on the neuroradiological definition of the 4th ed. and was diagnosed pathologically. These cases aged 46 to 73 years (median age: 55.5 years) consisted of 3 men and 5 women. The initial symptoms were mainly cognitive impairment and seizure. The symptoms of ordinary brain tumor, including increased intracranial pressure, as well as focal signs, including hemiparesis, were less frequent. The tumoral topography based on CT or MRI revealed that most of the lesions were diffused in the white matter, often extending to the basal ganglia, brain stem or cerebellum which is unlikely to be invaded by ordinary diffuse glioma. These lesions were characterized by bilateral progression accompanied by hypertrophy of the corpus callosum. Wide resection of tissue, including areas over the white matter and cortical regions, was considered preferable as the surgical procedure to obtain a reliable pathological diagnosis. Therefore, anterior temporal lobectomy and maximally possible tumor resection were performed. Pathological diagnosis was anaplastic astrocytoma (Grade III) in most of the cases. However, GC consisting of oligodendroglial tumor cells was found in 2 cases. Basic treatment was radiation therapy (30 Gy to whole brain and 30 Gy focal boost) combined with chemotherapy (ACNU, Temozolomide). Except for a patient who developed central brain herniation in the early phase after operation, patients receiving sufficient adjunctive therapy tended to maintain partial response or stable disease.

2.1 Case 2

A 46-year old woman. She was admitted with a 2-month history of clumsiness and numbness of the right hand as well as gradual development of disorientation and right hemiparesis. The head MRI on admission revealed a lesion arising primarily in the left corona radiata and extending to the right parietal lobe and frontal lobe white matter through the corpus callosum, showing no obvious contrast enhancement (Fig. 1 A-D). CT-guided stereotactic biopsy of the left frontal lobe white matter was performed to make a definite diagnosis. Infiltration of large cells with abundant cytoplasm and thick processes, suggestive of reactive astrocytes, was observed in the matrix of the edematous white matter. However, a diagnosis of neoplastic lesion was not reached. Triggered by status epileptics, her condition deteriorated. Two months after the operation, she died of brain herniation. Cerebral autopsy revealed a widespread edema over the region from the left corona radiata to the basal ganglia, further extending to the right frontal lobe and the temporal lobe white matter through the corpus callosum. KB staining, Bodian staining, Holtzer staining, etc. demonstrated the extent of the lesion (Fig. 2 A-D). The pathological features of each section showed infiltration of gemistocytic cells, forming parallel rows along the nerve fibers. Although lack of nuclear atypism was noted, most of the nuclei were MIB-1 positive. The degree of myelin destruction varied across sections, being the most severe in the corpus callosum. However, Bodian staining demonstrated that the involved axis cylinder was preserved even in the corpus callosum. (Fig. 2 E, F) The autopsy-based diagnosis was GC consisting of gemistocytic astrocytoma.

2.2 Case 8

A 47-year old women. She was admitted to the hospital because of having abrupt cognitive impairment 1 month previously and gradual development of ataxic gait and urinary incontinence thereafter. Head MRI showed a lesion with enlargement of the corpus callosum in the white matter of the bilateral frontal lobe. Although the lesion extended from the bilateral corona radiata to the white matter of the parietal lobe, no obvious contrast enhancement was observed (Fig. 3 A-D). The partial removal of the tumor was performed to

Case	Age/Sex	Initial symptom	Tumoral Topography	Surgery	Pathological Dx	Treatment	Prognosis
1	54/ Male	Headache, Depression	White matter, Basal ganglia, Brain Stem, Cerebellum	ATL	Anaplastic oligodendroglioma	RTx	D: 2 months
2	46/ Female	Disorientation, Heminumbness	White matter, Basal ganglia, Corpus callosum	Biopsy	Gemistocytic astrocytoma	None	D: 2 weeks
3	71/ Female	Seizure, Hemiparesis	White matter, Corpus callosum	Partial removal	Glioblastoma	none	D: 8 months
4	50/ Female	Seizure, Cognitive impairment	White matter, Basal ganglia	Biopsy	Anaplastic astrocytoma	RTx, Chemo Tx	D: 26 months
5	66/ Male	Cognitive impairment	White matter, Corpus callosum	Biopsy	Anaplastic astrocytoma	RTx, Chemo Tx	A: 49 months
6	73/ Male	Seizure	White matter, Basal ganglia	ATL	Anaplastic astrocytoma	RTx, Chemo Tx	D: 4 months
7	57/ Female	Cognitive impairment	White matter, Basal ganglia	ATL	Anapalstic astrocytoma	RTx, Chemo Tx	D: 20 months
8	47/ Female	Cognitive impairment	White matter, Corpus callosum	Partial removal	Anaplastic oligodendroglioma	RTx, Chemo Tx	A: 11 months

ATL: anterior temporal lobectomy, RTx: radiation therapy, Chemo Tx: chemotherapy, D: dead, A: alive

Table 1. Case summary

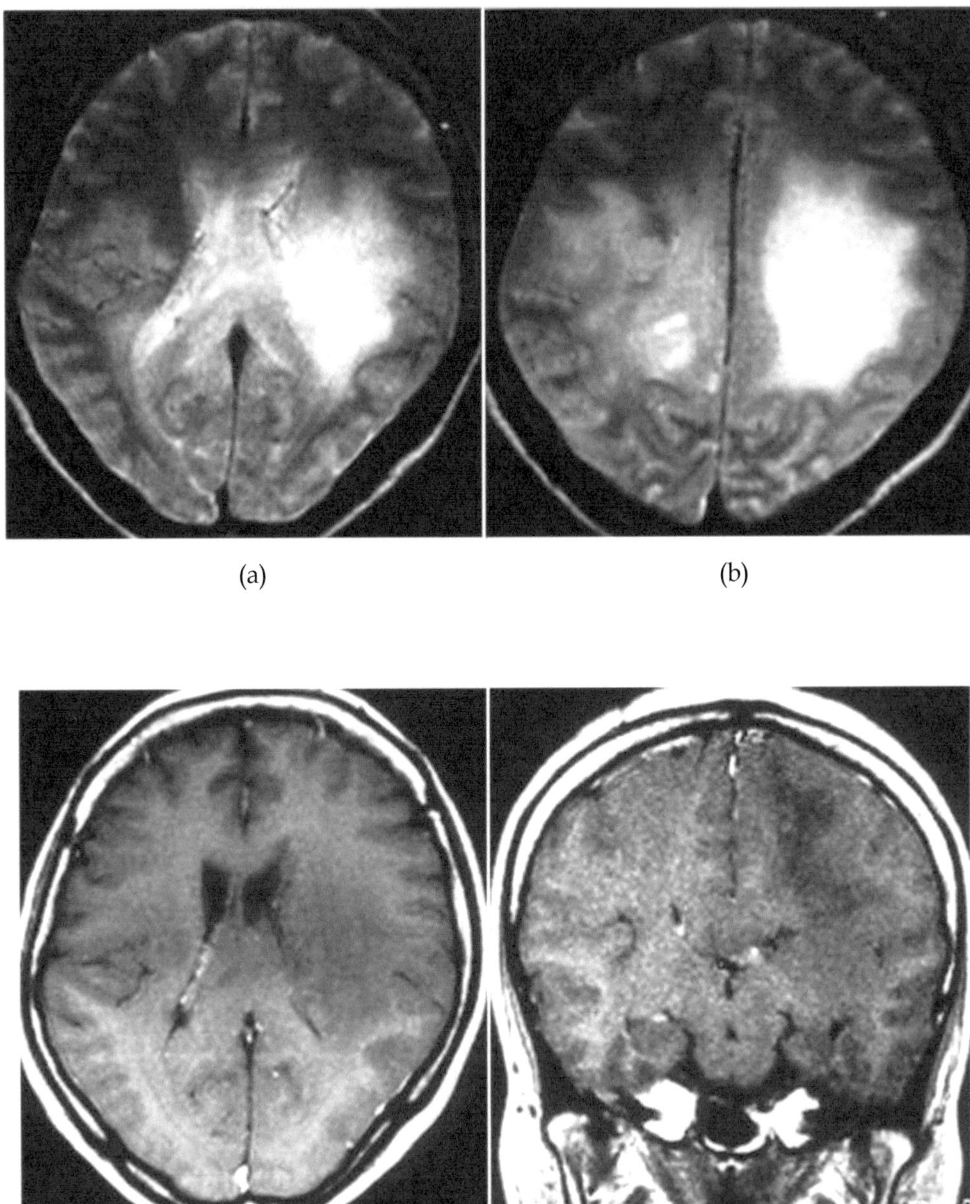

(a) (b)

(c) (d)

T2-weighted MRI (A, B) demonstrated diffuse high intensity in the white matter of both cerebral hemispheres, with enlargement of the corpus callosum. T1-weighted MRI with Gd-DTPA (C, D) demonstrated slightly low intensity in the white matter without enhancement.

Fig. 1. MRI on admission (A-D)

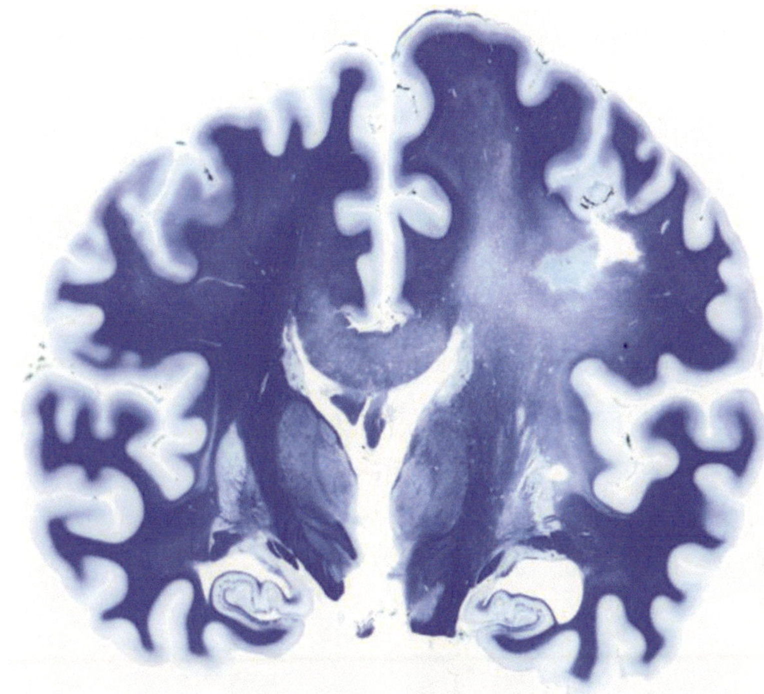

a

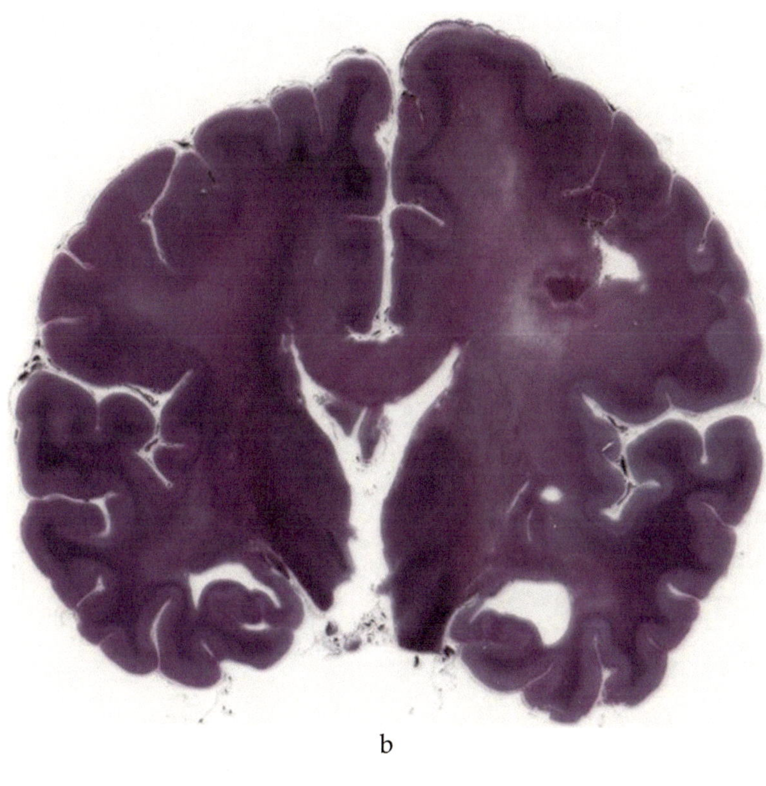

b

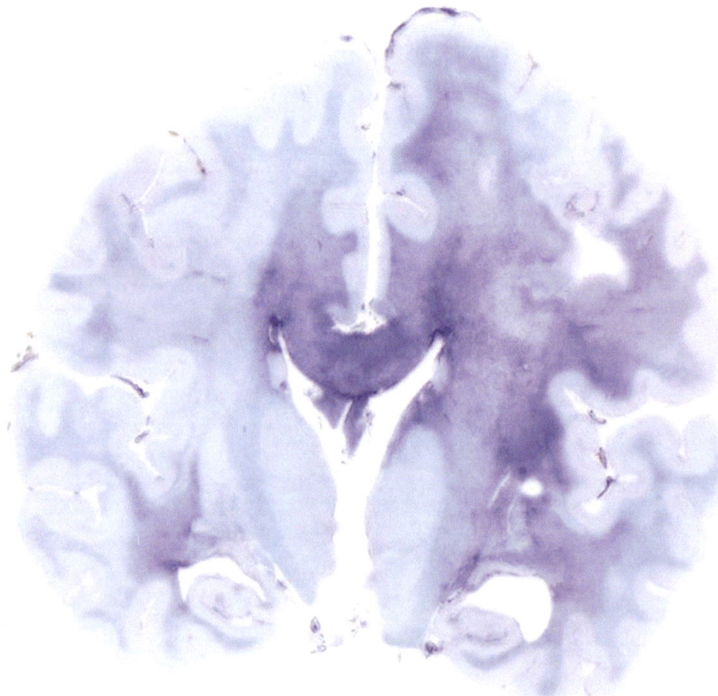

c

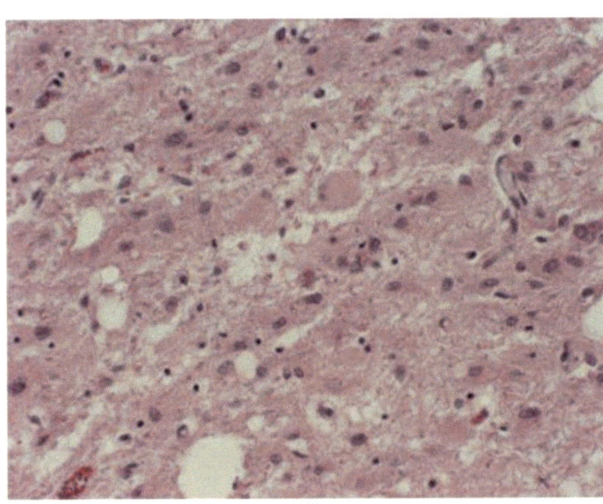

d

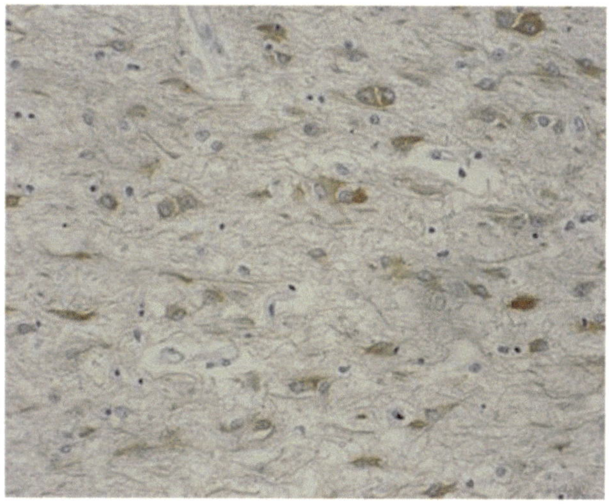

e

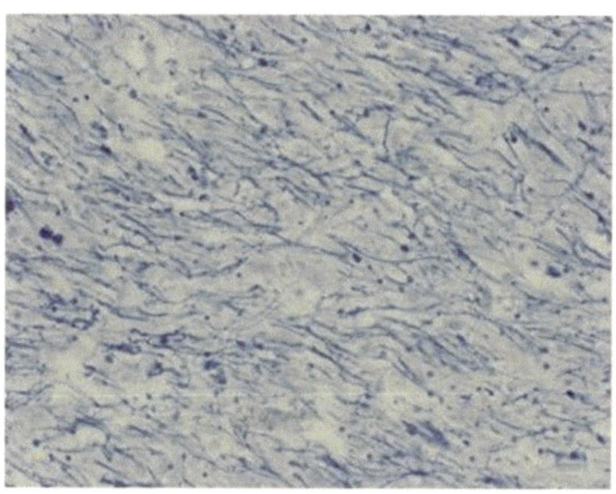

f

Klüver-Barrera stain (A) demonstrated the affected region to be a broad region of myelin destruction extending from the white matter of the left parietal lobe to the basal ganglia and to the corpus callosum and in a part of the right hemisphere. Bodian stain (B) demonstrated the preservation of axons, but the intensity of staining of the white matter and corpus callosum was slightly decreased owing to edematous change. Holzer stain (C) demonstrated the broad area of reactive gliosis. The region showed increased atypical gemistocyte-like cells of various sizes and forms [D: hematoxylin and eosin (HE) stain, ×100], Immunohistochemically, most tumor cells were positive for GFAP (E). Klüver-Barrera stain (F) showed extensive destruction of myelin.

Fig. 2. Coronal section of the autopsy brain (A-C) and microscopic appearance of autopsy material (D-F)

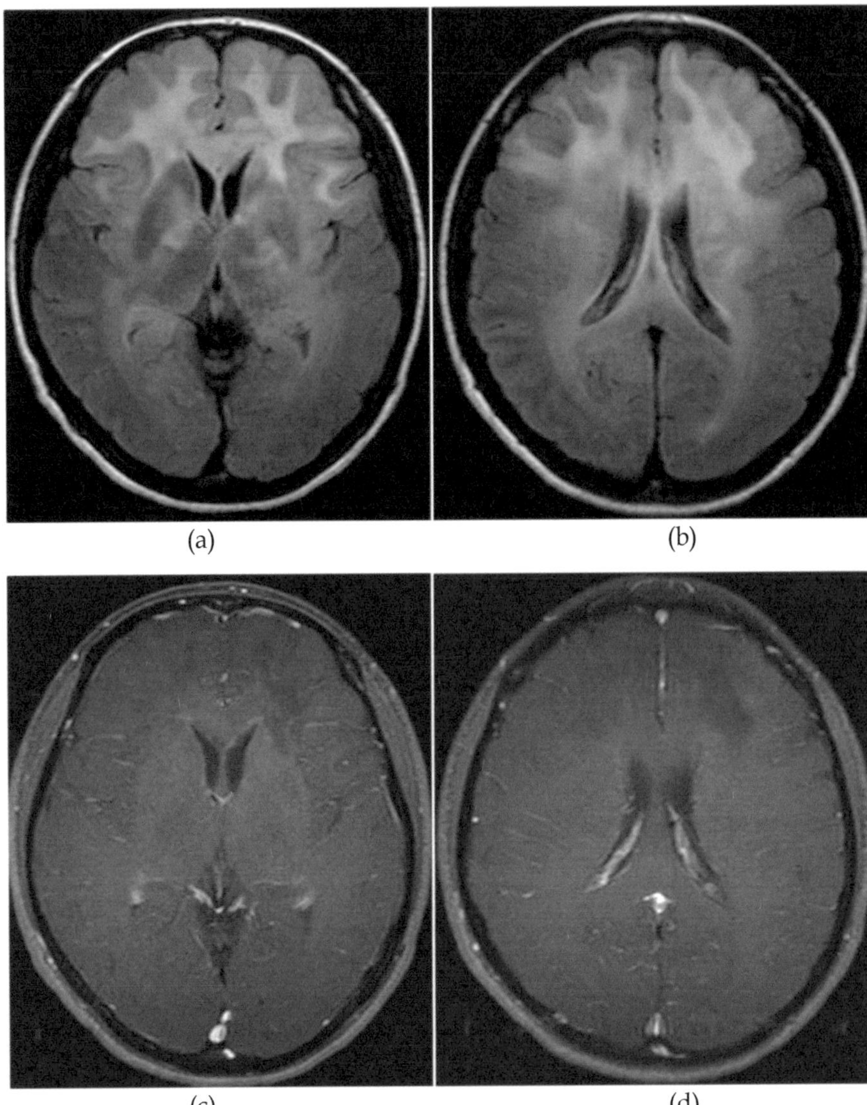

FLAIR MRI (A, B) demonstrated diffuse high intensity in the white matter of both frontal lobe and bilateral corona radiata, with enlargement of the corpus callosum. T1-weighted with Gd-DTPA (C, D) demonstrated low intensity in the white matter of the left frontal lobe without enhancement.

Fig. 3. MRI on admission (A-D)

make a definite diagnosis showed a dense proliferation of tumor cells with round nuclei, scant cytoplasm and perinuclear halo in the left superior frontal gyrus. The perineuronal satellitosis-like infiltration of tumor cells was observed even in the deep layer of the cerebral cortex. Myelin was preserved although partially destroyed by tumor cell infiltration (Fig. 4 A, B). The tumor cells were found to be Olig-2 positive, and the proportion of MIB-1 positive patients was also high. As a result of analysis using fluorescence in situ hybridization (FISH), she was found to be positive for 1pLOH (1p36) and 19qLOH (19q36) (Fig. 4 C, D). Based on these results, she was diagnosed with GC consisting of anaplastic oligodendroglioma cells. After the operation, she underwent radiation therapy (60 Gy) combined with chemotherapy using oral temozolomide. At 11 months post-operative, a reduction in the lesion size was observed, with an improvement in cognitive function.

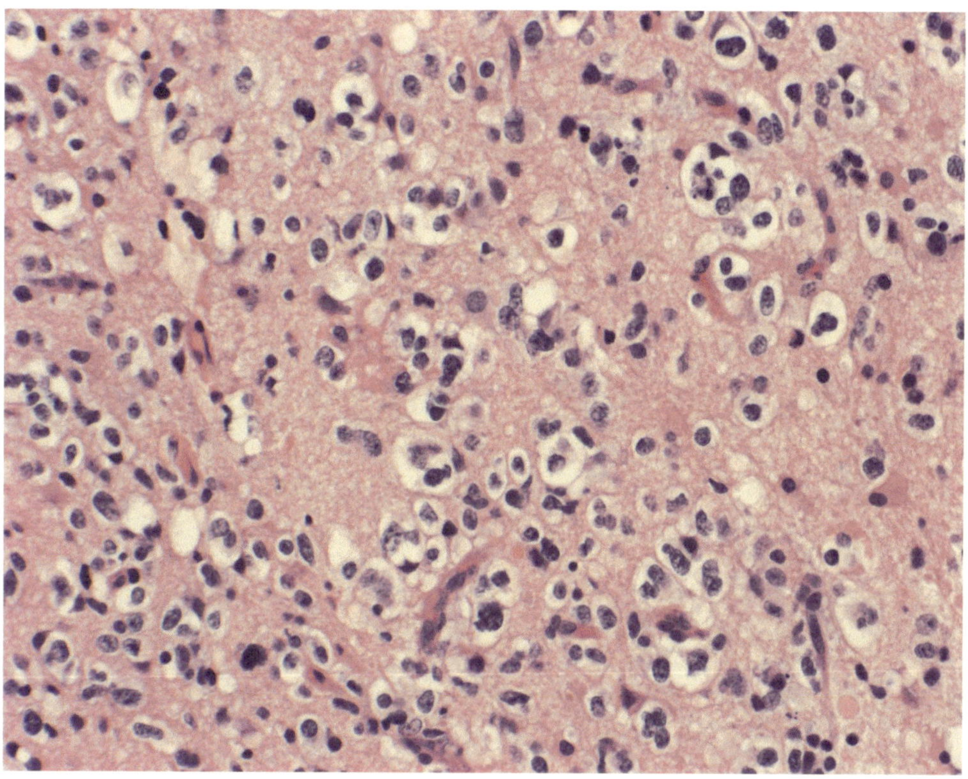

a

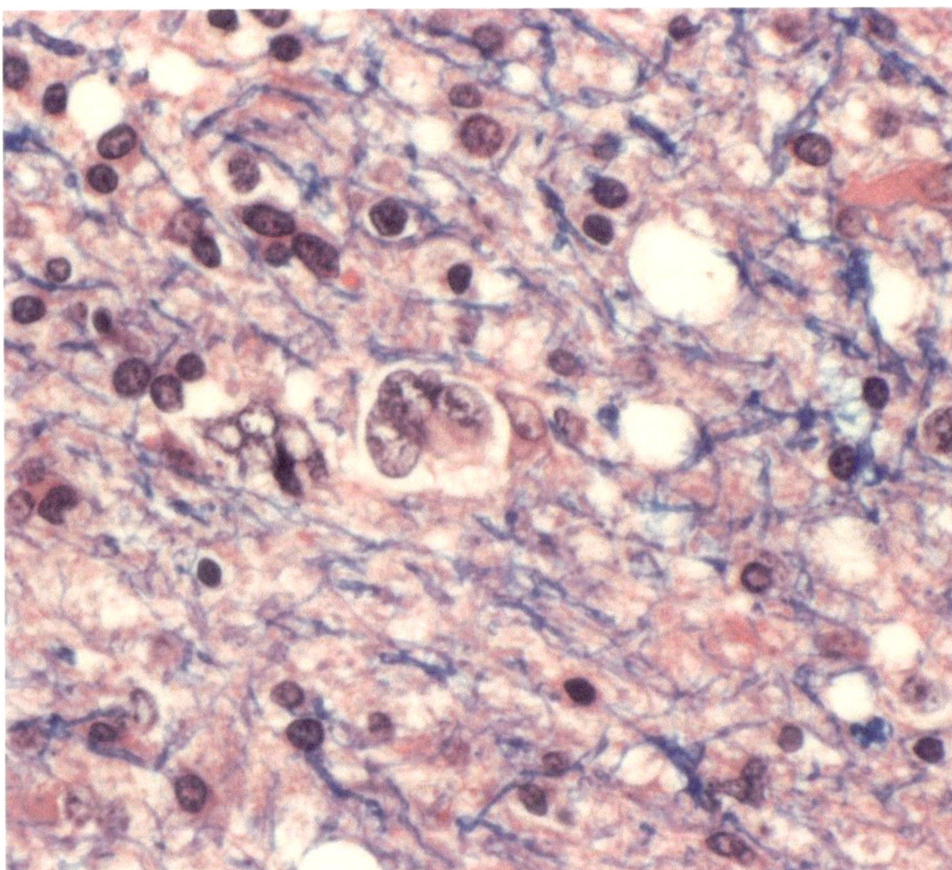

b

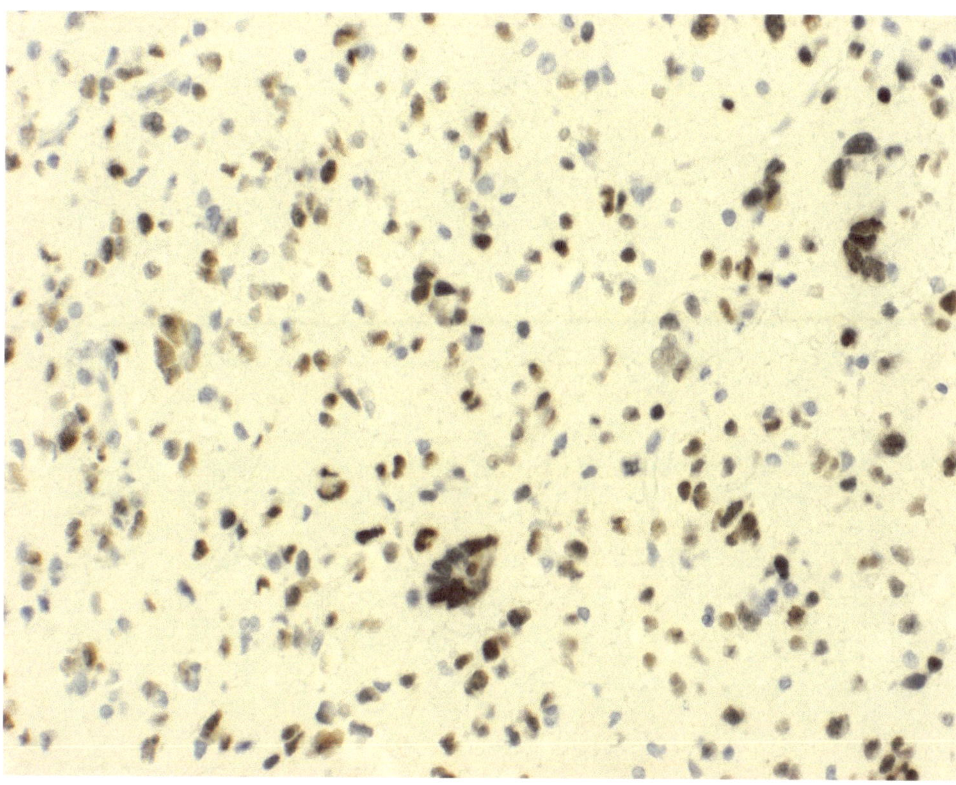

c

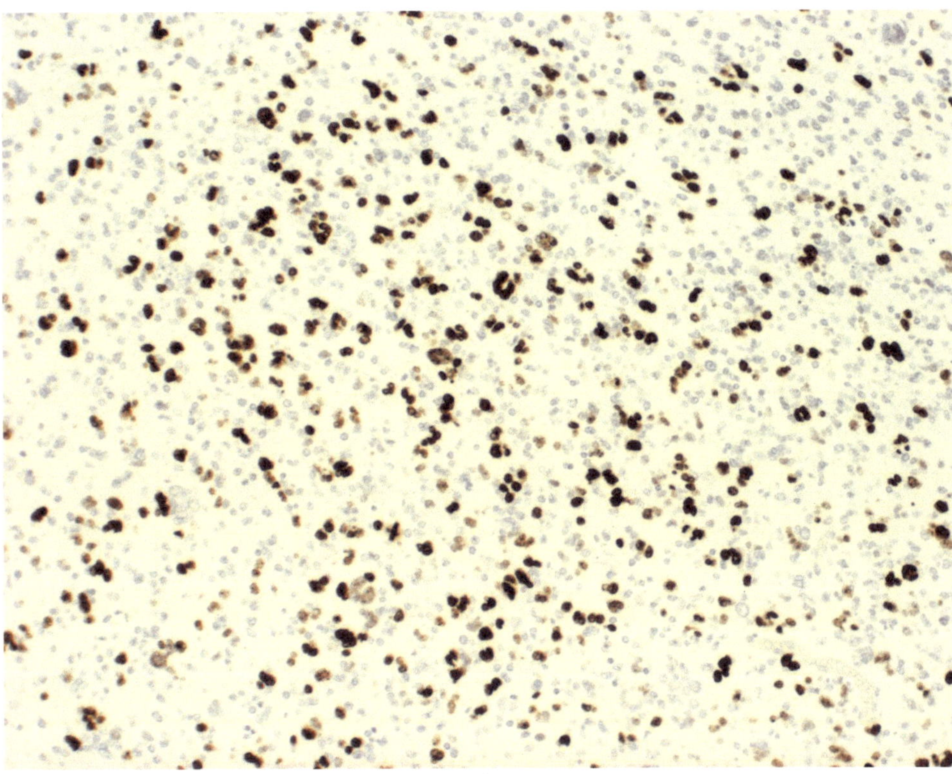

d

The region showed increased atypical oligodendroglial cells of various sizes and forms (A: HE stain, ×100). Luxol fast blue and HE stain showed extensive destruction of myelin (B, ×100). Immunohistochemically, most tumor cells were positive for olig2 (C) and MIB-1 (D).

Fig. 4. Microscopic appearance of resected tissue (A-D)

3. Discussion

3.1 Points to be noted in radiological diagnosis

Based on the definition of the 4th ed., confirmation of the presence of bilateral lesions over at least 3 lobes as well as the absence of an obvious focal tumor mass is considered essential to make an imaging-based diagnosis of GC. In addition, detection of infiltration of the basal ganglia, brain stem, cerebellum and spinal cord lends more confidence to the imaging-based diagnosis of GC. In other words, GC is considered a pathological condition where great emphasis is placed only on the invasive potential among the two growth mechanisms of ordinary glioma, i.e., the proliferative potential and invasive potential (Akimoto, 2004; Peretti-Viton, 2002; Saraf-Lavi, 2003). According to one report (Sanson et al., 2004), factors determining the diagnosis of GC based on MRI are: (1) a high signal area over at least 3 lobes on T2-weighted and FLAIR images; (2) absence of a contrast-enhanced tumor mass of 1 cm or greater; and (3) thickening of the corpus callosum or anterior commissure. These factors are the criteria adopted in the 4th ed. Such a clear definition may make it possible to suspect the presence of GC by performing MRI. However, these imaging findings are also obtained in white matter lesions other than tumors, such as demyelinating disease, encephalitis and venous sinus thrombosis (Essig, 2001; Saraf-Lavi, 2003). Therefore, it becomes necessary to confirm the presence of tumor cells by histological diagnosis. In recent years, studies evaluating GC by MR spectroscopy have been published (Bendszus, 2000; Galanaud, 2003; Saraf-Lavi, 2003). According to these studies, increased choline and decreased NAA levels, which are findings characteristic of glioma, are not necessarily observed in GC, but rather increased NAA levels are often observed. Increased myoinositol (m-Ins), which indicates increased activity of glia cells, has been reported as a finding characteristic of GC. Although the 4th ed. only states that multivoxel MRS is useful for determining the target of biopsy, it appears that biopsy of the sites with increased choline or m-Ins levels lends more confidence to the histological diagnosis of GC.

3.2 Points to be noted in pathological diagnosis

It is important to be faithful to the criteria for the pathological diagnosis of GC (Scheinker & Evans, 1943). More specifically, GC is basically defined as an invasive and tumoral lesion, with no tumor mass centered in the white matter, and the axis cylinder is preserved even when myelin destruction takes place (Akimoto, 2004; Peretto-Viton, 2002; Vates, 2003). To thoroughly carry out these evaluations, stereotactic biopsy sampling is often difficult. We previously reported the need to remove, as much as possible, the cerebral lobes with lesions detectable by imaging (Akimoto, 2004). In other words, not only the evaluation of tumor cells but also the evaluation of normal tissue is necessary for making the pathological diagnosis of GC. The cases presented in this article demonstrate the significance of the additional response evaluation for myelin by KB staining, axis cylinder by Bodian staining and reactive glia by Holtzer staining. The evaluation of tumor cells infiltrating between normal nerve fibers is by no means easy. In addition, the shape of the nuclei varies greatly from elongated-form or fusiform to round-form, and no consistency is found regarding the presence or absence of atypical cells. In fact, there are some reports on cases of GC consisting of oligodendroglioma-like cells, as shown in Case 8 (Akimoto, 2004; Balko, 1996; Benjelloun, 2001; Sanson, 2004; Vates, 2003). Confirmation of the preservation of the axonal structure after evaluation of the proliferative potential of infiltrating cells by MIB-1 and

AgNORs can contribute to the diagnosis of GC (Akimoto, 2004). In the 4th ed., the range of MIB-1 index is specified to be from not more than 1% to 30%, which is difficult to understand. However, it is also the fact that objective calculation of MIB-1 index is extremely difficult in tissues containing responsive glia cells due to normal tissue infiltration (Akimoto, 2004; Nishioka, 1996; Vates, 2003). Therefore, we consider it useful to evaluate the proliferative potential of each cell by AgNORs. However, there have only been two case reports on AgNORs in GC(Hara et al., 1991). A recent study has reported that L1, which is a cell adhesion factor, is expressed more abundantly in GC than in ordinary glioma (Suzuki et al., 2010). Since L1 is a glycoprotein that plays an important role in the migration of the immature neurons in the development stage, L1 might be significantly involved in the invasive potential of GC. In addition, it was reported that the control of L1-functions might contribute to the treatment of GC. Moreover, according to a study (Seiz et al., 2005) evaluating the mutation of IDH1 in GC, the frequency of IDH1 mutations is relatively high in the secondary GC, caused by the progression of diffuse astrocytoma, whereas no IDH1 mutation was observed in primary GC. This suggests the possibility that the evaluation of IDH1 mutations may become important for making the diagnosis of GC, as suggested in the molecular analysis of the development of glioblastoma.

3.3 Topics regarding treatment

According to the 3rd ed., GC has extremely poor prognosis, and 1-, 2- and 3-year survival rates are 48%, 37% and 27%, respectively, being similar to those in glioblastoma. The 3rd ed. specifies only MIB-1 as a prognostic factor. However, the 4th ed. is not intended to provide data, and states only that age, performance status and histological features, especially for grade and subtype (oligodendroglioma), are important as prognostic factors. The deletion of the description on MIB-1 suggests the difficulty of the evaluation (Akimoto, 2004; Nishioka, 1996; Vates, 2003). There are many reports discussing the extremely poor prognosis of GC (Taillibert, 2006; Vates, 2003). However, recent studies have reported some cases with relatively better prognosis due to greater sensitivity to adjuvant therapy (Levin, 2004; Sanson, 2004; Taillibert, 2006). Of these, one report (Taillibert et al., 2006) summarizing 296 cases from the literature showed that the overall survival (OS) in GC was 14.5 months. Examined for each prognostic factor, OS was 27 months and 9 months in KPS of ≥80 and ≤80, respectively, and 20 months and 8.5 months in Grade 2 and 4, respectively, showing significant differences. However, no significant difference was observed between cases with and without radiation therapy, and there was a trend for prolonged OS in patients receiving additional chemotherapy. The most noteworthy was the difference between cases of astrocytic tumor and oligodendroglial tumor: the OS was 11 months for the former and 36 months for the latter, showing a marked difference. Moreover, one study reported (Levin et al., 2004) that, in the use of temozolomide (TMZ), which is regarded as the standard treatment for ordinary glioma, the response rate was 45%, the median TTP to time to progression (TTP) was 13 months, with 1- and 2-year progression-free survival (PFS) rates of 55% and 23%, respectively. In another study (Sanson et al., 2004) where PCV and TMZ were used as first-line treatment in the 63 cases they encountered, no significant difference was observed in the response rate between the two treatment groups. In the study, no significant differences were observed in PFS and OS between patients stratified by age, tumor grade, KPS, etc.

However, in GC consisting of oligodendroglial tumor cells, significantly better responses were observed in both PFS and OS, with PFS of 21.2 months and OS of 33.9 months. Therefore, also for the treatment of GC, it is considered important to determine 1p, 19qLOH and the methylation status of MGMT by adequate tissue sampling in GC, for additional evaluation of the sensitivity to chemotherapy.

4. Conclusion

In terms of diagnosis, we are focusing on the application of chemical shift imaging MR spectroscopy with m-Ins, application of *in vivo* imaging technique using L1 and integrin as markers, and accurate detection of oligodendroglial GC by adequate tissue sampling and detailed evaluations of pathological morphology and gene mutations. In terms of treatment, focus is being placed on the evaluation of sensitivity to chemotherapy and the establishment of a treatment protocol for TMZ. The algorithm from the diagnosis of GC to treatment, we propose currently, is shown in Table 2. The pathological conditions for the diagnosis of GC have been specified in the 4th ed., but GC is still stated as an orphan disease. We believe that a multicenter study on the treatment of patients definitely diagnosed as having GC should be started.

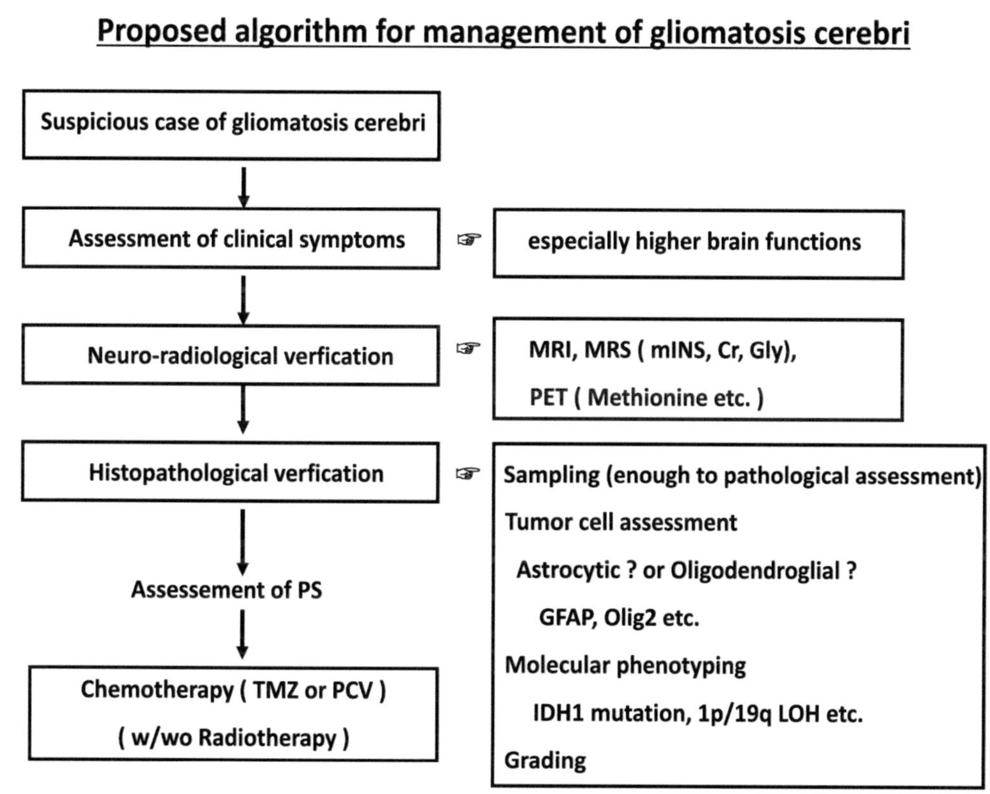

Table 2. Proposed algorithm of the management of gliomatosis cerebri

5. References

Akimoto J, Nishioka H, Miki T et al: Clinical diagnosis of gliomatosis cerebri. Brain Tumor Pathology 21, 87-95, 2004

Balko MG, Brisard KS, Samaha FJ: Oligodendoglial gliomatosis cerebri. Br J Neurosurg 10, 103-107, 1996

Bendszus M, Warmuth-Metz M, Klein R et al: MR spectroscopy in gliomatosis cerebri. Am J Neuroradiol 21, 375-380, 2000

Benjelloun A, Delavelle J, Lazeyras F et al: Possible efficacy of temozolomide in a patient with gliomatosis cerebri. Neurol 57, 1932-1933, 2001

Essig M, Schlemmer HP, Tronnier V et al: Fluid-attenuated inversion recovery MR imaging of gliomatosis cerebri. Eur Radiol 11, 303-308, 2001

Galanaud D, Chinot O, Nicoli F et al: Use of proton magnetic resonance spectroscopy of thebrain to differentiate gliomatosis cerebri from low-grade glioma. J Neurosurg 98, 269-276,2003

Hara A, Sakai N, Yamada H et al: Assessment of proliferative potential in gliomatosis cerebri. JNeurol 238, 80-82, 1991

Levin N, Gomori JM, Siegal T: Chemotherapy as initial treatment in gliomatosis cerebri. Neurol 63, 354-356, 2004

Nishioka H, Ito H, Miki T et al: Difficulties in the antemorten diagnosis of gliomatosis cerebri. Br J Neurosurg 10, 103-107, 1996

Peretti-Viton P, Brunel H, Chinot O et al: Histological and MR correlation in gliomatosis cerebri. J Neurooncol 59, 249-259, 2002

Sanson M, Caralat-Carel S, Taillibert M et al: Initial chemotherapy in gliomatosis cerebri. Neurol 63, 270-275, 2004

Saraf-Lavi E, Bowen BC, Pattany PM et al: Proton MR spectroscopy of gliomatosis cerebri: Case report of elevated myoinositol with normal choline levels. Am J Neuroradiol 24, 946-951, 2003

Seiz M, Tuettenberg J, Meyer J et al.: Detection of IDI1 mutations in gliomatosis cerebri, but only in tumors with additional solid component: evidence for molecular subtypes.Acta Neuropathol 2010, 120: 261-267

Scheinker IM, Evans JP: Diffuse cerebral glioblastomatosis. J Neuropathol Exp Neurol 2, 178-189, 1943

Suzuki T, Izumoto S, Fujimoto Y et al: Clinicopathological study of cellular proliferation and invasion in gliomatosis cerebri: important role of neural cell adhesion molecule L1 in tumour invasion. J Clin Pathol 58, 166-171, 2005

Taillibert S, Chodkiewitcz C, Laigle-Donadey F et al: Gliomatosis cerebri: a review of 296 cases from the ANOCEF database and the literature. J Neurooncol 76, 201-205, 2006

Vates GE, Chang S, Lamborn KR et al: Gliomatosis cerebri. A review of 22 cases. Neurosurg 53,261-271, 2003